REGENERATIVE ENGINEERING

REGENERATIVE ENGINEERING

CATO T. LAURENCIN, MD, PhD
YUSUF KHAN, PhD

Foreword by Robert S. Langer

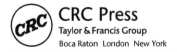

CRC Press
Taylor & Francis Group
Boca Raton London New York

CRC Press is an imprint of the
Taylor & Francis Group, an **informa** business

CRC Press
Taylor & Francis Group
6000 Broken Sound Parkway NW, Suite 300
Boca Raton, FL 33487-2742

First issued in paperback 2018

© 2013 by Taylor & Francis Group, LLC
CRC Press is an imprint of Taylor & Francis Group, an Informa business

No claim to original U.S. Government works

ISBN 13: 978-1-138-07517-7 (pbk)
ISBN 13: 978-1-4398-1412-3 (hbk)

Library of Congress Cataloging-in-Publication Data

Regenerative engineering / editors, Cato T. Laurencin and Yusuf Khan.
    p. ; cm.
Includes bibliographical references and index.
ISBN 978-1-4398-1412-3 (alk. paper)
I. Laurencin, Cato T. II. Khan, Yusuf, 1968-

[DNLM: 1. Tissue Engineering. 2. Biocompatible Materials. 3. Regenerative Medicine--methods. QT 37]
610.28'4--dc23   2012043347

Visit the Taylor & Francis Web site at
http://www.taylorandfrancis.com

and the CRC Press Web site at
http://www.crcpress.com

Contents

Foreword

IT IS A DISTINCT pleasure for me to write the foreword for the book *Regenerative Engineering* edited by Professor Cato T. Laurencin and Professor Yusuf Khan. This is an outstanding textbook. It describes a realistic view of the future where the technologies at our disposal today and technologies still in development will be applied to the regeneration of complex tissues. For some, this will be an invaluable reference book in the areas of biomaterials, tissue engineering, stem cell science, regenerative biology, and bionanotechnology. For others, the book will serve as a handbook describing pathways and ideas with clinically relevant applications that can be transformative to this field. The timeliness of the prodigious text cannot be overstated. The technologies we have seen developed in the past 25 years, and the new technologies being developed today—all described in this book—present countless possibilities for the development of next-generation solutions to the problems associated with the regeneration of tissues and organ systems. The book could be described as state of the art, but it also goes beyond this and helps show us a path to the future. I believe this textbook will be a part of homes, libraries, and classrooms throughout the world.

Robert S. Langer
David H. Koch Institute Professor
Massachusetts Institute of Technology
Cambridge, Massachusetts

Preface

THE FIELD OF REGENERATIVE ENGINEERING

The field of regenerative engineering has been defined as the integration of materials science and tissue engineering with stem and developmental cell biology and regenerative medicine toward the regeneration of complex tissues, organs, or organ systems. Regenerative engineering has elements of tissue engineering, regenerative medicine, and morphogenesis but is distinct from these individual disciplines in that it focuses specifically on the integration and subsequent response of stem cells to biomaterials and the regeneration of the interface between different tissue types. Further, regenerative engineering seeks to develop and evaluate biomaterials with the specific focus of stem cell interaction and response. The emergence of this field is similar to that of tissue engineering, which was formalized in the late 1980s and assessed by the National Science Foundation in 2003. The following is an excerpt from that report:

> Tissue engineering represents the confluence of a complex array of pre-existing lines of work from three quite different domains: the worlds of clinical medicine, engineering, and science… Landmark conceptual developments prerequisite for a concept of tissue engineering have emerged over a period of decades within the problem-solving traditions of clinical medicine. In some clinical domains, physicians and non-clinician researchers reached the stage of incorporating living cells into prototype tissue-engineered clinical solutions years before the emergence of a generalized concept of tissue engineering.*

Much like tissue engineering, the establishment of regenerative engineering as a distinct discipline does not mark the beginning of the integration of tissue engineering and regenerative medicine but serves to formalize the notion to give currently ongoing work a context and a framework from which to develop. Distinct from tissue engineering, which focused primarily on the *repair* of tissues, regenerative engineering focuses on the *regeneration* of tissues. This distinction, at first seemingly semantic, is important in that the lessons from regenerative engineering may be less applicable to spot repair of injured tissue elements but may lead to greater insight into the redevelopment or regeneration of intact multi-component complex tissues, limbs, and organs. The lessons from morphogenesis, namely,

---

* Taken from "The emergence of tissue engineering as a research field." http://www.nsf.gov/pubs/2004/nsf0450/start.htm

the importance of transitioning from individual cells to structured tissues, are a central point in regenerative engineering, but with the use of polymers and ceramics integrated.

The challenge of introducing a topic like regenerative engineering to undergraduate students lies, in part, in the breadth of information required to truly appreciate and begin to think about this field, which spans materials science, cell biology, stem cell biology, and clinical medicine. Students interested in these topics come from a spectrum of academic interests and have not always received the comprehensive background necessary to be adequately prepared for the growing complexity of this and related fields. It is not unusual for undergraduate students to develop an interest in biomaterials but have a background focused in either materials science or cell biology, but less frequently both. The goal of this textbook is to introduce the concept of regenerative engineering through the presentation of fundamental concepts of cell biology, stem cell science, materials science, and cell–material interactions, followed by an examination of specific organ and tissue types in which the fundamental lessons covered in the earlier chapters are used to present up-to-date examples of ongoing work, often in the context of a specific clinical need. The integration of (1) fundamental information, (2) up-to-date application of this information, and (3) clinical relevance of these applications provides a context within regenerative engineering that serves to reinforce the importance of each element in understanding the whole.

While this textbook covers many of the more widely studied tissue types within the fields of tissue engineering and regenerative medicine, it cannot cover all. Chapters have been included that discuss regenerative engineering of various organ tissues, vascular tissues, bone, ligament, neural tissue, and the interfaces between tissues. Chapter 1 provides a brief overview of many other tissue types that are currently the topic of regeneration and repair but were beyond the scope of this book.

Acknowledgment

W E WOULD LIKE TO acknowledge Raymond and Beverly Sackler for their vision to establish the Raymond and Beverly Sackler Center for Biomedical, Biological, Physical, and Engineering Sciences at the Institute for Regenerative Engineering, University of Connecticut, Storrs, Connecticut.

Editors

Cato T. Laurencin, MD, PhD, earned his BSE in chemical engineering from Princeton University, his PhD in biochemical engineering/biotechnology from the Massachusetts Institute of Technology, and his MD magna cum laude from Harvard Medical School. Dr. Laurencin is currently the chief executive officer of the Connecticut Institute for Clinical and Translational Science and director of the Institute for Regenerative Engineering at the University of Connecticut. He previously served as the vice president for health affairs and dean of the School of Medicine. He is a university professor and holds the Van Dusen Endowed Chair in the Department of Orthopaedic Surgery. He also holds an appointment as a professor of chemical, materials, and biomolecular engineering. Dr. Laurencin was the Lillian T. Pratt Distinguished Professor and Chair of the Department of Orthopaedic Surgery at the University of Virginia. In addition, he was designated as a university professor, one of the university's most prestigious titles, and held professorships in biomedical engineering and chemical engineering. Dr. Laurencin is an elected member of the Institute of Medicine of the National Academies and the National Academy of Engineering. In addition, he is an elected member of the African Academy of Sciences (AAS) and the Third World Academy of Sciences (TWAS). His research interests are in the fields of polymer synthesis, musculoskeletal tissue engineering, gene therapy, drug delivery, nanotechnology, and regenerative engineering.

Yusuf Khan, PhD, earned his master's degree and PhD in biomedical engineering from Drexel University. He is currently an assistant professor in the Institute for Regenerative Engineering and the Department of Orthopaedic Surgery at the University of Connecticut Health Center. He also has an appointment in the Department of Chemical, Materials, and Biomolecular Engineering and is part of the Department of Biomedical Engineering within the School of Engineering at the University of Connecticut. Dr. Khan was formerly an assistant professor in the Department of Orthopaedic Surgery and the Department of Biomedical Engineering at the University of Virginia. His research interests include musculoskeletal tissue regeneration using implantable biodegradable scaffolds, development of composite structures for bone regeneration, and the development of clinically relevant healing modalities using ultrasound.

Contributors

Shyam Aravamudhan, PhD
Joint School of Nanoscience and
  Nanoengineering
North Carolina Agricultural and Technical
  State University
The University of North Carolina at
  Greensboro
Greensboro, North Carolina

Anthony Atala, MD
Wake Forest Institute for Regenerative
  Medicine
Wake Forest School of Medicine
Winston-Salem, North Carolina

Ravi V. Bellamkonda, PhD
The Wallace H. Coulter Department of
  Biomedical Engineering
Georgia Tech
and
Emory University
Atlanta, Georgia

Edward A. Botchwey, PhD
The Wallace H. Coulter Department of
  Biomedical Engineering
Georgia Tech
and
Emory University
Atlanta, Georgia

Susan V. Bryant, PhD
Department of Developmental and Cell
  Biology
University of California
Irvine, California

James A. Cooper, Jr., PhD
Department of Biomedical Engineering
Musculoskeletal and Translational Tissue
  Engineering Research Laboratory
and
Center for Biotechnology and
  Interdisciplinary Studies
Rensselaer Polytechnic Institute
Troy, New York

Anusuya Das, PhD
Department of Biomedical Engineering
University of Virginia
Charlottesville, Virginia

Meng Deng, PhD
Institute for Regenerative Engineering
University of Connecticut Health Center
Farmington, Connecticut

Saadiq F. El-Amin III, MD, PhD
Southern Illinois University School of
  Medicine
Springfield, Illinois

David M. Gardiner, PhD
Department of Developmental and Cell
  Biology
University of California
Irvine, California

A. Jon Goldberg, PhD
Center for Biomaterials
Institute for Regenerative Engineering
University of Connecticut Health Center
Farmington, Connecticut

David J. Goldhamer, PhD
Department of Molecular and Cell Biology
Center for Regenerative Biology
University of Connecticut
Storrs, Connecticut
and
Stem Cell Institute
University of Connecticut Health Center
Farmington, Connecticut

Gloria Gronowicz, PhD
Department of Surgery
and
Department of Orthopaedic Surgery
University of Connecticut Health Center
Farmington, Connecticut

Ashim Gupta, MS
Department of Medical Microbiology,
  Immunology, and Cell Biology
Southern Illinois University School of
  Medicine
Springfield, Illinois

Ugonna N. Ihekweazu, MD
Department of Orthopaedics
Baylor College of Medicine
Houston, Texas

Yusuf Khan, PhD
Department of Orthopaedic Surgery
Institute for Regenerative Engineering
Raymond and Beverly Sackler Center for
  Biomedical, Biological, Physical, and
  Engineering Sciences
University of Connecticut Health Center
Farmington, Connecticut

Nora T. Khanarian, PhD
Biomaterials and Interface Tissue
  Laboratory
Department of Biomedical Engineering
Columbia University
New York, New York

Liisa T. Kuhn, PhD
Department of Reconstructive Sciences
School of Dental Medicine
University of Connecticut Health Center
Farmington, Connecticut

Sangamesh G. Kumbar, PhD
Department of Orthopaedic Surgery
Institute for Regenerative Engineering
Raymond and Beverly Sackler Center for
  Biomedical, Biological, Physical, and
  Engineering Sciences
University of Connecticut Health Center
Farmington, Connecticut

Cato T. Laurencin, MD, PhD
Institute for Regenerative Engineering
and
Connecticut Institute for Clinical and
  Translational Science
University of Connecticut Health Center
Farmington, Connecticut

Kristen L. Lee, BS
Musculoskeletal and Translational Tissue
  Engineering Research Laboratory
Department of Biomedical Engineering
and
Center for Biotechnology and
  Interdisciplinary Studies
Rensselaer Polytechnic Institute
Troy, New York

Nancy M. Lee, MEng
Biomaterials and Interface Tissue
  Laboratory
Department of Biomedical Engineering
Columbia University
New York, New York

Xue-Jun Li, PhD
Department of Neuroscience
and
Stem Cell Institute
University of Connecticut Health Center
Farmington, Connecticut

Helen H. Lu, PhD
Biomaterials and Interface Tissue
  Engineering Laboratory
Department of Biomedical Engineering
and
Columbia University College of Dental
  Medicine
Columbia University
New York, New York

Anil Magge, BS
School of Medicine
University of Connecticut
and
University of Connecticut Health Center
Farmington, Connecticut

Kristen Martins-Taylor, PhD
Department of Genetics and
  Developmental Biology
University of Connecticut Health Center
Stem Cell Institute
Farmington, Connecticut

Shaun W. McLaughlin, BS
Institute for Regenerative Engineering
University of Connecticut Health Center
Farmington, Connecticut

Benjamin R. Mintz, BS
Department of Biomedical Engineering
Musculoskeletal and Translational Tissue
  Engineering Research Laboratory
and
Center for Biotechnology and
  Interdisciplinary Studies
Rensselaer Polytechnic Institute
Troy, New York

Ken Muneoka, PhD
Department of Cell and Molecular
  Biology
Tulane University
New Orleans, Louisiana

Lakshmi S. Nair, MPhil, PhD
Department of Orthopaedic Surgery
Institute for Regenerative Engineering
Raymond and Beverly Sackler Center for
  Biomedical, Biological, Physical, and
  Engineering Sciences
University of Connecticut Health Center
Farmington, Connecticut

Rebekah A. Neal, PhD
Harvard-MIT Division of Health Sciences
    and Technology
Massachusetts Institute of Technology
Cambridge, Massachusetts

Jung Hyun Park, PhD
Biomaterials and Interface Tissue
    Laboratory
Department of Biomedical Engineering
Columbia University
New York, New York

Karen Sagomonyants, DMD
Division of Pediatric Dentistry
and
Department of Craniofacial Sciences
University of Connecticut Health Center
Farmington, Connecticut

Parimala S. Samuel, MS
Musculoskeletal and Translational Tissue
    Engineering Research Laboratory
Department of Biomedical Engineering
and
Center for Biotechnology and
    Interdisciplinary Studies
Rensselaer Polytechnic Institute
Troy, New York

Joylene W.L. Thomas, MD
Division of Orthopaedics
Southern Illinois University School of
    Medicine
Springfield, Illinois

Xiaofang Wang, MD, PhD
Department of Genetics and
    Developmental Biology
and
Stem Cell Institute
University of Connecticut Health Center
Farmington, Connecticut

Yong Wang, PhD
Department of Chemical, Materials, and
    Biomolecular Engineering
School of Engineering
University of Connecticut
Storrs, Connecticut

Mia D. Woods, MS
Department of Medical Microbiology,
    Immunology, and Cell Biology
Southern Illinois University School of
    Medicine
Springfield, Illinois

Michael N. Wosczyna, PhD
Department of Molecular and Cell Biology
Center for Regenerative Biology
and
Stem Cell Institute
University of Connecticut Health Center
Storrs, Connecticut

Ren-He Xu, MD, PhD
Department of Genetics and
    Developmental Biology
and
Stem Cell Institute
University of Connecticut Health Center
Farmington, Connecticut

CHAPTER 1

Regenerative Engineering

The Future of Medicine

Saadiq F. El-Amin III, MD, PhD; Joylene W.L. Thomas, MD; Ugonna N. Ihekweazu, MD; Mia D. Woods, MS; and Ashim Gupta, MS

CONTENTS

1.1 ORGAN AND TISSUE REGENERATION: THE CLINICAL NEED, EARLY STRATEGIES, AND THE FUTURE

Regenerative engineering is an interdisciplinary field that merges bioengineering, material science, and life science for the development of biological substitutes that will replace, restore, and/or regenerate tissue function. It combines cells, growth factors, and a synthetic scaffold to form a construct that will be functionally, structurally, and mechanically equivalent to or greater than that of the native tissue that has been damaged or lost. Great strides have been made in this area to meet the growing needs for regenerative strategies, but while there have been great accomplishments thus far, the field continues to rapidly evolve. Here in this chapter, we describe the trends and research in the areas of regenerative engineering, tissue engineering, and regenerative medicine.

The objective of regenerative engineering and regenerative medicine is to create living functional tissue that has the ability to replace organs that are dysfunctional due to age, disease, damage, or congenital defects (Orlando et al., 2010). The basic necessity within the field of regenerative medicine is to address two of the biggest dilemmas in transplant medicine: the shortage of donor organs and the toxicity of immunosuppression following transplantation. Regenerative medicine also possesses the potential for processing a patient's diseased tissue to correct its pathological constituents to further develop a healthy state.

1.1.1 Heart

Cardiovascular disease is one of the most common causes of morbidity and mortality in western society, and heart transplantation is an inevitable intervention for many of its conditions. As with other transplanted organs, donor heart shortages have forced researchers to find alternative donor sources. Tissue-engineered cardiovascular grafts (TECG) are being developed to compensate for the shortage in this area. In 1957, Akutsu and Kolff at Cleveland Clinic performed the first artificial heart transplant on a dog that survived for roughly 90 min. The artificial heart was fashioned from plastic polyvinyl chloride with its contractions driven by compressed air from an outside source. Following this experience, investigators devised further transplantation experiments in other animals culminating in its extrapolation to humans (DeVries et al., 1984). Since the 1980s, a number of whole artificial hearts have been developed, including—but not limited to—the Jarvik-7, HeartMate, CardioWest, and Novacor devices. These devices have yielded positive results by largely serving as a bridge to orthotopic transplantation. However, an ideal option for patients requiring heart transplantation is the creation of replacement cardiac tissue using the basic principles of tissue engineering (Figure 1.1).

Cardiac tissue is unique in that it has a high metabolic demand, has poor native regenerative potential, and must also possess sufficient thickness to maximize the tissue's nutritional and contractile properties. Over the previous two decades, methods to engineer cardiac tissue have evolved from simply seeding cardiomyocytes into a scaffold to a number of more elegant techniques (Tee et al., 2010). The engineered heart tissue (EHT) model, which uses neonatal cardiomyocytes, collagen I matrix, Matrigel™, and a mechanical stretching device to create independently contractile tissue, has shown promise in rat models

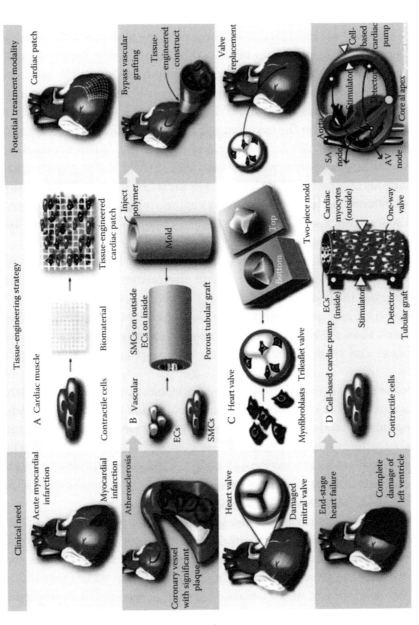

FIGURE 1.1 Tissue engineering can be applied to developing various aspects of the cardiovascular system. (A) Tissue-engineered cardiac patches can be applied to following acute myocardial infarction to improve the contractility of damage cardiac tissue. (B) Vascular graft can be engineered utilizing scaffolds or hydrogels to fabricate tubular structure seeded with smooth muscle cells and endothelial cells lining the lumen. (C) Trileaflet heart valves require a complex mold prototype to replicate the structural geometry accurately prior to seeding with myofibroblast that will result in functional heart valves. (D) Bioengineered cell-based cardiac pumps may be a viable substitute for mechanical left ventricular assist devices (LVADs) used to bypass the failing left ventricle in transplant patients. (Reproduced from Hecker, L. and Birla, R.K., *Regen. Med.*, 2(2), 125, 2007, with permission of Future Medicine Ltd.)

(Zimmermann et al., 2002). Alternatively, with a cell sheet technique, researchers utilize a thermosensitive cell culture surface coated with a polymer, poly(N-isopropylacrylamide) (PIPAAm), which changes properties with temperature, thus facilitating the separation of beating cells from the culture dish without disrupting vital gap junctions or the architecture of the engineered tissue construct (Shimizu et al., 2002). These cell sheets are then able to be stacked to create a 3D contractile cardiac tissue, as proven in rat models (Furuta et al., 2006). Another method of cardiac tissue engineering using biological cell assembly avoids the use of a porous scaffold for seeding of cells. This technique uses hydrogel-based scaffolds facilitating cardiomyocyte migration and assembly into contractile networks either *in vitro* with gravity-enforced techniques or *in vivo* with an arteriovenous loop embedded chamber for proper vascularization (Kelm et al., 2006). Finally, using a decellularized heart matrix allows for the use of a whole heart extracellular matrix scaffold that maintains the cardiac tissue's 3D architecture and vasculature. When neonatal rat cardiomyocytes and endothelial cells are seeded into this scaffold under physiological conditions, a spontaneous contractile whole heart can be created (Ott et al., 2008). Future efforts in the aforementioned routes of cardiac tissue engineering must address the need for an optimal cell source and ensure that the nutritional requirements of the tissue are met without compromising its contractile responsibilities.

Biodegradable polymer scaffolds seeded with vascular cells have been used to address diseased tissues and repair congenital defects within the cardiovascular system. The benefits of these materials include unlimited supply, durability, resistance to infection, decreased thrombogenicity, and lack of rejection. Thrombogenicity is countered via drug delivery systems, which allow the release of heparin directly to the graft site. In the same manner, growth factors can be delivered to promote revascularization and healing of damaged tissues.

Tissue-engineered heart valves (TEHV) hold promise as viable substitutes to outperform existing valve replacements. This thought is based on the idea that a defective valve will be replaced by living functional tissue. As with other areas of tissue engineering, the use of synthetic polymer scaffolds has the benefits of low cost and readily available supply along with decreased risks of tissue rejection and zoogenic infection. Reasonable short-term results have been seen using synthetic polymer scaffolds for tissue-engineered valves (Sutherland et al., 2005).

Under ordinary conditions, healthy heart valve tissue undergoes cyclic circumferential stretch, oscillating shear stress, and cyclic flexure. Not only will the artificial valve need to be able to match the biomechanical properties of the native valve that it replaces, but there is also a need for valves to grow and remodel in pediatric patients while maintaining these properties. The development of a bioreactor capable of testing these properties independently or in combination was described by Engelmayr et al. (2008). There is a need for a standard protocol by which TEHV will be conditioned to function at physiological levels. Future studies will involve the use of bioreactors to test cyclic stretch, flexure, and shear stress for the purpose of determining the ideal parameters *in vitro* prior to use *in vivo* (Berry et al., 2010).

1.1.2 Lungs

For lung transplants, efforts to ameliorate the difficulties that arise during transplantation of other organs, namely, a limited donor supply and the toxicity of immunosuppression, have led researchers to seek alternative supplies of lung. Since the 1960s, investigators have largely experimented with models of artificial lungs (Bodell et al., 1965); however, with the success of lung transplantation beginning in the 1990s, the necessity of bridging patients to transplantation and temporarily supporting the newly transplanted lung has further driven the field of artificial lung development and engineering. The current techniques of temporarily supporting patients with lung disease using extracorporeal membrane oxygenation (ECMO) and intravenacaval devices are limited in their potential for long-term or bridge-to-transplantation therapies. Animal models with intrathoracic oxygenator devices using the right heart as a pump have accomplished full basal O_2 and CO_2 transfer for up to 7 days (Cook et al., 1996; Witt et al., 1999). While research continues in these areas of artificial lung development, researchers are also exploring the principles of regenerative medicine to develop engineered lungs (Figure 1.2).

Using a whole-organ decellularization approach, researchers have demonstrated with *in vivo* rat models that for short-time intervals, engineered lungs have the capacity to participate in gas exchange (Ott et al., 2010; Petersen et al., 2010). In these studies, the lungs were decellularized in a manner that preserved the organ's native morphological

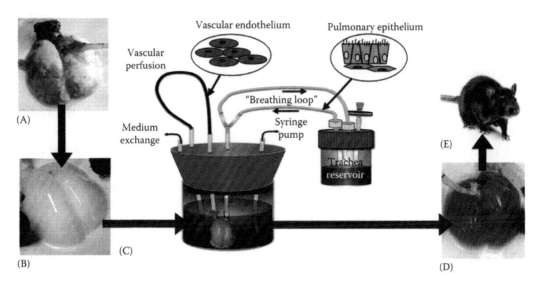

FIGURE 1.2   In this schematic, tissue engineering of the lung begins with (A) decellularization of a native adult rat lung. The pulmonary artery and trachea are cannulated for infusion of decellularization solutions, which remove all immunogenic cellular constituents. (B) This process leaves the lung matrix devoid of cells after 2–3 h of treatment, while retaining alveolar microarchitecture. (C) The acellular scaffold is mounted inside a biomimetic bioreactor for seeding of vascular endothelium into the pulmonary artery and pulmonary epithelium into the trachea. (D) The engineered lung is removed from the bioreactor after 4–8 days of culture and is suitable for implantation into (E) the syngeneic rat model. (Reproduced from Petersen, T.H. et al., *Science*, 329, 538, 2010.)

characteristics, vasculature, and architecture of its airways (including its alveoli). These scaffolds were then maintained in bioreactors and repopulated with both epithelial and endothelial tissues creating the engineered lung (Ott et al., 2010; Petersen et al., 2010). While these studies represent the initial stages of lung tissue engineering, their results do suggest that repopulation of a decellularized lung scaffold is a viable strategy for whole lung construction. Akin to the challenges faced with other engineered tissues, future research into lung tissue development must define the optimum source of cells for scaffold repopulation, its applicability to humans, and whether proper O_2 and CO_2 transfer can be adequately sustained with the engineered tissues.

1.1.3 Liver

The current deficit of available livers for patients requiring transplantation is 4000 (Punch et al., 2007). While hepatocyte transplantation is a considerable alternative to orthotopic liver transplantation, limited cell supply and low engraftment efficiency has limited its potential (Smets et al., 2008). Prior attempts at tissue-engineered liver have encountered the roadblocks of inadequate nutrition and oxygenation of the transplanted grafts. Using a perfusion decellularization method to preserve the liver-specific extracellular matrix, the 3D structural characteristics, and its microvascular network, Uygun et al. (2010) developed a transplantable liver graft. This technique allows for the recellularization of a liver matrix with adult hepatocytes. Most importantly, since the decellularized liver matrix grafts retain their native vascular network, the graft is readily connected to the circulation facilitating rapid oxygen and nutrient delivery when implanted (Uygun et al., 2010). Uygun et al. also found that the recellularized grafts support liver function: albumin secretion, urea synthesis, and cytochrome P450 expression comparable to the normal liver *in vitro*. A potential benefit of this technology is that the supply of whole livers can be derived from the cohort of donor livers that are currently unsuitable for orthotopic transplantation, e.g., following donor cardiac death (Safar, 1988).

Uygun et al. (2010) proposed two questions that may be answered with subsequent research: first, what is the role of non-parenchymal cells (e.g., liver sinusoidal endothelial cells, stellate cells, biliary epithelial cells, and Kupffer cells) in constructing an entire liver, and second, how is the responsibility of parenchymal cells defined in maintaining vascular integrity. Finally, these techniques must be able to be safely scaled up to humans.

1.1.4 Kidney

Patients with end-stage renal disease awaiting transplantation also face the dilemma of a growing list of patients requiring transplantation concurrent with a steady or dwindling supply of organs (Shrestha, 2009). As a result, a significant number of patients are forced to undergo dialysis, a therapy that is associated with a number of both medical and economic challenges. To combat the problem of organ shortage and morbidity of immunosuppression, investigators are exploring the principles of tissue engineering to construct and reconstruct kidney tissue. Current techniques in kidney engineering primarily utilize stem cell and scaffold technologies. Ross et al. have demonstrated that proliferation and differentiation of pluripotent embryonic stem cells are possible when seeded in a complex decellularized kidney scaffold (Ross et al., 2009). This technology has the potential to generate whole kidney organs. However, these studies are largely experimental as a viable cell source of kidneys and the extrapolation of this technique to humans has yet to be identified.

1.1.5 Pancreas

Diabetes mellitus is a major cause of morbidity and mortality for millions of U.S. citizens. Current treatment of type I diabetes revolves around a variety of insulin replacement methods. While there have been credible gains in the formulation and administration of insulin along with enhanced methods of glucose monitoring, a definitive cure for the disease remains elusive. Recently, pancreas and islet cell transplantation has emerged as a viable candidate in the pursuit for a cure as promising results have been observed when pancreata have been transplanted in conjunction with kidneys for well-selected diabetic patients with concurrent end-stage renal disease (Lipshutz and Wilkinson, 2007). Nevertheless, combined pancreas and kidney transplantation does not address the specific disease for the vast majority of diabetics, thus making it a nonviable treatment option for the general population.

Prior to the turn of the century, trials of islet cell transplantation failed to yield prolonged insulin independence for type I diabetics. Major roadblocks for the treatments were that researchers were unable to identify both the optimum islet cell mass for transplantation and determine an adequate non-diabetogenic immunosuppression protocol (Brendel et al., 1999). In 2000, Shapiro et al. showed that following islet cell transplantation, the use of a glucocorticoid-free immunosuppressive regimen resulted in sustained independence from exogenous insulin (Shapiro et al., 2000). However, a number of barriers to islet cell transplantation still exist including a limited donor supply, the need for lifelong immunosuppression, and the propensity for long-term graft dysfunction, returning the patient to insulin dependence (Yechoor and Chan, 2010). These challenges have led to the renewed interest in β-cell replacement therapy from tissue engineering technologies.

In vivo induction of β-cell neogenesis and *in vitro* conversion of pluripotent stem cells into β-cells are two emerging methods for creating ideal sources of transplantable β-cells. *In vivo* induction of β-cell neogenesis revolves around the principles of transdifferentiation and transdetermination. Transdifferentiation, the act of shifting a terminally differentiated cell from one lineage to another, is a desirable method for inducing β-cell neogenesis as terminally differentiated cells are readily abundant from many tissues. Zhou et al. (2008) has demonstrated that when three transcription factors (NgN$_3$, Pdx1, and MafA) are delivered via an adenovirus by direct injection into the exocrine pancreas of non-diabetic mice, the tissue is induced to create insulin-positive cells. Of the vector-infected cells, 20% were transdifferentiated into insulin-positive cells. When applied to diabetic mice, there is a partial correction of fasting hyperglycemia (up to 3 months). Ultimately, this study has achieved targeted differentiation, as terminally differentiated exocrine pancreas cells were able to be redirected into cells that achieved characteristics similar to β-cells with regards to morphology, gene expression, immunocytochemistry, and ultrastructure (Zhou et al., 2008).

Originally, transdetermination, the process of redirecting multipotent cells such as an adult cell of one lineage to a developmentally related yet differentiated cell lineage, has been described in *Drosophila* larvae (Maves and Schubiger, 1999). Embryologically, both the endocrine and exocrine portions of the pancreas are derived from the distal foregut endoderm. This portion of endoderm also happens to give rise to liver progenitors, showing that both liver and pancreatic progenitors are closely related. From this perspective, adult liver stem (oval) cells were induced to switch to an islet cell lineage using a single lineage-defining transcription factor, Ngn3 (Yechoor et al., 2009). This study illustrates the real potential of transdetermination and its likelihood for therapeutic organogenesis for the treatment of diabetes.

The *in vitro* conversion of pluripotent stem cells via use of a number of transcription factors is yet an additional option for inducing islet cell neogenesis (Blyszczuk and Wobus, 2004). The immediate future of β-cell transplantation therapy research faces the challenges of creating β-cells that are not only structurally similar to native β-cells but also functionally resemble the native β-cells. Specifically, the functional concern of ensuring disciplined secretion–stimulus behavior in the transplanted β-cells is of foremost importance as these cells are currently constitutive secretors of insulin. Additionally, further research into β-cell transplantation for treatment of diabetes must address a number of questions: (1) what is the preferred method of lineage programming, (2) how to measure the completeness of β-cell creation, (3) what is the oncogenic potential of the transplanted cells, (4) what is the prime location for transplantation, and (5) what is the optimum immunosuppression regimen (Yechoor and Chan, 2010).

1.1.6 Intestinal Tissue

Short gut syndrome is a collection of symptoms occurring after bowel resection as a result of nutritional and absorptive deficiencies of the remaining bowel. The current therapeutic approach is with total parenteral nutrition; however, this method is associated with many complications. Small bowel transplantation is an acceptable option but is limited by the high likelihood for transplant rejection, the need for immunosuppression, and a low donor pool (Warner and Chaet, 1993). Additional alternatives to treat short gut syndrome are the intestinal lengthening procedures. It is thought that by lengthening the remaining segment of bowel following resection, the intestinal transit time of food is prolonged, thereby maximizing the absorptive potential of those segments. Unfortunately, intestinal lengthening has experienced limited success as a treatment (Bianchi, 1999). As a result of these shortcomings, researches have begun exploring options methods of engineering neo-intestine.

In an animal model, researching the efficacy of engineered intestine in treating short gut syndrome (Grikscheit et al., 2004) obtained epithelial cells from neonatal rats organizing them into "organoid units." These organoid units were then seeded onto a tubular biodegradable scaffold to create intestinal epithelial tissues. Next, the tissues were then implanted on the adult rat omentum and over time became cyst-like structures that were both vascularized and confirmed by immunofluorescence and electrophysiology to be similar to native adult intestinal mucosa. After a period of time, the cysts were anastomosed with the remaining bowel to form a continuous intestinal system. The authors successfully illustrated that the rat's nutritional status as measured by weight and B12 absorption significantly improved and that the clinical picture of short gut syndrome was cured (Grikscheit et al., 2004).

A review paper by Rehman proposed that the following questions should be answered with future research: (1) Does this method have the capability of generating an adequate intestinal absorptive area in the human bowel? (2) What is the role of generating neural tissue in addition to bowel tissue to facilitate the ability of the engineered segment to peristalse? (3) What is the optimum cell source? (4) Does the engineered bowel actually have the capacity to absorb or does it simply lengthen the intestinal unit and prolong transit time? (5) In addition to using growth factors that promote gut development, what is the role of nerve growth factors as well as others that promote lymphogenesis and angiogenesis? (Rehman, 2008).

1.1.7 Spleen and Lymph Nodes

Secondary lymphoid organs such as spleen, peripheral lymph nodes, and mucosal-associated lymphoid tissues are responsible for the development of a number of vital immune responses. An improved understanding of the development and architecture of lymphoid tissue has enhanced attempts at generating artificial lymphoid tissue. Successful transplantation of engineered secondary lymphoid organs will be of great benefit to the immunodeficient, as it has the potential to augment immunoprotection and potentially prolong patient survival.

Suematsu and Watanabe (2004) have engineered secondary lymphoid tissue organoids that contain similar characteristics to native tissue by using a thymic stromal cell line TEL-2 embedded in a scaffold implanted into the renal subcapsular space in mice. When transplanted into either naive or SCID mice, the organoids have the capacity of inducing IgG antibodies following intravenous administration of antigen (Suemastu and Watanabe, 2004).

Investigators have also produced specific types of secondary lymphoid organs, such as mucosal-associated lymph tissues (Perez et al., 2002) and spleen. For the latter, Grikscheit et al. (2008) used multicellular components of juvenile spleen transplanted on a biodegradable polymer scaffold to regenerate functional spleen. Their technique was therapeutic against overwhelming postsplenectomy sepsis and demonstrated enhanced survival rates following splenectomy (Grikscheit et al., 2008). Future research in secondary lymphoid tissue engineering will need to determine its applicability to humans and further define its role in clinical immunotherapy (Tan and Watanabe, 2010).

1.1.8 Eyes

1.1.8.1 Retina

Much of the ophthalmic applications of tissue engineering have focused on developing retinal, corneal, and lens tissues. The mechanisms of retinal degeneration that cause blindness usually involve deterioration of the outer retina, specifically the photoreceptors and retinal pigment epithelial cells. With the exception of antiangiogenic medications that fight neovascular age-related macular degeneration, there are no treatments that address retinal-based vision loss. Our current understanding of these pathological mechanisms maintains that independent of the outer retinal deterioration, the inner retinal tissues maintain their architecture and functionality.

The current hope is that with engineering, the outer retinal cells, photoreceptors, and retinal pigment epithelial cells can be delivered with a material scaffold to the subretinal space for interaction with the functional inner retinal layer. As of now, there is no definitive technique for retinal repair. In a review, Hynes and Lavik (2010) suggest using a synthetic hydrogel to promote differentiation and migration of retinal pigment epithelial cells. An alternative approach may be to explore the use of induced pluripotent stem cells differentiated into retinal pigment epithelial cells (Buchholz et al., 2009). As it is clear that damage to either retinal progenitor cells or retinal pigment epithelial cells also induces the demise of the other cell type, yet an additional scheme has developed to transplant both cell types (Radtke et al., 2008). Further research into retinal tissue engineering will need to develop a combined tissue scaffold of retinal progenitor cell and retinal pigment epithelial cells (Hynes and Lavik, 2010).

1.1.8.2 Cornea

The cornea is a protective layer of the eye and also represents two-thirds of its refractive power. Pathology to the cornea may affect one or all of its layers and is currently treated with keratoplasty; however, the ideal treatment of corneal damage would be corneal transplantation. Currently, engineered corneas include prosthetic devices that simply replace damaged cornea and tissue-engineered hydrogels that facilitate regeneration of corneal tissue (De Miguel et al., 2010). Today, investigators are using corneal stem cells to regenerate corneal tissue; however, these efforts have been limited by the fact that these stem cell compartments are easily damaged. Furthermore, in order to generate adequate cell number for transplantation long *ex vivo* cultures are required. The hope is that in the future advanced biomaterials can be combined with cells from various sources such as oral mucosa, bone marrow, and adipose cells to engineer corneal tissues (De Miguel et al., 2010; Figure 1.3).

1.1.8.3 Lens

Engineering of the ocular lens was classically observed in studies with the Newt (Ito et al., 1999). Ito et al. found that when pigment epithelial cells are aggregated and implanted in the eye they not only transdifferentiate into lens tissue, but also build a lens of similar architecture to natural lenses. These results suggest that *in vitro* aggregated pigment epithelial cells can build a perfect lens when implanted *in vivo*.

1.1.9 Musculoskeletal Tissues

1.1.9.1 Bone and Ligament

Currently in orthopedic surgery, especially in the area of trauma, there is a shortage of opportunities for fixation of bone after a major bone defect (Bolander, 1992). One alternative therapy is to introduce tissue engineering as a means of restoring tissue after a defect. Tissue engineering is becoming a solution for the shortage in tissue regeneration

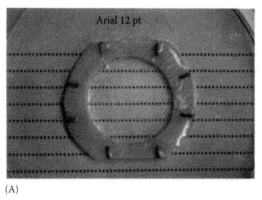
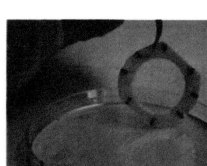

(A)   (B)

FIGURE 1.3 Proulx et al. have designed the tissue-engineered human cornea using three different cell types. (A) A series of dots typed in Arial 12 pt font are visualized well through the tissue-
engineered cornea. (B) This engineered cornea is shown to have a slight haze. (Reproduced from
Proulx, S. et al., *Mol. Vis.*, 16, 2192, 2010.)

and the repair of skeletal and congenital defects (Langer and Vacanti, 1993). Currently,
options for tissue regeneration rely heavily on autografts, allografts, and xenografts,
which are limited in supply and can be associated with disease transmission (Ibim
et al., 1997; Ignatius and Claes, 1996; Jackson and Simon, 1999). Tissue-engineered
applications offer biocompatibility, availability, and diversity when being applied to
various areas of bone and tissue regeneration (Figure 1.4). This topic is covered in detail
in Chapter 11.

Stability of the knee relies on the ligaments supporting the joint. Currently, anterior
cruciate ligament (ACL) tears are treated with surgical reconstruction using hamstring or
bone–patellar–bone autografts or allografts. Studies have shown that there are mesenchymal stem cells present in the injured ACL. In the proper environment, growth factors have
been shown to stimulate the morphological development of the pluripotent stem cells into
osteoblasts, chondrocytes, and tenocytes. While these studies have only been performed
in vitro, there is the promise of regenerating the ACL *in vivo* and eliminating the more
invasive procedures that are currently performed. Ligament regenerative engineering is
covered in detail in Chapter 14.

1.1.9.2 Cartilage

With the loss of supportive and protective structures such as the ACL and/or meniscus, the
risk of osteoarthritis is significantly increased. The absence of these structures allows for
increased motion at the joint that leads to wear and tear of the cartilage as well. Once cartilage
has been destroyed, the friction and pressure of bone on bone contact is a source of pain
for affected patients. At present, these defects are treated with microfracture, autologous
chondrocyte implantation (ACI), or osteoarticular transfer system (OATS) procedures.
Microfracture involves drilling small holes in the area of the defects, permitting increased
blood flow with delivery of the necessary growth factors to develop a new layer of cartilage.
The cartilage that is formed, however, is not the same as the native Type II hyaline cartilage,

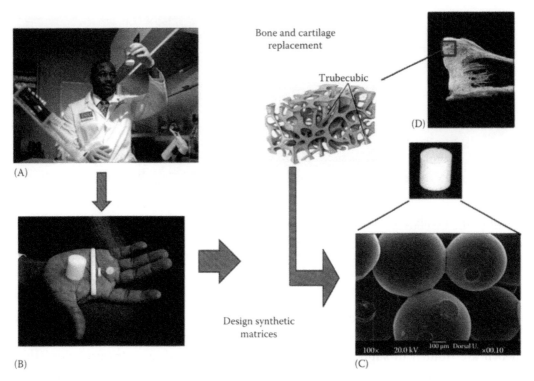

FIGURE 1.4 Tissue-engineered bone graft substitutes. The goal is to develop 3D matrices that have the ability to serve as bone graft substitutes for bone defects. (A) The process begins with a polymer in powder form. (B) Polymer solutions can be injected into molds to create a variety of different shaped scaffolds. (C) Scanning electron microscopy (SEM) imaging of the scaffold demonstrates a 3D structure with pore sizes similar to that of (D) trabecular bone.

but Type I fibrocartilage. Not only does this procedure depend on the body's natural ability to create a new cartilage layer, we do not know the integrity of the Type I cartilage that is formed. The main disadvantages of ACI are time, cost, and the fact that two procedures are required. The initial procedure involves the removal of the patient's own chondrocytes, which are then grown *in vitro* over a 6 week period. The patient then requires a second surgery for the chondrocytes to be implanted at the defect site. In the OATS procedure, a bone plug with the attached cartilage is removed from a non-weight-bearing region and transplanted to fill a defect in a weight-bearing region. Ideally, a less invasive procedure would allow the transfer of chondrocytes delivered in solution, in microspheres, or on a biodegradable scaffold, such as a polymer film layer enriched with growth factors that specifically target the production of cartilage.

Cui et al. have evaluated the histological findings, compressive properties, and GAG contents of tissue-engineered osteochondral composites (chondrocyte–polylactic-*co*-glycolic acid [PLGA] construct sutured to an osteoblast–tricalcium phosphate [TCP] construct with an absorbable suture) and tissue-engineered cartilage used to repair cartilage defects in the knees of pigs (Cui et al., 2011). Their findings showed a significantly better score on the International Cartilage Repair Society (ICRS) Visual Histological Assessment Scale for the osteochondral composite compared to the tissue-engineered cartilage and controls. Based on assessment of the compressive properties and GAG contents, the tissue-engineered osteochondral composite provided a better repair than the tissue-engineered cartilage.

A team of engineers from MIT have developed osteochondral scaffolds using what they describe as "liquid-phase cosynthesis" (Harley, 2006, part III). This concept enables the production of porous, multilayered scaffolds that simulate the composition and structure of articular cartilage on one side, subchondral bone on the other side, and the continuous, gradual or "soft" interface between these tissues: the tidemark of articular joints. With detailed design, the layered scaffolds can be implanted directly into the subchondral bone of an osteochondral defect site without the need for sutures, glue, or screws. It also allows for a highly interconnected porous network. An additional benefit is that the differential moduli of the osseous and cartilaginous compartments enable these layered scaffolds to exhibit compressive deformation behavior that mimics the behavior observed in natural articular joints (Harley, 2011; Harley et al., 2010a,b; Lynn et al., 2010).

1.1.9.3 Meniscus

The meniscus serves as a shock absorber between the femur and the tibia. Tearing or absence of this cushion can lead to accelerated and advanced osteoarthritis. At the present time, the standard treatment for a meniscal tear is a partial meniscectomy. Meniscal repairs are successful only in young patients. A variety of materials have been used for meniscal replacements including allografts, collagen, permanent synthetic scaffolds, and biodegradable scaffolds. These materials have been used both experimentally and clinically (van Tienen et al., 2009). Allografts for meniscus replacements are limited in supply. The use of an artificial meniscus with the same dimensions and biomechanical properties of a native meniscus would solve the shortage issue and decrease the advancement of osteoarthritis in the knee (Figure 1.5).

Collagen meniscus implants have been shown to support new tissue ingrowth sufficient to improve meniscal function in patients with chronic meniscal injuries (Rodkey et al., 2008). Zaffagnini et al. (2011) have reported a 10 year prospective study comparing 33 men (mean age 40 years) who received either a medial collagen meniscus implant (MCMI) or a partial medial meniscectomy (PMM). All patients were evaluated at time 0, 5 years, and a minimum of 10 years after surgery (mean follow-up, 133 months). This study showed that pain, activity level, and radiological outcomes were significantly improved with the use of the MCMI at a minimum 10 year follow-up compared with PMM alone. Future studies should include randomized controlled trials on a larger population (Zaffagnini et al., 2011).

1.1.9.4 Rotator Cuff

A massive rotator cuff tear is considered irreparable if it involves greater than 5 cm and more than one tendon. There is great difficulty in restoring a cuff to its original insertion after it has been retracted to that degree, especially if adhesions form following no repair for an extended period of time. Often, there may be either too much tension after such a repair or insufficient viable tissue for a solid repair. A bridge would need to be formed to reattach the rotator cuff. Ideally, a polymer-based artificial tendon would enable the gap to be filled

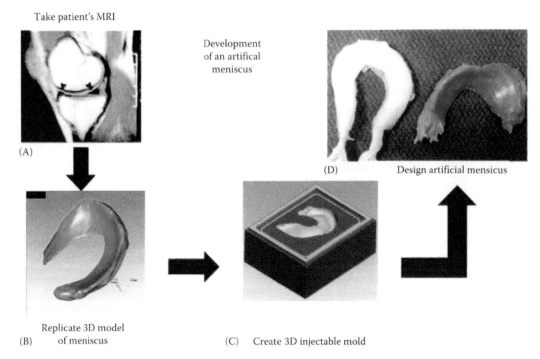

Take patient's MRI

(A)

Development of an artifical meniscus

(D)   Design artificial mensicus

Replicate 3D model
(B)   of meniscus

(C)   Create 3D injectable mold

FIGURE 1.5   A tissue-engineered meniscus was developed with the ability to serve as a meniscus substitute and spacer. (A) An MRI of the patient's knee is used to develop (B) a 3D model of the same dimensions. (C) From the model, a 3D mold is created into which a polymer hydrogel can be injected. (D) The artificial meniscus (left) is shown compared to a native meniscus (right).

restoring the function of the rotator cuff. This scaffold, embedded with mesenchymal stem cells and the necessary proteins to cause an ingrowth of tenocytes, has the potential to induce the formation of a new tendon that will gradually replace the biodegradable polymer.

There have been studies where bone marrow stromal cells isolated from the proximal humerus were able to differentiate into human osteoblasts and tenocytes (Rios et al., 2007). Ouyang et al. (2006) applied sheets of bone marrow–derived mesenchymal stem cells (BM-MSCs) to cryopreserved tendon allografts to revitalize nonviable dense grafts. The composites were cultured, and after 3 weeks, the MSCs had successfully infiltrated the tendon. Many of the MSCs were found to have a spindle-shaped appearance similar to tenocytes. Derwin et al. (2009) augmented the repair of an acute rotator cuff repair in a canine model using a poly-L-lactide repair device. The device that served as a tendon–bone bridge and scaffold for the deposition and ingrowth of host tissue provided improved functional and biomechanical outcomes. These findings suggest that scaffolds seeded with MSCs show potential earlier mobilization and faster recovery after surgery.

1.1.10 Neural Tissue

1.1.10.1 Spinal Cord Injuries

Gelain et al. (2011) have demonstrated anatomical and functional regeneration in chronic spinal cord injuries using transplanted multinanostructured composite scaffolds.

Fluid-filled cysts in postcontusion spinal cord were replaced with neuroprosthetics of electrospun nanofibers composed of blended polycaprolactone and PLGA. The PLGA seeded with neural stem cells have led to significant functional recovery (Teng et al., 2002), while the PCL foam implants have been shown to support axonal regrowth (Cai et al., 2007). Newly formed tissue comprised of neural and stromal cells replaced the cysts and resulted in improved activity in the ascending and descending motor pathways as well as the global locomotion score. These findings provide hope for axonal regeneration and neurological recovery for patients who have sustained chronically injured spinal cords (Gelain, 2010).

1.1.10.2 Parkinson's Disease

There have been advances in tissue engineering that have point to a potential cure for Parkinson's disease (PD). The pathology involved in PD is based on the degeneration of dopamine (DA)-producing neurons primarily in the substantia nigra. While treatment has been focused on replacing DA by the delivery of its precursor, L-dopa, the efficacy of this treatment relies on the presence of functioning DA neurons to produce and release DA. With time, as DA-releasing neurons continue to degenerate, this pharmacological treatment continues to decrease in its effect. As a result, alternative treatments have been pursued. Xi and Zhang (2008) wrote "at present, the fundamental issue ... is the generation of consistent, defined, and functional population of transplantable human DA neurons." The survival rate of dopaminergic neurons has been found to be higher in those with long culture periods. It is believed that this can be attributed to the presence of astrocytes, which appear at 6–8 weeks (Johnson, 2007; Roy, 2006).

Glial cell line–derived neurotrophic factor (GDNF) is a member of the transforming growth factor-β superfamily that has been found to provide a neuroprotective effect on DA neuron (Wu et al., 2010). "Cell replacement strategies combined with GDNF adjunctive therapy might provide the most beneficial effect for PD in the long-term, since GDNF has been proven to be potent neurotrophic on survival, neurite outgrowth, and differentiation toward DA neurons" (Dezawa et al., 2004). To gain the most benefit, a scaffold incorporating stems cells, the necessary growth factors to transform the cells into DA neurons, as well as the astrocytes and GDNF would allow for the regeneration of new DA neurons while maintaining the integrity of existing neurons. This combination provides the potential for both a preventative and curative approach to treating PD. The same concept could be applied to any neurogenerative disorder.

1.1.11 Vascularized Tissue Constructs

Survival of tissue-engineered constructs is often limited by insufficient vascularization. Poor blood supply can lead to insufficient nutrients and hypoxia, which result in failed cell integration and/or cell death. Improving the vascular supply to the tissue-engineered implants will increase the success rate. With this in mind, focus has been turned toward ways to increase both the number of functional blood vessels and the amount of blood carried through the vessels.

There are four main approaches: scaffold design, angiogenic factor delivery, *in vivo* prevascularization, and *in vitro* prevascularization. The scaffold itself must be designed in such a way that vascular ingrowth can be optimized. While pore size plays a role, the actual arrangement of the pores within the 3D structure is more critical for successful vascular ingrowth. Angiogenic factors, such as vascular endothelial growth factor (VEGF) and basic fibroblast growth factor (bFGF), incorporated within the scaffold have been shown to accelerate neovascularization of the implant. However, excess VEGF has resulted in severe vascular leakage and hypotension (Zisch et al., 2003). Stabilization of the vessels requires growth factors such as platelet-derived growth factor (PDGF), transforming growth factor β (TGF-β), and angiopoietin 1. A combination of VEGF and PDGF results in a high number of mature vessels within an implanted scaffold (Chen et al., 2007; Richardson et al., 2001).

Of the four approaches, *in vivo* prevascularization has the fastest vascularization rate. However, the biggest disadvantage is that this procedure requires two surgeries. The first step involves two options: (1) wrapping the graft in an axially vascularized tissue (e.g., muscle) or (2) implanting an artery in the graft. The graft has a temporary arterial supply until a microvascular capillary network can be formed within the graft over a several week period. The second step is a separate procedure where the graft is transferred from the vascularization site to the actual defect with surgical anastomosis providing immediate perfusion (Kneser et al., 2006).

1.2 REGENERATIVE ENGINEERING: FUTURE CHALLENGES

Applications for tissue engineering are broadening routinely. While significant strides have been made, there is still room for growth and improvements. The ideal cell sources have yet to be determined. Further investigations will be required to understand how these cells differentiate, proliferate, and adhere to the appropriate scaffolds. There are many options regarding the biomaterials that are used as scaffolds. The nanostructures, degradation rates, and biomechanical properties must be optimized to provide the best repair with the most efficient recovery. Ultimately, tissue engineering offers an amazing opportunity to combine basic science, medicine, and engineering to increase our knowledge of how the body functions with the goal of improving the health and lifestyles of current patients and future generations.

REFERENCES

Atala A, Bauer SB, Soker S, Yoo JJ, Retik AB. 2006. Tissue engineered autologous bladders for patients needing cystoplasty. *Lancet*. 367: 1241.

Attawia MA, Uhrich KE, Botchwey E, Langer R, Laurencin CT. 1996. *In vitro* bone biocompatibility of poly(anhydride-*co*-imides) containing pyromellitylimidoalanine. *J Orthop Res*. 14(3): 445–454.

Berry JL, Steen JA, Koudy Williams J, Jordan JE, Atala A, Yoo JJ. 2010. Bioreactors for development of tissue engineered heart valves. *Ann Biomed Eng*. 38(11): 3272–3279.

Bianchi A. 1999. Experience with longitudinal intestinal lengthening and tailoring. *Eur J Pediatr Surg*. 9: 256–259.

Blyszczuk P, Wobus AM. 2004. Stem cells and pancreatic differentiation *in vitro*. *J Biotechnol*. 113: 3–13.

Bodell BR, Head JM, Head LR, Formolo AJ. 1965. An implantable artificial lung. Initial experiments in animals. *JAMA*. 191: 301–303.

Bolander ME. 1992. Regulation of fracture repair by growth factors. *Proc Soc Exp Biol Med.* 200: 165–170.

Borden M, Attawia M, Khan Y, El-Amin SF, Laurencin CT. 2004.Tissue-engineered bone formation *in vivo* using a novel sintered polymeric microsphere matrix. *J Bone Joint Surg Br.* 86(8): 1200–1208.

Bostman OM, Pihlajamaki HK. 1998. Late foreign-body reaction to an intraosseous bioabsorbable polylactic acid screw. A case report. *J Bone Joint Surg Am.* 80: 1791–1794.

Brekke JH, Toth JM. 1998. Principles of tissue engineering applied to programmable osteogenesis. *J Biomed Mater Res.* 43: 380–398.

Brendel M, Hering B, Schulz A, Bretzel R. 1999. International Islet Tranplant Registry report. Giessen, Germany: University of Giessen, pp. 1–20.

Buchholz DE, Hikita ST, Rowland TJ, Friedrich AM, Hinman CR, Johnson LV, Clegg DO. 2009. Derivation of functional retinal pigmented epithelium from induced pluripotent stem cells. *Stem Cells.* 27: 2427–2434.

Cai J, Ziemba KS, Smith GM, Jin Y. 2007. Evaluation of cellular organization and axonal regeneration through linear PLA foam implants in acute and chronic spinal cord injury. *J Biomed Mater Res A.* 83: 512–520.

Chen RR et al. 2007. Spatio-temporal VEGF and PDGF delivery patterns blood vessel formation and maturation. *Pharm Res.* 24: 258–264.

Cook KE, Makarewicz AJ, Backer CL et al. 1996. Testing of an intrathoracic artificial lung in a pig model. *ASAIO J.* 42: M604–M609.

Cui W, Wang Q, Chen G, Zhou S, Chang Q, Zuo Q, Ren K, Fan W. 2011. Repair of articular cartilage defects with tissue-engineered osteochondral composites in pigs. *J Biosci Bioeng.* 111(4): 493–500.

De Miguel MP, Alio JL, Arnalich-Montiel F, Fuentes-Julian S, deBenito-Llopis L, Amparo F, Bataille L. 2010. Cornea and ocular surface treatment. *Curr Stem Cell Res Ther.* 5(2): 195–204.

Derwin KA, Codsi MJ, Milks RA, Baker AR, McCarron JA, Iannotti JP. 2009. Rotator cuff repair augmentation in a canine model with use of a woven poly-L-lactide device. *J Bone Joint Surg Am.* 91: 1159–1171.

DeVries WC, Anderson JL, Joyce LD, Anderson FL, Hammond EH, Jarvik RK, Kolff WJ. 1984. Clinical use of the total artificial heart. *N Engl J Med.* 310: 273–278.

Dezawa M, Kanno H, Hoshino M et al. 2004. Specific induction of neuronal cells from bone marrow stromal cells and application for autologous transplantation. *J Clin Invest.* 113(12): 1701–1710.

Engelmayr GC Jr, Soletti L, Vigmostad SC, Budilarto SG, Federspiel WJ, Chandran KB, Vorp DA, Sacks MS. 2008. A novel flex-stretch-flow bioreactor for the study of engineered heart valve tissue mechanobiology. *Ann Biomed Eng.* 36(5): 700–712.

Fan H, Liu H, Toh SL, Goh JC. 2009. Anterior cruciate ligament regeneration using mesenchymal stem cells and silk scaffold in large animal model. *Biomaterials.* 30(28): 4967–4977.

Furuta A, Miyoshi S, Itabashi Y et al. 2006. Pulsatile cardiac tissue grafts using a novel three-dimensional cell sheet manipulation technique functionally integrates with the host heart, *in vivo. Circ Res.* 98: 705–712.

Gelain F, Panseri S, Antonini S, Cunha C, Donega M, Lowery J, Taraballi F, Cerri G, Montagna M, Baldissera F, Vescovi A. 2011. Transplantation of nanostructure composite scaffolds results in the regeneration of chronically injured spinal cords. *ACS Nano.* 5(1): 227–236.

Grikscheit TC, Sala FG, Ogilvie J, Bower KA, Ochoa ER, Alsberg E, Mooney D, Vacanti JP. 2008. Tissue-engineered spleen protects against overwhelming pneumococcal sepsis in a rodent model. *J Surg Res.* 149: 214–218.

Grikscheit TC, Siddique A, Ochoa ER, Srinivasan A, Alsberg E, Hodin RA et al. 2004. Tissue-engineered small intestine improves recovery after massive small bowel resection. *Ann Surg.* 240: 748–754.

Harley BA, Lynn AK, Wissner-Gross Z, Bonfield W, Yannas IV, Gibson LJ. 2010a. Design of a multiphase osteochondral scaffold. II. Fabrication of a mineralized collagen-glycosaminoglycan scaffold. *J Biomed Mater Res A*. 92(3): 1066–1077.

Harley BA, Lynn AK, Wissner-Gross Z, Bonfield W, Yannas IV, Gibson LJ. 2010b. Design of a multiphase osteochondral scaffold III: Fabrication of layered scaffolds with continuous interfaces. *J Biomed Mater Res A*. 92(3): 1078–1093.

Hecker L, Birla RK. 2007. Engineering the heart piece by piece: State of the art in cardiac tissue engineering. *Regen Med*. 2: 125–144.

Hsu S-L, Liang R, Woo SLY. 2010. Functional tissue engineering of ligament healing. *Sports Med Arthrosc Rehabil Ther Technol*. 2: 12.

Hynes SR, Lavik EB. 2010. A tissue-engineered approach towards retinal repair: Scaffolds for cell transplantation to the subretinal space. *Graefes Arch Clin Exp Ophthalmol*. 248(6): 763–778.

Ibim SEM, Ambrosio A, Kwon MS, El-Amin SF, Allcock HR, Laurencin CT. 1997. Novel polyphosphazene/poly(lactide-*co*-glycolide) blends: Miscibility and degradation studies. *Biomaterials*. 18: 1565–1569.

Ignatius AA, Claes LE. 1996. *In vitro* biocompatibility of bioresorbable polymers: Poly(L,DL-lactide) and poly(L-lactide-*co*-glycolide). *Biomaterials*. 17: 831–839.

Ito M, Hayashi T, Kuroiwa A, Okamoto M. 1999. Lens formation by pigmented epithelial cell reaggregate from dorsal iris implanted into limb blastema in the adult newt. *Dev Growth Differ*. 41: 429–440.

Jackson DW, Simon TM. 1999. Tissue engineering principles in orthopaedic surgery. *Clin Orthop*. 367: S31–S45.

Javaid-Ur-Rehman, Waseem T. 2008. Intestinal tissue engineering: Where do we stand? *Surg Today*. 38(6): 484–486.

Kabatas S, Teng YD. 2010. Potential roles of the neural stem cell in the restoration of the injured spinal cord: Review of the literature. *Turkis Neurosurg*. 20(2): 103–110.

Kelm JM, Djonov V, Hoerstrup SP et al. 2006. Tissue-transplant fusion and vascularization of myocardial microtissues and macrotissues implanted into chicken embryos and rats. *Tissue Eng*. 12: 2541–2553.

Kobayashi D, Kurosaka M, Yoshiya S, Mizuno K. 1997. Effect of basic fibroblast growth factor on the healing of defects in the canine anterior cruciate ligament. *Knee Surg Sports Traumatol Arthrosc*. 5(3): 189–194.

Kneser, U. et al. 2006. Tissue engineering of bone: The reconstructive surgeon's point of view. *J Cell Mol Med*. 10: 7–19.

Kondo E, Yasuda K, Yamanaka M, Minami A, Tohyama H. 2005. Effects of administration of exogenous growth factors on biomechanical properties of the elongation-type anterior cruciate ligament injury with partial laceration. *Am J Sports Med*. 33(2): 188–196.

Langer R, Vacanti JP. 1993. Tissue engineering. *Science*. 260: 920–926.

Lipshutz GS, Wilkinson AH. 2007. Pancreas-kidney and pancreas transplantation for the treatment of diabetes mellitus. *Endocrinol Metab Clin North Am*. 36: 1015–1038.

Lynn AK, Best SM, Cameron RE, Harley BA, Yannas IV, Gibson LJ, Bonfield W. 2010. Design of a multiphase osteochondral scaffold. I. Control of chemical composition. *J Biomed Mater Res A*. 92(3): 1057–1065.

Maves L, Schubiger G. 1999. Cell determination and transdetermination in *Drosophila* imaginal discs. *Curr Top Dev Biol*. 43: 115–151.

Miyamoto S, Takaoka K, Okada T, Yoshikawa H, Hashimoto J, Suzuki S, Ono K. 1993. Polylactic acid–polyethylene glycol *block* copolymer. A new biodegradable synthetic carrier for bone morphogenetic protein. *Clin Orthop*. 333–343.

Murray MM, Spindler KP, Devin C, Snyder BS, Muller J, Takahashi M, Ballard P, Nanney LB, Zurakowski D. 2006. Use of a collagen-platelet rich plasma scaffold to stimulate healing of a central defect in the canine ACL. *J Orthop Res*. 24(4): 820–830.

Obaid H, Connell D. 2010. Cell therapy in tendon disorders: What is the current evidence? *Am J Sports Med.* 38: 2123–2132.

Orlandò G, Di Cocco P, D Angelo M, Clemente K, Famulari A, Pisani F. 2010. Regenerative medicine applied to solid organ transplantation: Where do we stand? *Transplant.* 42(4): 1011–1013.

Ott HC, Clippinger B, Conrad C, Schuetz C, Pomerantseva I et al. 2010. Regeneration and orthotopic transplantation of a bioartificial lung. *Nat Med.* 16: 927–933.

Ott HC, Matthiesen TS, Goh SK et al. 2008. Perfusion-decellularized matrix: Using nature's platform to engineer a bioartificial heart. *Nat Med.* 14: 213–221.

Ouyang HW, Cao T, Zou XH et al. 2006. Mesenchymal stem cell sheets revitalized nonviable dense grafts: Implications for repair of large-bone and tendon defects. *Transplantation.* 82: 170–174.

Perez A, Grikscheit TC, Blumberg RS, Ashley SW, Vacanti JP, Whang EE. 2002. Tissue-engineered small intestine: Ontogeny of the immune system. *Transplantation.* 74: 619–623.

Petersen TH, Calle EA, Zhao L, Lee EJ et al. 2010. Tissue-engineered lungs for *in vivo* implantation. *Science.* 329: 538.

Proulx S, d'Arc Uwamaliya J, Carrier P, Deschambeault A, Audet C, Giasson CJ, Guérin SL, Auger FA, Germain L. 2010. Reconstruction of a human cornea by the self-assembly approach of tissue engineering using the three native cell types. *Mol Vis.* 16: 2192–2201.

Punch JD, Hayes DH, LaPorte FB, McBride V, Seely MS. 2007. Organ donation and utilization in the United States, 1996–2005. *Am J Transplant.* 7: 1327–1338.

Radtke ND, Aramant RB, Petry HM, Green PT, Pidwell DJ, Seiler MJ. 2008. Vision improvement in retinal regeneration patients by implantation of retina together with retinal pigment epithelium. *Am J Ophthalmol.* 146: 172–182.

Richardson TP et al. 2001. Polymeric system for dual growth factor delivery. *Nat Biotechnol.* 19: 1029–1034.

Rios CG, McCarthy M, Arciero C, Spang JT, Arciero RA, Mazzocca AD. 2007. Biologics in shoulder surgery: The role of adult mesenchymal stem cells in tendon repair. *Tech Orthop.* 22: 2–9.

Rodeo SA, Delos D, Weber A, Ju X, Cunningham M, Fortier L, Maher S. 2010. What's new in orthopaedic research. *J Bone Joint Surg Am.* 92: 2491–2501.

Rodkey WG, DeHaven KE, Montgomery WH 3rd, Baker CL Jr, Beck CL Jr, Hormel SE, Steadman JR, Cole BJ, Briggs KK. 2008. Comparison of the collagen meniscus implant with partial meniscectomy. A prospective randomized trial. *J Bone Joint Surg Am.* 90(7): 1413–1426.

Ross EA, Williams MJ, Hamazaki T, Terada N, Clapp WL, Adin C, Ellison GW, Jorgensen M, Batich CD. 2009. Embryonic stem cells proliferate and differentiate when seeded into kidney scaffolds. *J Am Soc Nephrol.* 20(11): 2338–2347.

Rouwkema J, Rivron N, van Blitterswijk C. 2008. Vascularization in tissue engineering. *Trends Biotechnol.* 26(8): 434–441.

Royals MA, Fujita SM, Yewey GL, Rodriguez J, Schultheiss PC, Dunn RL. 1999. Biocompatibility of a biodegradable *in situ* forming implant system in rhesus monkeys. *J Biomed Mater Res.* 45: 231–239.

Safar P. 1988. Clinical death symposium. *Crit Care Med.* 16: 919–920.

Shapiro AM, Lakey JR, Ryan EA, Korbutt GS, Toth E, Warnock GL, Kneteman NM, Rajotte RV. 2000. Islet transplantation in seven patients with type 1 diabetes mellitus using a glucocorticoid-free immunosuppressive regimen. *N Engl J Med.* 343(4): 230–238.

Shimizu T, Yamato M, Isoi Y et al. 2002. Fabrication of pulsatile cardiac tissue grafts using a novel 3-dimensional cell sheet manipulation technique and temperature-responsive cell culture surfaces. *Circ Res.* 90: e40.

Shrestha BM. 2009. Strategies for reducing the renal transplant waiting list: A review. *Exp Clin Transplant.* 7: 173–179.

Suematsu, S, Watanabe, T. 2004. Generation of a synthetic lymphoid tissue-like organoid in mice. *Nat Biotechnol.* 22: 1539–1545.

Sutherland FW, Perry TE, Yu Y, Sherwood MC, Rabkin E, Masuda Y, Garcia GA, McLellan DL, Engelmayr GC Jr, Sacks MS, Schoen FJ, Mayer JE Jr. 2005. From stem cells to viable autologous semilunar heart valve. *Circulation*. 111(21): 2783–2791.

Tan JK, Watanabe T. 2010. Artificial engineering of secondary lymphoid organs. *Adv Immunol*. 105: 131–157.

Tee R, Lokmic Z, Morrison WA, Dilley RJ. 2010. Strategies in cardiac tissue engineering. *ANZ J Surg*. 80(10): 683–693.

Teng Y, Lavik E, Qu X, Park K, Ourednik J, Zurakowski D, Langer R, Snyder E. 2002. Functional recovery following traumatic spinal cord injury mediated by a unique polymer scaffold seeded with neural stem cells. *PNAS*. 99(5): 3024–3029.

Therin M, Christel P, Li S, Garreau H, Vert M. 1992. *In vivo* degradation of massive poly(alpha-hydroxy acids): Validation of *in vitro* findings. *Biomaterials*. 13: 594–600.

Uygun BE, Soto-Gutierrez A, Yagi H, Izamis ML, Guzzardi MA, Shulman C, Milwid J, Kobayashi N, Tilles A, Berthiaume F, Hertl M, Nahmias Y, Yarmush ML, Uygun K. 2010. Organ reengineering through development of a transplantable recellularized liver graft using decellularized liver matrix. *Nat Med*. 16(7): 814–820.

van Tienen TG, Hannink G, Buma P. 2009. Meniscus replacement using synthetic materials. *Clin Sports Med*. 28(1):143–156.

Wang G, Hu X, Lin W, Dong C, Wu H. 2011. Electrospun PLGA-silk fibroin-collagen nanofibrous scaffolds for nerve tissue engineering. *In Vitro Cell Dev Biol Anim*. 47(3):234–240.

Warner BW, Chaet MS. 1993. Nontransplant surgical options for management of the short bowel syndrome. *J Pediatr Gastroenterol Nutr*. 17: 1–12.

Wei XL, Lin L, Hou Y, Fu X, Zhang JY, Mao ZB, Yu CL. 2008. Construction of recombinant adenovirus co-expression vector carrying the human transforming growth factor-beta1 and vascular endothelial growth factor genes and its effect on anterior cruciate ligament fibroblasts. *Chin Med J (Engl)*. 121(15): 1426–1432.

Witt SA, Alpard SK, Lick SD, Deyo DJ, Montoya P, Zwischenberger JB. 1999. Total artificial lung perioperative management: A 7 day survival study in sheep. *Crit Care Med*. 27: A22.

Wu J, Yu W, Chen Y, Su Y, Ding Z, Ren H, Jiang Y, Wang J. 2010. Intrastriatal transplantation of GDNF-engineered BMSCs and its neuroprotection in lactacystin-induced Parkinsonian rat model. *Neurochem Res*. 35: 495–502.

Xi J, Zhang S-C. 2008. Stem cells in development of therapeutics for Parkinson's disease: A perspective. *J Cell Biochem*. 105(5): 1153–1160.

Yechoor V, Chan L. 2010. Minireview: Beta-cell replacement therapy for diabetes in the 21st century: Manipulation of cell fate by directed differentiation. *Mol Endocrinol*. 24(8): 1501–1511.

Yechoor V, Liu V, Espiritu C, Paul A, Oka K, Kojima H, Chan L. 2009. Neurogenin3 is sufficient for transdetermination of hepatic progenitor cells into neo-islets *in vivo* but not transdifferentiation of hepatocytes. *Dev Cell*. 16: 358–373.

Zaffagnini S, Marcheggiani Muccioli GM, Lopomo N, Bruni D, Giordano G, Ravazzolo G, Molinari M, Marcacci M. 2011. Prospective long-term outcomes of the medial collagen meniscus implant versus partial medial meniscectomy: A minimum 10-year follow-up study. *Am J Sports Med*. 39(5): 977–985.

Zhou Q, Brown J, Kanarek A, Rajagopal J, Melton DA. 2008. *In vivo* reprogramming of adult pancreatic exocrine cells to cells. *Nature*. 455: 627–632.

Zimmermann WH, Schneiderbanger K, Schubert P et al. 2002. Tissue engineering of a differentiated cardiac muscle construct. *Circ Res*. 90: 223–230.

Zisch AH, Lutolf MP, Hubbell JA et al. 2003. Biopolymeric delivery for angiogenic growth factors. *Cardiovasc Pathol*. 12: 295–310.

CHAPTER 2

Cell Biology

Gloria Gronowicz, PhD and Karen Sagomonyants, DMD

CONTENTS

2.1 INTRODUCTION

To be able to engineer tissues, a fundamental understanding of cell structure and function is essential. If we are to replace tissues with new biomaterials or tissue constructs, then basic cell processes must be understood so that we can engineer a biomaterial or a process that best simulates what is found in nature. The purpose of this chapter is to describe briefly the structure of macromolecules and organelles in the cell and to review several important processes for cell maintenance, survival, and proliferation.

2.2 MACROMOLECULES IN CELLS

2.2.1 Proteins

Proteins are the building blocks of the cell that catalyze chemical reactions, provide structure and rigidity, control membrane permeability, recognize and bind biomolecules, and regulate motility, metabolites, and gene function, among other activities. The building blocks of proteins are 20 different amino acids (Figure 2.1). They are joined together in many different combinations forming long linear chains. These amino acids are called standard amino acids and abbreviated by letters. An example is RGD, which represents the amino acids arginine, lysine, and aspartic acid. Each amino acid contains an amino group ($-NH_2$) and a carboxyl group ($-COOH$). An exception is proline, which only has a $-NH-$ group. Their monomeric structure is represented by a general chemical formula in which R represents a side group that gives each amino acid individuality.

Amino acids are connected by peptide bonds that are formed between an amino group of one molecule and the carboxyl group of another amino acid in a reaction called *condensation* that liberates water. Two connected amino acids ($n = 2$) form a *dipeptide*, three amino acids ($n = 3$) form a *tripeptide*, four amino acids ($n = 4$) form a *tetrapeptide*, and so on. If $n > 10$, molecule is called *polypeptide*. The word *protein* is generally used to refer to the complete biological molecule in a stable conformation, when $n > 30$–40.

In cells, typical proteins consist of 100–500 amino acids, and the longest known protein chain is built up more than 34,000 amino acids (titin). Most proteins fold into unique three-dimensional structures that can differ in size and shape (for example, rods or globular shapes). These protein architectures are stabilized by covalent (such as disulfide bonds) or non-covalent (ionic, van der Waals, and hydrophobic) interactions within the molecule.

In describing the structure of a polypeptide, scientists refer to the *primary structure*, which is the linear arrangement of amino acids along a polypeptide chain and its covalent bonds between chains. *Secondary structure* is described as the folding of parts of the chains into structures such as helices and β-pleated sheets, which form a *tertiary structure*

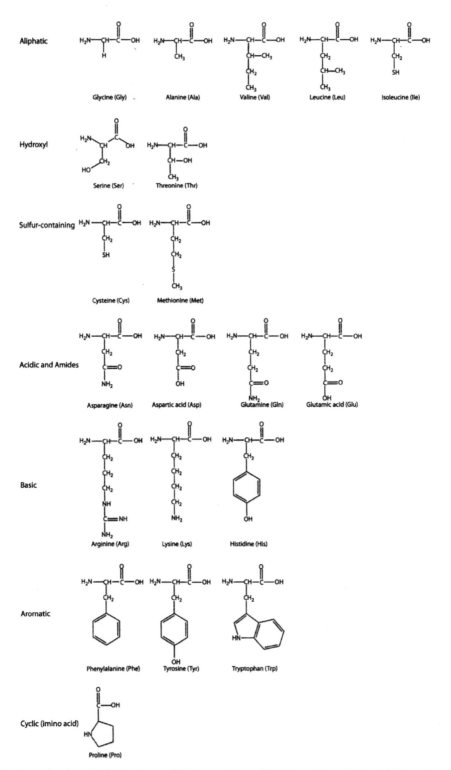

FIGURE 2.1   The chemical structure of the 20 amino acids. For each amino acid, there is a central carbon atom bonded to an amino group (or an imino group in proline), a carboxyl group, a hydrogen atom, and an R group that can vary depending on the amino acid.

through their interactions with each other to form compact shapes or domains. Finally, proteins can consist of multiple polypeptide chains held together by non-covalent or covalent bonds forming *quaternary structures*. The native structure of a protein can be denatured by heat, pH extremes, or chemicals.

Great structural diversity of proteins allows them to perform a myriad of cell functions carrying out the duties specified by the information encoded in genes. The major of these functions include structural functions (for example, structural protein *collagen* is the most abundant protein in mammals, making up about 25%–35% of the whole-body protein content) as well as enzymatic functions that are discussed in the next section.

2.2.2 Enzymes

Enzymes are proteins that catalyze chemical reactions. The chemical on which an enzyme acts is called a substrate, and often the enzyme's name has an -ase at the end of the substrate's name, such as proteases, which are enzymes that act on proteins, or phosphatases, which are enzymes that remove phosphate groups, etc. Enzymes are found mostly inside cells, often in particular types of cells and/or particular compartments of the cell or organelles, but some enzymes can be secreted outside the cell. Enzymes are characterized by their specificity of action between two closely similar substrates or reactions, and by their large catalytic potential. Their catalytic potential is an enzyme's ability to speed the rate of a reaction by 10^6–10^{12} times of an uncatalyzed reaction under otherwise identical conditions. Thus, enzymes need to be closely regulated by cells so that a specific metabolic pathway or specific synthetic reactions occur and then end. There are two important regions of an enzyme: the site where it recognizes and binds the substrate(s) and other site where it catalyzes the reaction. Together these two sites are called the active site and can be located near or far from each other in the amino acid sequence, but due to folding of the molecule can be brought in close proximity to initiate the reaction. The binding of the substrate usually involves the formation of non-covalent hydrogen, ionic, and hydrophobic bonds and van der Waals interactions. Sometimes covalent bonds between the substrate and enzyme are formed and then broken during the reaction, inducing a conformational change in the enzyme. Some enzymatic reactions require coenzymes, which are small molecules or prosthetic groups essential for the reaction. Many vitamins are converted into coenzymes.

Many enzymes have additional regulatory sites that bind to molecules in the cellular environment. The sites form weak, non-covalent bonds with these molecules, causing a change in the conformation of the enzyme. This change in conformation translates to the active site, which then affects the reaction rate of the enzyme.

2.2.3 Lipids

Lipids are a broad group of cellular molecules that includes fats, waxes, sterols, fat-soluble vitamins (such as vitamins A, D, E, and K), glycerolipids, phospholipids, and others. Lipids are the major structural components of biomembranes that separate cells from the extracellular environment, provide anchoring sites for some proteins, and form the boundaries of the organelles found in eukaryotic cells. Lipids are composed mainly of hydrogen and carbon atoms to form hydrocarbons. These hydrocarbons are hydrophobic so they segregate into a separate nonaqueous phase in aqueous environments, and thus are insoluble or slightly soluble in water. Fatty acids are the principal building blocks of lipids and membranes. They contain a long hydrocarbon chain attached to a carboxyl group, and can differ in length and in the extent and position of their double bonds. Fatty acids with no double bonds are termed saturated, and fatty acids with at least one double bond are called unsaturated. A double bond in an unsaturated fatty acid can be in *cis* or *trans* configurations (Figure 2.2); however, double bonds in most unsaturated fatty acids have the *cis* configuration.

Fatty acids are stored in cells as triacylglycerols and are highly hydrophobic. Triacylglycerols are a major form of energy storage in animals, and the complete oxidation of fatty acids provides high caloric content, about 9 kcal/g, compared with 4 kcal/g for breakdown of carbohydrates and protein. Figure 2.3 illustrates the process by which triacylglycerols are formed by esterification of fatty acids to each of the three hydroxyl

FIGURE 2.2   *Cis* and *trans* configurations of fatty acids.

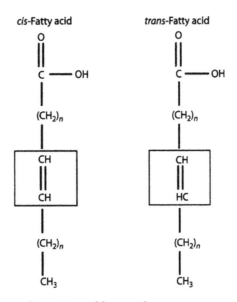

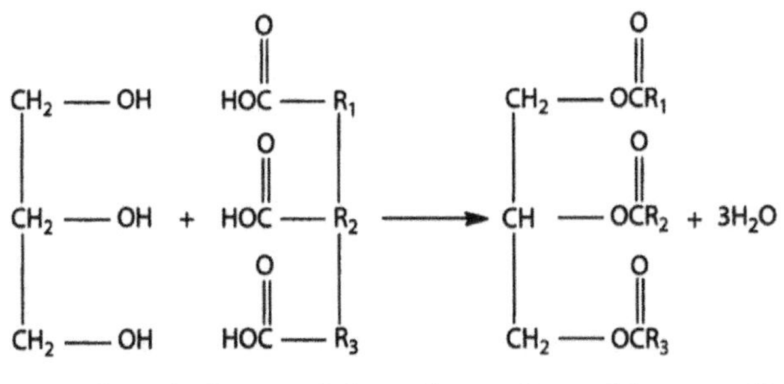

FIGURE 2.3   The process by which triacylglycerols are formed by esterification of fatty acids to each of the three hydroxyl groups in glycerol and the liberation of three molecules of water. Triacylglycerols are a storage form for fatty acids in the body.

groups in glycerol and the liberation of three molecules of water. The fatty acid part of the triacylglycerol is called an acyl group. Triacylglycerols are insoluble in water and salt solutions and form lipid droplets in cells. Fat cells termed adipose cells store these droplets of triacylglycerols as a source of energy. In response to particular hormones, adipose cells hydrolyze the triacylglycerols into free fatty acids that are released into the blood, whereupon cells remove them from circulation and degrade them for energy.

Long-chain fatty acid acyl groups are also found in membranes but they are linked usually by an ester bond to small hydrophilic groups. Due to this hydrophilic group, the membrane lipids orient themselves into sheets in which the hydrophilic groups are facing the aqueous environment while the hydrophobic region is concealed from the water creating a molecule that is termed *amphiphatic*.

Since amphiphatic molecules form organized structures in water, they are a key component of cell membranes. Phospholipids are the most abundant amphiphatic lipids of which phosphoglycerides are a major family that are illustrated in Figure 2.4. Phosphoglycerides contain a fatty acyl side chain forming ester bonds with two hydroxyl groups of glycerol and with the third hydroxyl group esterified to phosphate. In many phospholipids, the phosphate group is also esterified to a hydroxyl group on a hydrophilic molecule such as serine, choline, ethanolamine, or glycerol.

Phospholipids spontaneously form three different structures in aqueous solutions: micelles, liposomes, and bilayers (Figure 2.5). Which structure forms is dependent on the mixture of the phospholipids, the length and degree of saturation of the fatty acyl chains, temperature and ionic composition of the solution, and how the phospholipids are introduced into solution. Violent dispersal can create micelles (about 20 nm or less in diameter forming a sphere) with the hydrocarbon side chains facing within, and

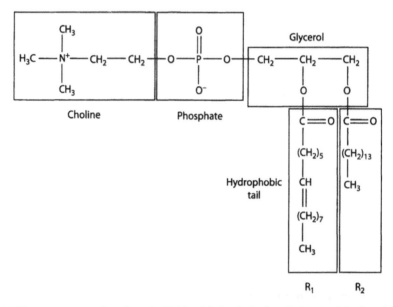

FIGURE 2.4 The structure of a phospholipid with both hydrophobic and hydrophilic regions creating an amphiphatic molecule. The example that is given is phosphocholine.

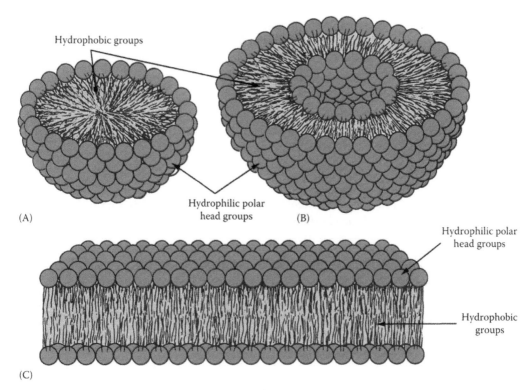

Hydrophobic groups

Hydrophilic polar head groups

(A)

(B)

Hydrophilic polar head groups

Hydrophobic groups

(C)

FIGURE 2.5   Micelles (A), liposome (B), and bilayer (C) that are formed by phospholipids in aqueous solutions. Bilayers are the basis of biological membranes.

polar groups facing the aqueous solution. Phospholipids can also spontaneously form symmetrical sheet-like structures termed phospholipid bilayers that are two molecules thick but can extend to large lengths. The hydrocarbon chains are in the center of the bilayer away from water and are tightly packed by van der Waals interactions. Electrostatic and hydrogen bonds stabilize the polar group's interactions with water. Liposomes can also artificially be prepared as spherical bilayers forming a vesicle, which can have an aqueous interior and contain drugs or other agents. Bilayers are the basis of biological membranes. Proteins are found within the biomembranes and interact specifically with the hydrophobic core. Through their interactions with the phospholipids, proteins can organize specific lipids around themselves.

Another important group of membrane lipids is steroids that are derived from cholesterol and its derivatives. The basic structure of the steroids is a four-ring hydrocarbon, which is illustrated in Figure 2.6. Cholesterol is shown as an example, and is a major steroid in animal tissues and also plant cell membranes. Steroids also have different biological roles as hormones and signaling molecules.

2.2.4 Carbohydrates

Carbohydrates are composed of carbon, hydrogen, and oxygen. The most simple carbohydrate is a monosaccharide with the formula $-(CH_2O)_n$, where $n = 3, 4, 5, 6,$ or 7. All monosaccharides contain hydroxyl groups and either an aldehyde or a keto group.

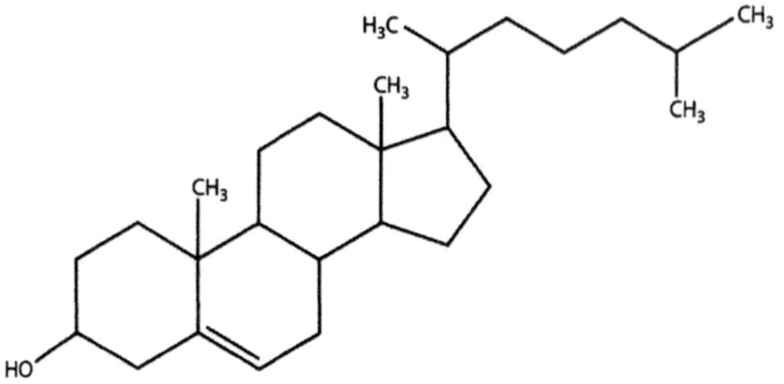

FIGURE 2.6 The general structure of a steroid with the same four hydrocarbon rings. Cholesterol is given as an example and is the major steroidal constituent of animal tissues.

The five-carbon sugars, pentose (ribose and deoxyribose), and the six-carbon sugars, hexose (glucose, fructose, and galactose), are very important in cells.

D-Glucose is the principal source of energy that is stored in a cell and it is also a hexose sugar, which is the structure of many biologically important sugars in cells. Therefore, Figure 2.7 illustrates the various configurations of glucose: D-glucose, the linear structure and the two different ring structures of glucose. Most sugars are D- rather than L-sugars

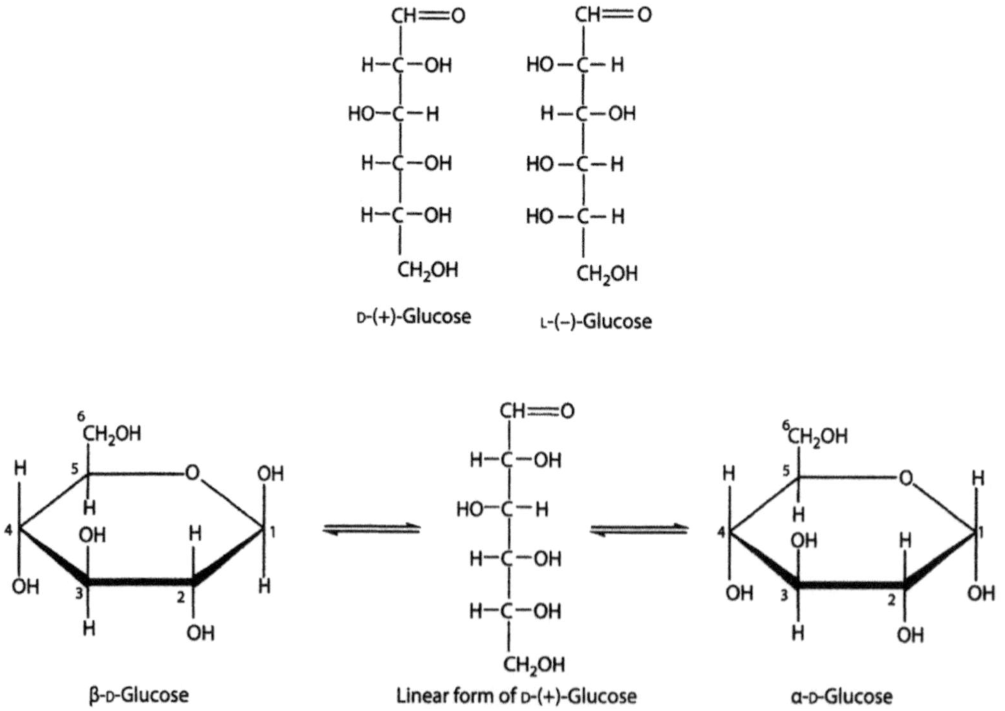

FIGURE 2.7 The alternate configurations of D-glucose, which is most commonly found in nature, and is often called dextrose.

in which D and L are mirror images of each other or stereoisomers. One of the set of isomers, the D-glucose is found in nature and is often referred to as dextrose. The ring structures are formed by the aldehyde group of one carbon reacting with the hydroxyl group on the five carbon to form a six-membered ring called glucopyranose. Each carbon atom in glucose is bonded to four different atoms or groups, and their spatial organization determines different types of sugars that are recognized by different enzymes and binding proteins. For example, mannose is identical to glucose except for the orientation of the group on the two carbon, while galactose is different from glucose only in the orientation of the hydroxyl group on the four carbon. Other modified molecules are N-acetylneuraminic acid (sialic acid), α-D-N-acetylglucosamine, α-D-N-acetylgalactosamine, and α-L-fucose, which are more common components of polysaccharides, glycoproteins, or glycolipids. N-Acetylneuraminic acid also called sialic acid is particularly prevalent in cells.

Monosaccharides are building blocks for more complex carbohydrates. Similar to amino acids within proteins, two different or identical monosaccharides can be linked together in condensation reaction forming a *glycosidic bond*, in which the one carbon of one sugar reacts with the hydroxyl group of another, liberating water (Figure 2.8). In cells, these reactions are catalyzed by specialized enzymes. Two joined monosaccharides are called a *disaccharide*. Examples include *sucrose* and *lactose*. Sucrose is composed of one glucose molecule and one fructose molecule. Sucrose is the main form in which carbohydrates are transported in plants. Lactose, a disaccharide composed of one galactose molecule and one glucose molecule, occurs naturally in mammalian milk.

Disaccharides can continue to join monosaccharides forming longer linear or branched chains. Carbohydrate chains containing dozens of monosaccharide units are called *oligosaccharides*, while *polysaccharides* contain hundreds and thousands of monosaccharide units. Polysaccharides represent an important class of biological polymers. *Starch* (a polymer of glucose) is used as a storage polysaccharide in plants. Glucose molecules are bound in starch by the easily hydrolyzed bonds, so starch can accumulate or liberate glucose depending on cell needs. In animals, the same function is executed by the structurally similar glucose polymer *glycogen*. *Cellulose* is another glucose polymer, but its glucose units are connected by a different kind of glycosidic bonds than in starch and glycogen and, therefore, cellulose has its specific physical–chemical properties. Cellulose is used as a structure-forming component of the cell walls in plants and is claimed to be the most abundant organic molecule on earth.

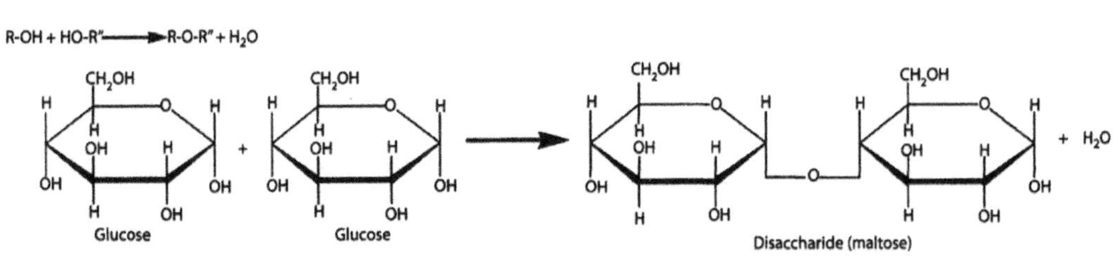

FIGURE 2.8 The enzymatic formation of glycosidic linkages to generate a disaccharide from two glucose molecules with the liberation of water.

2.2.5 Glycoproteins and Glycolipids

In the previous sections, monomeric building blocks such as amino acids, structural elements of lipids, and monosaccharides have been described, and a vast array of specialized cellular molecules are formed as a result of polymeric combinations of these building blocks. One more cellular strategy to get molecular species with new properties is to combine different types of molecules into chimeras. Examples of such hybrid molecules are *glycoproteins* and *glycolipids*.

Glycoproteins are proteins that contain oligosaccharide chains (*glycans*) covalently attached to polypeptide chain. Glycoproteins are frequently found in or associated with the cell membrane where they function as membrane proteins or as part of the extracellular matrix (ECM). They play a critical role in cell–cell interactions and they are involved in infection by bacteria and viruses. The carbohydrate chains contribute to the folding, stability, and solubility of the protein as well as to where the glycoproteins are synthesized and ultimately located in the cell.

There are three types of glycoproteins based on their structure and the mechanism of synthesis: N-linked glycoproteins, O-linked glycoproteins, and nonenzymatic glycosylated glycoproteins. N-linked glycoproteins have their sugars bound to the amide nitrogen of amino acid asparagine and are synthesized and modified within the rough endoplasmic reticulum (RER) and the Golgi apparatus (see later) of the cell. They are found in many membranes and secreted proteins. Many antibodies have these oligosaccharides attached to their serum proteins. In O-linked glycoproteins, the sugars are bound to the hydroxyl group of amino acids serine and threonine and, in collagen, to hydroxylysine. They are most often synthesized in the Golgi apparatus, and many O-linked glycoproteins are secreted by the cell to form the ECM. Nonenzymatic glycosylation or glycation creates glycoproteins by the chemical addition of sugars to polypeptides. In the human body, older proteins are more glycosylated. People with high levels of glucose, such as in diabetes, also have higher levels of nonenzymatic glycosylation. Some glycoproteins also serve as hormones.

Proteoglycans are glycoproteins that are heavily glycosylated. They have a core protein with one or more covalently attached *glycosaminoglycan* (GAG) chain(s), which are long, linear carbohydrate polymers that are negatively charged under physiological conditions, due to the occurrence of sulfate and uronic acid groups. Proteoglycans are a major component of the animal extracellular matrix, the "filler" substance existing between cells in an organism. Water sticks to GAGs and this allows connective tissues to resist pressure.

Glycolipids are very abundant in cell membranes and they are lipids to which carbohydrate chains are covalently linked. The simplest glycolipid is glucosylcerebroside, which contains a single glucose, and glycolipids containing *N*-acetylneuraminic acid are called gangliosides. Important human glycolipids and glycoproteins are the blood group antigens, which are involved in the immune response. The carbohydrates of the human blood groups, A, B, and O, are structurally related oligosaccharides that may be linked to either lipids or proteins. The ability of antibodies to distinguish these structures determines compatibility or rejection of blood transfusions.

2.2.6 Nucleotides

Nucleotides are simple building blocks of nucleic acids and also have additional functions in cells. Nucleotides are composed of a phosphate group, a pentose (a five-carbon sugar molecule), and an organic base. There are five bases: two *purines*, having a pair of fused rings, *adenine* (abbreviated A) and *guanine* (G), and three *pyrimidines*, having only one ring, *cytosine* (C), *thymidine* (T), and *uracil* (U) (Figure 2.9). To form a nucleotide, each base is linked to a sugar, which can be either ribose (in the case of A, G, C, and U) or deoxyribose (for A, G, C, and T), whose 1' carbon is attached to the 9' nitrogen of a purine or to the one nitrogen of a pyrimidine. The sugar is linked to a phosphate group by replacing its hydroxyl group on the 5' carbon atom with an ester bond to the phosphate group (Figure 2.10). Cells also can contain nucleosides, which are a base and sugar without a phosphate.

Nucleotides can have one, two, or three attached phosphate groups and are referred to as nucleoside monophosphates (NMP), diphosphates (NDP), and triphosphates (NTP), respectively, where N is any base. NTPs are numerous in cells and are necessary for the synthesis of nucleic acids. Thus, cells contain four ribonucleotide triphosphates (ATP, GTP, CTP, and UTP) that are building blocks of polymeric nucleic acid called *ribonucleic acid* (RNA) and four deoxyribonucleotide triphosphates (dATP, dGTP, dCTP, and dTTP) that are building blocks of deoxy*ribonucleic acid* (DNA).

When nucleotides polymerize to form nucleic acids, the hydroxyl group attached to the 3' carbon of the sugar of one nucleotide forms an ester bond to the phosphate of another

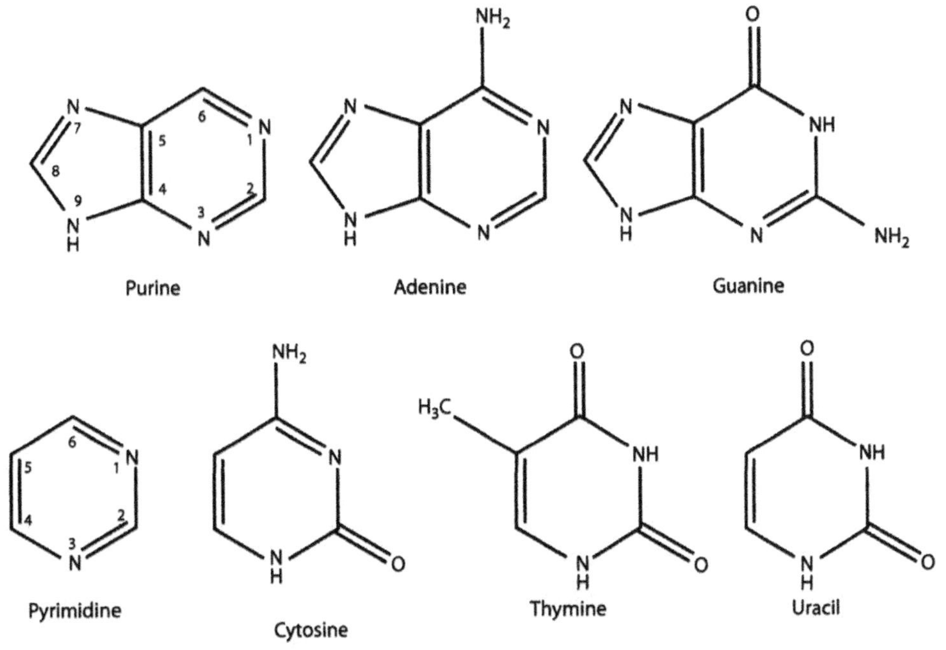

FIGURE 2.9 The basic chemical structure of the principal bases, purines and pyrimidines, in nucleic acids. Purines: adenine (A) and guanine (G). Pyrimidines: uracil (U), thymidine (T), and cytosine (C).

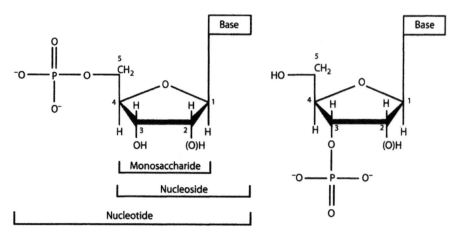

FIGURE 2.10 The chemical structure of a typical nucleotide, composed of a base, monosaccharide, and a phosphate group.

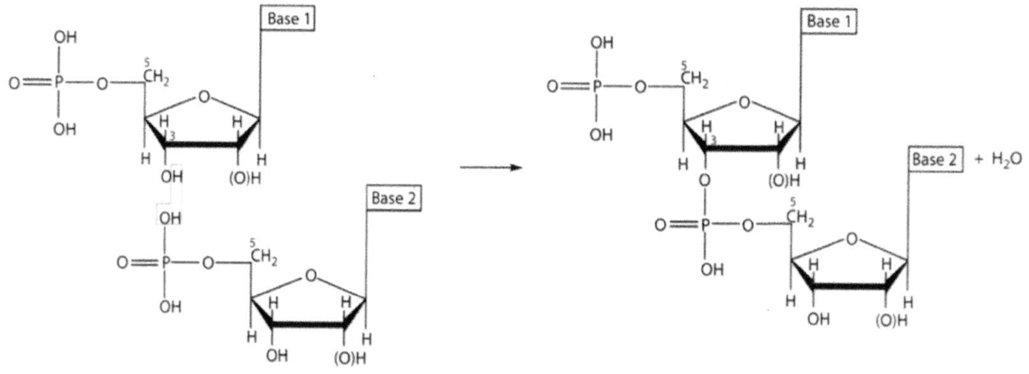

FIGURE 2.11 The condensation reaction for forming nucleic acids from multiple nucleotides with the release of water.

nucleotide, releasing water in the process, called condensation (Figure 2.11) similar to the aforementioned reaction for forming a peptide bond. A single nucleic acid strand is a phosphate–pentose polymer (a polyester) with purine and pyrimidine bases for side groups and phosphodiester bonds linking several nucleotides together. A nucleic acid strand is oriented with the 3′ end being the free hydroxyl group attached to the 3′ carbon of a sugar. The 5′ end has a free hydroxyl or phosphate group attached to the 5′ end of a sugar (Figure 2.12). This orientation is the convention for writing a polynucleotide sequence such as CAG in the 5′ → 3′ direction with 5′ C, followed by A and then G 3′.

Monomeric nucleotides have additional cellular functions. Adenosine triphosphate (ATP) serves as an ultimate source of chemical energy for almost all cellular needs. Guanosine triphosphate (GTP) also can provide energy for some cellular processes. Cyclic nucleotides (cAMP and cGMP) form when the phosphate group is bound to two of the sugar's hydroxyl groups and participate in cellular signaling (described later). In addition,

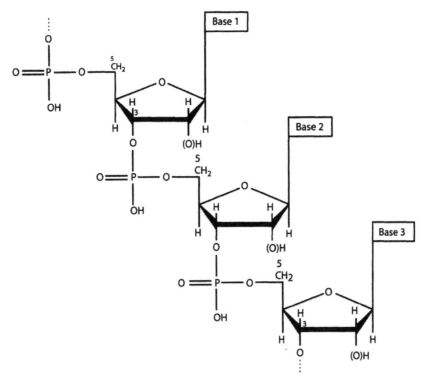

FIGURE 2.12 The chemical structure of a trinucleotide demonstrating the 3′ and 5′ ends of the trinucleotide. Hydrogen (H) binds to C4 in DNA and OH binds C4 in RNA.

adenine nucleotides are incorporated into important coenzymes (coenzyme A, flavin adenine dinucleotide, and nicotinamide adenine phosphate).

2.2.7 DNA, Nucleosomes, Chromosome, and RNA

The main role of DNA is long-term storage of genetic instructions for the development of an organism. These instructions are needed to construct other components of cells, such as proteins and RNA molecules. The DNA segments that carry this genetic information are called *genes*, but other DNA segments have structural purposes or are involved in regulating the use of this genetic information.

Cells can reproduce themselves and their duplication is based on DNA, which can be replicated to form copies of itself. Genetic information is expressed in cells by the mechanisms of *transcription* and *translation*. *Transcription* transfers the DNA-coded information to RNA molecules. *Translation* is the formation of specific proteins from these specific RNAs. Cells have two nucleic acids: DNA and RNA, which are polymers composed of monomers that form a chain varying in length from tens to thousands of units for RNA and millions of units for DNA. In cells, these polymerization reactions are catalyzed by specialized enzymes. Ribonucleotides and deoxyribonucleotides are never joined together, so RNA contains only ribonucleotides and DNA contains only deoxyribonucleotides. In RNA, the pentose is always ribose and for DNA it is deoxyribose. They also differ in one of

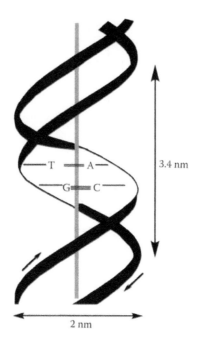

FIGURE 2.13   A model of double helix DNA. The x-ray diffraction pattern of DNA demonstrates that the stacked bases are regularly spaced 0.34 nm apart along the helix axis (shown as an imaginary line in gray through the double helix). The helix makes a complete turn every 3.4 nm, and the width of the DNA is about 2 nm.

their bases as discussed previously. The bases are adenine (A), guanine (G), and cytosine (C) for both RNA and DNA, while thymidine (T) is found only in DNA and uracil (U) is found only in RNA.

DNA molecules are composed of two strands of nucleotides (a polynucleotide) that wind around each other (Figure 2.13) to form a double helix. All DNA nucleotides consist of a deoxyribose (five-carbon sugar) with a phosphate group attached at one end and a base (a nitrogen-containing ring) at the other. The base pairs are stacked between the strands with the two strands running antiparallel to each other (their 5′ → 3′ directions are opposite). The strands are held together by hydrogen bonds and hydrophobic interactions so that the bases on opposite strands are across from each other with A paired to T and G paired to C. Thus, a purine must always pair with a pyrimidine but certain pairs are never found due to the fact that they would distort the helix (i.e., G–T and C–T are not normally found in DNA). Two polynucleotide strands can form either a right-handed or left-handed helix, but DNA is mainly right-handed due to the conformation of the sugar–phosphate backbone. Four bases (A, T, C, and G) are repeated millions times in the DNA molecule forming specific sequences that can be interpreted as genetic information. DNA molecules can be in linear or circular forms.

Before a cell divides, the strands of the helix separate, and each strand replaces the hydrogen-bonded complementary nucleotides with which it is no longer associated, with new nucleotides. Thus, two double helices identical to the original one are created. This process is called DNA replication and is described in Section 2.6.2.

In eukaryotes DNA is packaged into nucleosomes, which are particular segments of DNA wound around a histone protein core. There are five types of histone proteins in mammalian cells: H1, H2A, H2B, H3, and H4. The nucleosome core consists of ~147 base pairs of DNA wrapped in 1.67 superhelical turns around a histone octamer consisting of the core histones: H2A, H2B, H3, and H4. Linker DNA of ~80 base pairs connects the nucleosome core particles with each other. Linker histones such as H1 are involved in chromatin compaction and are found at the base of the nucleosome near DNA entry and exit to bind the linker region of DNA. Nucleosomes form the fundamental repeating unit of the chromatin and are folded through a series of highly ordered structures to form a chromosome. Non-condensed nucleosomes without the linker histone resemble "beads on a string."

RNA is quite similar to DNA in its structure forming double-stranded or single-stranded, linear or circular molecules but its sugar component is a ribose, and the base thymidine is replaced by uracil in RNA. Most RNA is single-stranded but local base pairing within some RNA segments can form short double helices. This leads to the formation of a RNA secondary structure with some recognizable domains like hairpin loops, bulges, and internal loops. The major function of RNA is protein synthesis in the cell in the process of translation described later. RNA can also act catalytically, similar to an enzyme. Some viruses use RNA as their genetic material instead of DNA.

2.3 TRANSCRIPTION AND TRANSLATION

The DNA in the chromosomes of the genome does not directly carry out protein synthesis but uses RNA as an intermediary. To create a protein, the nucleotide sequence in the DNA appropriate for that protein is copied into RNA, a process called transcription. This RNA is then used directly as a template to direct the synthesis of that protein in a process called translation.

2.3.1 RNA Synthesis

The term transcription is used to describe RNA synthesis leading to protein synthesis, because a particular portion of one strand of the DNA, a gene, is read and copied (or transcribed) into a RNA nucleotide sequence and thus serves as a template. Since this process is very complicated, and only a brief overview of the process will be given in this chapter, a better understanding of this topic can be obtained from two excellent cell biology books (Alberts et al. 2008; Lodish et al. 2008). The α-helix of the double-stranded DNA is "unzipped" by the enzyme helicase. The RNA polymerase with the help of an σ-factor must recognize a specific region of the DNA, the promoter region, where it can bind tightly and begin transcription, which is called the initiation phase. Transcription can be divided into three stages: initiation, elongation, and termination, regulated by specific transcription factors and coactivators. In the process of elongation, the RNA chain produced by transcription, the transcript, is created one nucleotide at a time and is complementary to the strand of DNA used as the template. The enzyme that performs this operation is called RNA polymerase II, and it unwinds the DNA and catalyzes the formation of the phosphodiester bonds that link the nucleotides together to form a single strand of RNA.

The DNA strand is read in the 3′ to 5′ direction and the mRNA is transcribed in the 5′ to 3′ direction by the RNA polymerase II using NTPs (ATP, CTP, UTP, and GTP) with the release of energy from these high-energy bonds. Termination signals are encoded in DNA, and many function by destabilizing the polymerase's hold of the DNA template and the newly made RNA chain.

In eukaryotes, the first product is called the primary transcript and it needs to be post-transcriptionally modified, such as capping with 7-methyl guanosine and the addition of a poly-A tail, to produce heterophil nuclear RNA (hnRNA). This hnRNA then undergoes splicing of introns (non-coding parts of the gene) via spliceosomes involving small nuclear RNA (snRNA) molecules and other proteins, to produce the final messenger RNA (mRNA). Most of the RNA in the cell is ribosomal RNA (rRNA), which has a specialized polymerase, RNA polymerase I that is dedicated to producing rRNA. A different RNA polymerase is used because its transcripts are neither capped or polyadenylated to help the cell distinguish between non-coding RNAs (such as rRNA) and mRNAs. The nucleolus is where the ribosome is processed and is characterized as a dense mass in the nucleus due to large aggregates of macromolecules such as rRNA genes, precursor and mature rRNA, enzymes for processing rRNA, small nucleolar RNAs (snoRNAs), ribosomal subunits, and partly assembled ribosomes. Transcription takes place in the nucleus, and the single strand of RNA leaves the nucleus through the nuclear pores into the cytoplasm.

2.3.2 Protein Synthesis

The synthesis of proteins is known as translation and occurs in the cytoplasm with the assistance of ribosomes. Since this process of translation is very complicated, and only a brief overview of the process will be given in this chapter, a better understanding of this topic can be obtained from two excellent cell biology books (Alberts et al. 2008; Lodish et al. 2008). It is called translation because the information in the RNA is converted into protein using an entirely different "language," i.e., the genetic code in which each group of three consecutive nucleotides in the RNA, a codon, specifies either one amino acid or a stop signal for the translation process. There are 20 amino acids in proteins but several different codons can specify a single amino acid. For example, alanine is specified by GCA, GCC, GCG, or GCU. The codon in an mRNA molecule does not directly recognize the amino acid it specifies, but uses transfer RNAs (tRNAs), each about 80 nucleotides in length, to create the amino acid. The anticodon is the region on the tRNA composed of a set of three consecutive nucleotides that pair with the complementary codon in the mRNA. RNA polymerase III helps to synthesize tRNAs. Recognition and attachment of the correct amino acids to each tRNA requires enzymes called aminoacyl-tRNA synthetases. To ensure that the RNA is decoded properly, protein synthesis occurs in the ribosome that contains about 50 different proteins and several RNA molecules. Ribosomes are made of a small and large subunit. In translation, mRNA is decoded to produce a specific polypeptide and involves four phases of translation: activation, initiation, elongation, and termination.

In activation, the correct amino acid binds to the correct tRNA. While this is not technically a step in translation, it is required for protein synthesis. The amino acid is joined by its carboxyl group to the 3′ OH of the tRNA through an ester bond. During initiation, the small subunit of the ribosome binds to the 5′ end of mRNA with the assistance of initiation factors (IF) and other proteins. During elongation, the next aminoacyl tRNA in line binds to the ribosome via GTP and an elongation factor. At termination, the A site of the ribosome encounters a stop codon (UAA, UAG, or UGA), which is not recognized by any tRNA, but a releasing factor recognizes the stop codon and the polypeptide chain is released. Since the synthesis of most proteins takes between 20 s and several minutes, multiple initiations take place on multiple complexes of ribosomes next to each other, making up a polyribosome.

2.3.3 Posttranslational Modifications of Proteins

Some proteins are made as a proprotein, which is an inactive protein, containing one or more inhibitory peptides linked to it. The inhibitory sequence is removed by proteolysis during posttranslational modification, when the active protein is needed. Thus some proteins can be stored as proproteins in the cell and then rapidly converted to active proteins by proteolysis. A preprotein can also be formed that contains a signal sequence (an N-terminal signal peptide) that specifies its insertion into or through membranes, i.e., targets it for secretion. The signal peptide is cleaved off in the endoplasmic reticulum. Also, the folding of proteins can be assisted by molecular chaperone proteins. Included in this class of proteins are the heat-shock proteins (hsp), hsp 60 and hsp 70. These events and others are termed posttranslational modifications and can also involve the formation of disulfide bridges, addition of other functional groups, such as acetates, phosphates, carbohydrates, and lipids. Or enzymes (kinases for phosphorylation, acetylases for acetylation, methyl transferases for methylation, etc.) can remove one or more amino acids or modify structures. It is not completely known when or where all these events occur during the synthesis of proteins. Other posttranslational modifications are opposite in that they involve dephosphorylation by phosphatases or phosphoryl transferases, deacetylation by deacetylases or acetyltransferases, demethylation by demethylases or methyl transferases, ubiquitination, biotinylation, etc. These are required for the specific activation of a protein or for deactivation followed by its total degradation of proteins that fail to properly fold or are not needed by the cell. Failed proteins are disposed by the proteosome, an ATP-dependent protease in the cytoplasm and nucleus that constitutes 1% of the cellular protein.

2.4 CELLULAR STRUCTURES/ORGANELLES

Cells are bound by the plasma membrane and contain a variety of membrane-bound organelles within the cellular cytoplasm. These organelles perform specific functions for cell maintenance and survival. Eukaryotic cells vary in size from 5 to 50 μm (Table 2.1) and contain varying numbers of specific organelles depending on cell type, developmental stage, and cell function. In the next section, a brief overview of the organelles mitochondria,

TABLE 2.1   Units of Measure for Tissues, Cells, Organelles, and Molecules

Units of Measure	Organic Structures in Cells
Centimeter (cm) = 0.394 in.	Macroscopic, seen by the naked eye
Millimeter (mm) = 0.1 cm	Some large cells
Micron (μ) = 0.001 mm	Light microscopy; limit of resolution = 0.2 μm
Micrometer (μm)	Most cells and larger organelles Cell size = 5–50 μm
Nanometer (nm) = 0.001 μm	Electron microscopy; limit of resolution = 0.05 nm Small organelles, largest macromolecules
Ångström (Å) = 0.1 nm	Electron microscopy, limit of resolution = 0.5 Å Molecules and atoms

ER (both rough and smooth ER), nucleus (including nucleolus), Golgi apparatus, lysosomes, peroxisomes, and centrosomes will be presented. The organelles of plant cells such as chloroplasts and the cell walls of plant cells will not be discussed.

2.4.1 Plasma Membrane

The plasma membrane is present on the surface of all cells and is the primary barrier that determines what can enter/leave or be excluded from the cell. Specific proteins are associated with the plasma membrane that have a myriad of functions: membrane-bound enzymes that catalyze reactions, receptor proteins that bind signaling molecules, membrane-spanning proteins that provide a pore to allow the passage of specific molecules, proteins that regulate fusion of the membrane with other cell membranes or other intracellular structures for instance in secretion, proteins that provide anchors for cytoskeletal fibers or for components of the ECM, etc. Every membrane has the same basic structure of a phospholipid bilayer with different membrane proteins for different tasks. The plasma membrane consists of two leaflets or layers of phospholipids forming the bilayer. The hydrophobic fatty acyl tails of the phospholipids form the middle of the bilayer, while the hydrophilic heads of the phospholipids are found on the surface. Figure 2.14 illustrates the basic structure of a biological membrane composed of phospholipid bilayer with integral proteins having one or more regions embedded in the lipid bilayer and peripheral proteins associated with the bilayer by specific protein–protein interactions. Both glycoproteins and glycolipids are found in the cell membrane. Some integral proteins are bound to the membrane by covalently attached lipids. Some transmembrane portions of integral membrane proteins pass through the entire plasma membrane several times. Different detergents are used to solubilize the membrane for the study of specific integral membrane proteins.

Subcellular fractionation techniques using centrifugation of disrupted cells in a gradient can partially separate and purify different biological membranes. When this is done, the composition of the different subcellular compartments and the plasma membrane can be analyzed. The protein:lipid ratio and the type of lipid differ depending on the organelle. For examples, the inner mitochondrial membrane contains ~76% protein and 5% cholesterol,

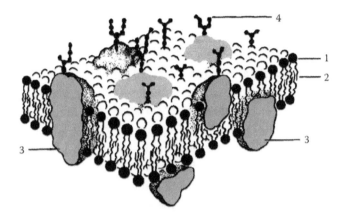

FIGURE 2.14 Plasma membrane. The basic structure of a biological membrane is a phospholipid bilayer with the phospholipid's hydrophobic fatty acyl tails forming the middle of the bilayer (1), and their hydrophilic heads (2) forming the surface of the membrane. The phospholipid bilayer has integral proteins (3) with one or more regions embedded in the lipid bilayer and peripheral proteins (3) associated with the bilayer by specific protein–protein interactions. Oligosaccharides (4) bind mainly to the membrane proteins to form glycoproteins or to the membrane lipid to form glycolipids.

and the plasma membrane of a mouse liver cell, hepatocyte, contains ~44% protein and 30% cholesterol. Phospholipids are prevalent in cell membranes. Both glycolipids and glycoproteins are abundant in the plasma membranes of eukaryotic cells but are absent from the inner mitochondrial membrane, for example.

Another property of the plasma membrane is that the phospholipid composition of the two leaflets differs in lipid composition, and each integral membrane protein has a single, specific orientation with respect to the cytoplasmic and extracellular faces of the cell membrane. The active site of every molecule of a particular membrane-bound enzyme is always located at the same face of the membrane. Thus, integral membrane proteins and glycolipids are asymmetrically located. Phospholipids and cholesterol are found in both leaflets but they are enriched in one leaflet or the other.

Another property of biomembranes is that most membrane proteins and lipids are laterally mobile in the membrane. This suggests that the membrane is somewhat fluid, as can be seen by watching fluorescence recovery after photobleaching (FRAP). Initially, the surface proteins or lipids are labeled with a fluorescent dye, followed by bleaching a very small area of the fluorescently labeled membrane with a laser. Then the diffusion of fluorescently labeled molecules back into the bleached region is analyzed to determine a diffusion coefficient (rate of diffusion of specific molecules).

Mobility in the plasma membrane can be restricted. Not all integral membrane proteins are mobile in the membrane due to interactions with other membrane proteins or due to cytoskeletal proteins that lie just under the plasma membrane. An extensive network of cytoskeletal proteins connects with the plasma membrane. The cytoskeleton will be discussed in Section 2.4.8. On the outer surface of the cell membrane, proteins and oligosaccharides sometimes can be found bound to the membrane. These form a coat or glycocalyx, which is negatively charged due to the propensity of sialic acid residues in the glycoproteins and glycolipids of the glycocalyx.

The plasma membrane can also exhibit specialized structures that contribute to the polarization of the cell. Polarization of the cells allows cells to perform different functions at specific ends of the cells, i.e., the apical and basal lateral surfaces. For example, the epithelium covers the body's internal and external surfaces, and, in different regions of the body, the epithelial cells perform different functions. In the lumen of the small intestine, the apical surface of the epithelial cells absorbs nutrients from the digested food in the lumen of the intestine, and then these sugars, amino acids, and lipids are transferred across the single layer of cells to the blood. To increase the surface area of the epithelial cells that are absorbing nutrients, the luminal or apical surface of the plasma membrane has numerous plasma membrane projections/finger-like extensions or microvilli forming a specialized structure, called the brush border. These microvilli increase the surface area of the plasma membrane for absorption, and also have enzymes associated with them to degrade compounds. They are rigid structures due to cytoskeletal components, actin microfilaments, running down the entire length of each microvillus, and these microfilaments are also anchored to the sides of the plasma membrane in specialized regions called desmosomes. In some cells, the plasma membrane is covered with enzymes and other glycoproteins to form glycocalyx on the outer surface of the apical membrane. The degraded components such as glucose, amino acids, small peptides, and oligosaccharides are then transported across the cell to the basolateral surface of the plasma membrane by another set of discrete proteins and vesicles. To maintain cell polarity, there are specialized structures between cells, such as tight junction, that do not allow molecules to pass freely between the cells.

2.4.1.1 Receptors for Growth Factors and Hormones

Many receptors for growth factors and hormones are found in the plasma membrane of cells. There are, however, other receptor proteins that are found in the nucleus and cytosol. Hormones and other molecules involved in cell-to-cell signaling can be of two types: lipid soluble or lipid insoluble. Lipid-soluble hormones such as steroids diffuse across the plasma membrane into the cytosol or nucleus where they interact with protein receptors that can either induce or repress specific genes. Lipid-insoluble hormones and peptide hormones such as insulin-like growth factor 1 bind to protein cell surface receptors. Receptors can be identified and quantified by their ligand binding of specific tagged agonists and antagonists, purified by affinity chromatography and then cloned.

There are a myriad of cell surface receptors, such as protein kinases and phosphatases, ligand-induced ion channels, and hormone or growth factor–binding receptors. Some surface receptors are coupled via a family of G proteins to the activation or inhibition of specific enzymes, or adenylate cyclase and the subsequent activation of $3',5'$-cAMP. Other hormones trigger activation of phospholipase C via other specific G proteins. Phospholipase C hydrolyzes the plasma membrane lipid phosphatidylinositol 4,5-bisphosphate, which generates 1,2-diacylglycerol and inositol 1,4,5-triphosphate. Then the 1,2-diacylglycerol activates protein kinase C, which phosphorylates several proteins involved in cell growth and metabolism. Activation of inositol 1,4,5-triphosphate releases Ca^{2+} into the cytosol via calmodulin. There are numerous signaling pathways that are activated by substrate binding to receptors at the plasma membrane and are too numerous to elaborate here but they have profound effects on cell growth and metabolism. Many of the signaling pathways converge in the cytoplasm to create a very complicated pattern of cell responses and gene activation.

The concentration of cell surface receptors in the cells is well regulated. Continuous exposure to a hormone can result in reduction of the receptor via a process called desensitization. Receptors can be reduced by several mechanisms: destroyed after internalization by endocytosis of the cell membrane, then degraded by lysosomes, or stored in an intracellular vesicle for future use or degradation. Some receptors stay on the cell surface but once activated are changed, such as via phosphorylation, so that they can no longer bind another ligand. Other receptors bind a ligand but form a complex that does not induce a normal hormone response. Receptors for hormones can also use multiple pathways for downregulation.

2.4.2 Mitochondria

A mitochondrion (plural mitochondria) is a membrane-enclosed organelle found in most eukaryotic cells and provides energy for the cell by generating ATP. Mitochondria are also involved in other important cell processes such as cell differentiation, cell death, signal transduction through the regulation of calcium, cell cycle regulation, and cell growth. Mitochondria range in size from 0.5 to 10 µm (Table 2.1) but are generally 0.5 µm. The mitochondria vary in number per cell with some cells having only one mitochondrion while other cells may have a few thousand, and they also differ in the number of proteins they contain depending on cell type. Each mitochondrion is composed of compartments that perform specialized functions: the outer membrane, the intramembranous space, the inner membrane, the cristae, and matrix (Figures 2.15 and 2.16). Although most of the genes for creating a mitochondrion are found in the cell nucleus, the mitochondrion also has its own genome, which is critical for its function. This mitochondrial genome is thought to have arisen from invasion of a primordial cell by bacteria, which through time and evolution developed a symbiotic relationship with the cell and became the mitochondrion. Thus, the mitochondrion's genome has some similarity to certain bacterial genes.

A major role of mitochondria is the production of ATP and the inner membrane of the mitochondrion is highly involved in this process. Glucose, the principal source of energy in animals, along with pyruvate and NADH, which are produced in the cytoplasm, is oxidized in the mitochondrion. The aerobic degradation of glucose to CO_2 and H_2O is coupled to the synthesis of ~32 molecules of ATP:

$$C_6H_{12}O_6 + 6O_2 \text{ and } 32P_i^{2-} + 32ADP + 32H^+ \qquad 6CO_2 + 32ATP + 38H_2O$$

This process is called cellular respiration or aerobic respiration since it is dependent on the presence of oxygen. Aerobic respiration takes place mostly in the matrix, and inner membrane of the mitochondrion, which is folded into cristae to increase the surface

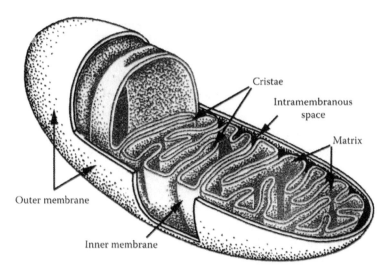

FIGURE 2.15 Mitochondrion. Each mitochondrion is composed of compartments that perform specialized functions: the outer membrane, the intramembranous space, the inner membrane, the cristae, and matrix. A major role of mitochondria is the production of ATP.

area for reactions and to maintain an electrochemical gradient. The outer membrane has many transmembrane channels and is mostly permeable to small molecules. When oxygen is limited, then anaerobic respiration occurs independent of mitochondria but this process is less efficient at producing ATP. ATP is needed by cells for fueling other energetically unfavorable process such as transport of molecules against a concentration gradient or muscle contraction. ATP is also required for the synthesis of nucleic acids and proteins.

Mitochondria also have other functions. They transiently store calcium and interact with the endoplasmic reticulum, the principal storage site for calcium, to maintain calcium homeostasis and provide calcium for particular signaling pathways. Mitochondria also have a role in programmed cell death or apoptosis, regulation of cellular proliferation and metabolism, and heme and steroid synthesis. In some cells, mitochondria have a specific function such as in liver cells where they contain enzymes that detoxify ammonia.

Both the mitochondria and the Golgi apparatus (Section 2.4.4) have a role in apoptosis, a programmed cell death process that most cells undergo without eliciting an inflammatory response. Several proteins of the Bcl-2 family of proteins, involved in protecting the cell from apoptosis or for promoting it, are found in the mitochondria and also in the Golgi apparatus.

2.4.3 Endoplasmic Reticulum

The ER is composed of an extensive network of cisternae or saclike structures of two types: rough endoplasmic reticulum (RER) or smooth endoplasmic reticulum (SER) that can interchange from one type to the other depending on the metabolic needs of the cell. The membranes of the RER and SER are also continuous with the outer layer of the nuclear envelope.

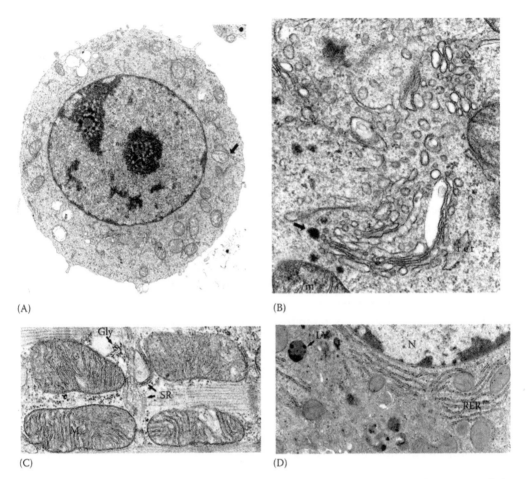

FIGURE 2.16 Transmission electron micrographs of cell organelles. Micrographs are provided to illustrate how organelles appear in the transmission electron microscope. One entire cell (A) with a nucleus (n), nuclear envelope (nu), and nucleolus (nuc) is shown. Mitochondria (m) and rough endoplasmic reticulum (rer) are also seen. In (B), the Golgi apparatus (g) is found near the nucleus (nu) with the rer at the *cis* face (c) of the Golgi and a secretory vesicle (arrow) at the *trans* face (t). In (C), four mitochondria (M) and glycogen granules (Gly) are present within a cell. In (D), the RER and a lysosome (LY) are found next to the nucleus (N) of a cell. (The transmission electron images are provided at the courtesy of Dr. A.R. Hand.)

The RER takes its name from the protein-manufacturing ribosome structures that decorate the cisternae and are constantly being bound and then released from the membrane (Figure 2.16). A ribosome binds to the membrane as it begins to synthesize a protein due to an ion linkage involving Mg^{2+} and the nascent polypeptide chain itself. The unfolded, growing protein chain passes from the ribosomal unit into and through the ER and is never exposed to the cytosol. The N-terminal signal sequence of the protein emerges from the ribosome and is bound by a signal recognition particle (SRP) that binds to the ER membrane through the SR receptor. Once the protein passes through the phospholipid bilayer, the SRP dissociates from the complex and is released into the cytosol where it is free to initiate insertion of another secretory protein. The signal sequence of the protein is cleaved in the ER lumen by a signal peptidase. Once the C terminus of the protein reaches the lumen, the protein folds into its final configuration at which times it is packaged into small transport vesicles that carry them to the Golgi apparatus, the *cis* face of the Golgi, for further modifications and packaging for secretion at the plasma membrane. Alternatively, integral membrane proteins remain in the membrane and are either transported to the Golgi or remain and function in the RER. Other processes occur in the lumen of the ER, carbohydrates are added by enzymes to the protein, two or more polypeptides are linked into oligomers, and disulfide bonds are made.

The SER is involved in the synthesis and metabolism of fatty acids and phospholipids. The SER is also the site for the regulation of calcium concentrations within the cell, carbohydrate metabolism, drug detoxification by converting chemicals into more water-soluble products for secretion from the body, and attachment of receptors to the cell membrane. The SER also contains the enzyme glucose-6-phosphatase that converts glucose-6-phosphate to glucose, a step in gluconeogenesis.

A special type of smooth ER is found in smooth and striated muscle and is called the sarcoplasmic reticulum, which serves to sequester, store, and then release calcium in response to electrical stimulation of the muscle.

2.4.4 Golgi Apparatus

The Golgi apparatus is involved in modifying, sorting, and packaging macromolecules for secretion or for delivery to other cellular compartments. The Golgi apparatus is characteristically located near the nucleus and centrosome of the cell. Similar to the ER, the Golgi apparatus is composed of multiple cisternae in the shape of flattened disks with a particular stacking of 4–8 cisternae. These cisternae are often linked by tubular connections forming a single complex. The localization and organization of the Golgi cisternae is maintained by microtubules. These stacks of cisternae are organized into *cis*, *medial*, and *trans* regions (Figure 2.17).

Macromolecules, sequestered in vesicles from the ER, fuse with the *cis* Golgi and progress through the stack to the *trans* Golgi network, where they are packaged for delivery to other sites in the cell such as for secretion. The *cis* and *trans* cisternae are linked to special sorting stations called the *cis* Golgi network and the *trans* Golgi network. New cisternae are also added to the *cis* face of the Golgi. Structural proteins for the maintenance of the Golgi are formed in the *cis* cisternae. The *trans* face of the Golgi is where vesicles leave for other cell compartments such as the cell membrane, late endosomes, and lysosomes. Each region contains different enzymes for selective modification of the macromolecules. The different functions of particular Golgi cisternae are maintained by a process that is not well understood.

The Golgi apparatus is the major site for carbohydrate synthesis. Proteoglycans composed of carbohydrates are mostly destined for the ECM but some proteoglycans remain anchored to the plasma membrane. Mucus that covers the epithelia also has proteoglycans as a major component. Glycoaminoglycans, long unbranched polysaccharides, are

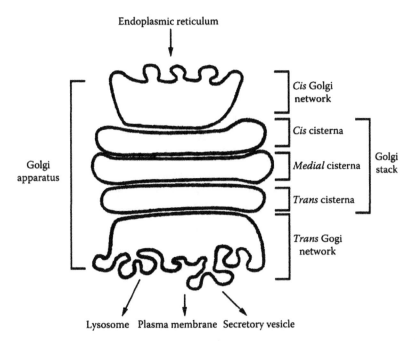

FIGURE 2.17 Golgi apparatus. The Golgi apparatus is involved in modifying, sorting, and packaging macromolecules for secretion or for delivery to other cellular compartments. The Golgi apparatus is composed of multiple cisternae that are stacked as flattened disks, which are often linked by tubular connections forming a single complex. These stacks of cisternae are organized into *cis*, medial, and *trans* regions. Macromolecules, sequestered in vesicles from the ER, fuse with the *cis* Golgi and progress through the stack to the *trans* Golgi network, where they are packaged for delivery to other sites in the cell, such as for secretion. The *trans* face of the Golgi is also where vesicles leave for other cell compartments such as the plasma membrane and lysosomes.

attached to proteins in the Golgi to form proteoglycans, often by Golgi enzymes that polymerize several of the GAGs via a xylose link to the protein core. Sulfotransferases also sulfate particular molecules, including the glycoaminoglycans of proteoglycans as well as the core proteins in the Golgi, so that they form negatively charged molecules. Some proteins have sugars added to the OH group of selected serine or threonine side chains in a process called O-linked glycosylation that is accomplished by glycosyl transferase enzymes in the Golgi. The N-linked oligosaccharides begin with the addition of a 14-sugar precursor to an asparagine in the polypeptide chain of the protein. In the Golgi, the high mannose oligosaccharides, which had been added to proteins in the ER, are often trimmed by removal of mannose, and then other sugars are added.

The Golgi is also involved in phosphorylation, the addition of phosphates to proteins and sugars. ATP is required and is therefore imported into the Golgi's lumen where kinases phosphorylate these substrates.

Another important function of the ER and Golgi apparatus is the synthesis of lysosomal hydrolases and membrane proteins for lysosomes that are essential for intracellular digestion of macromolecules. The Golgi apparatus adds mannose-6-phosphate (M6P) to N-linked oligosaccharides of soluble lysosomal enzymes as they pass through the lumen of the *cis* Golgi network. The M6P groups are recognized by transmembrane M6P receptor proteins in the *trans* Golgi. The receptors bind the lysosomal hydrolases on the lumen side of the membrane and to adaptins involved in assembling clathrin coats on the cytosolic side. Thus, hydrolases are packaged into clathrin-coated vesicles that bud from the *trans* Golgi so that they can deliver the hydrolases to a late endosome. Late endosomes are formed from macromolecules being taken up from the extracellular fluid by endocytosis, the pinching in or invagination of the plasma membrane. Some of the ingested molecules are selectively recycled to the plasma membrane while other are passed onto late endosomes for digestion (see Section 2.4.5).

The mechanism, by which proteins are sorted in the Golgi apparatus to be delivered to different cellular compartments, is not completely understood. All of the proteins retained within the Golgi complex are associated with the Golgi membrane according to their transmembrane domains rather than being soluble proteins within the lumen. In addition, signals in the cytoplasmic tails of some Golgi proteins mediate the retrieval of these proteins from subsequent compartments along the secretory pathway. Unregulated protein secretion is also found as a constitutive secretory pathway. However, in some cells, secretion is regulated by specific environmental signals, such as in response to hormones and neurotransmitters, and involves the recognition of signal factors shared by multiple proteins in the pathway. These secretory proteins selectively aggregate in the *trans* Golgi network and are then released by budding of secretory vesicles. For example, the digestive enzymes produced by pancreatic acinar cells are stored in secretory vesicles until food in the alimentary canal triggers their secretion.

The length of the transmembrane region of the Golgi-modified proteins also determines their location in the cell. Vesicles that leave the Golgi apparatus are rich in cholesterol. When cholesterol is added to the lipids in the bilayer it separates the lipid head groups of the two leaflets, thus causing the membranes to become thicker than the Golgi membranes themselves. Transmembrane proteins must have long transmembrane segments to span this thickness if they are to enter the cholesterol-rich transport vesicles budding from the *trans* face of the Golgi for destination to the plasma membrane. Proteins with shorter transmembrane segments are excluded. Thus, the Golgi apparatus is more prominent and larger in cells that are actively secreting macromolecules, such as osteoblasts, antibody-secreting cells of the immune system, etc.

As discussed earlier, the Golgi apparatus and the mitochondria have a role in apoptosis. Several proteins of the Bcl-2 family of proteins, involved in protecting the cell from programmed cell death (apoptosis) or for promoting it, are found in the Golgi apparatus. The Golgi anti-apoptotic protein (GAAP) is found only in the Golgi and protects the cell from apoptosis.

2.4.5 Lysosomes and Peroxisomes

Lysosomes are membrane-bound organelles that contain hydrolytic enzymes used for digestion of intracellular macromolecules (Figure 2.16). More than 40 acid hydrolases are found in lysosomes and they include proteases, glycosidases, lipases, phospholipases, phosphatases, nucleases, and sulfatases. These enzymes exhibit optimal activity near pH 5. The lysosomal membrane separates its lumen from the cytosol, which has a pH of ~7.2. The membrane of the lysosome contains a H$^+$ pump that uses ATP to pump H$^+$ into the lysosome to maintain a low pH. The lysosomal structural proteins are highly glycosylated to protect them from the proteases and low pH. The lysosomal membrane also has transport proteins that allow final digested products to escape and be reutilized or excreted by the cell. Newly synthesized lysosomal proteins are synthesized in the Golgi apparatus and then transported from the *trans* Golgi network to an intermediate compartment termed as endolysosome by transport vesicles (see Section 2.4.4 for the pathways for synthesizing lysosomal proteins through specific recognition molecules such as those containing M6P groups).

Endocytosis at the plasma membrane creates an invagination that becomes a specific type of vesicle called an endosome that can then fuse with the endolysosome for digestion of the endosome's contents. Two types of endocytosis are distinguished by the size of the endocytic vesicles formed. Phagocytosis involves the ingestion of large particles such as microorganisms or dead cells (usually greater that 250 nm in diameter), and this is often accomplished by specialized phagocytic cells (macrophages, neutrophils, and dendritic cells). Pinocytosis is a common process in eukaryotic cells and involves the ingestion of fluid and solutes/nutrients into small vesicles (about 100 nm in diameter).

Peroxisomes are membrane-bound organelles that are able to enlarge upon metabolic demand, divide, and self-replicate, but do not have their own genome. Peroxisome proteins are synthesized on free ribosomes in the cytoplasm and are transported via vesicles to the peroxisome. The role of the peroxisome is to metabolize fatty acids, and they also contain enzymes that get rid of toxic peroxides and other metabolites through the activity of their enzymes, such as catalase and D-amino acid oxidase. The peroxisome is a major site of oxygen utilization since they use oxygen and hydrogen peroxide to perform oxidative reactions, such as oxidizing phenols, formic acid, formaldehyde, and alcohol. About 25%–50% of the ethanol consumed by humans is oxidized to acetaldehyde. The peroxisome also breaks down fatty acids by a process called β-oxidation, which also occurs in the mitochondria. Fatty acids are converted to acetyl CoA, which is transported back to the cytoplasm for other use. Another role of peroxisomes is the production of bile acids and proteins. Peroxisomes are especially important in plants for photorespiration and in seeds for converting fatty acids to sugars for growth of seedlings.

2.4.6 Centrosome and Centriole

Centrosomes are organelles serving as the focal points for the spindle fibers of cell division. Spindle fibers are microtubules that attach to each end of the chromosome and pull apart the two copies of the chromosomal DNA during mitosis (Section 2.6.1). An integral part of each centrosome is a structure called the centriole. The centrioles are clusters of microtubules that help to organize the centrosomes and the spindle fibers. During the S phase of the cell cycle, the centrosome replicates and during prophase of mitosis the centrosomes migrate to either end of the cell. The mitotic spindle forms between the two centrosomes, and after division, each daughter cell receives one centrosome and its set of chromosomes.

Centrioles help to insure that cellular division evenly distributes the chromosomes of the parent cell to the two daughter cells.

2.4.7 Nucleus

The nucleus contains most of the cellular DNA organized in chromosomes (Figure 2.16). Chromosomes are long linear DNA molecules complexed with proteins, such as histones. The chromosome contains the genes that regulate cell activities in the cell. Therefore, the function of the nucleus is to regulate gene expression. There is a barrier around the nucleus that controls the transfer of DNA, RNA, and proteins between the nucleus and the cytosol called the nuclear envelope. The nuclear envelope is composed of two cellular membranes arranged parallel to each other with a 10–50 nm space. The outer nuclear membrane is often found to be continuous with the ER. A nuclear lamina, associated with the nuclear membrane and within the nucleus, forms a meshwork for mechanical support and is composed of specific intermediate fibers, such as lamins.

There are nuclear pores within the nuclear membrane, which allows small molecules and ions, and certain molecules to travel between the nucleus and cytoplasm. The nuclear pores have a specific structure composed of multiple proteins. Proteins and RNA need to be tagged with special sequences of amino and nucleic acids, respectively, or associate with carrier proteins in order to pass through the nuclear pores of the nuclear envelope. The interior of the nucleus is not uniform and it has several non-membrane-bound compartments made up of specific proteins and RNA molecules. One of the major compartments is the nucleolus discussed later.

Cellular DNA codes for all of the proteins found within the cytosol and extracellular matrix. The other source of DNA and proteins are the mitochondria. Two main proteins act upon the DNA in the nucleus: DNA polymerase and RNA polymerase. DNA polymerase replicates the DNA within the cell during interphase of the cell cycle so full copies of the genome can be inherited by each daughter cell. RNA polymerase is responsible for producing strands of RNA that eventually become transcribed into proteins. Both proteins are modulated by complex pathways that regulate their action.

2.4.7.1 Nucleolus

The nucleolus (Figure 2.16) is a non-membrane-bound structure that appears as a visible dark region within the nucleus. It is composed of proteins and nucleic acids that are involved in the synthesis of rRNA. The rRNA is exported through the nuclear pore to the cytoplasm to form the structures that are responsible for transcription: the ribosome on the RER.

2.4.8 Cytoskeleton

A cytoplasmic network of three protein polymers, actin filaments, intermediate filaments, and microtubules, are found throughout cells and are all involved in maintaining cell shape and modulating mechanical and other forces on the cells. The transport of proteins, vesicles, and organelles, cellular locomotion, and mitosis require actin filaments and microtubules. The cytoskeleton is a dynamic structure with rapid assembly and disassembly of its structure requiring numerous accessory proteins. Specific motor proteins either move the filaments or move **organelles** along filaments.

Microfilaments are composed of two intertwined chains of actin and are about 6 nm in diameter. Each actin subunit of the microfilament has an ATP-binding site for assembly of the filament that is then bundled with other filaments to form an even stronger structure. Microfilaments are found just beneath the cell membrane and are responsible for maintaining cell shape, interacting with cell receptors such as integrins, resisting tension, and forming cytoplasmic projections such as microvilli and pseudopodia. Pseudopodia, lamellipodia, and filopodia are structures that protrude from the cell so that the cell can explore and interact with the extracellular environment and also allow the cell to move. Along with myosin, actin filaments participate in muscle contraction.

Microtubules are dynamic structures, too, with a 23 nm diameter, mostly comprised of 13 protofilaments that are polymers of α- and β-tubulin monomers and a hollow center of about 15 nm. In nine triplet sets, they form centrioles and are thus involved in cell division and the mitotic spindle (see Section 2.6). When microtubules are organized in nine doublets around two central microtubules, they form cilia and flagella. Like actin, tubulin can bind a nucleotide, but GTP is the nucleotide involved in its polymerization. Microtubules are polarized and grow faster at one end than the other end. They are often organized by the centrosome (Section 2.4.6). Microtubules have a mechanical role, can resist compression, and are also involved in the transport of cytoplasmic particles along the microtubule by motor proteins, such as dyneins and kinesins, and they also transport organelles like mitochondria and vesicles.

Intermediate filaments are 10 nm in diameter and have different proteins associated with them depending on cell type. Vimentins are the structural support found in most cells, while lamin provides this support for the nuclear envelope. Keratin is found in hair, skin, and nails, and neurofilaments are associated with neural cells. They all have a central α-helical domain with successive amino acid side chains that are sevenfold, and two α-helices are twisted around each other to form a coiled coil. Intermediate filaments maintain cell shape, respond to tensile forces on the cell, anchor organelles, and support the nuclear envelope in all cells and sarcomeres in muscle. They also participate in some cell–cell and cell–matrix junctions.

2.5 CELL–MATRIX AND CELL–CELL INTERACTIONS

Cell surface receptors involved in cell–cell interactions and cell–matrix interactions are vital to the cell and play a role in many cellular processes such as growth, differentiation, embryogenesis, cancer metastasis, and immune cell responses. They also transmit information from outside the cell to the inside, thereby allowing the cell to respond to the ECM and other environmental factors. There are five major families of cell adhesion molecules (CAMs): integrins, cadherins, the immunoglobulin (Ig) superfamily CAMs, selectins, and mucins.

Prior to discussing these cell surface receptors for cell–cell and cell–matrix interactions, the ECM will be briefly described.

2.5.1 Extracellular Matrix

The ECM is produced and secreted by cells and determines the properties of tissues, which are held together by several different types of connective tissues. Connective tissue includes a number of seemingly diverse tissues that have certain structural and functional commonalities. Connective tissues serve the following purposes: provide mechanical support for cells, tissues, and organs; act as a selective barrier but allow for the diffusion of nutrients, gases, and waste products between blood vessels and other tissues; provide a substrate for cell migration; sequester growth factors and other molecules important for cell activities, such as growth and differentiation; and provide the sites where inflammatory reactions are carried out. Although many types of cells are found in connective tissues, these tissues are characterized mainly by the amount and nature of their ECM. The ECM of fibrous connective tissues contains different types and amounts of formed fibrous components, as well as glycoproteins, GAGs, and proteoglycans that make up the "ground substance."

Collagens are the most abundant class of ECM proteins in connective tissues of animals, especially in the connective tissue of mammals where it comprises about 25%–35% of the whole-body protein content. Collagens form a wide range of different structures with remarkable mechanical properties. The defining structural feature of collagen is a rod-shaped domain composed of a triple helix of protein chains. These triple helical domains have a repeating amino acid sequence: glycine–X–Y, where X is most often proline and Y is most often hydroxyproline. The size and shape of collagens vary according to their function and they are grouped as fibrillar, sheet forming, and connecting. The biosynthesis and assembly of collagens is complicated: the initial proteins, referred to as *procollagens*, translocate into the RER, where posttranslational modifications begin, which include several rounds of precise cleavage, glycosylation, and catalyzed folding. Then they pass through the Golgi apparatus and move in vesicles to the cell surface. Outside the cell, mature molecules are assembled into collagen structures reinforced by covalent crosslinking and can be further modified or interact with other types of collagens to form the final structure. Collagen is mostly found in fibrous tissues such as tendon, ligament, and skin, but it is also abundant in cornea, cartilage, bone, blood vessels, the gut, and intervertebral disk.

Elastic fibers are bundles of the protein elastin found in the ECM of connective tissue. They are produced by fibroblasts and smooth muscle cells in arteries. These fibers can stretch up to 1.5 times their length, and snap back to their original length when relaxed. Elastic fibers include elastin, elaunin, and oxytalan. Their elastic properties are very important in skin, the walls of arteries, and the lung. Elastic fibers are a composite material: a network of *fibrillin microfibrils* is embedded in amorphous core of cross-linked *elastin*. For better adaptation to particular functional requirements, cells also secrete many tissue- and age-specific proteoglycans into the ECM. To link all ECM components together, adhesive glycoproteins serve as adapters mediating many of the interactions.

Fibronectin is one of the most important adhesive glycoproteins in the ECM. Fibronectin is a high-molecular-weight (~440 kDa) ECM glycoprotein that binds to membrane-spanning receptor proteins called integrins and has multiple binding sites for collagens, proteoglycans, fibrin, heparan sulfate proteoglycans, and other adhesive glyco-proteins. Fibronectin exists as a dimer, with each monomer linked by a pair of disulfide bonds. Two types of fibronectin are present in vertebrates: one is a soluble form pro-duced by the liver and is a major component of blood plasma. The other fibronectin is an insoluble cellular fibronectin that is a major component of the ECM secreted by many cells but primarily by fibroblasts. Fibronectin plays a crucial role in wound healing and is necessary for normal embryonic development. It has major roles in cell adhesion, growth, migration, and differentiation of most cells.

The ECM is a dynamic structure, and many tissue-remodeling processes during embryogenesis, wound healing, and physiological changes (e.g., shedding of the uterine endometrium during menstruation) depend on the controlled degradation of the ECM. For this, cells secrete a set of special enzymes, matrix metalloproteinases, capable of degrading all kinds of ECM proteins.

The basal lamina, a special example of ECM, is a thin, planar assembly of ECM proteins supporting all epithelia, muscle cells, and nerve cells outside the central nervous system. This two-dimensional network of protein polymers forms a continuous rug under epithelia and a sleeve around muscle and nerve cells.

Due to the complexity and numerous ECM components that are particular to each tis-sue, bone will be used as another example to describe the various components of the ECM (Robey and Boskey 2008). Bone is unique in that its ECM is also composed of mineral deposits, which are highly substituted carbonated apatite, $[Ca_{10}(PO_4)_6(CO_3)]$, that changes with age. Type I collagen makes up 90% of the proteins of bone as a triple helix of two α_1-chains and one α_2-chain described as $[\alpha_1(I)]_2\alpha_2(I)$ with hydroxylation of 15%–20% of the lysine. It is secreted by osteoblasts as a larger molecule, procollagen, and then the pro-peptides are cleaved and excreted in urine to give the final Type I collagen fibers. Type III collagen is a minor collagen in bone and it is a triple helix of only one chain, $\alpha_1(III)_3$ that is thought to regulate the Type I collagen fiber diameter. Type V collagen $[\alpha_1(V)_2\alpha_2(V)]$ is another minor collagen in bone and also regulates collagen fiber diameter. Several glyco-proteins with different functions are found in bone: osteopontin, bone sialoprotein, and osteonectin. There are also numerous proteoglycans: decorin, biglycan, and osteoadherin. Then there are the RGD-containing proteins: fibronectin, thrombospondin, vitronectin, and fibrillin 1 and 2. The function of the RGD amino acid sequence will be discussed in more detail in the section on integrins (Section 2.3.2). In addition, there are the non-collagenous vitamin K–dependent proteins osteocalcin and matrix gla protein in the ECM of bone. There are other minor ECM proteins in bone, but refer to Robey and Boskey (2008) for further descriptions.

2.5.2 Cell Adhesion Involving Integrins

The integrins are a superfamily of cell adhesion receptors that bind to ECM proteins, and also mediate certain cell–cell interactions. Binding of ECM proteins to integrins triggers a series of intracellular signaling events that lead to changes in cell behavior and conformation such as adhesion, proliferation, survival or apoptosis, shape, motility, gene expression, and differentiation. Integrins have the ability to transduce signals from the ECM to the cytoplasm and to the nucleus of the cell and have been shown to be mechanotransducers of force on the cell through their interaction with the cytoskeleton and in particular the actin-based microfilaments making up the cytoskeleton of the cell. Integrins and their ligands have a critical role in development, immune responses, leukocyte traffic, and hemostasis but also are involved in cancer, other human diseases and can be receptors for many viruses and bacteria. Integrins are involved in a variety of biological processes, such as embryonic development, hemostasis, leukocyte homing and activation, bone formation and resorption, clot retraction, cellular response to mechanical stress, programmed cell death, tumor cell growth, metastases, and angiogenesis. Involvement of integrins in various normal and pathological processes has been demonstrated in various studies using genetically manipulated, integrin-knockout animals. Certain integrin peptide sequences have been used in tissue engineering. For bone tissue engineering, see referenced text for a more thorough discussion (Sagomonyants and Gronowicz 2011).

Integrins are transmembrane receptors composed of an α- and β-heterodimer and the combination of the α- and β-subunits determines the substrate specificity of the integrin, although many integrins can bind to the same substrate. In mammals, at least 19- and 8-integrin subunits can be combined to form at least 25 different receptors (Table 2.2). In terms of specificity of integrin–substrate binding, all mammalian integrins can be grouped into several categories: (1) laminin-binding integrins ($\alpha_1\beta_1$, $\alpha_2\beta_1$, $\alpha_3\beta_1$, $\alpha_6\beta_1$, $\alpha_7\beta_1$, $\alpha_9\beta_1$, $\alpha_v\beta_3$, $\alpha_6\beta_4$, and $\alpha_v\beta_8$), (2) collagen-binding integrins ($\alpha_1\beta_1$, $\alpha_2\beta_1$, $\alpha_3\beta_1$, $\alpha_9\beta_1$, $\alpha_{10}\beta_1$, $\alpha_{11}\beta_1$, and $\alpha_{11b}\beta_3$), (3) leukocyte integrins ($\alpha_L\beta_2$, $\alpha_M\beta_2$, $\alpha_X\beta_2$, and $\alpha_D\beta_2$), and (4) arginine–glycine–aspartic acid (RGD)-recognizing integrins ($\alpha_5\beta_1$, $\alpha_v\beta_1$, $\alpha_v\beta_3$, $\alpha_v\beta_5$, $\alpha_v\beta_6$, $\alpha_v\beta_8$, and $\alpha_{11b}\beta_3$). RGD was identified as the amino acid sequence in fibronectin and other cell adhesion proteins that modulate cell attachment by Pierschbacher in 1984. Integrins containing α_4, α_5, α_8, α_{11b}, and α_v subunits bind to ECM glycoproteins, mostly fibronectin and vitronectin that contain the RGD sequence. Proteoglycans, laminins, and collagens also contain RGD sequences but these RGD sequences are often inaccessible. In general, integrins of hematopoietic cells bind to counter-receptors on other cells or plasma proteins (for example, fibrinogen) and complement factors. Although most integrins are found in various tissues, some integrins have limited cell or tissue expression. For example, II_{b3} integrin is found in platelets, II_{64} is in keratinocytes (skin cells), and II_{E7} is in T cells (immune cells).

The structure of an integrin involves the non-covalent association of an α- and a β-subunit, both of which are type I glycoproteins consisting of large extracellular and short cytoplasmic domains (Figure 2.18). An overall shape of associated integrin subunits can be described by the presence of two long stalk regions containing C-terminal segments from both α- and β-subunits that connect extracellular ligand-binding globular headpiece to the transmembrane and cytoplasmic domains. Integrins require divalent cations such as Ca^{2+} or Mg^{2+} for binding their ligands to create a conformational change necessary for their function.

TABLE 2.2   Combinations of Integrin Subunits and Their Protein Ligands

Subunits		Ligands
β_1	α_1	Collagens, laminins
	α_2	Collagens, laminins, fibronectin
	α_3	Laminins, fibronectin, collagens, thrombospondin
	α_4	Fibronectin, VCAM, osteopontin
	α_5	Fibronectin, fibrinogen, ADAMs
	α_6	Laminin, ADAMs
	α_7	Laminins
	α_8	Fibronectin, tenascin
	α_9	Tenascin, collagen, osteopontin, laminin, VCAM, ADAMs
	α_{10}	Collagens
	α_{11}	Collagens
	α_v	Fibronectin, vitronectin, thrombospondin
β_2	α_L	ICAMs
	α_M	ICAM, fibrinogen. iC3b
	α_X	Fibrinogen, ICAM, iC3b
	α_D	VCAM, ICAMs
β_3	α_{IIb}	Collagens, fibronectin, vitronectin, von Willebrand factor
		Fibrinogen, thrombospondin, matrix metalloproteinase-2, disintegrins
	α_v	Fibronectin, vitronectin, fibrinogen, thrombospondin, von Willebrand factor, osteopontin, laminin, disintegrins, tenascin, bone sialoprotein, ADAMs
β_4	α_6	Laminins
β_5	α_v	Vitronectin, bone sialoprotein, fibronectin
β_6	α_v	Fibronectin, tenascin
β_7	α_4	Fibronectin, VCAM
	α_E	E-cadherin
β_8	α_v	Collagens, laminins, fibronectin

Sources: Plow, E.F. et al., *J. Biol. Chem.*, 275(29), 21785, 2000; van der Flier, A. and Sonnenberg, A., *Cell Tissue Res.*, 305(3), 285, 2001.

Abbreviations: ICAM, intracellular adhesion molecule; VCAM, vascular adhesion molecule; iC3b, inactivated complement component C3b; ADAM, a disintegrin and metalloproteinase.

2.5.3 Cadherins

The cadherins are the major CAMs responsible for calcium-dependent cell–cell adhesion. The three most common cadherins are neural (N) cadherin, placental (P) cadherin, and epithelial (E) cadherin. All three belong to the classical cadherin subfamily but there are a large number of nonclassical cadherins with more than 50 expressed in brain alone, the proto-adherins for instance. There are also desmosomal cadherins. In mature epithelial cells, E-cadherin is concentrated in the adherens junctions holding cells together and connecting to the actin cytoskeleton. Cadherins are found in vertebrates and invertebrates with almost all vertebrate cells expressing one or more cadherins. They are critical for embryological development and in tissue organization. Most cadherins are single-pass transmembrane glycoproteins about 700–750 amino acids in length. The extracellular domain is folded into 5–6 cadherin repeats and each is capable of binding calcium, which

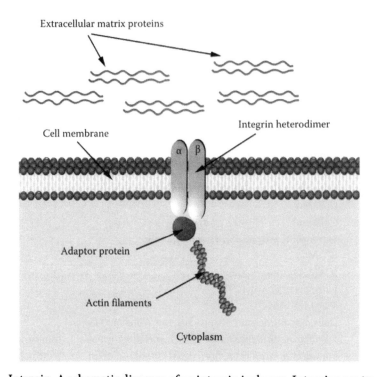

FIGURE 2.18 Integrin. A schematic diagram of an integrin is shown. Integrins are transmembrane receptors composed of an α- and a β-heterodimer with the combination of the different α- and β-subunits determining which specific extracellular matrix protein it will bind. The integrin heterodimer consists of a large extracellular domain and a short cytoplasmic domain, which can bind various adaptor proteins that connect to the actin-based cytoskeleton.

causes the extracellular domain to become rigid and rodlike. Cadherins strongly prefer homophilic binding, which describes the binding of cadherin of one cell to the same cadherin on another cell promoting the adhesion of like cells. Many cadherins interact with the cytoskeleton inside the cell. Adapter proteins link cadherins to actin filaments in many types of cells (through proteins such as catenins) and to intermediate filaments in other cells. These interactions provide mechanical continuity from cell to cell in muscles and epithelia, allowing them to transmit forces and resist mechanical disruption.

2.5.4 Immunoglobulin Superfamily Cell Adhesion Molecules

The immunoglobulin (Ig) superfamily CAMs are calcium-independent transmembrane glycoproteins and thus differ in their calcium independence from the other CAMs: cadherins, integrins, and selectins. They have received their name from their structure; each Ig superfamily CAM has an extracellular domain with several Ig-like intrachain disulfide-bonded loops with conserved cysteine residues. They also have a transmembrane domain, and an intracellular domain that interacts with the cytoskeleton. Typically, they bind integrins or other Ig superfamily CAMs. The Ig superfamily CAMs do not bind as strongly as cadherins but they are responsible for fine-tuning cell adhesion during development and tissue regeneration. Members of the Ig superfamily include the intercellular adhesion molecules (ICAMs), vascular CAM (VCAM-1), platelet–endothelial CAM (PECAM-1), and neural CAM (NCAM). Endothelial CAMs have a role in immune responses and inflammation. Neuronal CAMs have been implicated in neuronal patterning and appropriate cell recognition for synaptic connections.

2.5.5 Selectins and Mucin

The selectins are glycoproteins that mediate a variety of divalent cation-dependent, cell–cell interactions in the bloodstream. The three family members include E-selectin on activated endothelial cells, L-selectin on white blood cells, and P-selectin on platelets and endothelial cells that have been activated in the inflammatory response. Each selectin is a transmembrane protein with a highly conserved lectin domain that binds to specific oligosaccharides on another cell, an epidermal growth factor (EGF)-like motif, and varying numbers of a short repeat domain related to complement regulatory proteins (CRP). The selectins play an important role in the initial steps of leukocyte trafficking and binding to endothelial cells that line blood vessels, which enables them to migrate into a tissue in response to inflammation.

Selectins bind to another cell surface glycoproteins called *mucins*. Their extracellular segments are rich in amino acids serine and threonine, which are heavily modified with acidic oligosaccharide chains. Because of their strong negative charge, mucins extend like rods up to 50 nm from the surface. Although some mucins are membrane bound due to the presence of hydrophobic membrane-spanning domains that hold them in the plasma membrane, most mucins are secreted onto mucosal surfaces or secreted to become a component of saliva.

2.6 CELL DIVISION

All living organisms from bacteria to mammals arise from a process of cell growth and division to maintain the organism and its tissues. Cells are generated only from preexisting cells through cell division. Cells reproduce by duplicating their contents and dividing into two daughter cells with genetically identical material. The process of duplication and division is called the *cell cycle*.

2.6.1 Cell Cycle/Mitosis

The cell cycle consists of an orderly sequence of events involving DNA replication, segregation of the replicated chromosomes containing DNA, and duplication of the macromolecules and organelles within the cell to produce two cells of similar size and function. These events are highly regulated by the cell cycle control system that responds to signals from the inside and outside of the cell. Progression through the cell cycle within the cell occurs only when specific earlier events are completed and other events are delayed. The cell cycle control system depends on a family of protein kinases, cyclins, and cyclin-dependent kinases (cdks), and other proteins. The cell cycle control system also responds to outside signals that regulate cell number in a particular tissue, for example. Without this regulation, excessive growth would lead to cancer.

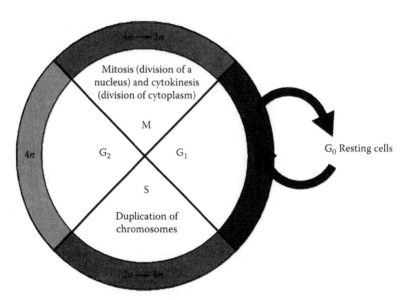

FIGURE 2.19 Cell cycle phases. There are four phases in the cell cycle: the S phase for DNA synthesis/replication, the M phase for mitosis (division of the nucleus) and two gap phases, GAP$_1$ (G$_1$), and GAP$_2$ (G$_2$), important for preparing the cell for the next phase and allowing for cell growth.

There are four phases in the cell cycle with the S phase for DNA synthesis/replication, the M phase for mitosis (division of the nucleus), and two gap phases, GAP$_1$ (G$_1$), and GAP$_2$ (G$_2$). Between M and S phases, G$_1$ involves processes in preparation for DNA synthesis. Between S and M, G$_2$ is necessary for preparing for mitosis. Thus, the sequence of the phases is G$_1$, S, G$_2$, and M (Figure 2.19). G$_1$, S, and G$_2$ are called *interphase* that can last 23 h with only 1 h for the mitosis (M) stage in a 24 h cycle. Also, the gap phases are essential for allowing time for growth, monitoring the internal and external environment to ensure the proper timing for cell division, and allowing checkpoints, important for monitoring DNA damage and arresting the cell cycle for DNA repair or other processes necessary for mitosis. These gap phases can vary in length. If conditions are not favorable, some cells delay progress through G$_1$ and enter a specialized resting state called G$_0$, which can last days, weeks, years, and even until the organism dies.

The two major phases of the cell cycle are M and S phases. During the S phase, chromosomal DNA is replicated into two DNA strands with the necessary proteins bound to them. In a typical mammalian cell, mitosis involves chromosome segregation and cell division and requires less than an hour of time but it dramatically affects the cell (Figure 2.20). Initially, the duplicated DNA strands are packaged into elongated chromosomes and then are condensed to ensure proper segregation of the chromosomes into the two daughter cells. Then the nuclear envelope breaks down and the sister chromatids are attached to the microtubules of the mitotic apparatus. During mitosis the chromosomes, aligned at the equator of the mitotic spindle, pause briefly in a state named *metaphase*, prior to their segregation. *Anaphase* is the next stage when the sister chromatids abruptly start to move to the opposite poles of the spindle where

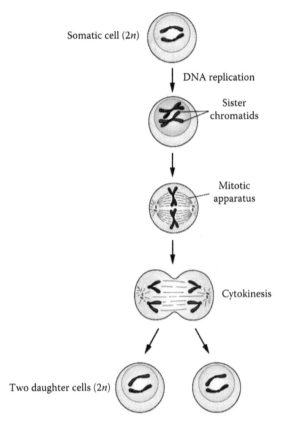

FIGURE 2.20 Mitosis. Mitosis involves chromosome segregation and cell division. The duplicated DNA strands are packaged, the nuclear envelope breaks down, and the sister chromatids are attached to the microtubules of the mitotic apparatus at the equator of the cell, followed by movement of the sister chromatids to the opposite poles of the spindle. Finally, separate nuclei form and the cell is divided by cytoplasmic division, cytokinesis.

they decondense, and the separate nuclei form. Finally, the cell is divided into two by cytoplasmic division in a process called *cytokinesis*.

2.6.2 DNA Replication and Recombination

The accurate duplication of the DNA must occur before the cell produces the two genetically identical daughter cells, and this process is called DNA replication. Also, there is a continued surveillance and repair of the DNA due to repeated damage by chemicals and radiation from the environment, or thermal variation and reactive molecules. A mutation is a DNA sequence that has been permanently damaged. Occasional mutations in DNA sequences can provide genetic diversity if the mutation does not have severe consequences. Some of these mutations may allow the organism to survive in changing environments and thus provide a new evolutionary step for the organism.

As previously described, the DNA double helix is very stable with numerous hydrogen bonds between bases. This double helix must be opened up into two separate strands to serve as a template. There are specialized sequences at which the DNA helix is first opened and these are called *replication origins*. In bacteria and simple eukaryotes, these replication origins are at a specific sequence of the DNA that is several nucleotide pairs long. Replication of the two strands of DNA can take only 40 min. In eukaryotes, these sequences are less well defined, are several thousand nucleotide pairs, with the process of replication taking 10 times longer if not more than in a bacterium, and occur only in the S phase of the cell cycle.

DNA replication requires an initiation site where proteins bind to DNA sequences at a replication origin to form an origin replication complex. In humans, the DNA sequences required for the origin extend over large distances along the DNA and the process is not completely identified or understood. A DNA polymerase catalyzes nucleotides polymerization in the 5′–3′ direction. Since the two strands of the DNA double helix are antiparallel, only one strand can be replicated continuously by the DNA polymerase. The lagging strand is completed by short strand replication of DNA fragments primed by short RNA primer molecules, Okazaki fragments, that are subsequently removed and replaced with DNA. Many proteins participate in the DNA replication process including (1) DNA polymerase and DNA primase to catalyze NTP polymerization, (2) DNA helicase and helicase loading factors to help open up the DNA helix so that it can be copied, (3) initiator proteins that bind to specific DNA sequences at the replication origin and catalyze the formation of the replication site, (4) for the lagging strand, a DNA ligase with an enzyme to degrade the RNA primers, is needed to combine the DNA fragments into one strand, and (5) DNA topoisomerases to relieve helical winding that can cause tangling.

In eukaryotes, the chromosomes are composed of both DNA and protein complexes called chromatin. Thus, chromosome duplication requires not only replication of the DNA but also the assembly of new chromosomal proteins behind the replication fork into nucleosomes. Different replication origins are activated in sequence determined in part by the chromatin structure so that chromosome duplication requires many replication origins to complete the synthesis in a typical 8 h S phase. Large amounts of new histone proteins are necessary to make the new nucleosomes and, therefore, multiple copies of the genes for each of the five histones in mammalian cells are synthesized mainly in S phase. The addition of the new histones into newly synthesized DNA is aided by chromatin assemble factors (CAFs). Also, old histones are directly inherited as nucleosomes by each daughter DNA molecule.

DNA polymerase polymerizes short DNA fragments at the replication fork. Since DNA polymerizes DNA only in the 5′–3′ direction, the last DNA fragment at the end of the chromosome needs to be replicated by a special procedure. The last DNA fragment has a special nucleotide sequence, which is incorporated into telomeres that are many tandem repeats of a short sequence with many G nucleotides (GGGTTA, this repeat in humans extends for about 100,000 nucleotides). The enzyme telomerase recognizes this sequence and elongate it in the 5′–3′ direction using an RNA template that belongs to the enzyme itself, which makes it a unique reverse transcriptase. After the telomerase has extended the parental DNA strand, replication of the lagging strand at the chromosome end can be completed by using these extensions as a template for synthesis of the complementary strand by a DNA polymerase molecule.

This telomere/telomerase process for replicating the terminal DNA sequence yields a protruding single-stranded end. Specialized proteins help to loop back the protruding end and tuck it into the duplex DNA of the telomeric repeat sequence, making this structure unique and protective from degradative enzymes and helps to distinguish it from any broken DNA in need of repair by the cell. In human somatic cells, the length of the telomeric repeat determines the number of replications and helps prevent unlimited proliferation. According to this hypothesis, somatic cells are born with a full complement of telomeric repeats, and each time a cell divides it loses 50–100 nucleotides from each of its telomeres. Once a cell has replicated numerous times, the descendent cells inherit defective chromosome and therefore will withdraw from the cell cycle, stop dividing, and enter a state of *replicative cell senescence*. For example, human fibroblasts normally proliferate for about 60 cell divisions in culture before undergoing replicative cell senescence. This process is also considered to be responsible for aging in some tissues of animals.

For an organism to survive their changing environment, the process of *genetic recombination* whereby the DNA is recombined to give different genes to the daughter cells is very important. In general recombination, two homologous DNA molecules break their double helix and the two broken ends join with the opposite DNA partners to reform two intact double helices. This process can involve more proteins in more advanced organisms but in *Escherichia coli* the RecA protein is required for this process. Usually, general recombination does not result in a rearrangement of the genes in the chromosome. The second recombination process, called *site-specific recombination*, alters the relative position of nucleotide sequences in chromosomes because extensive sequence homology between the two DNA strands is not required for recombination. Site-specific recombination is dependent on protein-mediated recognition of specific DNA sequences involving integrases and can often cause duplications in the DNA sequences.

2.6.3 Meiosis

In most eukaryote organisms, a special type of cell division, meiosis, occurs to produce haploid germ cells for heredity and procreation. The preparatory steps that lead up to mitosis are similar to the interphase of the mitotic cell cycle; however, meiosis is a "one-way" process leading to a haploid genome and therefore is not considered a part of the cell cycle. In animals, meiosis results in the formation of gametes while spores are produced in other organisms. An overview of meiosis is that the genome of a diploid germ cell, specific for sexual reproduction, undergoes DNA replication followed by two rounds of division producing four haploid cells. If meiosis produced gametes, then these cells must fuse during fertilization in eukaryotes to create a diploid cell, or zygote, eventually leading to a new individual.

Briefly, the interphase of meiosis involves a G_1 phase in which the cell synthesizes many proteins necessary for the next steps. At this point, human cells have 46 chromosomes or $2n$, identical to somatic cells (Figure 2.21). In the S phase of interphase, the DNA is duplicated so that each of the 46 chromosomes forms an identical sister chromatid. Because the cells still contain the same number of centromeres as in G_1, the cell is still considered diploid. Meiosis does not have an interphase G_2 stage. Instead, meiosis I occurs with

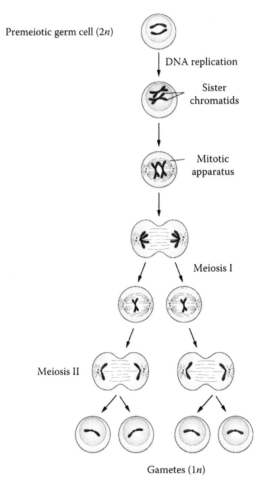

Premeiotic germ cell (2*n*)

DNA replication

Sister chromatids

Mitotic apparatus

Meiosis I

Meiosis II

Gametes (1*n*)

FIGURE 2.21   Meiosis. Meiosis is a process by which the genome of a diploid germ cell, specific for sexual reproduction, undergoes DNA replication followed by two rounds of division producing four haploid cells, important for sexual reproduction.

the separation of the pairs of homologous chromosomes into two cells that contain two sister chromatids. In the next stage of meiosis II, each of the chromosome's sister strands (chromatids) break apart and segregate the individual chromatids into haploid daughter cells, creating four haploid daughter cells. Both meiosis I and II have numerous stages but these will not be discussed here.

Genetic diversity is one of the major goals of meiosis. In the first meiotic division, the homologous chromosomes pairs align and separate independently creating gametes with individual characteristics. In addition to the other stages, homologous recombination of chromosomal regions produces new combinations of DNA within chromosomes. Another significant result of meiosis is that it allows different haploid cells (in humans: the sperm and the egg) to yield a normal diploid individual as a result of sexual reproduction and provides a stable process for survival of the organism.

ACKNOWLEDGMENTS

We would like to thank Drs. Bruce J. Mayer and Aleksandr Makeyev for their critical review of drafts of this chapter.

REFERENCES

Alberts B, Johnson A, Lewis J, Raff M, Roberts K, Walter P (eds.). 2008. *Molecular Biology of the Cell*, 5th edn. Garland Science, Taylor & Francis Group, New York.

Lodish H, Berk A, Kaiser CA, Kreiger M, Scott MP, Bretscher A, Ploegh H, Matsudaira P (eds.). 2008. *Molecular Cell Biology*, 6th edn. W.H. Freeman & Co., New York.

Pierschbacher, MD, Ruoslahti E. 1984. Variants of the cell recognition site of fibronectin that retain attachment-promoting activity. *Proc Natl Acad Sci USA*, 81(19):5988–8.

Plow EF, Haas TA, Zhang L, Loftus J, Smith JW. 2000. Ligand binding to integrins. *J Biol Chem* 275(29):21785–21788.

Robey G, Boskey A. 2008. The composition of bone. In *Primer on the Metabolic Bone Diseases and Disorders of Mineral Metabolism*, 7th edn. American Society for Bone and Medical Research, Washington, D.C., pp. 32–38.

Sagomonyants K, Gronowicz G. 2011. Biocompatibility: Integrin activated responses to metallic implant surfaces. In *Comprehensive Biomaterials*. Ducheyne P, Hultmacher DW, Kirkpatrick K, Healy K (eds.). Elsevier Limited, Oxford, U.K., Vol. 4, Chapter 9, pp. 101–113.

van der Flier A, Sonnenberg A. 2001. Function and interactions of integrins. *Cell Tissue Res* 305(3):285–298.

CHAPTER 3

Stem Cells and Tissue Regeneration

Kristen Martins-Taylor, PhD; Xiaofang Wang, MD, PhD;
Xue-Jun Li, PhD; and Ren-He Xu, MD, PhD

CONTENTS

3.1 INTRODUCTION

The *Superman* actor Christopher Reeve was a symbol of strength, not only for his famous role in the movie but more so for his courage in fighting a tragic spinal cord injury. He fought courageously for 9 years, from the moment that he was thrown from his horse in 1995 until he died in 2004 at the age of 52. Spinal cord injuries can occur not only from trauma, but also from many other causes, e.g., neurodegenerative diseases such as amyotrophic lateral sclerosis (ALS) and multiple sclerosis (AMS). Spinal cord injuries cause myelopathy or damage to nerve roots or myelinated fiber tracts that carry signals to and from the brain. Traumatic injury can also damage the gray matter in the central part of the cord, causing segmental losses of interneurons and motor neurons. Disappointingly, treatment options for acute, traumatic non-penetrating spinal cord injuries are still limited to the administration of anti-inflammatory agents or cold saline shortly after injury. Their effects are barely empirical and even disputable. The damaged nerves are barely repaired or regenerated due to scarring. Is there any way that they can be replaced with new, healthy neurons? The answer is yes given the discovery of neural stem cells (NSCs) and their regenerating power.

A stem cell is an undifferentiated cell that can continue dividing indefinitely, producing daughter cells, and has the capacity to differentiate into specific cell types. Stem cells are present almost in every organ in the body, and their ability to self-renew and differentiate provides the basis for tissue regeneration, permitting the body to naturally maintain homeostasis by replacing aged, damaged, and dysfunctional cells with new, healthy cells in the body. Stem cells can be classified based on their source (Figure 3.1). For example,

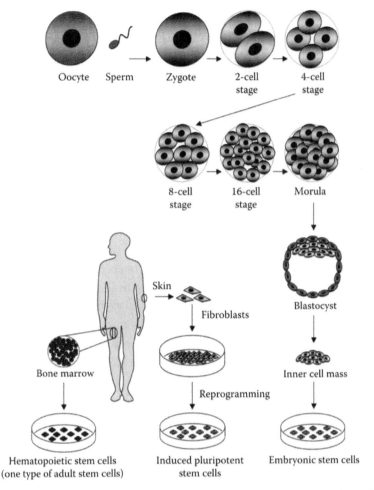

FIGURE 3.1 **Stem cell types based on their sources.** Embryonic stem cells are derived from early-stage embryos, while induced pluripotent stem cells are derived from somatic cells, such as skin fibroblasts, that are reprogrammed into ES cell–like cells. Adult stem cells are tissue-specific and can be isolated from various organs or tissues, such as the bone marrow.

embryonic stem (ES) cells are derived from early-stage embryos, and adult stem cells are tissue specific and can be isolated from almost any organ or tissue in the body. For instance, the brain is a source for NSCs, which can differentiate into many kinds of neural cells, including neurons, glial cells, and astrocytes. On the other hand, the bone marrow (BM) is a source for hematopoietic stem cells (HSCs), which can differentiate into all progeny of blood cells. Alternatively, stem cells can be categorized into totipotent, pluripotent, and multipotent stem cells, based on their differentiation ability. ES cells are pluripotent and can differentiate into any cell type in the body, whereas adult stem cells are multipotent and can usually differentiate into limited cell types for the organ or tissue from which they were isolated. In 2006, an ES-like stem cell type called induced pluripotent stem (iPS) cells was derived via the reprogramming of somatic cells with several defined factors identified from ES cells (Takahashi and Yamanaka 2006). Thus far, an increasing number of stem cell types have been identified and characterized (Martins-Taylor and Xu 2009). It is impossible to discuss all the stem cell types in one chapter. Therefore, we are going to use the neural (an ectodermal derivative) lineage, as well as hematopoietic, and mesenchymal (both mesodermal derivatives) lineages, as examples to introduce how scientists and physicians have been exploring the possibility of using stem cells to differentiate into or derive these lineages to treat neurological, hematopoietic, and connective tissue diseases.

3.2 ADULT NEURAL STEM CELLS

3.2.1 Location of NSCs in the Brain

In the 1960s, Drs. Joseph Altman and Gopal Das reported continuous stem cell activity in the hippocampus of the adult brain (Altman and Das 1965). As the first observation of ongoing stem cell activity in the adult brain, this finding refuted the dogma in the early twentieth century that no neurons could conceivably be generated in adulthood (Gross 2000). Subsequently, stem cell activity has also been observed in other brain regions (Altman 1969; Reynolds and Weiss 1992; Weiss et al. 1996). As shown in Figure 3.2, adult NSCs are located primarily in two regions: the subventricular zone (SVZ) of the lateral ventricle and the subgranular zone (SGZ) of the hippocampal dentate gyrus (Gage 2000). What is the potential for differentiation in these adult NSCs? Will these stem cells be activated after injury or under pathological conditions? Can they be used in therapies for brain disorders? These questions will be discussed in the following sections.

3.2.2 Differentiation Potential of Adult NSCs

NSCs can renew themselves and differentiate into multiple cell types of the neural lineage (Ming and Song 2005). Adult NSCs in the SVZ and SGZ are positive for GFAP and CD133. Under physiological conditions, NSCs in the SVZ develop into intermediate progenitors,

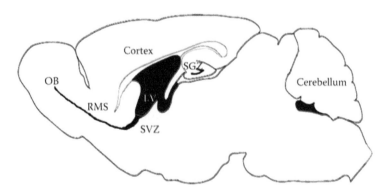

FIGURE 3.2 A schematic illustration showing the location of adult neural stem cells in a sagittal section of the mouse brain. (Modified from Paxinos, G and Franklin, K. (eds.) The mouse brain in stereotaxic coordinates. *Spiral Bound*, 2001) Adult neural stem cells are mainly located in the subgranular zone (SGZ) of the hippocampus and the subventricular zone (SVZ) of the lateral ventricle (LV), as indicated in blue color. Adult neural stem cells in the SVZ migrate to the olfactory bulb through the rostral migratory stream (RMS).

which then migrate to the olfactory bulb and differentiate into GABAergic interneurons (Lois et al. 1996; Curtis et al. 2007). In contrast, SGZ progenitors (also positive for Sox2), as shown in fate-tracing studies, give rise to neurons and astrocytes (Suh et al. 2007). Although NSCs in both areas are multipotent in Petri dish cultures, it is unclear whether a single NSC can give rise to multiple neural cell types in the brain under physiological conditions.

Adult NSCs can be isolated from the adult brain in animals (Morshead et al. 1994; Bonaguidi et al. 2008), brain biopsy and postmortem tissues in humans (Palmer et al. 2001), and expanded *in vitro* as free-floating clusters (neurospheres) in the presence of mitogens, such as bFGF and EGF. These cells have the two hallmarks of stem cells, in that they can self-renew and have the capacity to differentiate into multiple cell types in the neural lineage, such as neurons, astrocytes, and oligodendrocytes. At the clonal level, adult NSCs can form neurospheres and exhibit multipotency (Palmer et al. 1997). Adult NSCs give rise primarily to GABA interneurons and glutamatergic neurons but not other neuronal subtypes, such as spinal motor neurons (large projection neurons that form during early development) (Temple 2001). In addition to the SVZ and SGZ, neurospheres can also form after isolating cells from other regions of the brain (striatum and cortex) and spinal cord (Palmer et al. 1995; Weiss et al. 1996). Under physiological conditions, these areas do not undergo neurogenesis *in vivo*. However, after injury or under pathological conditions, endogenous stem cell activity is also observed in other areas of the brain, which will be discussed later. What is the niche for NSCs and how are the activation and differentiation of NSCs regulated? Insights into these questions will provide critical information for the application of NSCs in neurological diseases.

3.2.3 Therapeutic Applications of Adult NSCs in Neurological Disorders

The first step toward using adult NSCs for neurological diseases is to activate or recruit adult NSCs to replace the cells that have been lost. To a limited extent, the brain can replace and repair neurons that have been lost after injury (Emsley et al. 2005). In 2002, several groups examined the neurogenesis and generation of neuron after focal ischemia in rodents (Nakatomi et al. 2002; Parent et al. 2002; Kokaia and Lindvall 2003). Ischemia induces significant increases in the proliferation of the SGZ and SVZ. New neurons, such as hippocampal pyramidal neurons and striatal projection neurons that are lost in ischemia, were also generated in the ischemic region (Parent et al. 2002). One study also showed that infusing growth factors into the ventricle enhanced the generation of new neurons (Nakatomi et al. 2002). These newly generated neurons were electrophysiologically active and effected improvements in cognitive function after stroke.

Increases in SGZ neurogenesis have been observed after temporal lobe epilepsy, which usually leads to hippocampal cell damage; some NSCs in the SGZ migrated into the hilus and differentiated into mature granule neurons (Parent et al. 1997). It has also been shown that seizures promote synapse integration in nascent neurons (Overstreet-Wadiche et al. 2006). But, newly formed ectopic granule neurons might cause recurring seizures (Parent et al. 2006), suggesting that the proper synaptic connections and circuitry are important to experience functional improvements in seizures. Whether and how adult NSCs can give rise to certain neuronal subtypes and integrate into the circuitry *in vivo* remain to be elucidated and will be important for the development of endogenous cell replacement therapies for neurological diseases.

Another strategy for using NSCs in neurological diseases is the transplantation of NSCs from adult or, more likely, fetal brain (Lindvall and Kokaia 2006; Einstein and Ben-Hur 2008; Kim and de Vellis 2009). After transplanting the neurospheres that are formed from NSCs into the brain, these cells can also generate neuron and glial cells *in vivo* (Gage et al. 1995; Suhonen et al. 1996). NSCs have been transplanted into experimental models of Huntington disease (HD) (Kordower et al. 1997; Lee et al. 2005), ALS (Xu et al. 2006; Hwang et al. 2009), Parkinson disease (PD) (Love et al. 2005; Emborg et al. 2008), and stroke (Kim et al. 2008), etc. The survival of grafted cells and functional improvements has been reported.

3.2.4 Success and Limitations of NSC-Based Therapy

Some clinical trials are aimed at stimulating the differentiation of adult NSCs. For example, treatment with G-CSF and cistanche total glycosides is being assessed in ALS patients. Since the availability of adult NSCs from humans is limited, clinical trials that use transplanted adult NSCs are relatively difficult. In 2009, the Rajavithi Neuronal Adult Stem Cells Project (RNASc) in Thailand initiated a phase II clinical trial (clinicaltrials.gov). It is aimed at identifying unlimited human neuronal progenitor stem cells from the human brain from patient biopsies from either elective or emergency surgeries and generating oligodendrocytes progenitors, as well as other neuronal subtypes in the next phases, for treatment of Alzheimer's disease, multiple sclerosis (MS), and PD. Another strategy is to recruit or activate endogenous NSCs. However, success via this approach largely depends on more in-depth understanding of the mechanisms that regulate the activation and differentiation of NSCs and the functional integration of NSC-derived neurons. Due to the difficulty of obtaining NSCs from humans, scientists have been exploring other sources to procure human neural cells, as well as other therapeutic cells, in large quantity. Since ES cells can be *in vitro* differentiated into various cell types and be expanded without limitation, they are ideal for this purpose.

In February 2010, the United Kingdom Gene Therapy Advisory Committee announced that it had approved ReNeuron's phase I clinical trial for testing a stem cell–derived therapy on stroke patients (http://www.reneuron.com/news_events/news/document_178_237.php). This follows the approval from the UK Medicines and Healthcare Products Regulatory Agency. In developed countries, stroke is the third largest cause of death and the single largest cause of adult disability. The vast majority of strokes are ischemic, which is caused by a blockage of blood flow in the brain. As a result of the damage to the brain, stroke survivors are often left with permanent disabilities. Treating patients with anti-clotting agents within hours of the stroke is currently the major treatment for ischemic stroke patients. Unfortunately, most patients do not get to the hospital in time for the treatment. The late-phase treatment of ischemic stroke victims is rehabilitation measures. In this phase I clinical trial, safety and efficacy were assessed about injecting NSCs, derived from human fetal cortex at 14 week gestation, into disabled ischemic stroke patients between 6 and 24 months after their stroke. Preclinical testing in animal models of ischemic stroke has been promising in that many of the functional deficits associated with disabilities caused by strokes are reversed (reviewed in Gutierrez et al. 2009).

3.3 EMBRYONIC STEM CELLS

3.3.1 Early Embryogenesis

ES cells are derived from early-stage embryos. To understand the nature of the source cells, here we will briefly introduce the early embryogenesis (Figure 3.1). Upon fertilization, a mammalian embryo undergoes sequential cell divisions or cleavages, going through the 1-, 2-, 4-, and 8-cell stages. During these early stages, the cells, also called blastomeres, within the embryo are loosely stuck together. When the embryo undergoes cell division from the 8-cell to the 16-cell stage, the cells tightly compact to form a ball of cells called a morula. There are tight junctions between the cells that seal the interior of the morula from the external medium. As a result, an internal cavity forms, converting the morula into a blastocyst. The outer layer of cells of the blastocyst is called trophectoderm, which will give rise to extraembryonic tissue, including the amniotic sac and placenta. The amniotic sac and the placenta enclose and protect the embryo proper. Moreover, they supply the embryo proper with the metabolites required during development from the mother. These tissues are referred to as extraembryonic tissues, since they do not form any part of the adult and are discarded at birth. The cavity of the blastocyst contains an inner clump of cells called the inner cell mass (ICM) that is located to one side. The cells within the ICM differentiate to form the embryo proper and other extraembryonic tissues, such as the yolk sac. The individual cells within the ICM are pluripotent, meaning that they can give rise to any cells within the adult body, including germ cells.

The cells of the ICM differentiate to form the three primary, embryonic germ layers: ectoderm, mesoderm, and endoderm. The transformation from the sphere of cells of the ICM into a structure with a gut is called gastrulation. During gastrulation, the germ layers are positioned such that layers can develop into bodily systems. The ectoderm is the outermost layer and differentiates first, forming the precursor of the epidermis (external ectoderm) and the nervous system (neuroectoderm). The mesoderm forms the middle layer and can differentiate into a number of tissues, including bone, muscle, connective tissue, and the middle layer of the skin. The endoderm is the innermost layer and is the precursor to the gut and its appendages, including the liver and lung. In one form or other, this is the universal feature of animal development.

3.3.2 Derivation and Characterization of Mouse ES Cells

ES cells were first derived by Martin Evans and Gail Martin laboratories from mouse embryos in 1981 by isolating and culturing the ICM of mouse blastocysts in serum-containing medium on mitotically inactivated mouse embryonic fibroblasts (MEFs) as a feeder layer (Evans and Kaufman 1981; Martin 1981). Mouse ES cells have normal karyotype, although they can become unstable in extended culture. They highly express transcription factors Oct3/4, Nanog, and Sox2 among many other pluripotency-sustaining factors. Mouse ES cells also express cell surface antigen SSEA-1 and alkaline phosphatase.

It has been known that two cytokines, leukemia inhibitory factor (LIF) (Yoshida et al. 1994) and bone morphogenetic proteins (BMP) (Ying et al. 2003), in replacement of serum, can maintain the culture of mouse ES cells and prevent them from differentiation. Inhibitors of two signaling kinases ERK and GSK-3 (the 2i system), which presumably serve the same target as for LIF and BMP, can also maintain their undifferentiated expansion (Ying et al. 2008).

Mouse ES cells can be differentiated *in vitro* into cell types that represent all the three embryonic germ layers, through directed differentiation or formation of embryoid bodies (EBs). EBs are formed by dissociating the ES cell colonies into smaller clumps and culturing them using methods that prevent their attachment (i.e., in hanging drops or in low-attachment tissue culture flasks). ES cells start to differentiate with the EB to a limited extent by recapitulating embryonic development, which gives rise to precursors that can differentiate into cell types from the three germ layers, as well as extraembryonic lineages. ES cells can also form teratomas when injected into immunodeficient mice. Teratomas are encapsulated tumors that contain tissues from the three germ layers. Furthermore, they are capable of producing chimeras. Mouse ES cells can be injected into an early-stage embryo from a different strain of mice and develop into an adult chimeric mouse. The adult chimeric mouse is composed of cells from both strains. Coat color is often used as a marker for chimerism. Mouse ES cells are also capable of producing chimeras through germline transmission (i.e., transmission via gametes to offspring), which is the ultimate test of pluripotency. The derivation and characterization of mouse ES cells have set the basic methods and standards for the subsequent derivation of ES cells from other species, including human.

3.3.3 Derivation and Characterization of Human ES Cells

Seventeen years after mouse ES cells were first derived, James Thomson's laboratory derived ES cells from human blastocysts in 1998 (Thomson et al. 1998), based on their previous success in derivation of monkey ES cells from rhesus and Marmoset (Thomson et al. 1995, 1996). It is undoubtedly a breakthrough progress for this important research from animals to humans. Advances in the culture conditions for human embryos in *in vitro* fertilization clinics also contributed to the derivation of human ES cells (Gardner et al. 1998). Similar to other ES cells, human ES cells are capable of long-term self-renewal, maintain a normal karyotype, and can differentiate into cell types that represent the three germ layers via EB or teratoma formation. Like monkey ES cells, human ES cells express the surface markers SSEA-3, SSEA-4, TRA1-60, and TRA1-81.

The growth factors required for human ES cell self-renewal are distinct from those required for mouse ES cells. Human ES cells do not require LIF for the maintenance of self-renewal (Humphrey et al. 2004; Sumi et al. 2004). Moreover, BMPs induce human ES cell differentiation into trophectoderm and primitive endoderm (Xu et al. 2002; Pera et al. 2004). We (Xu et al. 2005, 2008) and others (reviewed in Okita and Yamanaka 2006; Watabe and Miyazono 2009) have shown that FGF signaling, as well as TGF-β/activin/nodal signaling, are required for human ES cell self-renewal. Ligands of these two signaling pathways can sustain long-term culture of human ES cells although, like mouse ES cells, human ES cells can also be derived and maintained on MEF as feeders and in medium conditioned by the feeders. These feeder cells have been shown to provide multiple ligands to activate these essential pathways and inhibitors to block the differentiation pathways.

3.3.4 Potential Applications of ES Cells to Treat Degenerative Diseases

Thus far, ES cells have been also derived from avian, monkey, rat, rabbit, and dog, but mouse ES cells are mostly used for modeling and treating human diseases both *in vitro* and *in vivo* (Martins-Taylor and Xu 2009). Thus, the derivation of ES cells from these species has created important resources for studying these diseases and for pharmaceutical research. These ES cell lines may be used for developing and testing potential therapies for treatment of human diseases. However, the therapeutic promises of ES cell progeny depend on our knowledge and our ability to drive ES cells differentiation into the particular cell types desired. Great efforts are being made to understand and recapitulate the niches that control differentiation into specific lineages. ES cells cannot be directly transplanted into patients due to their pluripotency that can cause teratomas in the host.

Progress has been made to differentiate ES cells into lineage-specific precursors that may be used in regenerative medicine applications. In particular, differentiation of ES cells into neuronal lineages has been extensively studied and thus, reproducible generation of different subtypes of neurons is possible. Degeneration of certain types of neurons is implied in many neurodegenerative disorders, such as PD, HD, and ALS. In addition to neurons, astrocytes and oligodendrocytes are two important cell types in the central nervous system. Congenital dysmyelinating and acquired demyelinating diseases are caused by degeneration of oligodendrocytes, the sole source of myelin in the central nervous system. Currently, there is no effective treatment or prevention for these diseases, partially due to the lack of a system to study these diseases and screen drugs. Thus, generation of neuronal progenitors from ES cells holds promise for studying human neurogenesis, developing assays for pharmacological and toxicological studies, and developing potential cell therapy applications.

3.3.5 Differentiation of Functional Neural Cells from ES Cells

During development, neural induction is initiated when BMP signaling is inhibited, as we (Xu et al. 1995) and others (Sasai et al. 1995; Dale and Jones 1999) first demonstrated in *Xenopus* embryo, or when FGF signaling is activated (Wilson and Edlund 2001). Administration of a BMP antagonist (Noggin), basic FGF, and other factors spurs efficient neural differentiation from mouse and human ES cells. The most commonly used methods of neural induction involve adherent cultures (Chambers et al. 2009), EB formation (Zhang et al. 2001; Li and Zhang 2006), and coculture with stromal cells (Tabar et al. 2005; Pomp et al. 2008). Because the latter promotes the development of neural cells with a midbrain/hindbrain identity, this technique has been used widely to generate midbrain neurons.

Of the approaches that entail EB formation (or the aggregation of ES cells), a chemically defined system established by the Su-Chun Zhang laboratory (Zhang et al. 2001; Li and Zhang 2006) has been widely used. Briefly, ES cell colonies are detached from their feeder layers or matrices to initiate differentiation. The ES cell aggregates are kept in suspension in ES cell medium for 4 days and in a neural induction medium for the next 2 days, which mimics gastrulation and induces the formation of ectodermal germ layers. These ES cell aggregates adhere to the culture surface and form columnar neuroectodermal cells that organize into neural tube-like rosettes after 14 days of differentiation. These neuroectodermal cells can be isolated through enzymatic treatment and adhesion. This approach not only generates neuroectodermal cells at high efficiency, but it also recapitulates early embryonic development with regard to timing and morphology.

Neuroectodermal cells further pattern into regional progenitors along the dorsal–ventral and rostral–caudal axes (Briscoe and Ericson 2001), which subsequently develop into distinct neuronal subtypes that have different biochemical functions including secretion of neurotransmitters. Because the mechanism by which neurons express certain neurotransmitters is unknown, the specification of neuronal subtypes from ES cells is based primarily on their positional identities (Zhang 2006). Several neuronal subtypes, including spinal motor neurons (Li et al. 2005; Singh Roy et al. 2005; Lee et al. 2007) and midbrain dopaminergic neurons, have been successfully specified from ES cells with retinoic acid (RA)/sonic hedgehog (SHH) and FGF8/SHH, respectively. RA and FGF8 promote the specification of cells in the spinal cord and midbrain, respectively. SHH, an important ventralizing factor, can be used to specify spinal motor neurons and midbrain dopaminergic in culture.

The identities of such neurons have been confirmed based on the expression of various markers of neuronal position and neurotransmitters. Moreover, these neurons are electrophysiologically active, release dopamine upon stimulation (for dopaminergic neurons) (Perrier et al. 2004; Yan et al. 2005), or make functional connections with target muscle cells (for motor neurons) (Li et al. 2005; Lee et al. 2007). Generation of other cell types, such as oligodendrocytes (Nistor et al. 2005; Hu et al. 2009), retinal photoreceptor (Osakada et al. 2008), GABAergic neurons (Chatzi et al. 2009), and forebrain glutamatergic neurons (Li et al. 2009b), has also been reported.

3.3.6 ES Cell–Derived Neuronal Cells for Treatment of Neurological Diseases in Animal Models

To explore the potential application of ES cell–derived neurons in regenerative medicine, these neurons have been transplanted into animal models to evaluate their survival and function in the hosts (Zhang et al. 2008). Most of these studies have focused on several common neurodegenerative diseases, e.g., PD, ALS, HD, and spinal cord injury.

3.3.6.1 Parkinson Disease

PD is characterized by selective loss of dopaminergic neurons in the substantial nigra, resulting in muscle rigidity, tremor, and a slowdown or loss of movement. Due to the highly selective cell loss in a restricted location, PD is an ideal target for cell replacement therapy. Ron Mckay laboratory transplanted normal mouse ES cells and Nurr1-overexpressing mouse ES cells into 6-OHDA-lesioned animals (a PD model), demonstrating that Nurr1-overexpressing ES cells differentiate into TH-positive dopaminergic neurons after transplantation, effecting functional improvements, based on behavioral changes in these animals. Subsequently, monkey ES cells were induced to assume the dopaminergic phenotype and were transplanted into MPTP-lesioned monkeys, where differentiation of dopaminergic neurons and functional improvement were observed after transplantation.

Although human ES cells can also differentiate into dopaminergic phenotype *in vitro*, the rates of survival and differentiation of TH+ dopaminergic neurons *in vivo* are low. Goldman laboratory cotransplanted human ES cells with midbrain astrocytes, which improved the survival and differentiation of dopaminergic neurons from human ES cells (Roy et al. 2006). Although the recipients exhibited a decrease in rotation on stimulation, some animals rotated in the opposite direction, which might have been caused by the over-release of dopamine by the transplanted cells.

3.3.6.2 Amyotrophic Lateral Sclerosis

Motor neurons are large projection neurons that control all muscle movements. The degeneration of motor neurons is implied in certain devastating disorders, such as ALS and spinal muscular atrophy (SMA). Mouse and human ES cells have been successfully differentiated into spinal motor neurons that can make synaptic connections with muscle cells *in vitro* (Wichterle et al. 2002; Li et al. 2005; Lee et al. 2007). Because the pathway toward motor neuron axons and the functional connection between muscle cells and motor neurons are controlled precisely during embryonic development, it has been difficult for grafted motor neurons to grow out of the boundary between central and peripheral nervous systems (CNS–PNS) and home to the correct targets (the distance can be 1 m in adults compared with several millimeters in developing embryos).

After transplantation into chick embryos at the stage in which endogenous motor neurons are developed, mouse ES cell–derived motor neurons survive and grow axons out of the spinal cord that make functional connections with muscle cells (Wichterle et al. 2002). Upon combined treatment with an inhibitor of CNS–PNS boundary formation and a target-derived factor, mouse ES cell–derived motor neurons sprout several axons (Harper et al. 2004). A subsequent study by the same group improved this method and used an additional inhibitor to overcome the myelin-mediated repulsion during transplantation, which resulted in the recovery from paralysis in adult rats that were grafted with mouse stem cells (Deshpande et al. 2006).

Although motor neurons are specifically lost in ALS, the loss of motor neurons in ALS is not cell autonomous, and glial cells (both astrocytes and microglial cells) regulate the development and acceleration of the pathogenesis in these patients. Within the affected glial cells, transplanted motor neurons may not survive. Recently, a group reported the survival and functional improvement of ES cell–derived glial cells after transplantation (Lepore et al. 2008). Considering the difficulties in the outgrowth and homing of motor neuron axons, transplantation of glial cells might be a more effective and practical method to protect the remaining motor neurons in patients (Nayak et al. 2006).

3.3.6.3 Huntington Disease

HD is an inherited, autosomal dominant, neuropsychiatric disease that is caused by expansion of a polyglutamine tract in the Huntingtin protein, which results in significant neuronal loss and atrophy in the brain. The striatal projection neuron (spiny medial

GABAergic neuron) is the most important cell type that degenerates in HD. A recent study differentiated human ES cells into neurons that had striatal GABAergic neuronal phenotypes and transplanted them into the quinolinic acid–lesioned nude rats whose striatal neurons were injured and depleted, mimicking HD pathology (Aubry et al. 2008). Striatal progenitors generated many NESTIN+ early neural progenitors 4–6 weeks after transplantation. A small population of cells differentiated further into DARPP32+ striatal GABAergic neurons in rat brain 3–5 months after transplantation. However, the functional and behavioral changes in these rats were not examined.

3.3.7 Transplantation of ES Cell–Derived Oligodendrocyte Progenitors

ES cell–based therapy has also been applied to animal models of CNS injuries, such as spinal cord injury (Coutts and Keirstead 2008). Human ES cell–derived oligodendrocyte progenitors were transplanted into injured adult rat spinal cords, which resulted in improved locomotor ability and movement recovery (Keirstead et al. 2005). Oligodendrocytes supply myelin in the CNS, and enhanced remyelination was observed in these animals after transplantation. In addition to spinal cord injury, ES cell–derived oligodendrocytes also represent a source of myelin in myelin-related diseases, such as congenital hypomyelination and MS (Goldman 2005; Windrem et al. 2008).

Based on the success of the transplantation studies in animal models with spinal cord injury, the first clinical trial of human ES cells, which will be conducted by Geron Corporation, was approved by the U.S. Food and Drug Administration in January 2009 (http://www.geron.com/media/pressview.aspx?id=1148). In this phase I clinical trial, Geron Corporation will implant human ES cell–derived oligodendrocyte progenitors into 8–10 paraplegic patients who can use their arms but cannot walk. These patients have no other alternative methods available to regain the functions lost by their injuries. Patients with injuries in the middle of the spinal cord between the third and tenth vertebrae will receive injections at the site of the injury. Moreover, these patients must have sustained their injuries with 7–14 days to be included in this groundbreaking clinical trial. The primary goal of this study, according to Geron, is to determine whether injecting ES cell progeny into humans is safe, and also to monitor sensation and movement in the legs of the patients.

3.3.8 Challenges and Perspectives

Although several neuronal subtypes have been successfully specified from ES cells and functional improvements have been observed after transplanting these cells into animal disease models, many challenges still remain in this field. The most important issue is the safety of ES cell transplantation. Because ES cells can differentiate into any cell type, they can form teratomas after transplantation. Although most transplantation studies have used differentiated cells, proliferation of grafted cells has been observed several months after transplantation in many studies. To circumvent this potential, one can purify the transplanted cells or eliminate pluripotent stem cells by using flow cytometry–based cell sorting or drug selection.

In addition, there are other problems that need to be solved, such as how to improve and achieve the survival and integration of transplanted cells into the host environment and how to encourage the outgrowth and homing of motor neuron axons after transplantation.

Studies in these areas will provide important insights and facilitate the success of stem cell–based therapies for neurological diseases. Another challenge of ES cell–based therapy is immunorejection, because it is impossible to develop personalized ES cells. The use of early-stage human embryos is ethically disputable, although they are donated to research by infertility patients after treatment is completed. Recent advances in generating iPS cells by reprogramming somatic cells may provide solutions to overcome these hurdles.

3.4 INDUCED PLURIPOTENT STEM CELLS

Following the first derivation of human ES cell lines, scientists began seeking alternative approaches to deriving ES-like cells from cells that carry the same genotype as a patient, without using embryos, in order to circumvent the ethical concerns surrounding the disputable use of donated early human embryos for the derivation of ES cells. This was elegantly achieved by Yamanaka and Takahashi in 2006, who discovered that four essential transcription factors that are highly expressed in ES cells can be used to reprogram somatic cells into an embryonic-like state. This led to the creation of another new pluripotent stem cell type, known as iPS cells (Takahashi and Yamanaka 2006). This new technology has been quickly recapitulated in human (Takahashi et al. 2007; Yu et al. 2007) and many other species including monkey (Liu et al. 2008; Wu et al. 2010), pig (Esteban et al. 2009; Ezashi et al. 2009; Wu et al. 2009), rat (Li et al. 2009a; Liao et al. 2009), and canine (Shimada et al. 2010).

3.4.1 Derivation of iPS Cells

The first differentiated source cells for iPS cell derivation were MEFs and mouse adult tail fibroblasts (Takahashi and Yamanaka 2006). Retroviral transduction was used to express the reprogramming factors Oct4, Sox2, Klf4, and c-Myc. To sustain their pluripotency, mitotically inactivated MEFs were used as feeders in the derivation and maintenance of mouse iPS cells. The iPS cells exhibit similar features as mouse ES cells, including staining positive for alkaline phosphatase and SSEA-1. Moreover, they can be differentiated *in vitro* into cell types that represent all the three embryonic germ layers, through directed differentiation or formation of EBs, and form teratomas when injected into SCID mice. Furthermore, they are capable of producing chimeras with germline transmission (Maherali et al. 2007; Okita et al. 2007; Wernig et al. 2007).

Two independent groups using partially different combinations of reprogramming factors derived the first human iPS cell lines. Thomson group used OCT4, SOX2, NANOG, and LIN28 via lentiviral transduction (Yu et al. 2007), whereas Yamanaka group used the reprogramming factors and retroviral transduction (Takahashi et al. 2007), the same factors that were used for the mouse iPS cells (Takahashi and Yamanaka 2006). Similar to human ES cells, human iPS cells are derived on MEF feeders and cultured under the same conditions. Moreover, human iPS cells express the same cell surface markers as human ES cells, which include SSEA-3, SSEA-4, TRA1-60, and TRA1-81. Cell types from all three germ layers can be differentiated *in vitro* from human iPS cells. Furthermore, when injected into immunodeficient mice, they form teratomas. Thus, iPS cells appear to have the same developmental potency as ES cells.

3.4.2 Methodological Improvement

Since these groundbreaking reports, iPS cells have been generated from various tissues such as keratinocytes, B lymphocytes, BM cells, liver cells, NSCs, and meningiocytes (reviewed in Feng et al. 2009). One or more viral factors can be replaced and reprogramming efficiency can be enhanced through the use of pharmaceutical inhibitors that specifically target epigenetic modifiers or pluripotency regulators (reviewed in Feng et al. 2009). Virus-free methods have been developed for the derivation of iPS cells. To prevent transgene integration in the genome, adenoviral transduction (Stadtfeld et al. 2008), transient transfection (Okita et al. 2008), and the *piggyBac* (PB) transposon gene-delivery systems (Kaji et al. 2009; Woltjen et al. 2009; Yusa et al. 2009) have been used for reprogramming mouse cells. Moreover, iPS cells can be generated from mouse and human differentiated cells via the transduction of recombinant OCT4, SOX2, KLF4, and c-MYC proteins, free of any DNA delivery (Bru et al. 2008; Zhou et al. 2009). Furthermore, human iPS cells can be generated using serial RNA transfections with mRNA that was synthesized *in vitro* cloned from the cDNA of OCT4, SOX2, KLF4, and c-MYC (Yakubov et al. 2010). These are remarkable progresses for preserving the integrity of the host genome, but the cost of the derivation appears very high while the efficiency being extremely low.

iPS cells have been recently derived and maintained in the completely defined medium mTeSR1 (Stem Cell Technologies, Vancouver, Canada) (Ludwig et al. 2006) from human adipose stem cells with the Yamanaka factors via lentiviral transduction (Sun et al. 2009). Furthermore, iPS cells have been derived from rat, monkey, porcine, and canine, creating important resources for studying human disease and pharmaceutical research. These animal models are used to study numerous human diseases, especially in the development and testing of potential therapies.

3.4.3 Potential Clinical Applications of iPS Cells

There is great potential for the use of iPS cells in therapeutic applications for regenerative medicine. Proof-of-principle experiments have been done using mouse iPS cells in a humanized sickle cell anemia mouse (Hanna et al. 2007). Sickle cell anemia or sickle cell disease is a painful genetic disorder that affects the shape of red blood cells, resulting in a loss of elasticity. The red blood cells change shape or sickle in low oxygen conditions. However, these cells fail to return to normal shape when normal oxygen tension is restored. These rigid red blood cells are unable to pass through narrow capillaries, resulting in blood vessel blockages and restriction in the blood supply, which can damage tissues. Moreover, the sickled red blood cells are destroyed in the spleen, causing anemia. This disease is caused by mutations in the hemoglobin gene. In these experiments, gene targeting and reprogramming were coupled to correct the mutation in the hemoglobin gene. When hematopoietic progenitors that were derived from the iPS cells were transplanted into the mouse model, the sickle cell phenotype can be rescued. Proof-of-principle experiments have also been done using iPS cell–derived dopaminergic neurons in a rat model of PD (Wernig et al. 2008). The transplanted dopaminergic neurons were able to improve behavior of the rats. These findings demonstrate the therapeutic potential of iPS cells in regenerative medicine. The progeny of patient-specific iPS cells may also be used as a tool for diagnostic testing of disease and screening for drugs most effective for the patient.

3.4.4 Challenges and Perspectives

Although the iPS cell technology has eliminated the need for human embryos and avoided immunorejection of stem cell progeny by recipients, there are still some preexisting and new challenges. For example, the iPS cell derivation efficiency is still very low, especially for virus-free methods. The efficiency for iPS cells to differentiate into desired cell lineages for therapy appears to be even lower than that for ES cells (Choi et al. 2009; Feng et al. 2010; Hu et al. 2010; Kim et al. 2010; Kulkeaw et al. 2010). Teratoma-forming risk remains if any therapeutic cells are mixed with residual, undifferentiated pluripotent stem cells. There is also risk of oncogenesis due to the disruption of the host genome or reactivation of the reprogramming factors in iPS cell progeny, if the iPS cells were reprogrammed via viral transduction. In-depth study is necessary to understand the fate of the iPS cell progeny *in vivo*, for example, their survival, integration, and functionality. Finally, we must continue to develop various animal-free conditions for lineage-specific differentiation of the stem cells so that their differentiated cells are directly at clinical grade.

Earlier, we used application of stem cell–differentiated neurogenic cells to treat neurological diseases as an example. Obviously, ES or iPS cells and many other stem cell types have been studied or used for therapy of non-neurological diseases. We will introduce some of them later to broaden our knowledge of these additional aspects.

3.5 HEMATOPOIETIC STEM CELLS

HSCs are multipotent stem cells that can differentiate into all blood cell types including myeloid (monocytes and macrophages, neutrophils, basophils, eosinophils, erythrocytes, megakaryocytes/platelets, dendritic cells) and lymphoid lineages (T cells, B cells, NK cells). HSCs also have plasticity to transdifferentiate into other cell types such as muscle, endothelial cells, and bone cells (Hombach-Klonisch et al. 2008). HSC transplantation is the earliest stem cell-based therapy that started in 1950s and has been widely used to treat cancers, as well as many blood and immune system disorders. Currently, human BM, mobilized peripheral blood, and umbilical cord blood (UCB) represent the major sources of transplantable HSCs (Copelan 2006). However, there are many drawbacks to the current sources of all these cells. The availability of these cells is dramatically limited due to the limited number of tissue-derived HSCs, the limited expansion of the HSCs *in vitro*, rare histocompatibility or match of human leukocyte antigen (HLA) types between donors and recipients, and the risk of transmission of infectious diseases. Thus, sources with robust, continuous supply of hematopoietic cells are highly desired. Human ES and iPS cells provide great promise for this purpose.

3.5.1 Differentiation of HSCs from Human ES Cells

For treatment of hematopoietic diseases, human ES cells must be first differentiated into hematopoietic cells. Differentiation methods can be categorized into two main approaches: coculture on supportive stromal cell layers and the formation of EBs. Cell lines have been used in stromal coculture systems. One benefit of differentiating human ES cells using these stromal cell lines in coculture is the ability to control the specific elements needed to provide a microenvironment or anatomical niche that supports lineage-specific development. Specific stromal cell lines can be selected to generate a desired progenitor type. Moreover, the stromal cell lines also can be genetically engineered to enhance progenitor quality and number. For example, expression of Wnt1 in S17 cells increases hematopoietic differentiation from human ES cells (Woll et al. 2008). OP9-DL1 cell line, which expresses a Notch ligand, promotes the differentiation into lymphoid lineages (Schmitt et al. 2004). However, the involvement of animal-derived stromal cells and the variation of yield limit the use of these methods. Three-dimensional EB differentiation cultures have also been used to differentiate human ES cells into hematopoietic cells (Chadwick et al. 2003). This method yields more consistent and efficient results; however, appropriate EB sizes are critical (Ng et al. 2005).

To characterize human ES cell–derived hematopoietic cells, common markers such as CD34, CD45, c-Kit, and Lin can be used for characterization of HSCs. Many studies suggest that from human ES cell–derived HSCs have a similar profile of the markers and can reconstitute certain lineages in immunodeficient mice. However, long-term reconstitution of multilineage hematopoietic cells in mouse models has not yet succeeded for human ES cell–derived HSCs, in comparison with HSCs derived from BM or umbilical blood (Kaufman 2009).

3.5.2 Lineage-Specific Differentiation of Human ES Cell–Derived HSCs

Human ES cell–derived HSCs have been successfully differentiated *in vitro* into several mature blood cell lineages, which hold great potential for applications in regenerative medicine.

3.5.2.1 Erythroid Cells

Although the current red blood cell supply is adequate and relatively safe, the need for rare blood groups and the risk of contamination by new pathogens cannot be completely eliminated. Thus, derivation of erythroid cells from human ES cells may translate into a new and safer source of red blood cells for transfusions. Recently, Advanced Cell Technology, Inc. has successfully produced large amounts of red blood cells from human ES cells, using a procedure that involves a combination of EB formation and the ectopic expression of the HoxB4 transcription factor (Lu et al. 2008). Through the amplification and maturation of hematopoietic and erythroid precursors, they were able to obtain enucleated red blood cells on a feeder layer. This is a great progress toward the application of human ES cell–derived erythroid cells in potential therapies.

3.5.2.2 T, B, and Natural Killer Cells

OP9 coculture and EB formation can also be used to derive T and B cells from human ES cell–derived HSCs, using cocktails of cytokines at multiple steps within differentiation. T cells can be differentiated by coculture with the OP9-DL1 stroma cell, while B cells can be differentiated by adding FLT-3 ligand to the culture during the early lymphopoietic progenitor stage (Cho et al. 1999). However, the engraftment of these cells in the immunocompromised SCID mice is typically 1% or less (Wang et al. 2005; Narayan et al. 2006). In contrast, T cells derived from human BM, UCB, or fetal liver have much higher levels of engraftment in SCID mice. This indicates that T and B cells derived from these various sources may carry intrinsic differences.

The *in vitro* differentiation of human ES cell–derived HSCs into NK cells is less difficult, which was first demonstrated by Dan Kaufman laboratory. Functional NK cells can be efficiently generated from human ES cells, using a two-step culture method (Woll et al. 2005). The human ES cells are first cocultured with the stromal cell line S17. The resulting human ES cell–derived HSCs are then cocultured with AFT024 cells. Interestingly, these NK cells can kill multiple cancers both *in vitro* and *in vivo* and the *in vivo* killing is more effective for NK cells derived from human ES cells than those from UCB cells (Woll et al. 2009).

3.5.2.3 Macrophages and Dendritic Cells

Macrophage and dentritic cells have very important immune functions and are good candidates for cell therapy to treat cancer and immune diseases. Multiple groups have reported the derivation of macrophage and dentritic cells from human ES cells, mainly by using the stromal cell coculture system to first generate HSCs (Slukvin et al. 2006). Subsequently, these HSCs are induced to differentiate into macrophages upon the addition of the cytokines M-CSF and GM-CSF, or dentritic cells upon the addition of the cytokines GM-CSF and IL-4 (Slukvin et al. 2006).

3.5.3 Challenges and Perspectives

Human ES cell–derived hematopoietic progenitors and immune cells have several advantages for potential clinical application. First, unlimited numbers of HSCs can be generated from self-renewing human ES cells, in contrast to the limited source from BM and UCB. Second, the transplantation of human ES cell–derived HSCs, along with other cell lineages such as islet cells, neurons, and muscle cells derived from human ES cell lines, may help HSCs to engraft and function by reducing transplantation rejection and inducing immune tolerance (Priddle et al. 2006). Finally, the derivation of HSCs derived from human ES cells may provide opportunities to genetically engineer or modulate antigens at different stages of hematopoietic development, which may be used to treat certain genetic diseases or immune disorders.

However, several challenges are predictable for cell therapy–based applications using human ES cell–derived hematopoietic cells. First, for some hematopoietic cell therapies such as the development of red blood cells for transfusion, the number of cells needed is enormous. Novel bioengineering methods need to be developed in order to produce the cells on a larger scale. Second, the risk remains for development of teratomas from human ES cell–derived hematopoietic cells if any pluripotent cells are mixed in the transfusion. Thus, the safety of these cells must be strictly assessed, if these cells are to reach their therapeutic application. Finally, host immune cells may reject allergenic human ES cell–derived hematopoietic cells, and the foreign cells may also induce graft versus host disease. The last challenge can now be overcome by using iPS cells to obtain patient-specific hematopoietic cells as described earlier for iPS cell–derived neural cells.

3.5.4 Differentiation of Hematopoietic Cells from Human iPS Cells

In 2009, the OP9 coculture system was used by the Slukvin laboratory at the University of Wisconsin to direct the differentiation of human iPS into hematopoietic progenitors (Choi et al. 2009). Although the hematopoietic differentiation potential of the human iPS cell lines is very similar to potential of human ES cell lines, there are some variations in the efficiency of hematopoietic differentiation between different human iPS cell lines. Other laboratories have also observed these differences. Advanced Cell Technologies, Inc. found that the hematopoiesis efficiency of the various iPS cells is much lower than that of ES cells (Feng et al. 2010). Some possible reasons for this decrease in efficiency are increased apoptosis, severely limited expansion capability, and early aging (Feng et al. 2010). It could also be caused by the differences between tissue sources, reprogramming extensiveness, etc.

3.6 MESENCHYMAL STEM CELLS

Mesenchymal stem cells (MSCs) are multipotent, and can differentiate into multiple cell types, including adipocytes, cartilage, bone, tendons, muscle, and skin. MSCs have been used in preclinical models for tissue engineering of bone, cartilage, muscle, marrow stroma, tendon, fat, and other connective tissues (Caplan 2005). MSCs have also been used to treat heart failure and acute heart infarction due to their ability to differentiate into cardiomyocytes and vascular endothelial cells and to secrete angiogenic and anti-apoptotic factors (Ohnishi and Nagaya 2007). It has also been shown that MSCs have immune suppressive function, which is being used to treat autoimmune disease (Uccelli et al. 2007).

3.6.1 MSCs Isolated from Adult Tissues

MSCs are traditionally isolated from BM (Friedenstein et al. 1966). Now, they can also be isolated from many other sources such as UCB, peripheral blood, fallopian tube, and fetal liver and lungs. However, the MSCs derived from the adult tissues have very low percentages in their source tissues, limited capacity to proliferate (Bianchi et al. 2003), and quickly have reduced multipotency and viability during aging (Kretlow et al. 2008). Thus, use of ES cells may overcome some of the limitations, perhaps permitting them to become a reliable source of cells for various therapeutic applications.

3.6.2 *In Vitro* Differentiation of MSC from ES Cells

MSCs can also be derived from human ES cells, which can be done in several ways. One method cocultures human ES cells with the OP9 stroma cell line (Barberi et al. 2005). Following 40 days of coculture, the cells can be harvested and sorted for CD73$^+$ cells to purify the MSCs. Other cell surface markers such as CD105, CD90, Stro-1, CD106, CD29, CD44, CD43, and CD166 are used to further characterize the purified MSCs. Since these cells are grown in culture systems similar to that for HSC differentiation, the CD34, CD45, and CD14 markers are used to rule out the presence of HSCs. A method that can be used is a stroma-free differentiation system, which just uses gelatin-coated plates to culture the ES cells in DMEM/F12 medium supplemented with insulin, transferrin, and selenium (ITS medium) (Barberi et al. 2007). These cells are further cultured in α-MEM to increase the percentage of MSCs. MSCs derived from both methods can be differentiated into bone, cartilage, fat, and muscle cells. In addition, ES cells can also spontaneously differentiate into MSCs on the feeder MEF (Olivier et al. 2006). These MSCs can be scraped off, replated into a new dish, and cultured in DMEM for another 4 weeks to yield a population of cells with uniform morphology. The advantage of this method is that it yields high percentage of CD73$^+$ cells without requiring further purification.

3.6.3 Functional Differentiation of Human ES Cell–Derived MSCs

Myogenesis, osteogenesis, adipogenesis are most commonly used assays for characterization of MSCs. For myogenesis, the skeletal muscle marker NCAM is used to purify the myogenic potential of MSCs. N2 medium is used for the terminal differentiation of these cells into myocytes. For osteogenesis, β-glycerophosphate method can be used. In brief, the cells are cultured for 21 days in osteogenic medium containing dexamethasone, ascorbic acid, and β-glycerophosphate (Colter et al. 2001). For adipogenesis, both classic 3-isobutyl-methylxanthine method (21 day culture in medium containing hydrocortisone, isobutyl-methylxanthine, and indomethacin) (Pittenger et al. 1999) and serum withdrawal/hypoxia (SWH) methods (21 day culture in hESC medium in 5% O_2) (Olivier et al. 2006) have produced consistent results.

3.6.4 Immunosuppression of Human ES Cell–Derived MSCs

It has been shown that human ES cell–derived MSCs have even stronger immunosuppressive activity than the BM-derived MSCs, according to a recent report (Yen et al. 2009). The authors found that human ES cell–derived MSCs do not express HLA-DR and costimulatory molecules, but express HLA-G, a nonclass MHC I protein involved in mediating maternal–fetal tolerance. Human ES cell–derived MSCs can suppress CD4 and CD8 T cell proliferation, and the cytotoxic effects of NK cells. Thus, it may be possible in the future to use MSCs to treat multiple autoimmune diseases such as MS, diabetes, arthritis, Alzheimer's, and AMS (El-Badri et al. 2004).

3.6.5 Challenges and Perspectives

Use of human ES cell–derived MSCs may have several advantages for potential clinical applications. First, unlimited number of MSCs can be generated from self-renewing human ES cells. Second, MSCs isolated from adult tissues have been widely used in clinical trial to treat many diseases, and one of the major mechanisms for the MSC activities is their capability of cytokine secretion rather than tissue regeneration. Thus, it is possible to mitotically inactivate MSCs differentiated from human ES cells and use them for clinical trials to avoid the possible tumorigenicity by residual undifferentiated human ES cells. Lastly, human ES cell–derived MSCs can also be genetically modified via gene targeting on human ES cells.

3.7 ESSENTIAL ROLE OF BIOENGINEERING IN STEM CELL RESEARCH

Despite the remarkable potential clinical applications of the stem cell types described earlier, how to best mimic the physiological environments for these stem cells or their derivatives remains a daunting question. Bioengineering has come to play as a vital approach to optimizing both *in vitro* and *in vivo* conditions for stem cell culture and therapy. Biomaterials approaches, in combination with other bioengineering technologies such as microfabrication and microfluidics, are well suited to assist studies of stem cell biology through the creation of evolving systems that allow key variables to be systematically altered and their influence on stem cell fate analyzed.

Specifically, bioengineering can facilitate optimization of stem cell culture condition, especially toward the development of current good manufacturing practice (cGMP) system. cGMP is a quality assurance that is used in the pharmaceutical industry to define the quality and traceability of raw materials used in validated standard operating procedures. In order for stem cell research to reach its clinical potential, everything used for stem cell research must be cGMP grade. Mechanical methods, instead of the traditional enzymatic methods, have allowed the derivation of human ES cell lines under animal-free condition. Xeno-free defined media such as the TeSR medium series and xeno-free extracellular matrices such as CellStart (which replaces the mouse tumor–derived Matrigel) have assured the complete animal-free conditions for culture of human ES/iPS cells. Nevertheless, many animal-derived and unidentified materials such as fetal bovine serum and differentiation-inducing stromal cells are still used for *in vitro* differentiation of human ES/iPS cells, thus unqualified for the cGMP grade. More research is needed to develop and validate additional xeno-free materials to be used in protocols to direct the differentiation of human ES/iPS cells into specific cell types for potential therapeutic applications for patients.

3.8 CONCLUSION

In this chapter, we have discussed the regeneration of neural, hematopoietic, and mesenchymal tissues as examples to elucidate how various types of stem cells including multipotent (fetal or adult) stem cells (e.g., NSCs, HSCs, and MSCs) and pluripotent stem cells (e.g., ES and iPS cells) can differentiate into functional cells of these lineages.

3.8.1 Multipotent Stem Cells

There are many advantages to use fetal or adult multipotent stem cells in regenerative medicine. Immunocompatible autologous cells can be derived from adult stem cells. Moreover, adult stem cell can be easily differentiated into specific lineages. However, despite the ability of adult stem cells to self-renew and differentiate *in vivo* throughout an entire human lifetime, scientists have not been able to expand or differentiate adult stems *ex vivo* as effectively. Great effort is being made to understand and recapitulate the niches that mediate the self-renewal and differentiation of adult stem cells. Greater understanding at the molecular level of stem cell biology is needed in order to allow engineers to design better scaffolds that can retain the regenerative capacity of the stem cells and direct their fate. In addition, more cell surface markers need to be elucidated in order to isolate these rare stem cells. Another hurdle that must be overcome is the loss of their regenerative capacity during their *ex vivo* expansion. Better culture conditions need to be developed that more closely mimic the cell–cell interactions and cell–matrix interactions found within the stem cell niches.

3.8.2 Pluripotent Stem Cells

The pluripotency of ES and iPS cells is a double-edge sword, which allows the cell differentiation into any lineage of therapeutic value provided the appropriate experimental protocol can be developed. On the other hand, it also potentially causes teratomas in the host if residual undifferentiated cells are mixed in the transplanted therapeutic cells. ES cells hold the golden standard for pluripotency as indicated by their differentiation ability. However, the ability of iPS cells to differentiate into neural and hematopoietic cells varies among different cell lines, and is generally lower than that of ES cells (Choi et al. 2009; Feng et al. 2010; Hu et al. 2010; Kim et al. 2010; Kulkeaw et al. 2010). This may result from varying levels of reprogramming of the epigenome of their parental somatic cells.

In addition, an ES cell line carries a genotype identical to that of the original embryo, so their progeny will express a HLA type irrelevant to most potential recipient patients. Whereas, an iPS cell line carries a patient-specific genome, so their progeny will express a HLA type identical to that of the donor patient. Thus, unlike ES cells, iPS cells avoid the concern of immunorejection by the recipient of their progeny.

The extremely low efficiency of iPS cell derivation via protein transduction remains a hurdle, although this best preserves the genomic integrity of the cells and avoids oncogenesis that would otherwise happen in iPS cells reprogrammed via DNA delivery. Finally, some common questions for both ES and iPS cells include how to determine and obtain ideal population(s) of therapeutic cell types for specific disease, and how to improve and achieve the survival, integration, and long-term functions of transplanted cells in the host environment. Solving these questions will certainly expedite the realization of the great promise of stem cell–based therapy.

REFERENCES

Altman, J. 1969. Autoradiographic and histological studies of postnatal neurogenesis. IV. Cell proliferation and migration in the anterior forebrain, with special reference to persisting neurogenesis in the olfactory bulb. *J Comp Neurol* 137(4): 433–457.

Altman, J. and Das, G.D. 1965. Autoradiographic and histological evidence of postnatal hippocampal neurogenesis in rats. *J Comp Neurol* 124(3): 319–335.

Aubry, L., Bugi, A., Lefort, N., Rousseau, F., Peschanski, M., and Perrier, A.L. 2008. Striatal progenitors derived from human ES cells mature into DARPP32 neurons *in vitro* and in quinolinic acid-lesioned rats. *Proc Natl Acad Sci U S A* 105(43): 16707–16712.

Barberi, T., Bradbury, M., Dincer, Z., Panagiotakos, G., Socci, N.D., and Studer, L. 2007. Derivation of engraftable skeletal myoblasts from human embryonic stem cells. *Nat Med* 13(5): 642–648.

Barberi, T., Willis, L.M., Socci, N.D., and Studer, L. 2005. Derivation of multipotent mesenchymal precursors from human embryonic stem cells. *PLoS Med* 2(6): e161.

Bianchi, G., Banfi, A., Mastrogiacomo, M., Notaro, R., Luzzatto, L., Cancedda, R., and Quarto, R. 2003. *Ex vivo* enrichment of mesenchymal cell progenitors by fibroblast growth factor 2. *Exp Cell Res* 287(1): 98–105.

Bonaguidi, M.A., Peng, C.Y., McGuire, T., Falciglia, G., Gobeske, K.T., Czeisler, C., and Kessler, J.A. 2008. Noggin expands neural stem cells in the adult hippocampus. *J Neurosci* 28(37): 9194–9204.

Briscoe, J. and Ericson, J. 2001. Specification of neuronal fates in the ventral neural tube. *Curr Opin Neurobiol* 11(1): 43–49.

Bru, T., Clarke, C., McGrew, M.J., Sang, H.M., Wilmut, I., and Blow, J.J. 2008. Rapid induction of pluripotency genes after exposure of human somatic cells to mouse ES cell extracts. *Exp Cell Res* 314(14): 2634–2642.

Caplan, A.I. 2005. Review: Mesenchymal stem cells: Cell-based reconstructive therapy in orthopedics. *Tissue Eng* 11(7–8): 1198–1211.

Chadwick, K., Wang, L., Li, L., Menendez, P., Murdoch, B., Rouleau, A., and Bhatia, M. 2003. Cytokines and BMP-4 promote hematopoietic differentiation of human embryonic stem cells. *Blood* 102(3): 906–915.

Chambers, S.M., Fasano, C.A., Papapetrou, E.P., Tomishima, M., Sadelain, M., and Studer, L. 2009. Highly efficient neural conversion of human ES and iPS cells by dual inhibition of SMAD signaling. *Nat Biotechnol* 27(3): 275–280.

Chatzi, C., Scott, R.H., Pu, J., Lang, B., Nakamoto, C., McCaig, C.D., and Shen, S. 2009. Derivation of homogeneous GABAergic neurons from mouse embryonic stem cells. *Exp Neurol* 217(2): 407–416.

Cho, S.K., Webber, T.D., Carlyle, J.R., Nakano, T., Lewis, S.M., and Zuniga-Pflucker, J.C. 1999. Functional characterization of B lymphocytes generated *in vitro* from embryonic stem cells. *Proc Natl Acad Sci U S A* 96(17): 9797–9802.

Choi, K.D., Yu, J., Smuga-Otto, K., Salvagiotto, G., Rehrauer, W., Vodyanik, M., Thomson, J., and Slukvin, I. 2009. Hematopoietic and endothelial differentiation of human induced pluripotent stem cells. *Stem Cells* 27(3): 559–567.

Colter, D.C., Sekiya, I., and Prockop, D.J. 2001. Identification of a subpopulation of rapidly self-renewing and multipotential adult stem cells in colonies of human marrow stromal cells. *Proc Natl Acad Sci U S A* 98(14): 7841–7845.

Copelan, E.A. 2006. Hematopoietic stem-cell transplantation. *N Engl J Med* 354(17): 1813–1826.

Coutts, M. and Keirstead, H.S. 2008. Stem cells for the treatment of spinal cord injury. *Exp Neurol* 209(2): 368–377.

Curtis, M.A., Kam, M., Nannmark, U., Anderson, M.F., Axell, M.Z., Wikkelso, C., Holtas, S. et al. 2007. Human neuroblasts migrate to the olfactory bulb via a lateral ventricular extension. *Science* 315(5816): 1243–1249.

Dale, L. and Jones, C.M. 1999. BMP signalling in early *Xenopus* development. *Bioessays* 21(9): 751–760.

Deshpande, D.M., Kim, Y.S., Martinez, T., Carmen, J., Dike, S., Shats, I., Rubin, L.L. et al. 2006. Recovery from paralysis in adult rats using embryonic stem cells. *Ann Neurol* 60(1): 32–44.

Einstein, O. and Ben-Hur, T. 2008. The changing face of neural stem cell therapy in neurologic diseases. *Arch Neurol* 65(4): 452–456.

El-Badri, N.S., Maheshwari, A., and Sanberg, P.R. 2004. Mesenchymal stem cells in autoimmune disease. *Stem Cells Dev* 13(5): 463–472.

Emborg, M.E., Ebert, A.D., Moirano, J., Peng, S., Suzuki, M., Capowski, E., Joers, V., Roitberg, B.Z., Aebischer, P., and Svendsen, C.N. 2008. GDNF-secreting human neural progenitor cells increase tyrosine hydroxylase and VMAT2 expression in MPTP-treated cynomolgus monkeys. *Cell Transplant* 17(4): 383–395.

Emsley, J.G., Mitchell, B.D., Kempermann, G., and Macklis, J.D. 2005. Adult neurogenesis and repair of the adult CNS with neural progenitors, precursors, and stem cells. *Prog Neurobiol* 75(5): 321–341.

Esteban, M.A., Xu, J., Yang, J., Peng, M., Qin, D., Li, W., Jiang, Z. et al. 2009. Generation of induced pluripotent stem cell lines from Tibetan miniature pig. *J Biol Chem* 284(26): 17634–17640.

Evans, M.J. and Kaufman, M.H. 1981. Establishment in culture of pluripotential cells from mouse embryos. *Nature* 292(5819): 154–156.

Ezashi, T., Telugu, B.P., Alexenko, A.P., Sachdev, S., Sinha, S., and Roberts, R.M. 2009. Derivation of induced pluripotent stem cells from pig somatic cells. *Proc Natl Acad Sci U S A* 106(27): 10993–10998.

Feng, B., Ng, J.H., Heng, J.C., and Ng, H.H. 2009. Molecules that promote or enhance reprogramming of somatic cells to induced pluripotent stem cells. *Cell Stem Cell* 4(4): 301–312.

Feng, Q., Lu, S.J., Klimanskaya, I., Gomes, I., Kim, D., Chung, Y., Honig, G.R., Kim, K.S., and Lanza, R. 2010. Hemangioblastic derivatives from human induced pluripotent stem cells exhibit limited expansion and early senescence. *Stem Cells* 28(4): 704–712.

Friedenstein, A.J., Piatetzky, S. II, and Petrakova, K.V. 1966. Osteogenesis in transplants of bone marrow cells. *J Embryol Exp Morphol* 16(3): 381–390.

Gage, F.H. 2000. Mammalian neural stem cells. *Science* 287(5457): 1433–1438.

Gage, F.H., Coates, P.W., Palmer, T.D., Kuhn, H.G., Fisher, L.J., Suhonen, J.O., Peterson, D.A., Suhr, S.T., and Ray, J. 1995. Survival and differentiation of adult neuronal progenitor cells transplanted to the adult brain. *Proc Natl Acad Sci U S A* 92(25): 11879–11883.

Gardner, D.K., Vella, P., Lane, M., Wagley, L., Schlenker, T., and Schoolcraft, W.B. 1998. Culture and transfer of human blastocysts increases implantation rates and reduces the need for multiple embryo transfers. *Fertil Steril* 69(1): 84–88.

Goldman, S. 2005. Stem and progenitor cell-based therapy of the human central nervous system. *Nat Biotechnol* 23(7): 862–871.

Gross, C.G. 2000. Neurogenesis in the adult brain: Death of a dogma. *Nat Rev Neurosci* 1(1): 67–73.

Gutierrez, M., Merino, J.J., de Lecinana, M.A., and Diez-Tejedor, E. 2009. Cerebral protection, brain repair, plasticity and cell therapy in ischemic stroke. *Cerebrovasc Dis* 27(Suppl 1): 177–186.

Hanna, J., Wernig, M., Markoulaki, S., Sun, C.W., Meissner, A., Cassady, J.P., Beard, C., Brambrink, T., Wu, L.C., Townes, T.M., and Jaenisch, R. 2007. Treatment of sickle cell anemia mouse model with iPS cells generated from autologous skin. *Science* 318(5858): 1920–1923.

Harper, J.M., Krishnan, C., Darman, J.S., Deshpande, D.M., Peck, S., Shats, I., Backovic, S., Rothstein, J.D., and Kerr, D.A. 2004. Axonal growth of embryonic stem cell-derived motoneurons *in vitro* and in motoneuron-injured adult rats. *Proc Natl Acad Sci U S A* 101(18): 7123–7128.

Hombach-Klonisch, S., Panigrahi, S., Rashedi, I., Seifert, A., Alberti, E., Pocar, P., Kurpisz, M., Schulze-Osthoff, K., Mackiewicz, A., and Los, M. 2008. Adult stem cells and their trans-differentiation potential—Perspectives and therapeutic applications. *J Mol Med* 86(12): 1301–1314.

Hu, B.Y., Du, Z.W., Li, X.J., Ayala, M., and Zhang, S.C. 2009. Human oligodendrocytes from embryonic stem cells: Conserved SHH signaling networks and divergent FGF effects. *Development* 136(9): 1443–1452.

Hu, B.Y., Weick, J.P., Yu, J., Ma, L.X., Zhang, X.Q., Thomson, J.A., and Zhang, S.C. 2010. Neural differentiation of human induced pluripotent stem cells follows developmental principles but with variable potency. *Proc Natl Acad Sci U S A* 107(9): 4335–4340.

Humphrey, R.K., Beattie, G.M., Lopez, A.D., Bucay, N., King, C.C., Firpo, M.T., Rose-John, S., and Hayek, A. 2004. Maintenance of pluripotency in human embryonic stem cells is STAT3 independent. *Stem Cells* 22(4): 522–530.

Hwang, D.H., Lee, H.J., Park, I.H., Seok, J.I., Kim, B.G., Joo, I.S., and Kim, S.U. 2009. Intrathecal transplantation of human neural stem cells overexpressing VEGF provide behavioral improvement, disease onset delay and survival extension in transgenic ALS mice. *Gene Ther* 16(10): 1234–1244.

Kaji, K., Norrby, K., Paca, A., Mileikovsky, M., Mohseni, P., and Woltjen, K. 2009. Virus-free induction of pluripotency and subsequent excision of reprogramming factors. *Nature* 458(7239): 771–775.

Kaufman, D.S. 2009. Toward clinical therapies using hematopoietic cells derived from human pluripotent stem cells. *Blood* 114(17): 3513–3523.

Keirstead, H.S., Nistor, G., Bernal, G., Totoiu, M., Cloutier, F., Sharp, K., and Steward, O. 2005. Human embryonic stem cell-derived oligodendrocyte progenitor cell transplants remyelinate and restore locomotion after spinal cord injury. *J Neurosci* 25(19): 4694–4705.

Kim, D.S., Lee, J.S., Leem, J.W., Huh, Y.J., Kim, J.Y., Kim, H.S., Park, I.H., Daley, G.Q., Hwang, D.Y., and Kim, D.W. 2010. Robust enhancement of neural differentiation from human ES and iPS cells regardless of their innate difference in differentiation propensity. *Stem Cell Rev* 6(2): 270–281.

Kim, S.U., Nagai, A., Nakagawa, E., Choi, H.B., Bang, J.H., Lee, H.J., Lee, M.A., Lee, Y.B., and Park, I.H. 2008. Production and characterization of immortal human neural stem cell line with multipotent differentiation property. *Methods Mol Biol* 438: 103–121.

Kim, S.U. and de Vellis, J. 2009. Stem cell-based cell therapy in neurological diseases: A review. *J Neurosci Res* 87(10): 2183–2200.

Kokaia, Z. and Lindvall, O. 2003. Neurogenesis after ischaemic brain insults. *Curr Opin Neurobiol* 13(1): 127–132.

Kordower, J.H., Goetz, C.G., Freeman, T.B., and Olanow, C.W. 1997. Dopaminergic transplants in patients with Parkinson's disease: Neuroanatomical correlates of clinical recovery. *Exp Neurol* 144(1): 41–46.

Kretlow, J.D., Jin, Y.Q., Liu, W., Zhang, W.J., Hong, T.H., Zhou, G., Baggett, L.S., Mikos, A.G., and Cao, Y. 2008. Donor age and cell passage affects differentiation potential of murine bone marrow-derived stem cells. *BMC Cell Biol* 9: 60.

Kulkeaw, K., Horio, Y., Mizuochi, C., Ogawa, M., and Sugiyama, D. 2010. Variation in hematopoietic potential of induced pluripotent stem cell lines. *Stem Cell Rev* 2010: 17.

Lee, S.T., Chu, K., Park, J.E., Lee, K., Kang, L., Kim, S.U., and Kim, M. 2005. Intravenous administration of human neural stem cells induces functional recovery in Huntington's disease rat model. *Neurosci Res* 52(3): 243–249.

Lee, H., Shamy, G.A., Elkabetz, Y., Schofield, C.M., Harrsion, N.L., Panagiotakos, G., Socci, N.D., Tabar, V., and Studer, L. 2007. Directed differentiation and transplantation of human embryonic stem cell-derived motoneurons. *Stem Cells* 25(8): 1931–1939.

Lepore, A.C., Rauck, B., Dejea, C., Pardo, A.C., Rao, M.S., Rothstein, J.D., and Maragakis, N.J. 2008. Focal transplantation-based astrocyte replacement is neuroprotective in a model of motor neuron disease. *Nat Neurosci* 11(11): 1294–1301.

Li, X.J., Du, Z.W., Zarnowska, E.D., Pankratz, M., Hansen, L.O., Pearce, R.A., and Zhang, S.C. 2005. Specification of motoneurons from human embryonic stem cells. *Nat Biotechnol* 23(2): 215–221.

Li, W., Wei, W., Zhu, S., Zhu, J., Shi, Y., Lin, T., Hao, E., Hayek, A., Deng, H., and Ding, S. 2009a. Generation of rat and human induced pluripotent stem cells by combining genetic reprogramming and chemical inhibitors. *Cell Stem Cell* 4(1): 16–19.

Li, X.J. and Zhang, S.C. 2006. *In vitro* differentiation of neural precursors from human embryonic stem cells. *Methods Mol Biol* 331: 169–177.

Li, X.J., Zhang, X., Johnson, M.A., Wang, Z.B., Lavaute, T., and Zhang, S.C. 2009b. Coordination of sonic hedgehog and Wnt signaling determines ventral and dorsal telencephalic neuron types from human embryonic stem cells. *Development* 136(23): 4055–4063.

Liao, J., Cui, C., Chen, S., Ren, J., Chen, J., Gao, Y., Li, H., Jia, N., Cheng, L., Xiao, H., and Xiao, L. 2009. Generation of induced pluripotent stem cell lines from adult rat cells. *Cell Stem Cell* 4(1): 11–15.

Lindvall, O. and Kokaia, Z. 2006. Stem cells for the treatment of neurological disorders. *Nature* 441(7097): 1094–1096.

Liu, H., Zhu, F., Yong, J., Zhang, P., Hou, P., Li, H., Jiang, W. et al. 2008. Generation of induced pluripotent stem cells from adult rhesus monkey fibroblasts. *Cell Stem Cell* 3(6): 587–590.

Lois, C., Garcia-Verdugo, J.M., and Alvarez-Buylla, A. 1996. Chain migration of neuronal precursors. *Science* 271(5251): 978–981.

Love, S., Plaha, P., Patel, N.K., Hotton, G.R., Brooks, D.J., and Gill, S.S. 2005. Glial cell line-derived neurotrophic factor induces neuronal sprouting in human brain. *Nat Med* 11(7): 703–704.

Lu, S.J., Feng, Q., Park, J.S., Vida, L., Lee, B.S., Strausbauch, M., Wettstein, P.J., Honig, G.R., and Lanza, R. 2008. Biologic properties and enucleation of red blood cells from human embryonic stem cells. *Blood* 112(12): 4475–4484.

Ludwig, T.E., Levenstein, M.E., Jones, J.M., Berggren, W.T., Mitchen, E.R., Frane, J.L., Crandall, L.J. et al. 2006. Derivation of human embryonic stem cells in defined conditions. *Nat Biotechnol* 24(2): 185–187.

Maherali, N., Sridharan, R., Xie, W., Utikal, J., Eminli, S., Arnold, K., Stadtfeld, M. et al. 2007. Directly reprogrammed fibroblasts show global epigenetic remodeling and widespread tissue contribution. *Cell Stem Cell* 1(1): 55–70.

Martin, G.R. 1981. Isolation of a pluripotent cell line from early mouse embryos cultured in medium conditioned by teratocarcinoma stem cells. *Proc Natl Acad Sci U S A* 78(12): 7634–7638.

Martins-Taylor, K. and Xu, R.H. 2009. Determinants of pluripotency: From avian, rodents, to primates. *J Cell Biochem* 109(1): 16–25.

Ming, G.L. and Song, H. 2005. Adult neurogenesis in the mammalian central nervous system. *Annu Rev Neurosci* 28: 223–250.

Morshead, C.M., Reynolds, B.A., Craig, C.G., McBurney, M.W., Staines, W.A., Morassutti, D., Weiss, S., and van der Kooy, D. 1994. Neural stem cells in the adult mammalian forebrain: A relatively quiescent subpopulation of subependymal cells. *Neuron* 13(5): 1071–1082.

Nakatomi, H., Kuriu, T., Okabe, S., Yamamoto, S., Hatano, O., Kawahara, N., Tamura, A., Kirino, T., and Nakafuku, M. 2002. Regeneration of hippocampal pyramidal neurons after ischemic brain injury by recruitment of endogenous neural progenitors. *Cell* 110(4): 429–441.

Narayan, A.D., Chase, J.L., Lewis, R.L., Tian, X., Kaufman, D.S., Thomson, J.A., and Zanjani, E.D. 2006. Human embryonic stem cell-derived hematopoietic cells are capable of engrafting primary as well as secondary fetal sheep recipients. *Blood* 107(5): 2180–2183.

Nayak, M.S., Kim, Y.S., Goldman, M., Keirstead, H.S., and Kerr, D.A. 2006. Cellular therapies in motor neuron diseases. *Biochim Biophys Acta* 1762(11–12): 1128–1138.

Ng, E.S., Davis, R.P., Azzola, L., Stanley, E.G., and Elefanty, A.G. 2005. Forced aggregation of defined numbers of human embryonic stem cells into embryoid bodies fosters robust, reproducible hematopoietic differentiation. *Blood* 106(5): 1601–1603.

Nistor, G.I., Totoiu, M.O., Haque, N., Carpenter, M.K., and Keirstead, H.S. 2005. Human embryonic stem cells differentiate into oligodendrocytes in high purity and myelinate after spinal cord transplantation. *Glia* 49(3): 385–396.

Ohnishi, S. and Nagaya, N. 2007. Prepare cells to repair the heart: Mesenchymal stem cells for the treatment of heart failure. *Am J Nephrol* 27(3): 301–307.

Okita, K., Ichisaka, T., and Yamanaka, S. 2007. Generation of germline-competent induced pluripotent stem cells. *Nature* 448(7151): 313–317.

Okita, K., Nakagawa, M., Hyenjong, H., Ichisaka, T., and Yamanaka, S. 2008. Generation of mouse induced pluripotent stem cells without viral vectors. *Science* 322(5903): 949–953.

Okita, K. and Yamanaka, S. 2006. Intracellular signaling pathways regulating pluripotency of embryonic stem cells. *Curr Stem Cell Res Ther* 1(1): 103–111.

Olivier, E.N., Rybicki, A.C., and Bouhassira, E.E. 2006. Differentiation of human embryonic stem cells into bipotent mesenchymal stem cells. *Stem Cells* 24(8): 1914–1922.

Osakada, F., Ikeda, H., Mandai, M., Wataya, T., Watanabe, K., Yoshimura, N., Akaike, A., Sasai, Y., and Takahashi, M. 2008. Toward the generation of rod and cone photoreceptors from mouse, monkey and human embryonic stem cells. *Nat Biotechnol* 26(2): 215–224.

Overstreet-Wadiche, L.S., Bromberg, D.A., Bensen, A.L., and Westbrook, G.L. 2006. Seizures accelerate functional integration of adult-generated granule cells. *J Neurosci* 26(15): 4095–4103.

Palmer, T.D., Ray, J., and Gage, F.H. 1995. FGF-2-responsive neuronal progenitors reside in proliferative and quiescent regions of the adult rodent brain. *Mol Cell Neurosci* 6(5): 474–486.

Palmer, T.D., Schwartz, P.H., Taupin, P., Kaspar, B., Stein, S.A., and Gage, F.H. 2001. Cell culture. Progenitor cells from human brain after death. *Nature* 411(6833): 42–43.

Palmer, T.D., Takahashi, J., and Gage, F.H. 1997. The adult rat hippocampus contains primordial neural stem cells. *Mol Cell Neurosci* 8(6): 389–404.

Parent, J.M., Elliott, R.C., Pleasure, S.J., Barbaro, N.M., and Lowenstein, D.H. 2006. Aberrant seizure-induced neurogenesis in experimental temporal lobe epilepsy. *Ann Neurol* 59(1): 81–91.

Parent, J.M., Vexler, Z.S., Gong, C., Derugin, N., and Ferriero, D.M. 2002. Rat forebrain neurogenesis and striatal neuron replacement after focal stroke. *Ann Neurol* 52(6): 802–813.

Parent, J.M., Yu, T.W., Leibowitz, R.T., Geschwind, D.H., Sloviter, R.S., and Lowenstein, D.H. 1997. Dentate granule cell neurogenesis is increased by seizures and contributes to aberrant network reorganization in the adult rat hippocampus. *J Neurosci* 17(10): 3727–3738.

Paxinos, G and Franklin, K. (eds.) The mouse brain in stereotaxic coordinates. *Spiral Bound*, 2001.

Pera, M.F., Andrade, J., Houssami, S., Reubinoff, B., Trounson, A., Stanley, E.G., Ward-van Oostwaard, D., and Mummery, C. 2004. Regulation of human embryonic stem cell differentiation by BMP-2 and its antagonist noggin. *J Cell Sci* 117(Pt 7): 1269–1280.

Perrier, A.L., Tabar, V., Barberi, T., Rubio, M.E., Bruses, J., Topf, N., Harrison, N.L., and Studer, L. 2004. Derivation of midbrain dopamine neurons from human embryonic stem cells. *Proc Natl Acad Sci U S A* 101(34): 12543–12548.

Pittenger, M.F., Mackay, A.M., Beck, S.C., Jaiswal, R.K., Douglas, R., Mosca, J.D., Moorman, M.A., Simonetti, D.W., Craig, S., and Marshak, D.R. 1999. Multilineage potential of adult human mesenchymal stem cells. *Science* 284(5411): 143–147.

Pomp, O., Brokhman, I., Ziegler, L., Almog, M., Korngreen, A., Tavian, M., and Goldstein, R.S. 2008. PA6-induced human embryonic stem cell-derived neurospheres: A new source of human peripheral sensory neurons and neural crest cells. *Brain Res* 1230: 50–60.

Priddle, H., Jones, D.R., Burridge, P.W., and Patient, R. 2006. Hematopoiesis from human embryonic stem cells: Overcoming the immune barrier in stem cell therapies. *Stem Cells* 24(4): 815–824.

Reynolds, B.A. and Weiss, S. 1992. Generation of neurons and astrocytes from isolated cells of the adult mammalian central nervous system. *Science* 255(5052): 1707–1710.

Roy, N.S., Cleren, C., Singh, S.K., Yang, L., Beal, M.F., and Goldman, S.A. 2006. Functional engraftment of human ES cell–derived dopaminergic neurons enriched by coculture with telomerase-immortalized midbrain astrocytes. *Nat Med* 12(11): 1259–1268.

Sasai, Y., Lu, B., Steinbeisser, H., and De Robertis, E.M. 1995. Regulation of neural induction by the Chd and Bmp-4 antagonistic patterning signals in *Xenopus*. *Nature* 377(6551): 757.

Schmitt, T.M., de Pooter, R.F., Gronski, M.A., Cho, S.K., Ohashi, P.S., and Zuniga-Pflucker, J.C. 2004. Induction of T cell development and establishment of T cell competence from embryonic stem cells differentiated *in vitro*. *Nat Immunol* 5(4): 410–417.

Shimada, H., Nakada, A., Hashimoto, Y., Shigeno, K., Shionoya, Y., and Nakamura, T. 2010. Generation of canine induced pluripotent stem cells by retroviral transduction and chemical inhibitors. *Mol Reprod Dev* 77(1): 2.

Singh Roy, N., Nakano, T., Xuing, L., Kang, J., Nedergaard, M., and Goldman, S.A. 2005. Enhancer-specified GFP-based FACS purification of human spinal motor neurons from embryonic stem cells. *Exp Neurol* 196(2): 224–234.

Slukvin, II, Vodyanik, M.A., Thomson, J.A., Gumenyuk, M.E., and Choi, K.D. 2006. Directed differentiation of human embryonic stem cells into functional dendritic cells through the myeloid pathway. *J Immunol* 176(5): 2924–2932.

Stadtfeld, M., Nagaya, M., Utikal, J., Weir, G., and Hochedlinger, K. 2008. Induced pluripotent stem cells generated without viral integration. *Science* 322(5903): 945–949.

Suh, H., Consiglio, A., Ray, J., Sawai, T., D'Amour, K.A., and Gage, F.H. 2007. *In vivo* fate analysis reveals the multipotent and self-renewal capacities of Sox2+ neural stem cells in the adult hippocampus. *Cell Stem Cell* 1(5): 515–528.

Suhonen, J.O., Peterson, D.A., Ray, J., and Gage, F.H. 1996. Differentiation of adult hippocampus-derived progenitors into olfactory neurons *in vivo*. *Nature* 383(6601): 624–627.

Sumi, T., Fujimoto, Y., Nakatsuji, N., and Suemori, H. 2004. STAT3 is dispensable for maintenance of self-renewal in nonhuman primate embryonic stem cells. *Stem Cells* 22(5): 861–872.

Sun, N., Panetta, N.J., Gupta, D.M., Wilson, K.D., Lee, A., Jia, F., Hu, S., Cherry, A.M., Robbins, R.C., Longaker, M.T., and Wu, J.C. 2009. Feeder-free derivation of induced pluripotent stem cells from adult human adipose stem cells. *Proc Natl Acad Sci U S A* 106(37): 15720–15725.

Tabar, V., Panagiotakos, G., Greenberg, E.D., Chan, B.K., Sadelain, M., Gutin, P.H., and Studer, L. 2005. Migration and differentiation of neural precursors derived from human embryonic stem cells in the rat brain. *Nat Biotechnol* 23(5): 601–606.

Takahashi, K., Tanabe, K., Ohnuki, M., Narita, M., Ichisaka, T., Tomoda, K., and Yamanaka, S. 2007. Induction of pluripotent stem cells from adult human fibroblasts by defined factors. *Cell* 131(5): 861–872.

Takahashi, K. and Yamanaka, S. 2006. Induction of pluripotent stem cells from mouse embryonic and adult fibroblast cultures by defined factors. *Cell* 126(4): 663–676.

Temple, S. 2001. The development of neural stem cells. *Nature* 414(6859): 112–117.

Thomson, J.A., J. Kalishman, et al. 1995. Isolation of a primate embryonic stem cell line. *Proc Natl Acad Sci USA* 92(17): 7844–7848.

Thomson, J.A., J. Kalishman. et al. 1996. Pluripotent cell lines derived from common marmoset (callithrix jacchus) blastocysts. *Biol Reprod* 55(2): 254–259.

Thomson, J.A., Itskovitz-Eldor, J., Shapiro, S.S., Waknitz, M.A., Swiergiel, J.J., Marshall, V.S., and Jones, J.M. 1998. Embryonic stem cell lines derived from human blastocysts. *Science* 282(5391): 1145–1147.

Uccelli, A., Pistoia, V., and Moretta, L. 2007. Mesenchymal stem cells: A new strategy for immunosuppression? *Trends Immunol* 28(5): 219–226.

Wang, L., Menendez, P., Shojaei, F., Li, L., Mazurier, F., Dick, J.E., Cerdan, C., Levac, K., and Bhatia, M. 2005. Generation of hematopoietic repopulating cells from human embryonic stem cells independent of ectopic HOXB4 expression. *J Exp Med* 201(10): 1603–1614.

Watabe, T. and Miyazono, K. 2009. Roles of TGF-beta family signaling in stem cell renewal and differentiation. *Cell Res* 19(1): 103–115.

Weiss, S., Dunne, C., Hewson, J., Wohl, C., Wheatley, M., Peterson, A.C., and Reynolds, B.A. 1996. Multipotent CNS stem cells are present in the adult mammalian spinal cord and ventricular neuroaxis. *J Neurosci* 16(23): 7599–7609.

Wernig, M., Meissner, A., Foreman, R., Brambrink, T., Ku, M., Hochedlinger, K., Bernstein, B.E., and Jaenisch, R. 2007. *In vitro* reprogramming of fibroblasts into a pluripotent ES-cell-like state. *Nature* 448(7151): 318–324.

Wernig, M., Zhao, J.P., Pruszak, J., Hedlund, E., Fu, D., Soldner, F., Broccoli, V., Constantine-Paton, M., Isacson, O., and Jaenisch, R. 2008. Neurons derived from reprogrammed fibroblasts functionally integrate into the fetal brain and improve symptoms of rats with Parkinson's disease. *Proc Natl Acad Sci U S A* 105(15): 5856–5861.

Wichterle, H., Lieberam, I., Porter, J.A., and Jessell, T.M. 2002. Directed differentiation of embryonic stem cells into motor neurons. *Cell* 110(3): 385–397.

Wilson, S.I. and Edlund, T. 2001. Neural induction: Toward a unifying mechanism. *Nat Neurosci* 4(Suppl): 1161–1168.

Windrem, M.S., Schanz, S.J., Guo, M., Tian, G.F., Washco, V., Stanwood, N., Rasband, M. et al. 2008. Neonatal chimerization with human glial progenitor cells can both remyelinate and rescue the otherwise lethally hypomyelinated shiverer mouse. *Cell Stem Cell* 2(6): 553–565.

Woll, P.S., Grzywacz, B., Tian, X., Marcus, R.K., Knorr, D.A., Verneris, M.R., and Kaufman, D.S. 2009. Human embryonic stem cells differentiate into a homogeneous population of natural killer cells with potent *in vivo* antitumor activity. *Blood* 113(24): 6094–6101.

Woll, P.S., Martin, C.H., Miller, J.S., and Kaufman, D.S. 2005. Human embryonic stem cell-derived NK cells acquire functional receptors and cytolytic activity. *J Immunol* 175(8): 5095–5103.

Woll, P.S., Morris, J.K., Painschab, M.S., Marcus, R.K., Kohn, A.D., Biechele, T.L., Moon, R.T., and Kaufman, D.S. 2008. Wnt signaling promotes hematoendothelial cell development from human embryonic stem cells. *Blood* 111(1): 122–131.

Woltjen, K., Michael, I.P., Mohseni, P., Desai, R., Mileikovsky, M., Hamalainen, R., Cowling, R. et al. 2009. piggyBac transposition reprograms fibroblasts to induced pluripotent stem cells. *Nature* 458(7239): 766–770.

Wu, Z., Chen, J., Ren, J., Bao, L., Liao, J., Cui, C., Rao, L. et al. 2009. Generation of pig-induced pluripotent stem cells with a drug-inducible system. *J Mol Cell Biol* 3: 3.

Wu, Y., Zhang, Y., Mishra, A., Tardif, S.D., and Hornsby, P.J. 2010. Generation of induced pluripotent stem cells from newborn marmoset skin fibroblasts. *Stem Cell Res* 2010: 6.

Xu, R.H., Chen, X., Li, D.S., Li, R., Addicks, G.C., Glennon, C., Zwaka, T.P., and Thomson, J.A. 2002. BMP4 initiates human embryonic stem cell differentiation to trophoblast. *Nat Biotechnol* 20(12): 1261–1264.

Xu, R.H., Kim, J., Taira, M., Zhan, S., Sredni, D., and Kung, H.F. 1995. A dominant negative bone morphogenetic protein 4 receptor causes neuralization in *Xenopus* ectoderm. *Biochem Biophys Res Commun* 212(1): 212–219.

Xu, R.H., Peck, R.M., Li, D.S., Feng, X., Ludwig, T., and Thomson, J.A. 2005. Basic FGF and suppression of BMP signaling sustain undifferentiated proliferation of human ES cells. *Nat Methods* 2(3): 185–190.

Xu, R.H., Sampsell-Barron, T.L., Gu, F., Root, S., Peck, R.M., Pan, G., Yu, J., Antosiewicz-Bourget, J., Tian, S., Stewart, R., and Thomson, J.A. 2008. NANOG is a direct target of TGFbeta/activin-mediated SMAD signaling in human ESCs. *Cell Stem Cell* 3(2): 196–206.

Xu, L., Yan, J., Chen, D., Welsh, A.M., Hazel, T., Johe, K., Hatfield, G., and Koliatsos, V.E. 2006. Human neural stem cell grafts ameliorate motor neuron disease in SOD-1 transgenic rats. *Transplantation* 82(7): 865–875.

Yakubov, E., Rechavi, G., Rozenblatt, S., and Givol, D. 2010. Reprogramming of human fibroblasts to pluripotent stem cells using mRNA of four transcription factors. *Biochem Biophys Res Commun* 394(1): 189–193.

Yan, Y., Yang, D., Zarnowska, E.D., Du, Z., Werbel, B., Valliere, C., Pearce, R.A., Thomson, J.A., and Zhang, S.C. 2005. Directed differentiation of dopaminergic neuronal subtypes from human embryonic stem cells. *Stem Cells* 23(6): 781–790.

Yen, B.L., Chang, C.J., Liu, K.J., Chen, Y.C., Hu, H.I., Bai, C.H., and Yen, M.L. 2009. Brief report—Human embryonic stem cell-derived mesenchymal progenitors possess strong immunosuppressive effects toward natural killer cells as well as T lymphocytes. *Stem Cells* 27(2): 451–456.

Ying, Q.L., Nichols, J., Chambers, I., and Smith, A. 2003. BMP induction of Id proteins suppresses differentiation and sustains embryonic stem cell self-renewal in collaboration with STAT3. *Cell* 115(3): 281–292.

Ying, Q.L., Wray, J., Nichols, J., Batlle-Morera, L., Doble, B., Woodgett, J., Cohen, P., and Smith, A. 2008. The ground state of embryonic stem cell self-renewal. *Nature* 453(7194): 519–523.

Yoshida, K., Chambers, I., Nichols, J., Smith, A., Saito, M., Yasukawa, K., Shoyab, M., Taga, T., and Kishimoto, T. 1994. Maintenance of the pluripotential phenotype of embryonic stem cells through direct activation of gp130 signalling pathways. *Mech Dev* 45(2): 163–171.

Yu, J., Vodyanik, M.A., Smuga-Otto, K., Antosiewicz-Bourget, J., Frane, J.L., Tian, S., Nie, J. et al. 2007. Induced pluripotent stem cell lines derived from human somatic cells. *Science* 318(5858): 1917–1920.

Yusa, K., Rad, R., Takeda, J., and Bradley, A. 2009. Generation of transgene-free induced pluripotent mouse stem cells by the piggyBac transposon. *Nat Methods* 6(5): 363–369.

Zhang, S.C. 2006. Neural subtype specification from embryonic stem cells. *Brain Pathol* 16(2): 132–142.

Zhang, S.C., Li, X.J., Johnson, M.A., and Pankratz, M.T. 2008. Human embryonic stem cells for brain repair? *Philos Trans R Soc Lond B Biol Sci* 363(1489): 87–99.

Zhang, S.C., Wernig, M., Duncan, I.D., Brustle, O., and Thomson, J.A. 2001. *In vitro* differentiation of transplantable neural precursors from human embryonic stem cells. *Nat Biotechnol* 19(12): 1129–1133.

Zhou, H., Wu, S., Joo, J.Y., Zhu, S., Han, D.W., Lin, T., Trauger, S. et al. 2009. Generation of induced pluripotent stem cells using recombinant proteins. *Cell Stem Cell* 4(5): 381–384.

CHAPTER 4

Introduction to Materials Science

Sangamesh G. Kumbar, PhD
and Cato T. Laurencin, MD, PhD

CONTENTS

4.1 INTRODUCTION

The importance of materials and materials science to regenerative engineering cannot be overstated. It is literally the basis upon which tissues are formed and having a comprehensive understanding of what materials are, how they are formed and degraded, and how they are described and characterized is essential. This chapter does not seek to provide a comprehensive overview of materials science but rather provide the reader the fundamental information necessary to begin to understand what materials are. The information given here applies to all materials but when possible is presented in the context of biomaterials. Several excellent introductory materials science texts are available should the reader wish to delve deeper into any of the categories discussed.

4.2 ATOMIC STRUCTURE AND INTERATOMIC BONDING

Materials are built by the small structural units called atoms. These atoms are held together by interatomic bonds such as primary (strong) or secondary bonds (weak) to create a three-dimensional (3D) network. In an atom, the nucleus is made of protons (positive charge) and neutrons (neutral charge), and electrons (negative charge) that revolve around the nucleus in circular orbits (Bohr's atomic model). An example of carbon atom is presented in Figure 4.1. In solid materials, atoms or ions (charged atoms) are held together by strong interatomic bonds (primary bonds). Most of the physical

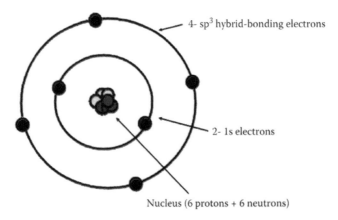

4- sp^3 hybrid-bonding electrons

2- 1s electrons

Nucleus (6 protons + 6 neutrons)

FIGURE 4.1   Bohr's atomic model: an example of carbon atom.

properties of materials are dependent on these bonds. The three different types of primary bonds are ionic, covalent, and metallic.

4.2.1 Primary Bonds

4.2.1.1 Ionic Bond

Ionic bonds are electrostatic attractive forces between two charged atoms formed by the transfer of one or more electrons from an atom to another. The metal atom that loses electrons gains positive charge (cation) and the electron-accepting atom (nonmetal) gains a negative (anion) charge, resulting in the creation of an ionic bond. Ionic compounds in general are solids with high melting and boiling points, are water soluble, and conduct electricity in molten or aqueous states. Examples include sodium chloride (NaCl), calcium carbonate ($CaCO_3$), and ferric sulfate ($Fe_2(SO_4)_3$).

4.2.1.2 Covalent Bond

Covalent bonds are formed by an equal (nonpolar) or unequal (polar) sharing of one or more pairs of electrons between two atoms. Unlike ionic bonding, neither atom completely loses or gains electrons. Covalent bonds are formed between either two different nonmetal atoms or two identical nonmetal atoms. A hydrogen molecule (H_2) is an example of a nonpolar covalent molecule where each hydrogen atom contributes one electron for the covalent bond formation. Hydrogen chloride (HCl) and hydrocarbons are examples of polar covalent molecules.

4.2.1.3 Metallic Bond

Metallic bonds are formed by sharing electrons between two metal atoms. The ease with which electricity and heat conduct through metals suggests that electrons are delocalized and freely move in all directions. Hence, electrons involved in metallic bond formation may be shared between many surrounding metal atoms. Often metallic bonding is described as "positive ions in a sea of electrons."

4.2.2 Secondary Bonds

Primary bonds are stronger than secondary bonds such as *hydrogen* and *van der Waals forces of attraction*. Hydrogen atoms that are covalently bonded to an electronegative atom such as chlorine, oxygen, and nitrogen in a chemical group are often involved in hydrogen bond formation. The electronegative atom pulls the shared pair of electrons toward itself and thus creates partial positive charge on the hydrogen atom. These oppositely charged atoms are involved in the formation of hydrogen bonds within the molecule (intramolecular) or between different molecules (intermolecular). For example, hydrogen bonds are quite common in macromolecules, proteins, DNA, polysaccharides, HF, NH_3, and water.

The van der Waals forces include attractions between atoms, molecules, and surfaces. The random motion of electrons around the nucleus converts a nonpolar molecule to polar. During that time, the atom acts as a very weak dipole. The van der Waals electrostatic attractive forces include the contributions from the polar and nonpolar molecules and result in weak bonding. Hydrogen bonds are the strongest weak bonds and hence result in higher melting and boiling points than those materials with van der Waals forces of attraction.

4.3 STRUCTURE OF MATERIALS

4.3.1 Crystalline Structures

All crystalline solids are composed of orderly arrangements of atoms, ions, or molecules. In crystalline solids, atoms, ions, or molecules are arranged in symmetrical shapes and contribute toward material properties. Atoms, ions, or molecules are specially arranged in lattice points. In the crystal lattice, the smallest structural repeat unit is called a unit cell.

4.3.1.1 Unit Cells

A unit cell is characterized by the three edges (a, b, and c) and the angles between the edges, α (between b and c), β (between a and c), and γ (between a and b). There are 14 different types of unit cells also known as Bravais lattices. The 14 Bravais lattices include three different cubic types (simple, face centered, and body centered), two different tetragonal types (simple and body centered), four different orthorhombic types (simple, face centered, body centered, and base centered), two different monoclinic types (simple and base centered), one rhombohedral, one hexagonal, and one triclinic. Table 4.1 summarizes the different types of unit cells and the associated seven crystalline structures. The cubic unit cell is one of the most common and simplest crystal shapes found in minerals. There are three main types of cubic crystal systems: simple cubic (SC), body-centered cubic (BCC), and face-centered cubic (FCC) (see Figure 4.2). In simple cubic crystals, the lattice points only occur at the corners. The points at the corner of the cell are shared by the surrounding unit cells. In the case of a simple cube, 8 unit cells share each corner atom and hence its contribution forms one-eighth of the structure. In body-centered and face-centered cubes, lattice points in addition to corners in middle of cube (BCC) and middle of each face (FCC) form the structure. In the case of FCC, each face-centered atom is shared by 2 unit cells, which accounts for ½ per unit cell. Hence, total number of atoms in different cubic crystals are SC 8(1/8) = 1, BCC 8(1/8) + 1 = 2, FCC 8(1/8) + 6(1/2) = 4.

4.3.1.2 Crystal Lattice

A lattice is an array of points in space with identical environment. In a crystal, atoms are arranged in a regular fashion on each of the lattice points. Lattice parameters such as the length of the cell edges (a, b, c) and the angles (α, β, γ) between them are used to define the unit cell. The atoms within the unit cells are defined by the set of atomic positions (x_i, y_i, z_i). The orientation of a plane or set of planes within a lattice in relation to the unit cell is defined by Miller indices. For instance, consider a plane that intercepts the x axis at a/2, y axis at b/3, and z axis at c/1. Reciprocals of these intercepts give the Miller indices, i.e., (2 3 1). In general, the Miller indices for intercepts on x-, y-, and z-axes 1/h, 1/k, and 1/l are (h k l). Miller indices are also used to denote a set of planes that are parallel. For instance,

TABLE 4.1   Unit Cells and Associated Crystalline Structures

Crystal System	Axial Lengths and Angles	Unit Cell Geometry
Cubic	$a=b=c, \alpha=\beta=\gamma=90$	
Tetragonal	$a=b\neq c, \alpha=\beta=\gamma=90$	
Orthorhombic	$a\neq b\neq c, \alpha=\beta=\gamma=90$	
Rhombohedral	$a=b=c, \alpha=\beta=\gamma\neq90$	
Hexagonal	$a=b\neq c, \alpha=\beta=90, \gamma=120$	
Monoclinic	$a\neq b\neq c, \alpha=\gamma=90\neq\beta$	
Triclinic	$a\neq b\neq c, \alpha\neq\beta\neq\gamma\neq90$	

the plane (2 0 0) is parallel to (1 0 0). These indices are useful in explaining crystal shapes, material microstructure, and x-ray diffraction (XRD) pattern interpretation.

4.3.2 Metal Structures

Many material properties of metals such as density, deformation processes, and alloying behavior depend upon the crystal structure of the material. Thus, it is important to understand metal structures. The majority of common metals are formed from BCC, FCC unit cells, or a hexagonal closely packed structure (HCP) as presented in Figure 4.2.

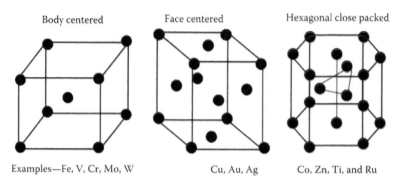

Body centered   Face centered   Hexagonal close packed

Examples—Fe, V, Cr, Mo, W   Cu, Au, Ag   Co, Zn, Ti, and Ru

FIGURE 4.2   Examples of cubic crystal systems: SC, BCC, and FCC found in metals.

The bulk properties of the metals are greatly dependent on the unit cell from which they are formed. For instance, FCC metals such as Cu, Au, and Ag are ductile and hence can be bent and shaped easily. BCC metals such as Fe, V, and Cr are stronger but less ductile. HCP metals such as Co, Zn, Ti, and Ru are usually brittle and are difficult to bend without breaking. In some metals, the structural arrangement also depends on the temperature. For instance, iron is a BCC crystal at room temperature while rearranges into FCC at a temperature of 910°C.

4.3.3 Polymeric Structures

Polymers in general are either amorphous or semicrystalline. Unlike metals, the degree of crystallinity in polymers varies between 10% and 90%. Polymer crystallinity refers to packing of polymer chains in an ordered atomic array. For instance, a simple polymer molecule such as polyethylene (PE) assumes an orthorhombic unit cell arrangement. Details of polymer structure property relations are discussed in more depth under Section 4.4.

4.3.4 Ceramic Structures

Ceramics contain metallic and nonmetallic elements connected by both ionic and covalent bonds. Ceramics are partially crystalline due to two different classes of elements. For instance, metals are ductile due to a densely packed regular arrangement of atoms. Ceramics differ from metals in elemental arrangement as well as bonding type and hence are brittle. The basic unit cell in ceramic crystals is either cubic or hexagonal. Silica (SiO_2), for example, is the basic component for many ceramics and glass. In silica, one silicon atom is surrounded by four equidistant oxygen atoms and assumes a tetrahedron structure. Silica is an example of an FCC crystal type. Silicate structural frameworks are created by sharing the corner oxygen atoms of the tetrahedron. The same chemical composition of silica makes either quartz or glass, depending on the material cooling process during its fabrication. For instance, slow cooling of silica from its melt results in a regular arrangement of tetrahedral structures, and hence makes quartz. Rapid cooling results in a random arrangement of structures and hence makes glass.

4.3.5 Polycrystalline Materials

In reality the vast majority of common metals and ceramics are polycrystalline. Polycrystalline materials are made up of many randomly oriented single crystals that are held together by thin layers of an amorphous solid. Noncrystalline materials, also referred to as amorphous materials, lack the long-range atomic order seen with metals and ceramics. Examples of purely noncrystalline materials include water and air. Other materials such as glass, plastics, and rubber have both crystalline and noncrystalline domains in their structures.

4.4 STRUCTURE AND PROPERTIES OF POLYMERS

Polymers are characterized by their high molecular weight ranging from several thousands to few million atomic mass units (amu). Polymers are made of several basic structural units that are repeatedly joined by covalent linkages to form long, branched, or cross-linked chains. Because of their high molecular weight, polymers are also known as macromolecules. Polymers present several diverse properties in their physical, chemical, and mechanical characteristics when compared to low-molecular-weight materials. For instance, sodium chloride, an inorganic salt of low molecular weight, dissolves in water instantaneously and attains saturation at a particular concentration. A polymer, on the other hand, while soluble in solvents, takes time to absorb solvent toward its eventual dissolution as polymer chains start freely moving in the solvent. Polymers, however, do not have a saturation point as seen with inorganic salts. Properties of polymers rather are dependent on the basic structural unit composition, chain length, extent of chain branching, and cross-linking. Consider the structure of the PE molecule (Figure 4.3), which is made of many ethylene repeat units joined together by a covalent bond to form a long polymer chain. In this linear structure, the highlighted portion of Figure 4.3 represents the smallest repeat unit of the polymer, called "mer." The term "mer" is defined as the group of atoms that constitutes a polymer chain repeat unit. A single repeat unit of a polymer chain is called *monomer*. Similarly, a chain with a number of mer units such as two, three, and four is called a dimer, trimer, and tetramer, respectively. A relatively small number of "mer" units present in a chain is termed an oligomer. Hence dimers, trimers, and tetramers are oligomers. So in summary, polymers can be defined as solid, nonmetallic compounds of very high molecular weight, the structure of which is composed of several "mer" units.

4.4.1 Polymer Classification

Polymers can be broadly classified into two main categories based on their functional behavior: elastomers and plastics. Figure 4.4 provides the general stress–strain behavior of elastomers, plastic, and rigid plastic materials. Flexible or rubbery polymers that can be readily stretched and return to their original shape and size upon the release of applied stress are called elastomers. Some of the examples of elastomers are silicone rubber, fluoroelastomers, ethylene vinyl acetate, and elastin (protein). Plastics, due to higher

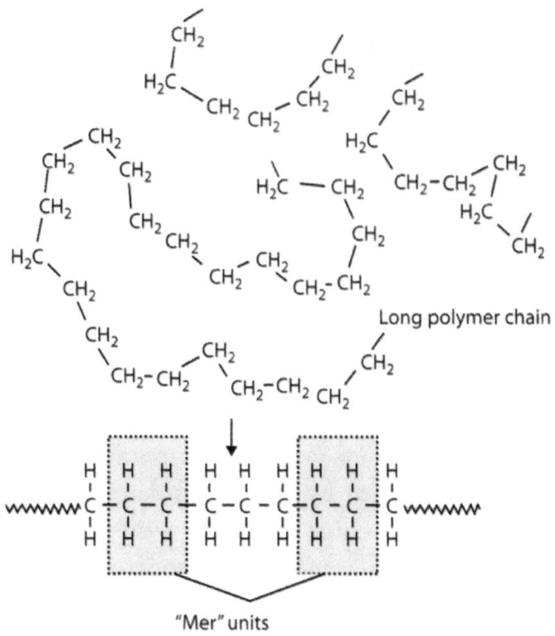

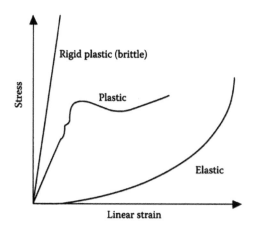

FIGURE 4.3   Example of long polymer chain, polyethylene.

FIGURE 4.4   General stress–strain behaviors of polymers.

stiffness, deform permanently under the applied stress and fail to return to their original shape and size. Plastics can be further divided into thermoplastics and thermosets, based on their processability. Thermoplastics can be recycled and reused and melt when exposed to sufficient heat. Examples include poly(methyl methacrylate) (PMMA), polycaprolactone (PCL), polystyrene (PS), and polyvinyl chloride (PVC). Thermosets are cross-linked polymer networks that resist melting once they are processed. Some resins like phenol formaldehyde, melamine formaldehyde, urea formaldehyde, epoxies, and certain polyesters are thermosets. Since thermosets are cross-linked rigid networks, they generally cannot be recycled or reprocessed. Elastomers can be both thermosets (such as vulcanized rubber used in tires and rubber band) and thermoplastics (such as the material used for the soles of tennis shoes).

Polymers can be classified as synthetic or natural. The majority of commonly used plastics are synthetic polymers while proteins and polysaccharides are examples of natural polymers. Synthetic polymers are subcategorized into several families based on the monomer linkages found in long polymer chains. For example, the polyolefin family of polymers is made of olefin (alkene) monomers. Some of the popular examples of polyolefin polymer family include PE, polypropylene (PP), PS, PVC, PMMA, and polytetrafluoroethylene (PTFE) (see Figure 4.5). In a polymer chain, mer units can be connected by ester, amide, imide, or urethane linkages. Polymers can be further classified into different families such as polyesters, polyamides, polyimides, and polyurethanes, based on the linkages between monomers. Some of the popular examples of polyester family presented in Figure 4.6 include poly(lactic acid) (PLA), poly(glycolic acid) (PGA), their copolymer poly(lactic acid-*co*-glycolic acid) (PLAGA), and PCL. Figure 4.7 provides few general examples of amides, imides, and urethane family polymers. Figure 4.8 provides few examples of natural polysaccharide polymers such as cellulose and chitosan.

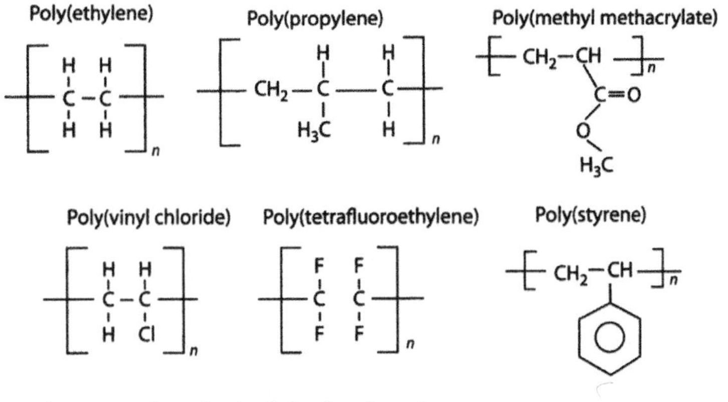

FIGURE 4.5 Popular examples of polyolefin family polymers.

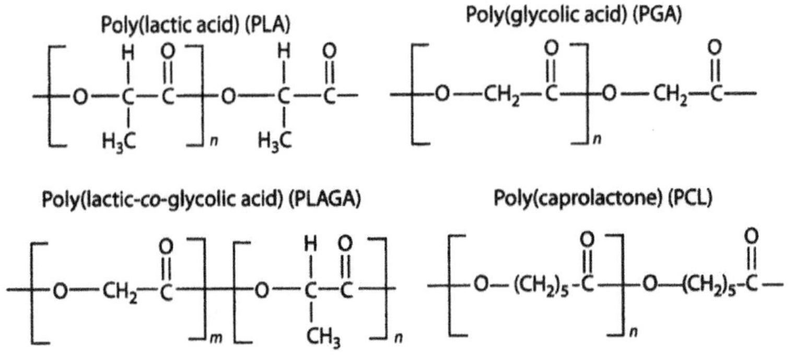

FIGURE 4.6 Popular examples of polyester family polymers.

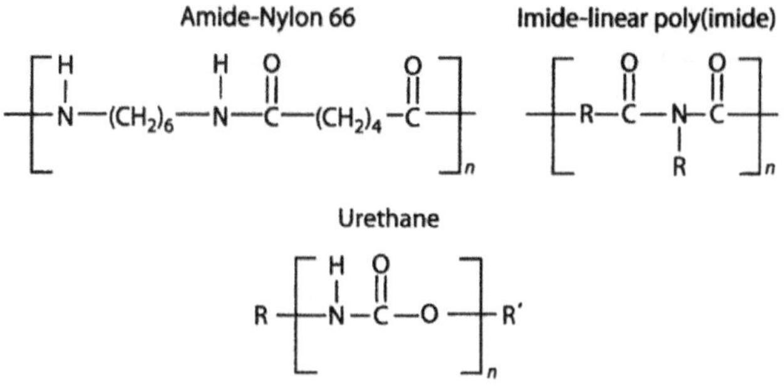

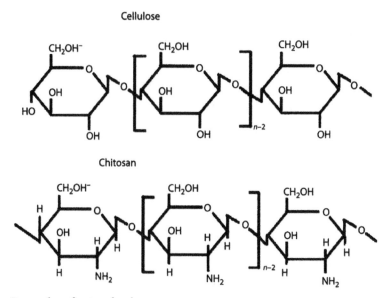

FIGURE 4.7 Popular examples of poly(amide), poly(imide), and poly(urethane) family polymers.

FIGURE 4.8 Examples of natural polymers.

Polymers are further classified into homo-, hetero-, and copolymers, based on the arrangement of mer units in the polymer chain. If the polymer chain is composed of only one type of monomer repeat unit, it is called a homopolymer. Some examples of homopolymers are presented in Figures 4.6 through 4.8. Polymers derived from two or more different repeat units or monomers are called heteropolymers or copolymers. In a copolymer, it is possible to have a different arrangement of each type of monomer units. Based on the arrangement of each type of monomer, copolymers are categorized into random, alternating, block, and graft copolymers. Figure 4.9 shows schematics of different copolymer types. In a random copolymer chain, monomer units are randomly arranged. In an alternating copolymer, each monomer type appears in an alternating fashion in the polymer chain. In a block copolymer, each type of monomer appears in a block on a polymer chain. In a graft copolymer, polymer backbone is made of one monomer type while the side chain is made of different monomer type.

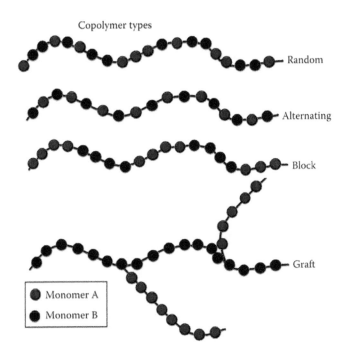

FIGURE 4.9   Schematics of copolymer types.

Polymer architecture contributes to polymer strength, toughness, thermal properties, and degradation stability. For example, two forms of PE, high-density PE (HDPE) and low-density PE (LDPE), offer altogether different mechanical properties due to the difference in polymer architecture. HDPE is comprised of long polymer chains with higher molecular weight and greater stiffness and is often used to fabricate milk containers. Due to its branched architecture, LDPE attains comparatively lower molecular weights and offers flexibility often used to fabricate plastic films. Polymers can be classified into four categories based on polymer chain arrangement: linear, branched, cross-linked, and network. In a linear chain polymer, monomer units are joined end-to-end in single chains (see Figure 4.10). Some of the popular examples used as biomaterials include PE, PVC, PS, PMMA, and nylon. A branched polymer network consists of a long polymer backbone to which one or more side chains or branches are attached. Some of the examples of this architecture used commonly in drug delivery applications include dendrimers, micelles, and liposomes. Cross-linked polymers are produced by linking adjacent linear polymer chains to one another at various positions with covalent bonds. Hydrogels commonly used for drug delivery and tissue engineering are ideal examples of cross-linked polymers. Network polymers are created by the use of trifunctional mer units. Such multifunctional units readily create three active sites for covalent bond formation in a polymer chain and hence result in 3D polymer networks. Epoxies, urea formaldehyde and phenol formaldehyde, are examples of network polymers. Figure 4.10 presents the schematics of all the four polymer chain architectures.

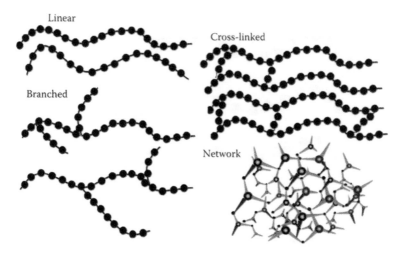

FIGURE 4.10 Schematics of polymer chain arrangement.

4.4.2 Polymer Molecular Weights

Polymers are macromolecules with the molecular weight in the order of 10^3 to 10^6. Polymer properties such as viscosity, stiffness, strength, viscoelasticity, glass transition temperatures, and degradation behavior are mainly dependent on the polymer molecular weight. For example, polymers with high molecular weight offer higher mechanical properties as compared to lower molecular weights of the same polymer. In general, higher-molecular-weight polymers take more time to degrade than lower molecular weights of the same polymer. Unlike a small molecule, a polymer molecular weight cannot have one unique value. That is, all polymers are mixtures of many large polymer chains with variable chain lengths and molecular weights. Hence, polymers have a distribution of molecular weights. The breadth of this distribution will depend on the polymerization technique and extent of control over polymerization. For instance, polymers synthesized in controlled reaction conditions tend to have a narrower molecular weight distribution than one synthesized in less controlled conditions. Due to the distribution of molecular weights in a polymer, it is customary to report the molecular weight as either weight average molecular weight or number average molecular weight. The weight average is most commonly used to account for the contributions of different polymer chains to the overall polymer physical properties.

Number average molecular weight, $\overline{Mn}$, is the distribution of molecular weight over the number of molecules. In other words, it is the average of the molecular weights of the individual macromolecules:

$$\overline{Mn} = \frac{\sum NiMi}{\sum Ni}$$

where Ni is the number fraction of polymer weight Mi.

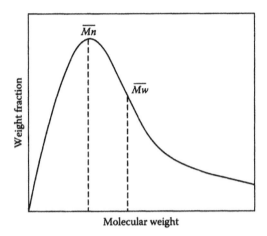

FIGURE 4.11 Example of molecular weight distribution pattern of a polymer.

Weight average molecular weight, $\overline{Mw}$, is the distribution of molecular weight over the weight of each chain:

$$\overline{Mw} = \frac{\sum NiMi^2}{\sum NiMi}$$

where *Ni* is the number fraction of polymer weight *Mi*.

Experimentally, polymer molecular weights are determined using techniques such as gel permeation chromatography (GPC), dynamic light scattering, and viscometry. A typical molecular weight distribution for a polymer is presented in Figure 4.11.

Polydispersity index (PDI) is the ratio of $\overline{Mw}$ to $\overline{Mn}$ and provides information about the breadth of weight distribution. For a well-controlled polymer synthesis, the PDI is close to 1. Such polymer systems are considered monodisperse. For the majority of commercial polymers, the PDI value ranges between 1.5 and 2. A degradable polymer PDI value begins to rise as the polymer begins to degrade, as the bonds between monomers are broken, and as the long polymer chains become smaller fragments. Hence, PDI values provide useful information about the polymer and changing properties over time.

4.4.3 Polymer Synthesis

Polymerization is the process of stitching mer units together to form a long covalently bonded polymer chain. Based on the monomer units, different polymerization techniques can be applied to produce polymers, such as addition polymerization, condensation polymerization, and ring opening polymerization. Two monomeric units are joined together by condensation polymerization which generally occurs by the elimination of a small molecule. Ring opening polymerizations are commonly used for cyclic monomers.

Addition polymerization is the process by which unsaturated hydrocarbon (alkene and alkyne) monomers are joined together to form a long polymer chain. This particular

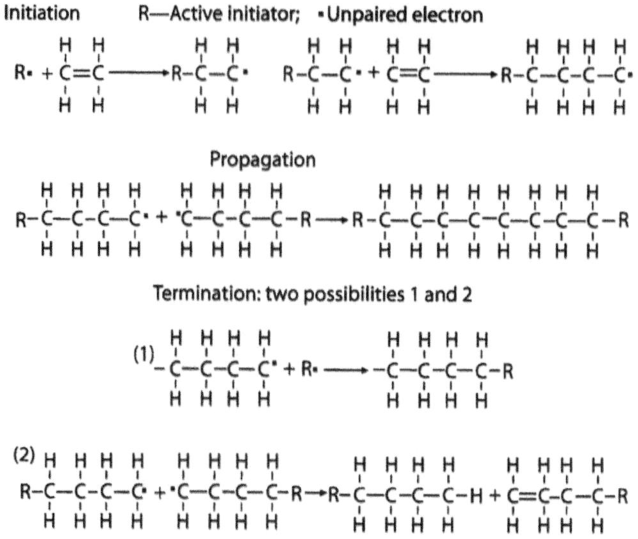

FIGURE 4.12 Addition polymerization schematics.

polymerization process involves three stages: initiation, propagation, and termination (see Figure 4.12).

Initiation: An active center capable of chain propagation is formed by a reaction between an initiator species and the monomer unit as presented in Figure 4.12. In addition to a chemical initiator, it is also possible to create a free radical by heat and radiation energy (UV light or γ-ray).

Propagation: In this step, free radicals created in the initiation step attach to one another in succession to produce the polymer chain as presented in Figure 4.12.

Termination: Theoretically, propagation reaction can continue until all the monomer in a reaction is utilized. However, the polymerization may terminate much earlier by the use of a termination reaction. Termination can occur by combination or disproportionation (exchange of a proton). In combination, the reactive ends of two propagating chains may react or link together to form a nonreactive molecule thus terminating the growth of each chain. The illustration in Figure 4.12 depicts the chain termination by combination process. An active chain end may react with an initiator, or strip a hydrogen atom from an active chain, or the presence of another chemical species with a single active bond can lead to termination of chain growth.

Condensation polymerization: Two monomers react to form a covalent bond usually by a small molecule such as water, hydrochloric acid, methanol, or carbon dioxide. Figure 4.13 illustrates the synthesis of Nylon 6,10 by condensation polymerization.

Ring opening reaction: Cyclic monomers such as lactide, glycolide, ε-caprolactone upon treatment with a catalyst and heat initiate ring opening and create a reactive center at the chain terminal. Polymerization occurs quite similarly to addition polymerization following the ring opening. Examples of ring opening polymerization are presented in Figure 4.14.

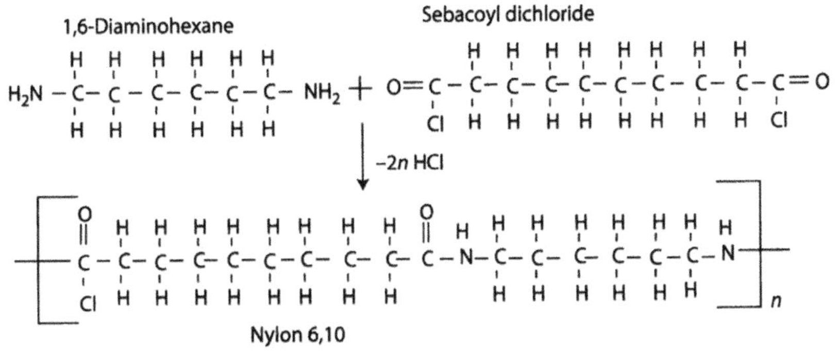
1,6-Diaminohexane
Sebacoyl dichloride
-2n HCl
Nylon 6,10

FIGURE 4.13 Condensation polymerization schematics, synthesis of Nylon 6,10.

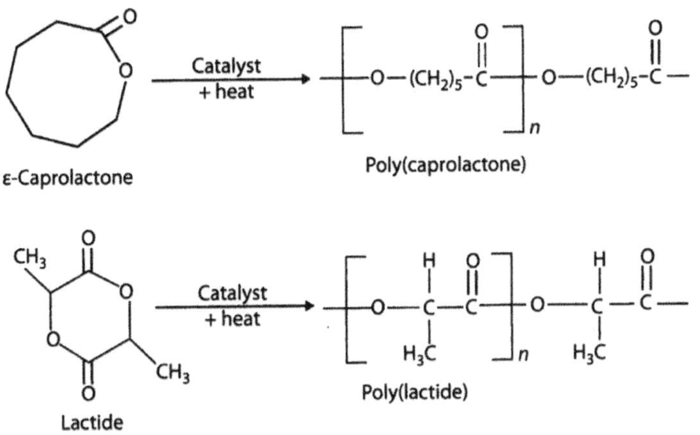
Catalyst
+ heat
ε-Caprolactone
Poly(caprolactone)
Catalyst
+ heat
Lactide
Poly(lactide)

FIGURE 4.14 Examples of ring-opening polymerization.

4.4.4 Tacticity

In a polymer chain, monomeric units can be arranged in various possibilities through the rotation of a valence bond. Tacticity refers to the way monomeric units are arranged along the polymer backbone. Polymerization of vinyl monomers such as ethylene and styrene gives rise to three different kinds of monomer arrangements: isotactic (same side), syndiotactic (alternating), and atactic (irregular), based on the polymerization technique used. Tacticity dictates physical properties of a polymer such as its rigidity, flexibility, crystallinity, and melting points. For example, a regular monomer arrangement along the polymer chains allows better crystal packing than an irregular arrangement and hence results in a crystalline polymer rather than one randomly arranged. It is possible to control the arrangement of monomeric units along the polymer chain by using special polymerization techniques and catalysts. Figure 4.15 summarizes the isotactic, syndiotactic, and atactic arrangement of pendent groups in PS.

In isotactic polymers, all of the pendent groups of a polymer chain are arranged on one side. For example, isotactic PP is produced by Ziegler–Natta catalysis. Usually, isotactic polymers are semicrystalline. In syndiotactic polymers, the pendent groups are arranged

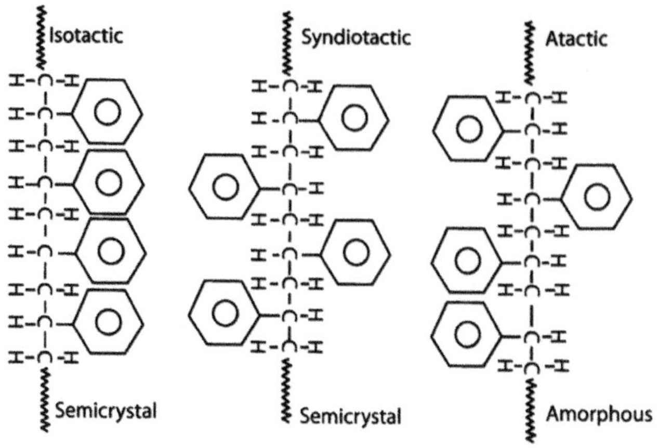

FIGURE 4.15 Examples of isotactic, syndiotactic, and atactic arrangements of pendent groups in polystyrene.

in an alternating pattern. Syndiotactic PS is produced by metallocene catalysis and it is a semicrystalline polymer. In atactic polymers, the pendent groups are randomly arranged along the length of a polymer chain. Free radical polymerization often leads to atactic polymers. For example, PMMA, better known as bone cement, is an atactic polymer. Because of the disorderliness of their pendent group arrangement, these molecules do not pack well and thus result in amorphous polymers.

4.4.5 Polymer Crystallinity

Polymer crystallinity refers to the packing of polymer chains in an ordered atomic array. As seen with the earlier examples of isotactic and syndiotactic polymers, because of the orderliness in the arrangement of pendent groups the molecules can pack well to form ordered regions. The majority of synthetic polymers are semicrystalline, meaning they contain both crystalline and amorphous regions (see Figure 4.16). For polymers, the semicrystallinity is expressed as a percent crystallinity, with most polymers ranging between 10% and 90% crystallinity. Crystallization of polymers can occur upon cooling from the melt, from mechanical deformation, and solvent evaporation. Rate of cooling can also dictate degree of crystallinity. For instance, faster polymer cooling from the melt does not give enough time for polymer chains to arrange in ordered structures and hence results in less crystalline polymers. The degree of crystallinity is measured by various methods including density measurement, differential scanning calorimetry (DSC), XRD, infrared spectroscopy, and nuclear magnetic resonance (NMR). In general, linear and more simple structured polymers are more crystalline than copolymers. Highly crystalline polymers are strong but brittle. Semicrystalline polymers are generally tougher due to amorphous regions within their structure and hence they are more ductile, or more likely to bend without breaking. The stress–strain behavior of different polymers is presented in Figure 4.4.

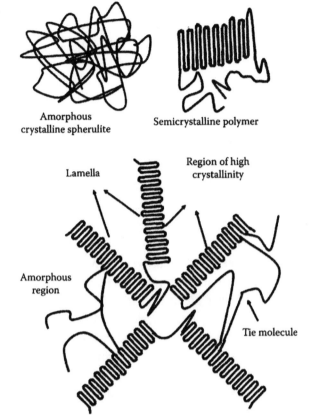

Amorphous
crystalline spherulite

Semicrystalline polymer

Lamella

Region of high
crystallinity

Amorphous
region

Tie molecule

FIGURE 4.16 Schematics of amorphous and crystalline domains in semicrystalline polymers.

4.4.6 Nondegradable Polymers

Polymers such as poly(ethylene terephthalate) (PET), PTFE, PE, and PMMA have been used as biomaterials to fabricate various implants for clinical use. These materials were primarily chosen based on their material properties to serve the intended purpose. For instance, ultrahigh-molecular-weight PE (UHMWPE) is used in the manufacture of hip and knee components due to its toughness and superior wear performance. These materials have shown excellent biocompatibility with little to no immune response. However, these polymers are nondegradable and remain in the body for life or until they are removed.

PE is a simple nondegradable polymer made of ethylene monomer units and has been used in the manufacture of articulating surfaces such as hips and knees due to its mechanical properties and wear resistance. Between LDPE and HDPE, HDPE is an obvious choice for the manufacture of articulating surfaces due to its mechanical properties. For instance, LDPE is a branched flexible amorphous polymer with molecular weight ~4,000–50,000. HDPE is a linear tough semicrystalline polymer with molecular weight ~50,000–200,000. However, in the manufacture of hip and knee articulating surfaces, ultrahigh-molecular-weight PE (>1,000,000) is used due to its improved mechanical performance, with better wear resistance than HDPE and an implantation life as long as 20 years.

Poly(aryl-ether-ether-ketone) (PEEK) is another nondegradable polymer that has been used to make a variety of orthopedic implants for load-bearing applications. PMMA has been used as contact lenses, dentures, maxillofacial prostheses, and bone cements.

4.4.7 Degradable Polymers

Degradation is process in which materials break down into smaller fragments that are soluble in aqueous environment so that they can be removed from the body. Degradation is uncommon in metals while ceramics degrade to a certain extent in the physiological environment. Polymers with carbon–carbon backbone tend to resist degradation due to their hydrophobic nature. However, degradable polymers can be synthesized by introducing hydrolytically labile linkages such as such as ester, anhydride, and amide bonds to promote hydrolysis. The usual mechanism for degradation is by hydrolysis or enzymatic cleavage of these labile linkages, resulting in a scission of the polymer backbone. As a result, decrease in polymers' molecular weight ($\overline{Mw}$ and $\overline{Mn}$), strength, and mass is observed. In general, amorphous polymers break down easily than the crystalline polymers. It is possible to synthesize polymers with a predictable degradation pattern for a variety of biomedical applications. Several physicochemical factors also influence polymer degradation. Polymer degradation can be promoted by introducing hydrophilic backbone, hydrophilic end groups, and reactive hydrolytic groups in the backbone. Further less crystalline polymers with increased porosity and smaller device size tend to degrade faster. Biodegradable polymers are attractive in the design of biomedical implants as they provide tissue-compatible mechanics and do not need a second surgery for removal; additionally, bioactive factors and drugs can be released from them to promote tissue healing.

4.4.7.1 Degradation Mechanism

Polymers undergo degradation either by bulk or surface erosion mechanism based on the polymer nature. Hydrophilic polymers undergo bulk degradation. In bulk degradation mechanism, water penetration into material exceeds rate at which material breaks down. As a result, entire polymer degrades roughly at the same time and hence molecular weight and mechanical properties decrease. Throughout the degradation process, polymer maintains its general shape and material crumbles (fails) as the mechanical properties decrease following polymer degradation. The degradation schematics are presented in Figure 4.17. Some of the popular polyesters such as PLA, PGA, and PLAGA degrade via bulk degradation mechanism. Hydrophobic polymers undergo degradation via surface erosion mechanism. Due to its hydrophobic nature, only the surface that comes in contact with aqueous media starts degrading which resembles much like peeling an onion. As surface erodes polymer becomes thinner, smaller with time, visible structural changes. Such polymers that undergo surface erosion are highly desirable for drug delivery applications as they provide a zero-order (constant) release profile of encapsulated bioactive factor. Gliadel® wafer, a drug delivery implant made of a poly(anhydride), namely, poly(1,3-bis-(*p*-carboxyphenoxy propane)-*co*-(sebacic anhydride) (CPP:SA), undergoes degradation by surface erosion mechanism.

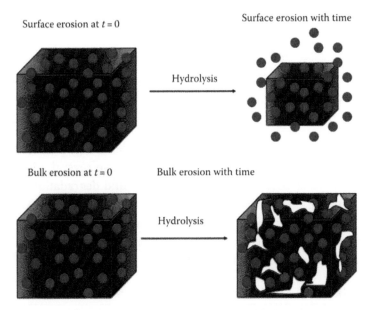

Surface erosion at $t = 0$

Surface erosion with time

Hydrolysis

Bulk erosion at $t = 0$

Bulk erosion with time

Hydrolysis

FIGURE 4.17 Schematics of surface erosion and bulk degradation mechanisms in polymers.

Among the biodegradable polyesters, PLA, PGA, and their copolymers PLAGA have been widely used for a variety of biomedical applications including biodegradable sutures, orthopedic fixation devices, and drug delivery. PLA, a semicrystalline hydrophobic polymer with an elastic modulus of 2.7 Gpa, takes more than 24 months to degrade. PGA, a hydrophilic polymer with more crystalline domains, has an elastic modulus of 7 Gpa and degrades within 6–12 months. Commercially, PLAGA is available in various PLA/PGA ratios such as PLAGA 50:50, 65:35, 85:15, and 10:90 with predictable mechanical properties and degradation profile. For instance, higher PLA content copolymer is amorphous with reduced modulus and takes longer time to degrade. Higher PGA content copolymer is relatively crystalline with higher modulus and takes shorter time to degrade. These polymers degrade into their monomeric units such as lactic acid and glycolic acid, which are known to increase acidity in the tissue microenvironment and can elicit inflammatory response and foreign body reaction.

Polyphosphazenes are inorganic–organic hybrid polymers. Polyphosphazene inorganic backbone is made of phosphorous and nitrogen atoms and to each of phosphorus atom two organic side groups. This family constitutes more than 700 different polymers with varied mechanical properties and degradation profiles. The general polyphosphazene structure is presented in Figure 4.18. R represents the side groups. In particular, polyphosphazenes with amino acid ester, glyceryl, glycosyl, glycolic, or lactic acid ester side groups have been synthesized for a variety of tissue engineering and drug delivery applications. Bulkier hydrophobic side groups such as methyl phenoxy or phenyl phenoxy substitution improves the mechanical strength and decelerates polymer degradation. These polymers undergo hydrolytic degradation via surface or bulk erosion based on the nature of the side groups. Polyphosphazene backbone degrades into ammonium hydroxide and phosphates that constitutes a natural buffer and corresponding side groups.

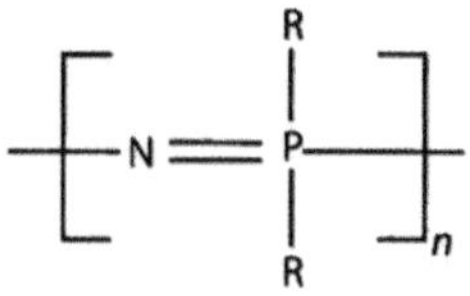

$$\left[-N = \overset{\overset{\displaystyle R}{|}}{\underset{\underset{\displaystyle R}{|}}{P}} - \right]_n$$

FIGURE 4.18 The general polyphosphazene structure.

Polymers such as collagen, starch, alginates, plant-derived gums, chitin, and chitosan are examples of natural polymers. Natural polymers have several advantages: they are abundant in nature, cost-effective, and biodegradable and degradation products are easily absorbed due to the chemical similarity with extracellular matrix (ECM) components. Further, these polymers have excessive presence of functional groups such as OH, COOH, and NH_2 readily available for chemical and surface modification. These polymers have been used for a variety of tissue engineering and drug delivery applications.

4.5 STRUCTURE AND PROPERTIES OF METALS

Metals are characterized by high melting and boiling points, electrical and thermal conductivity due to strength of metallic bonds and delocalized electrons. Metals are malleable (can be beaten into sheets) and ductile (can be pulled out into wires) due to the ability of constituent atoms to roll over each other into new positions without breaking the metallic bonds. Imperfections in metals where the atoms are not in good contact with each other are referred to as grain boundaries. The hindrance to rows of atoms from slipping over each other following mechanical load makes the metal to fail at grain boundaries. Thus, presence of more number of grain boundaries makes metals harder and brittle. It is possible to control the grain size by the application of heat. For instance, heating the metals allows the atomic rearrangement that decreases the grain boundaries and converts the metal softer. Majority of the metals are either too soft, brittle, or chemically reactive for practical use. However, these properties can be altered by breaking the regular atomic arrangement in pure metals by inserting atoms of different sizes and structures. For instance, brass an alloy of copper (copper and zinc mixture) is harder than the original metals due to atomic irregularities in the arrangement that hinders the rolling of layers of atoms over each other.

4.5.1 Metal Alloys

An alloy is a mixture of two or more elements in solid solution in which the major component is a metal. Alloys produced by combining different ratios of metals offer superior strength and corrosion resistance as compared to parent metals. Alloys can be broadly classified into two ferrous (iron based) and nonferrous alloy categories. Ferrous alloys are alloys with iron as its main constituent. Iron alloyed with various proportions of carbon gives low-, mid-, and high-carbon steels, with increasing carbon levels reducing ductility and toughness. Steel is an alloy of iron produced with low, mid, and high carbon contents. Higher carbon levels in the steel reduce ductility and toughness. Based on the carbon content, ferrous materials are classified into steels and cast irons. Carbon content in steels can be up to 2.14% while cast iron contains higher amount of carbon. Cast iron is brittle due to higher carbon content in the form of iron carbide and hence manufactured through casting technique. The brittle nature limits cast iron usage in engineering applications. To improve mechanical properties, steel is alloyed with a variety of elements. Based on the other element content alloy, steels are categorized into low-alloy steel and high-alloy steel. The difference between the two is defined somewhat arbitrarily. High-alloy steel contains more than 8% of other elements beside iron and carbon. Some of the commonly used other alloying elements include manganese, nickel, chromium, molybdenum, vanadium, silicon, and boron. Majority of the ferrous alloys are low-alloy steels that offer greater hardness, durability, corrosion resistance, or toughness as compared to carbon steel. High-alloy steel such as stainless steel produced by alloying with a minimum of 10% chromium is more resistant to stains, corrosion, and rust than ordinary steel. Nonferrous metal alloys do not contain iron as a major constituent. Nonferrous alloys offer several properties such as reduced weight, higher strength, nonmagnetic properties, higher melting points, higher electrical and thermal conductivities, resistance to chemical and atmospheric corrosion, which make them attractive for a variety of structural applications. Nonferrous alloys of Al, Cu, Mg, Ti, noble metals (Au, Ag, Pt), and refractory metals (Nb, Mo, W, and Ta) are designed for specific applications. Titanium and cobalt–chromium alloys are extensively used in constructing biomedical implants due to their biocompatibility, improved mechanical properties (high tensile strength and toughness), and corrosion resistance.

4.5.2 Metal Fabrication

Metals and alloys are fabricated into desired size and shape by applying one of the four basic fabrication techniques such as casting, forming, machining, and joining. In casting, molten metals are poured into a mold of the required shape and allowed to harden at ambient conditions. Forming involves application of hydraulic pressure to metals to achieve desired shapes. Machining is used to convert bulk materials into desired shape and joining involves connecting prefabricated parts by various means. Powder metallurgy utilizes mixing and pressing of fine metal powders into a desired shape followed by heating the compressed material in a controlled atmosphere to sinter the particles together.

Thermal processing is also known as heat treatment. Metals and alloys upon heat treatment undergo atomic reorientation and improve several material properties. Heat treatment is used to improve ductility, strength, toughness, and machinability by refining grain sizes and relieving internal stresses. In thermal processing, material properties are greatly dependent on process parameters such as processing temperature, duration of material at the elevated processing temperature, rate of cooling, and the surrounding atmosphere.

4.5.3 Corrosion Mechanisms

Degradation of metals in general is termed as corrosion. Metals undergo corrosion primarily due to oxidation–reduction (redox) reactions quite similar to an electrochemical process. During oxidation, electrons are liberated and consumed during reduction process.

For instance, oxidation of a metal M with n valence electrons liberates electrons and acts as an anode:

$$M \rightarrow M^{n+} + ne^-$$

The corresponding reduction reaction where these electrons are consumed depends on the environment surrounding the metal. Some of the common scenarios include the presence of acidic, alkaline, or neutral aqueous environment as well as the dissolved oxygen. The representative reduction reactions are as follows:

$$\text{Acidic solution: } 2\,H^+ + 2e^- \rightarrow H_2$$

$$\text{Alkaline or neutral acidic solution: } O_2 + H_2O + 4e^- \rightarrow H_2$$

$$\text{Dissolved } O_2\text{: } O_2 + 4H^+ \rightarrow 2H_2O$$

Redox reactions represent an electrochemical battery or galvanic battery. Metallic implant corrosion in the human body is facilitated by the presence of ions in the physiological aqueous environment. Redox reactions damage the metal surfaces and typically produce corresponding metal oxides and/or salts. A thin oxide layer formed on the metal surface acts as a barrier and prevents further metal corrosion.

4.6 COMPOSITE MATERIALS

Polymer–polymer composites have been developed to achieve combinations of physical properties that make them ideal for specific applications. In general, polymer composites will have a continuous polymer phase where ceramic or polymeric particles or fibers are dispersed. Composite materials can be custom tailored to give desirable combinations of physical properties for certain applications. Composite materials offer superior elongation, modulus, strength, flammability, abrasion resistance, barrier properties, impact resistance, and creep resistance as compared to neat materials. Bone is an example of natural composite material composed on collagen and hydroxyapatite in a 3D network. Collagen provides bone with a structural framework, high tensile strength, and flexibility, while crystalline hydroxyapatite accounts for the stiffness and high compressive strength of bone. For instance, polymers are often flexible and ceramics are brittle. Polymer–ceramic composites offer mechanical properties that are intermediate to both the material class. Mechanical properties of the polymer–ceramic composite can be altered by varying the ceramic composition to meet the biomechanical loads for bone repair and regeneration application. Various compositions of biodegradable polymers such as PLA, PLAGA, and PCL with HA or β-tricalcium phosphate (TCP) have been explored as artificial bone graft substitutes. Polymers such as polyolefins, PVC, polyamides, polyimides, epoxy, polyurethanes, PEEK, and PTFE have been utilized in the manufacture of composite materials for high technology applications. Traditionally, calcium carbonate, mica, silica, carbon black, glass fibers, and talc were used as fillers for composite perpetration. High-performance fiber-based fillers include graphite, carbon, and ceramic fibers. In recent days, surface-modified polymer particles and fibers have gained interest in the manufacture of polymer–polymer composites. Surface modification introduces functional groups that promote interaction between two phases of a composite to achieve better compatibility and bonding. Mechanical properties of microfibrillar-reinforced PE and PET composites are superior to blends of the same material. PEEK–carbon fiber composites offer enhanced mechanical properties in terms of stiffness, strength, and creep resistance that are ideally suited for creating nondegradable orthopedic fixation devices. The CF-PEEK-OPTIMA and Endolign™, carbon fiber–reinforced composite materials with bone-like modulus, are currently used as alternatives to metal fixation devices in clinics.

4.7 MECHANICAL BEHAVIOR AND PROPERTIES OF MATERIALS

Mechanical properties dictate the suitability of a class of material for certain applications. Mechanical properties are also used to help classify and identify material. Basic modes of deformation of a material include extension, contraction, and shearing. A stress–strain curve presented in Figure 4.19 is unique for each material and is constructed by record-ing the amount of deformation (strain) at distinct intervals of tensile or compressive loading. Materials can be tested in tension, compression, torsional, and bending modes.

Normal stress is defined as $\sigma = F/A$ where σ is normal stress (N/m^2), F is applied force (N), and A is cross-sectional area (m^2). In the normal stress, applied force acts perpendicular to cross-sectional area. Shear stress (τ) is analogous normal stress σ; however, the applied force acts in the plane of cross-sectional area. *Strain* is defined as $\varepsilon = \Delta l / l_o$, where ε is normal strain (unit less), Δl is change in length (m), and l is initial length (m). Shear strain (γ) is analogous to normal strain; however, the deformation is perpendicular to the applied force. Schematics presented in Figure 4.20 illustrate the differences between normal stress and shear stress.

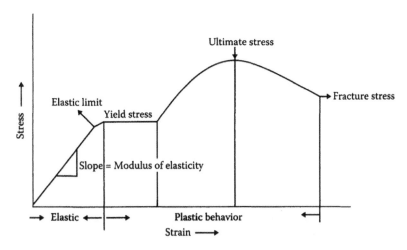

FIGURE 4.19   General stress–strain curve of a material.

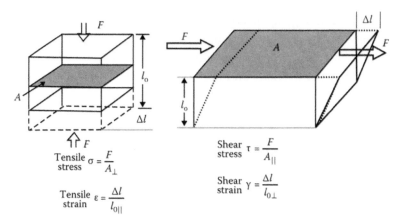

FIGURE 4.20   Schematics of stress and strain.

4.7.1 Modulus of Elasticity (Young's Modulus or Tensile Modulus)

Stress–strain curve presented in Figure 4.19 has two distinct elastic and plastic regions. Majority of the materials to a certain extent follow Hooke's law where the displacement is directly proportional to applied load. The slope on the linear portion of the curve in elastic region is defined as modulus of elasticity (E):

$$E = \frac{\text{Stress}}{\text{Strain}} = \frac{(F/A)}{(\Delta l/l_{o})} \text{ expressed in the units as Pa}$$

Shear modulus or modulus of rigidity is the ratio of shear stress to shear strain within elastic limits. It is given by $G = \tau/\gamma$, where G is shear modulus (Pa), τ is shear stress (N/m^2), and γ is shear strain (unit less).

Increase in applied load beyond the elastic limits increases the stress and material undergoes permanent deformation called plastic deformation. Yield stress (σ_y) is defined as the stress at which material undergoes plastic deformation. The maximum load material can handle prior to failure is defined as the ultimate load and corresponding stress is called ultimate stress (σ_u). At ultimate stress material looses the ability to sustain the load and further increase in load leads to material failure. Fracture stress (σ_f) is defined as the point where material breaks.

Toughness of a material is defined as the ability of the material to absorb energy to undergo plastic deformation prior to failure. It is the amount of energy per volume prior to material failure. Area under the stress–strain curve gives the material toughness. A unit for toughness in the SI system is Joules per cubic meter (J/m^3). Metals in general are tough and undergo greater deformation (ductile) as compared to brittle ceramic materials. Hence area under curve for metals will be more than ceramics. As seen with the earlier discussions, steel can have varied degree of toughness based on the carbon content. For instance, 0.1% carbon content steel is the most ductile form while 0.2% is the toughest form and 0.6% carbon content steel has the highest strength.

Materials can be classified into elastic, plastic, and brittle based on their stress–strain pattern presented in Figure 4.4. An elastic material deforms and reverts back to original shape and size following load removal. A plastic material permanently deforms (yields) and does not return to original size following load removal. A brittle material fails immediately after elastic region of stress/strain curve, with little or no deformation before failure. A ductile material deforms considerably before failure.

Viscoelasticity is the dual nature of a material to exhibit both viscous properties as a liquid and elasticity as a solid during deformation. Majority of the polymers and tissues are viscoelastic in nature and exhibit creep and relaxation properties. Viscoelastic materials with an applied constant load continue to deform over time even without increasing the load. Such an extension under constant load is referred to as creep. Further, viscoelastic materials held at a constant extension tend to drop the original applied load with time. The decrease in load over time at constant stretch is referred to as relaxation.

4.8 MATERIAL STERILIZATION

Prior to implantation in the human body all materials have to be free from pathogenic microorganisms, or sterilized. Sterilization is a process that kills microorganisms or destroys their cellular material (DNA or RNA) and metabolic components necessary for their replication. Sterilization can be achieved by applying the proper combinations of heat, chemicals, irradiation, and filtration. Some of the conventionally used sterilization techniques include moist heat, ethylene oxide gas, γ-ray, and electron beam sterilization. Moist-heat sterilization involves exposure of the implant to saturated heat at 121°C–125°C for 15–30 min in an autoclave chamber. Thermally stable polymers and metallic implants are good candidates for this technique. Exposure to ethylene oxide, another sterilization method that requires the exposure of the material to highly toxic gas, kills the microorganisms by attacking their DNA/RNA. However, residual gas in the implants and porous structures can cause significant problems. In γ and electron beam sterilization, exposure of implants to these radiations ionizes DNA/RNA and kills microorganisms. γ-rays can penetrate deep into the sample; however, electron penetration is limited. Hence, electron beam sterilization is limited only to sterilizing surfaces. Thus, based on the material properties, suitable sterilization techniques are chosen since material properties after sterilization can change depending on the techniques used. PE wear is also affected by the sterilization method adopted for implant sterilization. PE exposure to γ and electron beam irradiation results in the formation of free radicals, oxidation, and polymer chain breakage (decrease in molecular weight) from the ambient oxygen during the sterilization process. Alternatively, carrying out sterilization in the absence of oxygen (evacuated packaging) results in the cross-linked polymer networks and increased wear resistance of UHMWPE.

ACKNOWLEDGMENT

The authors would like to acknowledge financial support from the Institute of Regenerative Engineering and the Center for Science and Technology Commercialization, University of Connecticut.

CHAPTER 5

Biomaterials

A. Jon Goldberg, PhD and Liisa T. Kuhn, PhD

CONTENTS

5.1 INTRODUCTION

Over the last 60 years, modern biomaterials have evolved from industrial materials with an inert surface to sophisticated designs that recognize and influence biological response. While cell-free biomaterials are not the physiological tissue replacement that is the goal of regenerative engineering, they do represent an ever-improving standard of care against which engineered tissues must be judged. This chapter describes the fundamental clinical problems that drive the need for biomaterials in musculoskeletal, cardiovascular, ophthalmic, dental, neural, and skin diseases and injury. Design criteria for biomaterials in each area are described. A summary of the historical and current biomaterials used in each clinical application is provided. Overall, this chapter explains how biomaterials have been applied in contemporary therapy. Only the future will determine if the current use of biomaterials becomes a historical phase in the transition to regenerative engineering or, with continuing sophistication of designs, remains a mainstay of treatment.

5.2 CARDIOVASCULAR BIOMATERIALS

Cardiovascular disease is a broad term encompassing diseases of the heart and blood vessels. The most common forms are coronary heart disease, stroke, high blood pressure, and heart failure. Cardiovascular diseases are the number one cause of death worldwide. These diseases are responsible for 40% of all deaths in the United States (Mayo Clinic 2010) and atherosclerosis accounts for almost half of all deaths in Europe (Stehouwer et al. 2009). Over the last 50 years, biomaterials have played a central and increasingly important role in the management of cardiovascular disease.

5.2.1 Clinical Problem

The primary cardiovascular clinical problem is atherosclerosis, an accumulation of plaques of lipids, calcium, cells, and cellular debris on the luminal surfaces of arteries (Figure 5.1). Arteries consist of three layers that perform various biological functions: the intima, media,

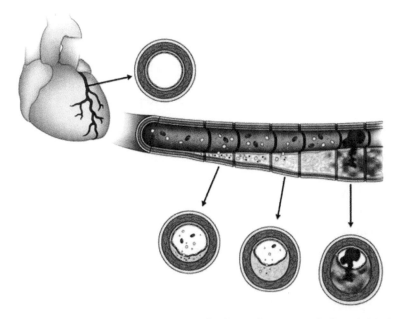

FIGURE 5.1 Layers of the artery and stages of atherosclerosis, including initiation, progression, and thrombotic complications. (From Springer Science+Business Media: *Essential Atlas of Cardiovascular Disease*, 2009, Gaziano, J.M. and Libby, P.)

and adventitia. The thickness of the layers varies with different types of vessels. The intima is the interior surface of the blood vessel and has a nonthrombogenic surface—it prevents blood contact with the thrombogenic media tissue. The intima is comprised of endothelial cells, which produce an array of biomolecules, including growth factors, vasoactive molecules, and adhesion molecules. The media or parenchymal tissue is the middle muscular layer. It is primarily smooth muscle cells (SMCs) and provides the required strength while maintaining elasticity. The outer adventitia layer is primarily fibroblast cells and acts as a stiff sheath that protects the smooth muscle media layer from biomechanical overload or overdistention. The primary components of the blood vessel extracellular matrix (ECM) are collagen and elastin.

One model of the etiology of atherosclerosis suggests that lipids accumulate on the inner walls of arteries as we age. Macrophages then accumulate as they ingest the lipids to remove them and in so doing further damage the intima layer. This injury attracts platelets, which triggers the release of proteins that form an overall matrix to the plaque. The plaque decreases blood flow, but the larger problem is the fragile nature of the plaque. It can break off, creating blood clots (embolism), which flow to the small arteries, blocking blood flow, and causing a heart attack if in the coronary artery or stroke if the artery is in the brain. Every year in the United States, more than 30,000 people undergo coronary artery bypass graft surgery (CABG) to bypass an occluded artery and another 640,000 undergo percutaneous transluminal coronary angioplasty (PTCA) to collapse plaque in an artery (Johns Hopkins Medicine Health Alters 2009).

Biomaterials and regenerative engineering play significant roles in cardiovascular therapy because much of the treatment involves devices to mechanically collapse accumulated plaque or replacement of diseased tissue. The procedures that rely on effective biomaterials are placement of stents, vessel replacement, and heart valve replacement.

5.2.2 Biomaterials for Cardiovascular Repair and Replacement

5.2.2.1 Stents

Because of the significant mortality and morbidity associated with atherosclerosis, there has been significant effort toward developing effective and improved procedures. Plaques primarily occur in limited, specific anatomic locations in the large coronary arteries just before the heart muscle. Accordingly, the restrictions in the blood vessels can be treated locally with angioplasty. Angioplasty, or PTCA, involves the use of a long catheter to position an inflatable balloon at the site of the restriction. The balloon is inflated, collapsing the plaque against the vessel wall. Angioplasty is initially successful, but vessels may lose patency within a few months mainly due to smooth muscle proliferation and new fibrous formations in the artery. Stents, and particularly those that deliver drugs, significantly reduce restenosis.

Stents are expandable metallic mesh tubes that are placed in the artery as part of the angioplasty (Figure 5.2). Most patients undergoing coronary angioplasty receive a stent and the subject has been recently reviewed (Hanawa 2009). As with all cardiovascular biomaterials, the main design criterion is the ability to resist thrombosis and accumulation of proteins and cellular debris. Because stents are essentially coil springs, their elasticity, modulus, and strength are the primary mechanical properties of interest. Additional desirable features include radiopacity and the ability to retain a polymer coating used to provide release of drugs. Mainly because of the mechanical property requirements all stents are fabricated from metals. The first clinically available coronary stents were made with a 40Co–20Cr–15Ni–7Mo–Mn alloy (Elgiloy™) (Sigwart et al. 1987). This Cr–Co–Ni alloy has been widely used in the field of biomaterials because of its high mechanical properties and biocompatibility. Today, stents are fabricated from stainless steel, Co–Cr, tantalum,

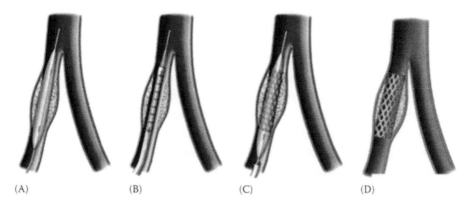

(A)   (B)   (C)   (D)

FIGURE 5.2 Angioplasty with stent placement. (A) Initial standard balloon angioplasty. (B) Positioning of stent on a balloon catheter. (C) Balloon inflated to expand stent. (D) Balloon removed. (From Springer Science+Business Media: *Essential Atlas of Cardiovascular Disease*, 2009, Creager, M.)

or Ni–Ti alloys, most coated with polymers for delivery of drugs (Puskas et al. 2009). The stainless steel stents are generally 316L. Ni–Ti alloys are candidate stent materials because their high elasticity and shape memory characteristics make them particularly useful in the self-expanding stent design. One brand of stent (Cordis™) is an alloy made from tantalum and Mg is currently being evaluated (Erbel et al. 2007).

Without a stent, a significant problem is the potential for almost immediate collapse of the artery following angioplasty and about 30% of coronary arteries experience luminal restriction as a result of cellular proliferation (Puskas et al. 2009). The bare metal stents significantly reduce these problems. However, about 20%–30% of patients with bare metal stents still experience artery closure due to excessive tissue response (Serruys et al. 1994). The drug-eluting stent significantly reduces restenosis (Morice et al. 2002). These devices are fabricated by coating the metal stent with a polymer that releases agents that have several effects, including mediation of cell proliferation (Weber et al. 2004). The controlled-release polymer coatings are rather sophisticated systems. Two current systems are based on poly(ethylene-co-vinyl acetate) and poly(n-butyl methacrylate) and poly(styrene-b-isobutylene-b-styrene), with several other systems under investigation.

5.2.2.2 Blood Vessel Replacement

When indicated, instead of angioplasty, occluded or diseased arteries are bypassed with graft surgery (Johns Hopkins Medicine Health Alerts 2009). The preferred graft is one of the patient's own arteries or veins. However, when not available, bypass surgery is accomplished with a polymeric synthetic graft. The topic of synthetic grafts has been recently reviewed (Chlupac et al. 2009). As with other cardiovascular biomaterials, the primary criterion is resistance to thrombogenicity and biocompatibility. In addition, the polymer must have sufficient mechanical properties and stability. The two most widely used biomaterials for vascular bypass are expanded polytetrafluoroethylene (ePTFE) and polyethylene terephthalate (PET). However, various polyurethanes and polyurethane copolymers have been evaluated over the past 30 years and recent results with this class of polymers for vascular grafts are more promising (Soldani et al. 2010; Theron et al. 2010).

As with angioplasty, the major problem with artificial blood vessel replacements is loss of patency over the long term. The problem is particularly acute for small diameter vessels. Synthetic grafts for arteries greater than 6 mm in diameter generally maintain their patency (Riccotta 2005). However, smaller diameter bypass grafts or those used in areas of low blood flow may lose patency within a few years (Faries et al. 2000; Klinkert et al. 2004). The length of the synthetic graft is also a factor in outcome (Georgiadis et al. 2005). The process of lumen restriction sequentially involves immediate absorption of proteins, platelet adhesion, and then endothelial and SMC migration (Chlupac et al. 2009). This hyperplastic growth occurs primarily where the graft is attached to the artery. There are several causes for this excessive growth, with the biomaterial factors involving the surface properties of the graft as well as a mismatch in mechanical compliance of the graft and the natural artery.

5.2.2.3 Heart Valve Replacement

There are several types of heart valve disease, but the most common cause of valve replacement is calcification and degeneration of the aortic valve, resulting in restricted blood flow and causing regurgitation of blood which can lead to heart failure. In 2006, there were ~100,000 valve replacements in the United States and about 200,000 in the rest of the world (Friedewald et al. 2007). There are two types of heart valve replacements currently in use. Bioprosthetic valves use acellular bovine pericardium or porcine valve tissue retained on a plastic or metal ring. These valves allow central flow of blood and are more hemodynamic and hemocompatible, but have limited mechanical durability (Kidane et al. 2009). Mechanical valves are typically of the ball-in-cage or leaflet design, have greater mechanical durability, but require daily anticoagulant therapy because of increased risk of thrombosis and thromboembolism (Kidane et al. 2009). Clinical use of replacements is about equally divided between tissue and mechanical types of heart valves.

Polymeric heart valve replacements have been attempted since the 1950s. A wide range of polymers have been evaluated, including silicones, PTFE, and PVA, but due to limited durability, thrombogenicity, and nonhemolytic properties none of these biomaterials have become clinically viable alternatives to the tissue and mechanical valves (Ghanbari et al. 2009). More recent studies of polyurethanes toughened or strengthened through copolymerization with PDMS (Dabagh and Al 2005) or POSS (Kannan 2007) have shown more promise.

5.3 MUSCULOSKELETAL BIOMATERIALS

The principal function of musculoskeletal tissues is to provide a framework to protect and support the organs and, in concert with nerves, to enable movement and locomotion. Bone, cartilage, tendons, ligaments, and muscles are all part of the musculoskeletal group of tissues; however, each has different functions and different biological properties. Due to the diversity of musculoskeletal tissues, each tissue must be considered individually in terms of scaffold design and biomaterials selection; thus this section is divided into subsections on bone, cartilage, ligament, tendon, and muscle. Where two tissue types meet, such as at the bone–cartilage, muscle–tendon, or tendon–bone interface, the biomaterial device or product must meet the requirements of both tissues with the proper function on each side. Composite biomaterials, biomaterials with gradients within them, or multicomponent devices are current strategies used to meet this challenge in musculoskeletal tissue repair. This topic is addressed in detail in Chapter 11.

5.3.1 Bone: The Clinical Problem

Bone provides mechanical and structural support to the human body, protecting soft tissues and playing a vital role in locomotion. There are many different shapes and sizes of bones in the human body. Bones are made of a complex fibrous composite material that contains primarily Type I collagen and calcium phosphate mineral crystals arranged in fibers or fibrils at many length scales (Figure 5.3). Long bones, such as the femur, have a different structure than membranous bones, such as the skull (calvaria). The midsection of the femur has a dense outer shell known as cortical bone with bone marrow on the inside.

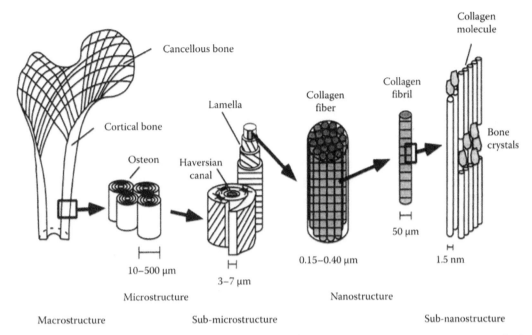

FIGURE 5.3 Hierarchical structural organization of bone. (From *Introduction to Biomedical Engineering*, 2nd edn., Enderle, J., Blanchard, S., and Bronzino, J., Copyright 2005, Elsevier.)

The ends of the long bones are covered with cartilage and contain a spongy bone inside known as cancellous or trabecular bone that assists with shock absorption and structural support. The calcium phosphate mineral crystals of bone serve as an ion reservoir maintaining blood homeostasis through dissolution and formation of the crystals that can store calcium and other ions such as magnesium and lead. Bone mineral is carbonated apatite, which resembles hydroxyapatite (HA), but has carbonate substitutions for the hydroxyl groups (Rey et al. 2009).

Bone is constantly in a state of remodeling, and several cell types work in concert to continuously optimize its chemical and physical structure to best meet the needs of the body. Bone is capable of undergoing spontaneous regeneration and thus microscopic fractures that often occur are rapidly healed without medical intervention. Larger bone fractures require some medical assistance to heal and are among the most common medical problems, with about 6.8 million patients seeking medical attention each year in the United States for bone fractures. Broken collar bones (clavicles), ribs, wrists, and tibias are common among younger patients. Craniofacial bones are often broken in automobile accidents. In those over the age of 75 years, hip fractures become the most common type of broken bones. Bone healing in the elderly is much slower than that in the younger patient. Degeneration of bones due to osteoporosis leads to bone frailty and increased risk for fracture of the spine and wrist. If two ends of the bone are not rigidly stabilized during the healing phase, incomplete healing known as a nonunion may result. Some cartilage starts to form in a nonunion and further inhibits the healing. Osteonecrosis is bone death that initiates from a poor blood supply to the area.

High doses of corticosteroids and chronic alcohol use are a few of the possible causes of osteonecrosis. The inflammation that results from the body attempting to clean out the dead bone further reduces the chance of healing. Birth defects such as osteogenesis imperfecta lead to a high occurrence of bone fractures. As can be seen, there are many clinical problems that occur with bone and hence research into bone healing remains an active area.

5.3.1.1 Design Criteria for Bone Repair Materials

For biomaterial scaffolds that are used for the repair of load-bearing bones, such as a femur or tibia, it is useful to have a compressive strength approximating that of cancellous bone (5–15 MPa). External fixation with metal pins and rods is typically used to provide the primary structural support while a bone fracture heals, thus the bone graft scaffold can have minimal strength. It is important to have a porous graft material that will bridge the defect and allow infiltration of the cells that will make the new bone. Previous studies have shown a porosity of 200–500 μm is needed to support bone cell and blood vessel infiltration. When a biomaterial supports bone cell infiltration and new bone growth near the edges of existing bone, the biomaterial is called "osteoconductive." When the biomaterial is combined with certain growth factors, the combination can actually stimulate new bone formation even when not adjacent to existing bone. This is known as "osteoinductivity." Both osteoconductive and osteoinductive biomaterials are currently used in bone repair.

5.3.1.2 Biomaterials Currently Used for Bone Repair and Regeneration

Depending on the type of bone injury and the surgical procedure selected by the orthopedic surgeon to repair the fracture, a variety of biomaterials may be used. Bone from the patient, known as autograft, remains the number one choice of orthopedic surgeons. Autograft has been used since the 1800s (Sanan and Haines 1997). Due to its limited availability, which requires another surgical procedure and thus pain and another wound to the patient, bone from another human, known as allograft, is also commonly used. To avoid immune rejection of the allograft by the patient, and to enhance its osteoinductivity, acid demineralization is used to remove the calcium phosphate phase and leave the Type I collagen matrix and other bone matrix proteins. Research on the calcification of demineralized bone matrix led to the discovery of the family of bone morphogenetic proteins (BMP) by Dr. Marshal Urist (Urist and Mikulski 1979). Purified BMPs, such as BMP-2, are now used clinically for spine repair (INFUSE, Medtronic Corp.) and require the use of a biomaterial scaffold to retain biologically relevant concentrations of the drug in the area where new bone regeneration is desired. BMP-2 delivered from a scaffold is even more effective than allograft in regenerating new bone, yet there are side effects such as soft tissue calcification from high doses of BMP-2 which is motivating more research on new scaffolds for BMP-2 delivery that allow lower doses to be more effective.

Metals, ceramics, and polymers, including natural ceramics and natural polymers are all currently used in the bone repair field (Table 5.1). Both nondegradable biomaterials and degradable biomaterials are used successfully. The degradable biomaterials listed in Table 5.1 make excellent choices for scaffolds for regenerative engineering of bone since

TABLE 5.1 Currently Used Biomaterials for Human Bone Repair

Category of Restorative Material	Biomaterials Used
Fixation and stabilization hardware including bone plates, rods, and screws	Metals: stainless steel, titanium, cobalt–chrome and Ti–6Al–4V alloys Polymers: polyesters, e.g., poly-L-lactic acid (PLLA), poly-L-glycolic acid (PLGA), polyetheretherketone (PEEK), Kevlar fibers or carbon fibers for reinforcement, polysulfone, polycaprolactone, polyethylene
Bone grafts and substitutes including bone cements	Natural tissues: bone autograft and bone allograft, demineralized bone allograft Ceramics: calcium phosphate, calcium sulfate, bioactive glasses, coral-derived calcium carbonate Polymers: collagen, polymethylmethacrylate
Total joint replacements, e.g., hip or knee implant	Metals: Ti alloy, Co–Cr alloy, tantalum Polymers (acetabular cup wear surface): ultrahigh-molecular-weight polyethylene (UHMWPE) Ceramics: alumina, zirconia ball and cups, hydroxyapatite coatings on the metal stems

they are already known to be compatible with, and even assist, the process of bone regeneration. Many other biomaterials are currently under investigation as bone grafts, but do not yet have regulatory approval for human clinical use.

Total joint replacements, such as hip implants, are made of a ball and stem component that inserts into the femur and a matching cup that encompasses the ball and provides for rotation in all directions. The biomaterials in a hip implant must replace bone as well as cartilage. Two different types of biomaterials are used in this case to best match the properties of the two different natural tissues, such as low-friction ultrahigh-molecular-weight polyethylene (UHMWPE) for the bearing surface/cartilage replacement and strong, non-corroding titanium alloys for the ball and stem/bone replacement. A highly porous structure made up of sintered beads and meshes is often included near the top of the hip implant to enhance bone ingrowth that stabilizes the bone-to-implant connection. A bone cement may be used to ensure a tight initial fit of the prosthesis. A high proportion of patients that receive total hip replacements go on to live active, pain-free lives, but loosening of the prosthesis may eventually occur over time. If the loosening is significant, it becomes painful and a revision of the joint replacement may be needed. Loosening is often triggered by wear particles from the UHMWPE-bearing surface that irritate the adjacent bone (Bhatt and Goswami 2008). Longer-lasting ceramic-on-ceramic designs are now available with alumina or zirconia acetabular cups and balls. With ceramic on ceramic-bearing surfaces, less wear is regenerated as compared to metal on plastic and thus there is less eventual bone resorption (osteolysis) and implant loosening due to wear debris. A metal stem is still used in joint replacements since ceramics are too stiff with too low a fracture resistance for the high bending forces experienced at the neck of the hip implant.

5.3.2 Cartilage: The Clinical Problem

There are different types of cartilage found throughout the body including fibrocartilage and hyaline cartilage. Fibrocartilage is found in the knee meniscus and spine vertebral disks. Hyaline cartilage is a few millimeter thick coating found at the ends of long bones, such as the femur, that meet at a joint. Hyaline cartilage is a highly organized, low-friction surface that allows for easy motion of two adjacent bones such as those found at a knee, shoulder, elbow, ankle, hip, finger, or wrist joint. Adult cartilage has minimal regenerative capacity due to a low number of progenitor cells in the tissue and a lack of blood supply to bring in other progenitor cells. The cartilage cells in articular cartilage receive their nutrients from the synovial fluid rather than blood vessels. Arthritis, osteoarthritis, sports injuries, and normal wear and tear lead to cartilage destruction. The joint then becomes stiff and painful and the pain and inflammation may be so severe that a person will avoid using the joint, which weakens the muscles and makes it even more difficult to move. Surgical procedures are then needed to alleviate the pain and restore function and range from cartilage repair procedures to total joint replacement procedures.

For superficial cartilage lesions, the surface may be smoothed using arthroscopic techniques. Because the knee joint is more readily accessible than the hip joint, arthroscopic cartilage repair techniques were pioneered in the knee joint. During arthroscopic surgery of the knee, a few small incisions are made around the knee to allow for a video camera and surgical instruments to be inserted and used within the joint. Removing bits of torn cartilage provides relief to the patient by alleviating some of the pain and discomfort, but it does not heal the defect. For deeper lesions including full thickness lesions that penetrate to the bone below, there are four commonly used surgical techniques: autologous osteochondral transfer, osteochondral allografting, microfracture, and autologous chondrocyte implantation (Farr et al. 2011). During the osteochondral transfer or allografting procedure, cylindrical plugs of structurally intact osteochondral tissue from a remote, relatively non-load-bearing site are transplanted into the load-bearing defect site. Osteochondral tissue is a piece of bone with intact hyaline cartilage. Autologous and allograft transplants survive within the site and have been shown to be successful for at least 10 years. There is a report of viable chondrocytes as long as 29 years after transplantation. However, one drawback to this approach of grafting tissue from one location in the body into another is that the location where the graft tissue was taken must also heal. Similar to bone autografting, donor site healing does not always occur uneventfully and patients may have pain or issues with the donor site for years after the surgery.

The microfracture procedure for cartilage repair involves removing the damaged cartilage and then making a series of small holes in the subchondral plate, which leads to bleeding, clot formation, as well as the introduction of marrow-derived stem cells to the site. These marrow-derived cells from the patient help to mediate a fibrocartilaginous repair of the defect. Autologous chondrocyte implantation is another new option for cartilage repair and starts with the harvest of a small piece of cartilage from the patients themselves. The cells from that piece of harvested cartilage are separated from the matrix and then the cells are grown on a plastic dish outside the body in a medium that causes the cells to increase in number to a large enough quantity that they can be implanted into the defect site, under a flap of tissue, also from the patient. These cells, similar to the marrow cells of the microfracture technique, initiate a fibrocartilaginous repair of the defect. Fibrocartilage is less durable, less organized, and has a higher proportion of Type I collagen than hyaline articular cartilage, but when formed within a defect, it does alleviate pain and may last up to 5 years. It eventually degrades because it does not have the mechanical strength of hyaline cartilage to survive the high stresses of the joint, thus hyaline cartilage remains a goal of regenerative engineering.

The meniscus is a small crescent-shaped piece of cartilage that maintains space between the femur and the tibia and helps transfer the load more uniformly to the articular cartilage. While mostly avascular, it does have a blood supply at the edges closest to the joint capsule. Due to this blood supply, partial repairs are possible, and accomplished by tacking or suturing the torn pieces together with polymeric biomaterials. Conduits into the avascular portions of meniscus tissue are sometimes surgically created to allow the influx of healing cells.

When joint destruction has proceeded beyond repair, with damaged articular cartilage extending over areas larger than several square centimeters, then the entire joint must be removed and replaced with an artificial joint, a prosthesis, also known as a total joint replacement. The design of a total hip replacement was described in Section 5.3.1. Designs for total knee replacement and other joints are described in the following sections.

5.3.2.1 Design Criteria for Cartilage Replacement

The replacement for articular cartilage must be of a shape that does not impede joint motion, have a smooth surface, be able to make contact and slide without friction, and yet be able to withstand high compressive forces. The joint capsule should be intact after surgery to allow for synovial fluid to bathe living cartilage tissue and provide lubricants and nutrients. For partial repairs, the areas of integration of the new cartilage with the existing cartilage should be of an even height and tightly adherent. Replacement cartilage for use in the ears or nose should be durable, flexible, and yet maintain its shape.

5.3.2.2 Historical and Current Biomaterials Used for Cartilage Repair

As an alternative to articular cartilage surgery, injections of a hyaluronic acid biomaterial into the joint capsule can provide temporary (5–12 weeks) relief for a patient with osteoarthritis and degraded cartilage. Hyaluronan is found naturally in the synovial fluid that surrounds the joints. It is a thick fluid that cushions the joint but becomes thin in patients with osteoarthritis. Injections temporarily restore more lubricity and shock absorption to the joint. When surgery is unavoidable, yet the lesions are still small, cartilage allograft and autograft remain the primary choices for the surgeon and lead to relatively good outcomes. The sutures used to stabilize allo- or autograft cartilage components during healing are made of polymeric biomaterials, such as poly-L-lactic acid or poly-D,L-lactic acid (PDDLA). Complete and total joint replacements require multicomponent devices and the use of biomaterials that mimic properties of bone and cartilage in order to restore function. As described earlier, UHMWPE is a type of polymer that is commonly used as the cartilage replacement component in a total joint replacement. Since it eventually wears and generates wear debris that causes adjacent bone to become inflamed and eventually degrade, there is still active research on wear-resistant polymers for total joint wear surfaces.

For the replacement of small joints, such as finger or toe joints, silicone is the biomaterial of choice for the prosthesis. Silicone has also been used since the 1950s for facial cartilage implants, such as ears and noses since it is solid, yet flexible, and very durable. Expanded ePTFE implants are softer than the harder silicone implants, so they are also used for ear and nose prostheses. ePTFE is not suitable for bearing surfaces such as knee or mandible joints though since it wears rapidly, releasing fragments that cause inflammation and tissue destruction within the joints. Porous foams of polyethylene are also currently used for successful ear reconstruction procedures.

Cartilage is one of the few tissues for which a cell-based therapy is already in clinical use. Rather than using any biomaterials, the patient's own cells accomplish the repair. Autologous cells, harvested from another location on the articular cartilage, are implanted back into the cartilage defect. The new cartilage tissue that is formed does not have the correct structure of hyaline articular cartilage and thus fails within about 5 years. Regenerative engineering techniques that grow multicomponent tissues with the correct structure and function may one day overcome these problems.

5.3.3 Tendon and Ligament: The Clinical Problem

Ligaments and tendons are dense, fibrous, connective tissues that are responsible for joint movements and stability. Ligaments connect different bones together, while tendons connect muscle to bone. Common areas of ligament damage, known as a sprain, include the ankle, wrist, and knee. The injury may vary from a mild to a severe sprain. A mild sprain is when a ligament is stretched or slightly torn, and a severe sprain is when a ligament tears completely. Mild sprains will heal on their own with rest, ice, compression, and elevation in about 6–8 weeks. When a ligament or tendon tears completely, it must be surgically reattached in order to reestablish stability and movement of the joint. In the knee, a ligament that often ruptures is the anterior cruciate or ACL, or the lateral collateral or LCL. The four most common areas of tendon rupture are the quadriceps, the Achilles, the rotator cuff, and the biceps.

Ligament and tendon repair represent a significant medical problem. Around 200,000 Americans required reconstructive ligament surgery in 2002, with a total expenditure of over $5 billion (Pennisi 2002; Vunjak-Novakovic et al. 2004). This estimate does not take into account those costs that were incurred due to loss of working abilities, healthcare, and social benefits. Reconstruction of the ACL is challenging and is the most difficult ligament to repair. There was about one ACL injury for every 3000 U.S. citizens in 1999 and this rate increases every year (Fu et al. 1999).

5.3.3.1 Design Criteria for Tendon and Ligament Replacement

When the tendon or ligament is irreparably damaged and must be completed replaced, the replacement materials must have the necessary mechanical strength to support the five times body weight they bear without much elastic deformation. Human ACL, for example, has an ultimate tensile strength of ~38 MPa and a Young's modulus of 110 MPa (Ge et al. 2006). Both ligaments and tendons have attachment points into bone and thus have gradients of mechanical properties through the tissue as a function of distance from the bone. Close to the bone, both tissues are highly calcified and resemble bone. Further away they are flexible, yet maintain a high strength due to the highly organized tissue structure. Ideally, tissue replacements for tendon and ligament would also have biochemical and biophysical gradients like the natural tissue to best accomplish load transfer and flexibility. Ligaments may appear on the surface to be easier to replace than tendons due to their "simple" function, but they are not simply passive joint restraints; they also provide electromechanical signals for joint-stabilizing muscle contractions.

5.3.3.2 Historical and Currently Used Biomaterials for Tendon and Ligament Repair

Depending on the extent of the damage, different strategies and different biomaterials are currently utilized for the repair of tendon and ligament. Surgical reattachment of a tendon or ligament into the bone involves tacking the tendon or ligament using titanium or polyetheretherketone (PEEK) bone anchors and a suturing process. For example, for rotator cuff repair, the frayed ends of the tendon are sutured to one or more bone anchors during arthroscopic surgery. Sometimes a patch of a natural ECM material is used to mechanically reinforce the repair site, particularly when successful reattachment was not achieved after the first surgery. ECM materials that have been tried for tendon repair include human dermis, porcine dermis, pig small intestine submucosa, and human rotator cuff tendon allograft. Porcine dermis and freeze-dried human dermis have had the most favorable results.

In current clinical practice for ACL reconstruction, autografts, including the bone-patellar tendon-bone grafts and hamstring tendons, have been the most popular and successful surgical replacements for the ACL. The bone-patellar tendon-bone graft has excellent bone-to-bone repair capabilities; yet, donor site morbidity is a major concern. The use of allograft avoids donor site morbidity, reduces surgical time, and minimizes postoperative pain; however, the decrease in tensile properties due to adverse effects of sterilization and preservation, as well as a risk of inflammatory reaction, are two major concerns associated with allograft use. Synthetic ligament prostheses like braided PTFE fibers (Gore-Tex), woven PET (Dacron), polypropylene, or PET polypropylene are used in patients, but only when autogenous tissue reconstruction has failed. Autogenous hamstring tendons implants lack a bony region as compared to the bone-patellar tendon-bone grafts and thus they do not integrate as well with bone. Synthetic biomaterials also have a high rate of clinical failures because it is difficult to get the synthetic tendons to form a strong mechanical bond with the bone. During surgery, the implants are placed into a bony tunnel and anchored down, but soft tissue forms, rather than the original calcified bone-like structure. Inflammatory reactions to the synthetic biomaterials typically cause joint swelling and graft rupture. These limitations continue to drive ongoing research to address the deficiencies of existing therapies. The regenerative engineering of ligament tissue is discussed in detail in Chapter 13.

5.3.4 Muscle: The Clinical Problem

Muscle consists of bundles of fibers in a hierarchical design (Figure 5.4), meaning each fiber bundle is composed of smaller fiber bundles and so on, down to the level of the

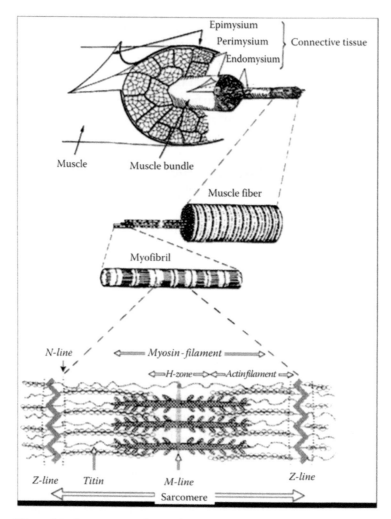

FIGURE 5.4   Hierarchical structure of muscle. (From Springer Science+Business Media: *Game Meat Hygiene in Focus*, 2011, Hofbauer, P. and Smulders, F.J.M.)

myofibril, made up of muscle cells, or myocytes. When muscle is overstrained through use or trauma, tears may develop in various levels of the muscle fibers, from a few cells up to the entire muscle. Skeletal muscle has an impressive ability to regenerate itself which it does on a daily basis, as well as in response to injury; however, complete rupture of muscle requires surgical reattachment. Muscle repair activity is initiated by progenitor cells known as satellite cells that reside within the muscle tissue. They are capable of proliferating and differentiating to myocytes and then eventually myofibrils. There are also acquired or genetic neuromuscular ailments (e.g., muscular dystrophy) that lead to muscle degeneration that require medical intervention.

5.3.4.1 Design Criteria for Muscle Repair and Replacement

The primary function of muscle is to provide a contractile or expansion force to move the skeleton. Thus there should be both mechanical and muscle cell conductivity across the wound or defect for normal synchronized function. There should be sufficient mechanical strength to accomplish the motion.

5.3.4.2 Historical and Currently Used Biomaterials for Muscle Repair/Replacement

Muscle can be reattached if it has been completely separated from itself or torn off from the tendon interface with the use of biomaterials such as sutures and staples. Sutures are usually made of a polymer such as polyester, either as a monofilament or multiple filaments braided together. The surgical technique for closing muscle incisions with sutures involves a careful balance between overtightening the sutures, which can cause necrosis, and leaving them too loose, which can cause the muscles to rip further apart during loading.

Autograft muscle transplants are used to replace nonskeletal muscles with poor function, such as sphincters, associated with either urinary or fecal incontinence. Silicone biomaterials are an alternative to muscle autograft and are injected to augment existing muscle tissue that is no longer capable of contracting or of insufficient size. A new fiber technology device comprising bundles of poly(ethylene terephthalate) fibers has been reported to couple muscles to bones in a superior manner to sutures (Franklin et al. 2009). The fibers are placed across the defect and new tissue grows into the fibers to form a strong tissue–prosthetic fiber composite.

5.4 DENTAL BIOMATERIALS

Worldwide, dental diseases are the most common of all the infectious diseases. In 2004, dental care represented 7.4% of total U.S. healthcare expenditures (Sommers 2007) and is expected to total $108 billion in 2010 (National Health Expenditure Projections 2010). The primary dental diseases are caries of the hard, mineralized structures and periodontal disease of the ligament that attaches the teeth to the mandibular and maxillary bones. Examining Figure 5.5 helps to explain the etiology of dental diseases.

Figure 5.5 is a schematic diagram through the cross section of a molar tooth. The outer layer is enamel, a highly mineralized structure (about 97% mineral) that is the hardest tissue in the body. The brittle enamel is supported by the tougher, less mineralized dentin. The pulp houses the nerves and vascular supply. Below the soft tissue of the gingival, the outer mineralized surface of the tooth is the cementum. The tooth is connected to the supporting bone by the periodontal ligament.

5.4.1 Clinical Problem

In the development of the biting (occlusal) surface, the cusps may not completely fuse, resulting in the creation of a pit or fissure as shown in Figure 5.6. The bacteria *Streptococcus mutans* can produce an adhesive ECM that allows the colonization of locations, such as the pits and fissures, which are not readily self-cleaning. The proximal smooth surfaces of teeth are self-cleaning. The products of the *S. mutans* colonies are highly acidic and if provided sufficient nutrients, the bacterial colony will irreversibly demineralize the enamel. If left untreated, this process will likely continue eroding the enamel and dentin. Once it reaches the pulp, the infectious disease can become systemic leading to an abscess of the pulp or worse.

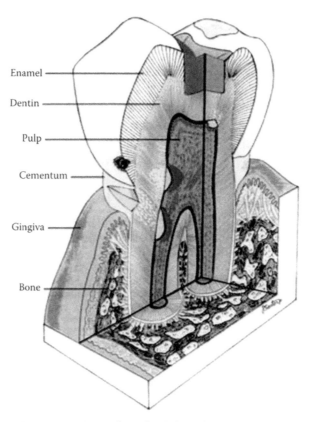

Enamel

Dentin

Pulp

Cementum

Gingiva

Bone

FIGURE 5.5 Schematic cross section of tooth with occlusal restoration. (From Summitt, J.B. et al., *Fundamentals of Operative Dentistry*, 2nd edn., Quintessence Publishing Co, Inc., Chicago, IL, 2001.)

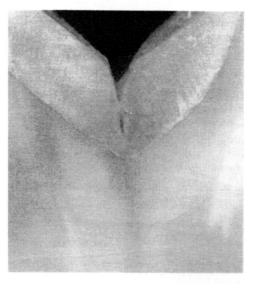

FIGURE 5.6 Cross section of a fissure. (From Summitt, J.B. et al., *Fundamentals of Operative Dentistry*, 2nd edn., Quintessence Publishing Co, Inc., Chicago, IL, 2001.)

Dental caries can be prevented by eliminating the organism, the nutrients, or the protected location. While all three strategies have been examined, interestingly use of an appropriate biomaterial to seal off the developmental pits and fissure locations has been the most effective in practice. Pit and fissure sealants are bisphenol-A-glycidyl methacrylate (Bis-GMA) resins. They are applied to newly erupted molars and have been shown to reduce caries 86% at 12 months (Ahovuo-Saloranta et al. 2004).

If caries develops and is detected in the very early, "white spot" stage, the lesion may not proceed or may be reversed with topical fluoride treatments (Hausen 2004). However, once the lesion has begun to undermine the enamel the only treatment is to remove the effected tooth structure and restore it with an appropriate dental biomaterial. The dentist will remove the diseased tissues creating a preparation or "cavity" that is then filled with a restorative material. An occlusal restoration is shown in Figure 5.5. An inherent problem with restorative dental materials is that they create an interface with the remaining tooth structure and this interface itself can be susceptible to secondary or recurrent dental carious lesions.

The region between the gingival tissues and the cementum is another location that can be colonized by oral bacteria. The organisms associated with periodontal disease are predominantly gram-negative anaerobic bacteria (Lovegrove 2004). These organisms can destroy the periodontal ligament and adjacent tissues, leading to recession of the gingiva, bone loss, and eventual loosening and loss of the tooth. Treatment primarily involves maintenance of oral hygiene and if necessary surgery to allow access for more effective hygiene by the patient. With more advanced disease, a number of surgical approaches are available to augment periodontal and bone tissue, although regenerative engineering strategies are being actively investigated (Chen and Jin 2010).

In summary, dental diseases develop when particular bacteria colonize protected locations on the teeth. The products produced by the bacteria demineralize or destroy the adjacent tissues. Once initiated, there are no physiological healing processes, leaving removal of the infected tissue and replacement with synthetic materials as the only current treatments.

5.4.2 Design Criteria for Dental Biomaterials

Several clinical factors make dental restoratives unique among the various classes of biomaterials. First, depending upon when it is detected the extent of the carious lesion can be small or large relative to the overall tooth. Larger restorations require higher mechanical properties. While biting forces may range from about 70 to 300 N (16–67 lb force), the *stresses* on dental restorative materials can exceed several thousand megapascals (pounds per square inch) because of the small cross-sectional area of the cusps. Second, many dental materials are placed while in a soft, pliable form and cured or hardened in the mouth. This *in situ* clinical usage requires materials that can cure with biocompatible components and catalysts, in a moist environment and in short periods of time. Third, dental restoratives have the unique requirement of needing to be aesthetic. This combination of requirements has resulted in a wide range of materials used in dentistry to restore carious lesions or trauma.

5.4.3 Historical and Current Dental Biomaterials

The practice of dentistry and the advent of dental biomaterials date back to almost 3000 BC, with the use of hand-carved ivory or bone teeth held in place by gold bands or wires. Through the sixteenth and seventeenth centuries, teeth were prepared and restored with a range of natural materials including stones, ivory, natural resins, cork, and metals. Many consider the use of pure gold foils in the eighteenth century as the beginning of contemporary dentistry. When properly handled, pure gold can be compressed into tooth preparations to form a biocompatible, mechanically competent restoration. The procedure is still practiced today in some regions. However, the needs for higher mechanical properties to restore large sections of the tooth and the ability to bond to the remaining tooth structure, as well as the demand for less operator-sensitive and aesthetic materials, continue to drive improvements in dental materials.

Today, small restorations are usually restored with a composite of acrylate-based resin and micron-sized glass or ceramic particles (Table 5.2). The most popular resin is Bis-GMA. The neat resin is transparent and can be pigmented to match the wide range of tooth shades. Generally, 50–70 vol% filler is added to reduce polymerization shrinkage and to achieve the necessary strength, modulus, and hardness. The composites are provided to the dentist in paste form. Following removal of the carious lesion and preparation of the tooth, the cavity is treated to provide bonding to the enamel and dentin. An unfilled, acrylate-based "bonding resin" is applied, followed by the more viscous, high strength composite. The system can be either light or chemically cured. Dental composites provide very good service, but technique sensitivity, polymerization shrinkage, wear in high stress bearing locations, and long-term stability of the bond to dentin remain concerns.

Larger restorations that include multiple cusps require restoration with materials that have higher mechanical properties than dental composites. Such clinical situations are often restored with dental amalgam. Dental amalgam is supplied to the dentist in premeasured capsules containing ~50% particles of amalgam alloy, Ag–Sn–Cu, and 50% liquid mercury. The capsules are vibrated to break the separating seal and mix the

TABLE 5.2   Types of Dental Biomaterials

Type of Dental Restoration	Category of Dental Material	Primary Components
Small restorations	Composite	50% Acrylate resin, 50% ceramic or glass particles
	Amalgam	Ag, Cu, Sn, Hg
Large restorations	Gold casting alloys	Au–Ag–Cu–Pd–Pt
	Base metal alloys	Cr–Co–Ni
	All-ceramic	Strengthened ceramic
Tooth replacement	Fix partial denture	Au–Ag–Cu–Pd–Pt Cr–Co–Ni
	Removable partial denture	Cr–Co–Ni
	Complete denture	Methacrylates
	Implant	CP titanium

components. The resulting plastic mix is placed in the cavity and hardens through a chemical reaction. While having provided excellent clinical service over the years, amalgam use continues to decline, being replaced with the more aesthetic, higher strength composites and ceramic materials.

When dental disease leaves too little remaining tooth structure to mechanically support a restorative cavity, most of the coronal portion of the tooth is removed and replaced. The high mechanical properties required for this clinical situation dictate the use of metal casting alloys or high-strength ceramics. To fabricate the restoration in metal, a gypsum cast of the prepared tooth is sent to a dental laboratory, where a wax model of the restoration is cast in either a noble or base metal alloy. The casting is usually veneered with porcelain for aesthetic purposes (Figure 5.7a).

The advent of high-strength, machinable ceramics has allowed the introduction of all-ceramic restorations (Figure 5.7b) as an alternative to traditional metal casting and porcelain-fused-to-metal restorations. Several fabrication methods are available, including the use of computer-assisted design, computer-assisted machining (CAD/CAM). The all-ceramic restorations can be very aesthetic because they are translucent with no underlying, dark metal casting.

If dental disease becomes extensive, it may not be possible to repair a tooth, but extraction and replacement may become necessary. Depending on the number of teeth to be replaced and the condition of the remaining teeth and bone, tooth replacement is accomplished with a cast metal fixed partial denture, a removable partial denture, a methacrylate removable complete denture, or a dental implant. The use of dental implants is rapidly expanding because of growing long-term clinical experience, improving techniques and the ability of implants to replace an individual tooth without involving adjacent teeth. Most dental implants are fabricated from commercially pure (CP) titanium. Bone grows into direct contact with the titanium oxide surface, a process referred to as osseointegration, providing the necessary functional support. Current research is directed toward improving the rate, extent, and stability of osseointegration with various implant designs and coatings.

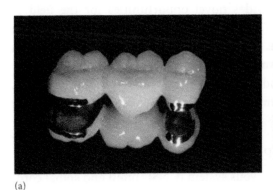
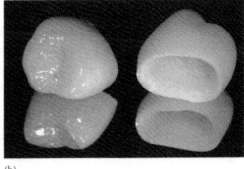

(a) (b)

FIGURE 5.7 Porcelain-fused-to-metal (a) and all-ceramic prostheses (b) for restoration of coronal portions of teeth. (Courtesy of Dr. P. Rungruanganunt.)

5.4.4 Regenerative Engineering of Dental Tissues

While the various dental restorative and implant biomaterials described earlier continue to be improved, there remains the fundamental problems that the treatments do not result in a physiological repair and a potentially problematic interface remains between the restoration or prosthesis and the natural tissues. Regenerative engineering of diseased or traumatized tissue remains the ultimate goal and progress in this area is accelerating.

Regenerative engineering of the pulp and hard dental tissue is a critical goal and recent discoveries demonstrate this can be achieved. Adult stem cells have been identified in the dental pulp and there is substantial evidence for the regenerative potential of the dentin and pulp by these cells.

Dentin is formed by odontoblast cells. Strong noxious stimuli including deep caries that lead to destruction of existing odontoblasts is followed by formation of reparative dentin secreted by a new generation of odontoblast-like cells derived from a precursor population in dental pulp (Sloan and Smith 2007). Potential populations of cells in dental pulp capable of giving rise to the new generation of odontoblasts are many (Sloan and Waddington 2009). A growing number of new studies have implicated a unique population of postnatal dental pulp stem cells (DPSC) as a potential precursor to the new generation of odontoblast-like cells (Jepsen et al. 1997). This subset of undifferentiated cells represent as little as 1% of the total cell population in the pulp; were clonogenic, pluripotent, highly proliferative; and were capable of regenerating a dentin pulp–like complex when mixed with HA–tricalcium phosphate (HA–TCP) powder and transplanted into immunocompromised mice. Furthermore, it was shown that treatment of DSPC with mineralization-inducing media (β-glycerophosphate and ascorbic acid) and/or ethylenediaminetetraacetic acid (EDTA)-soluble dentin extract (DE) resulted in the formation of odontoblast-like cells *in vitro* (Nakashima 1994). The same group has also identified a potential mesenchymal stem cell population derived from exfoliated deciduous human teeth (SHED), capable of extensive proliferation and multipotential differentiation.

The regenerative potential of the dentin and pulp together with the identification of different groups of stem/progenitor cell populations in dental pulp capable of differentiating into odontoblast-like cells provides novel opportunities for the field of dental tissue engineering. Several studies have shown that various scaffolds including polyglycolic acid (PGA), hydrogel, alginate, collagens, a porous ceramic, and a fibrous titanium mesh can support proliferation and differentiation of mineralized tissues by dental pulp stem/progenitor cells (Sloan and Smith 2007; Sloan and Waddington 2009). Efforts continue to identify appropriate stem/progenitor cells, scaffolds, and factors for dental regenerative engineering.

5.5 BIOMATERIALS FOR NEURAL REPAIR AND REPLACEMENT

The nervous system consists of the central nervous system (CNS) (brain and spinal cord) and the peripheral nervous system (sensory receptors and neurons, and motor neurons) that carry messages to and from the CNS, such as sensations of touch and taste, and activities including sight and motion. In addition to the brain and the spinal cord, principal organs of the nervous system include the following: eyes, ears, sensory organs of taste, sensory organs of smell, and sensory receptors located in the skin, joints, muscles, and other parts of the body. It is a complex, sophisticated system that regulates and coordinates the body's basic function and activities and is vulnerable to various disorders.

5.5.1 Clinical Problem

The nervous system can be damaged by many things including trauma, infections, degeneration, and tumors. Acute spinal cord injury (SCI) is a common cause of permanent disability and death in children and adults. About 11,000 people a year sustain a SCI from falls, motor vehicle accidents, and sports injuries. About 247,000 people in the United States are living with a SCI. More than half of all SCIs occur among young people between the ages of 16 and 30 years. The majority of SCI victims (78%) are males (Rush University Medical Center 2012).

Generally, the higher up the level of the injury to the spinal cord, the more severe the symptoms, with quadriplegia resulting from an injury of the spine close to the brain. Currently, there is no treatment to repair a damaged or bruised spinal cord, although researchers are actively seeking means of stimulating spinal cord regeneration. The peripheral nervous system on the other hand has a regenerative capacity and there are clinically successful repair strategies for small defects. This subchapter will therefore focus on peripheral nerve repair.

Peripheral nerves have a tubular anatomy with a sheath of loose fibrocollagenous tissue holding many nerve cell axons that conduct electrical impulses. Just as electrical wires need to be wrapped to prevent short circuiting, the nerve cells are wrapped by Schwann cells that produce a nonconductive myelin sheath. Many myelinated axons are clustered together into fascicles that are further bound together by the loose fibrocollagenous tissue into a larger tubular structure that is known as a peripheral nerve. Small blood vessels or capillaries are also found in the nerve. Damage to the peripheral nervous system in the form of a gap can occur due to trauma (saw, knife, bullet, and glass accidents) that leads to crushing or severing of the peripheral nerve. Electrical conduction is broken and sensation is lost. In 1995, there were in excess of 50,000 peripheral nerve repair procedures performed.

Surgically assisted peripheral nerve gap regeneration is possible as long as there is accurate alignment of the original fascicles. The microsurgical repair of peripheral nerves involves bringing the two ends of the nerve together and suturing them together. If the two ends are unable to be joined without tension, then a bridging section of nerve autograft taken from the back of the leg (sural nerve) is used. As with all autograft harvest procedures, there is loss of function at the donor site and often pain, thus alternatives to using nerve autograft in the gap have been developed. By surrounding a peripheral nerve gap of 3–10 mm in length with a tubular nerve guide, the nerve can regenerate within the tube because the tube creates a microenvironment for the Schwann cells to secrete neurotropic factors and form cellular tracks for the regenerating axons to follow and connect to the severed end (Van Blitterswijk 2008). New nerve growth occurs in humans at a rate of about 1 mm/day, thus significant injuries can take many months to heal and typically heal incompletely. A brief historical background of nerve repair strategies is given here but is covered in depth in Chapter 12.

5.5.2 Design Criteria for Nerve Repair and Replacement

Healthy nerve tissue has the ability to generate and conduct electrical signals, called nerve impulses, thus this is the primary outcome desired of the regenerated tissue. Since nerve cells in the peripheral nervous system have the capability to regenerate, the use of tubular biomaterials has been examined. The ideal graft material should have physical and biochemical characteristics similar to those of native nerve. The structure of the artificial graft may need to simulate the architecture of native nerve ECM, containing a series of longitudinally aligned channels with finely controlled diameters and interconnective structures.

5.5.3 Historical and Currently Used Biomaterials for Nerve Repair and Replacement

While there are no materials currently suitable for repair of the CNS, the use of biomaterials as peripheral nerve conduits has a long experimental and clinical history. The first nerve conduit was attempted as early as the late nineteenth century, but then abandoned until the 1980s when silicone tubing was discovered as a useful biomaterial for nerve conduits. Now silicone, collagen, PGA, and poly(lactic acid-*co*-caprolactone) tubing (Figure 5.8) are all used clinically as alternatives to autologous nerve grafting (Meek and Coert 2002; de Ruiter et al. 2009). Nonbiodegradable PTFE nerve tubes (GORE-TEX or Teflon) have been used in patients for median and ulnar nerve (Stanec and Stanec 1998) and inferior alveolar/lingual nerve lesions.

Luminal fillers, factors introduced into these nerve conduits, were later developed to enhance the nerve regeneration through the conduits. For example, a chitosan tube with internal oriented filaments of PGA has been used in patients as well as combinations of PGA tubes with collagen sponges. Although these synthetic grafts may avoid the problems

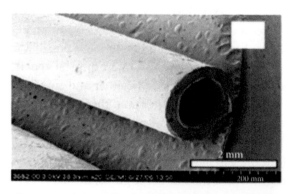

FIGURE 5.8 Scanning electron micrograph of poly(caprolactone fumarate) nerve conduit. (From *Acta Biomater.*, 5, Wang, S., Yaszemski, M.J., Knight, A.M., Gruetzmacher, J.A., Windebank, A.J., and Lu, L., Photo-cross-linked poly(epsilon-caprolactone fumarate) networks for guided peripheral nerve regeneration: Material properties and preliminary biological evaluations, 1531–1542, Copyright 2009, Elsevier.)

of availability, donor-site morbidity, and immune rejection, they do not possess an architecture similar to that of native nerve ECM, which may be necessary to provide precise directional guidance for axonal regeneration. Ongoing biomaterials research is thus focused on enhancing the inner architecture of the tubular nerve guide, as well as incorporating the use of growth factors and cells.

5.6 OPHTHALMIC BIOMATERIALS

5.6.1 Clinical Need

Biomaterials play a critical role in addressing several ophthalmic clinical conditions. Polymeric biomaterials are used as corneal implants, surgical adhesives, and implants for glaucoma and detached retinas (Refojo 2004). However, the major applications of ophthalmic biomaterials are for contact lenses and intraocular lens implants, the subjects of this section.

5.6.2 Biomaterials for Ophthalmic Repair and Replacement

5.6.2.1 Contact Lenses

Contact lenses are used widely throughout the world, although there is variation in the types of lenses used between countries. In the United States, about 30 million people wear contact lenses or about 20% of the people require vision correction. Worldwide there are ~125 million contact lens users (Barr 2005).

As biomaterials, contact lenses require an unusual combination of mechanical and physical properties. The materials need to have sufficient mechanical characteristics to resist tearing and permanent deformation, but soft contact lenses with modulus values of about 0.3 MPa are preferred for comfort (Opdahl et al. 2003). Additionally, the materials must be optically transparent, biocompatible, and chemically and thermally stable. However, most of the materials developed in the last 10 years has focused on engineering materials that additionally are highly wettable (hydrophilic), highly permeable to oxygen and electrolytes, and resistant to protein absorption (Goda et al. 2009). The cornea has no blood vessels, so it obtains oxygen from the air and from tears. Insufficient oxygen will result in corneal edema and other complications (Goda et al. 2009). Increasing the transport of oxygen and electrolytes, while resisting protein accumulation, allows contact lenses to be worn for extended periods of time. Oxygen permeability is generally expressed by the parameter Dk, which is measured in barrer units. A permeability of greater than 125 barrer is believed to be necessary in an extended use of contact lens to avoid adverse physiological effects due to oxygen depletion (Harvitt and Bonanno 1999).

The concept of a contact lens can be traced back to Leonardo da Vinci (Heitz and Enoch 1987). The method was reduced to practice with glass lenses in the late 1800s but was not fully commercialized until the 1940s with the use of poly(methyl methacrylate) (PMMA) (Nicolson and Vogt 2001). PMMA has excellent optical properties, biocompatibility, and acceptable surface wettability and can be readily machined. Of course, PMMA is rigid, so most patients require a period of adjustment. Additionally, the low oxygen permeability and protein accumulation of PMMA lenses required more frequent removal and cleaning. Rigid contact lens were made more permeable to oxygen by copolymerizing the methyl methacrylate with methacrylate-functionalized siloxanes and fluoromethacrylates, which increase the Dk permeability values to 10–30 and 30–160 barrer, respectively (Lloyd et al. 2001). However, silicone components also increase hydrophobicity and protein absorption.

A major advancement in the field came with the introduction of "soft" contact lenses based on hydrogels (Wichterle et al. 1961). The original contact lens hydrogels were lightly cross-linked poly(2-hydroxyethyl methacrylate) or polyHEMA. The network hydrophilic polymer structure with less than 1% cross-linking can retain water and the first formulations contained 38% water. Later formulations incorporated up to 50% water. The low modulus of the hydrated hydrogels makes the lenses more comfortable to wear and provides almost immediate patient acceptance. Nevertheless, two problems with the original hydrogels were dehydration and reliance on the water in the hydrogel to transport the oxygen. The oxygen permeability of water itself is limited to about 80 Dk barrer units, so higher permeability would be needed for extended use. This need leads to the use of polydimethylsiloxane (PDMS) for soft contact lenses (Lloyd et al. 2001). PDMS has very high oxygen permeability, with Dk values of up to 600 barrer, but siloxanes are very hydrophobic and bind proteins. The effect of water content on the oxygen permeability of acrylate and silicone is shown in Figure 5.9.

Accordingly, much of the research in the last 10 years has involved investigating approaches for combining the favorable oxygen transportation characteristics of silicones with the favorable hydrophilic characteristics of acrylate-based hydrogels. Simply blending these two components is problematic because they are immiscible. This phase

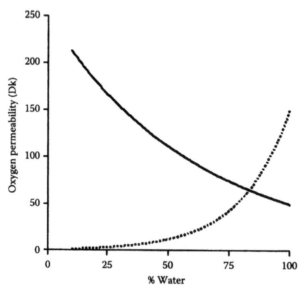

FIGURE 5.9 Effect of water content on oxygen permeability of acrylate (dashed line) and silicone (solid line) hydrogels. (From *Biomaterials*, 22, Lloyd, A.W., Faragher, R.G., and Denyer, S.P., Ocular biomaterials and implants, 769–785, Copyright 2011, Elsevier.)

separation can interfere with light transmission, so heterogeneous systems have generally been avoided in contact lens design. However, this problem was overcome by limiting the size of the phase regions to less than that of the wavelength of light (Nicolson and Vogt 2001). The resulting silicone hydrogels are very sophisticated biomaterials involving design of both the chemistry and the microstructure. A remaining problem is that the silicone component can still migrate to the surface so plasma surface treatments are sometimes used to maintain surface hydrophilicity (Olah et al. 2005). Silicone hydrogels were first commercially available in 1998. Their excellent balance of oxygen permeability, hydrophilicity, and mechanical properties makes them currently the most popular materials system for contact lenses.

5.6.2.2 Intraocular Lenses Implants

The lens of the eye is located in the posterior chamber immediately behind the iris. With age the lens becomes opaque reducing clarity, a process that eventually leads to blindness. This clouding of the lens is called a cataract and it is the leading cause of blindness worldwide (World Health Organization 2009). In the developed countries, the cataractous lens are removed and replaced with polymeric intraocular lens (IOLs) in a short surgical procedure that is now routine. The origination and development of the procedure over the past 60 years is a result of improved, less traumatic procedures to remove the cataractous lens and improvement of synthetic polymeric lenses that satisfy the requirements of biocompatibility, translucency, stability, and mechanical compliance.

In what is now one of the classic observations in biomaterials, Ridley (1951) noted that fragments of PMMA from damaged canopies of World War II airplanes remained stable in the pilots' eyes without excessive inflammation or foreign body reaction. This led to the concept of replacement IOLs and PMMA was successfully employed for many years. However, the early procedures placed the IOL in the anterior chamber of the eye in front of the iris. The evolution of IOLs was closely tied to the development of surgical techniques that required smaller incisions to remove the cataractous lens and placement of the polymeric IOL in its natural position behind the iris. A major improvement was the introduction of elastomeric IOLs that could be folded and inserted into the smaller incision, opening to their functional shape once in position. Polysiloxanes were the first foldable IOLs and with modification remain popular today. A second major category of IOLs in use are based on hydrophobic acrylates.

5.7 BIOMATERIALS FOR SKIN/WOUND HEALING AND REPLACEMENT

Skin is the largest organ of the body. It covers and protects everything in the body. Skin plays a vital role in maintaining homeostasis, preventing evaporation of body fluid, providing immunity, and supporting sensory feedback. Macroscopically, skin is a dual-layer organ consisting of the outer epidermis layer and the inner dermis layer (Figure 5.10).

The epidermis is made up of many layers of cells that are continually growing upward and shedding. The dermis is the layer containing nerve endings, sweat glands, hair follicles, and capillaries. The capillaries satisfy nutritional needs of the cells in the dermis and help the skin perform its body cooling function.

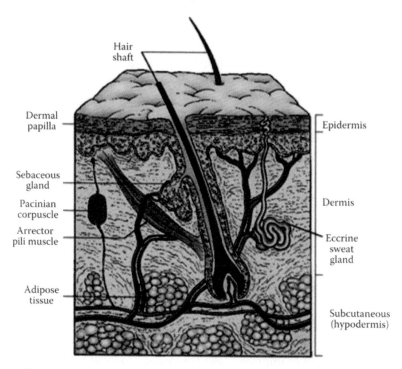

Hair
shaft

Dermal
papilla

Epidermis

Sebaceous
gland

Pacinian
corpuscle

Dermis

Arrector
pili muscle

Eccrine
sweat
gland

Adipose
tissue

Subcutaneous
(hypodermis)

FIGURE 5.10 Skin is made of multiple layers and contains glands and hair follicles in addition to the epithelial cells that make up the outer layer known as the epidermis. (From Springer Science+Business Media: *Textbook of Aging Skin*, 2010, Farage, M.A., Miller, K.W., and Maibach, H.I.)

The dermis, owing to its Type I collagen component, is mostly responsible for the structural integrity of the skin. In addition, dermal cells, specifically fibroblasts, produce chemical factors that are essential for the proper proliferation and differentiation of the epidermis. Between the dermal and epidermal layers lies a well-defined basal lamina. A proteinaceous extracellular layer, the basal lamina serves as the substrate upon which basal cells of the epidermis adhere and proliferate. Indeed, one common way to evaluate artificial skin is to assay for the presence of the basal lamina, as this would indicate dermal–epidermal integration. Basal keratinocyte cells form the first layer adjacent to the basal lamina. These cells undergo a program of proliferation and differentiation to form the full epidermal layer. The differentiated forms of epidermal cells from inner to outermost include basal, spinous, and granular keratinocytes (Figure 5.11). The stratum corneum, a highly cross-linked layer of packed keratinocytes, serves as the outermost barrier and provides the ultimate protection against desiccation.

5.7.1 Clinical Problem

There are a number of ways in which the skin becomes wounded. Smaller wounds to the skin, or bed sores, develop in the elderly due to lack of mobility and constant pressure on certain skin areas. Diabetic patients have delayed healing that leads to chronic leg skin

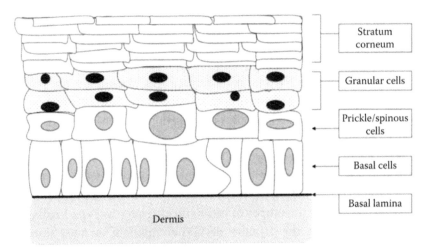

FIGURE 5.11 Skin is comprised of two layers, the dermis, which mainly contains fibroblast cells, and the epidermis, mainly containing keratinocytes at various stages of differentiation. (Illustration by V. Seetharaman from *Introduction to Biomedical Engineering*, 2nd edn., Enderle, J., Blanchard, S., and Bronzino, J., Copyright 2005, Elsevier.)

ulcers. Motorcycle or bicycle accident victims may have large areas of abraded skin requiring treatment. Large wounds to the skin, such as that resulting from burns, reduce its ability to maintain critical functions and make dehydration and infection much more of a threat. According to the American Burn Association (2008), in the United States, there are 500,000 patients per year requiring treatment for burns, with 40,000 hospitalizations/year for burn injury. Over one-third of admissions (38%) exceeded 10% total body surface area burned, and 10% exceeded 30% total body surface area burned. Most included severe burns of such vital body areas as the face, hands, and feet. Seventy percent of the patients were males and 30% females. The depth of the injury is the most important feature in determining the innate ability of the epidermis to undergo self-regeneration and thus achieve wound closure.

Traditionally, surgeons have used allogenic skin grafts as a primary means of treatment for most large-scale skin injuries. Because of additional wounding that results from skin grafts, considerable research has been devoted to the development of a skin equivalent and tissue-engineered skin is now available clinically to patients from several manufacturers. As will be seen, biomaterials are vital to the formation of skin substitutes that can truly act as replacements for the original.

5.7.2 Design Criteria for Skin Repair and Replacement

The primary goals of skin replacement are to prevent evaporation and to be a flexible material preventing infection. In the biomimetic tradition, it has been thought that effective skin substitutes should mimic the layered natural skin structure. In addition, well-designed skin substitutes should possess the proper physical integrity to withstand the environment and, at the same time, support the ingrowth of the cells.

5.7.3 Historical and Currently Used Biomaterials for Skin Repair and Replacement

Conventional autologous split thickness skin autografts still represent the gold standard to resurface large wounds. However, depending on the extent of lost skin, the donor sites may be limited. In patients with a 5% total body surface area wound, it is not possible to take skin from another area of the patient without increasing the mortality rate.

The possibility of tissue-engineered skin began with the discovery of the ability to culture epithelial cells under controlled *in vitro* conditions. Another catalyzing discovery was that epithelial cells would form the natural layers of skin when cultured at the air–water interface. A schematic drawing of a bilayered living artificial skin is shown in Figure 5.12. Biomaterials, in addition to providing the proper substrates for cellular growth, are excellent sources of mechanical strength. Type I collagen, a cross-linked polymer, is used as the primary dermal component of most skin substitutes. When cross-linked, collagen provides a mechanically sound matrix upon which to grow an epidermal layer and can even be impregnated with fibroblasts to provide chemical factors that diffuse through the porous collagen and allow for proper epidermal cell differentiation and proliferation.

To complete the dual-layer skin substitute, epidermal keratinocytes are seeded on the dermis and allowed to differentiate into the proper epithelial cellular arrangement. Some skin substitutes actually use a thin layer of silicone as a functional epithelial barrier while the dermal layer integrates into the wound site. A subsequent procedure replaces the silicone with an epidermal matrix, thus completing the skin. Both collagen and silicone are examples of how biomaterials can be used to recreate the functionality of normal skin.

Despite the advances, there are still problems with tissue-engineered skin that need further research and development. For example, the artificial skin cannot prevent infection since it lacks immune cells such as dendritic cells. Tissue rejection also eventually occurs. While allogeneic keratinocytes survive for long periods after transplantation

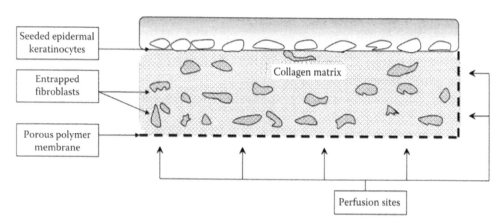

FIGURE 5.12 Drawing of biomimetic artificial skin showing the dual-layer structure similar to natural skin. (Illustration by V. Seetharaman from *Introduction to Biomedical Engineering*, 2nd edn., Enderle, J., Blanchard, S., and Bronzino, J., Copyright 2005, Elsevier.)

into a skin wound, rejection eventually occurs along with infiltration and growth of the patient's own skin cells. Since the rejection is so slow in the skin setting, it was not realized until recently.

ACKNOWLEDGMENT

The authors gratefully acknowledge technical and administrative assistance from Cheryl Gomillion for identifying some of the images used in this chapter and for accomplishing the significant task of obtaining copyright permissions and appropriate quality images.

REFERENCES

Ahovuo-Saloranta, A., Hiiri, A., Nordblad, A., Worthington, H., and Makela, M. 2004. Pit and fissure sealants for preventing dental decay in the permanent teeth of children and adolescents (review). *Cochrane Database of Systematic Reviews, 3.*

American Burn Association. 2008. Burn incidence and treatment in the US: 2007 fact sheet. http://www.ameriburn.org/resources_factsheet.php (accessed on December 19, 2012)

Barr, J., 2005. 2004 Annual Report—Contact lens spectrum. http://www.clspectrum.com (accessed on April 30, 2012)

Bhatt, H. and Goswami, T. 2008. Implant wear mechanisms—Basic approach. *Biomed Mater*, 3, 042001.

Chen, F.-M. and Jin, Y. 2010. Periodontal tissue engineering and regeneration: Current approaches and expanding opportunities. *Tissue Eng Part B*, 16, 219–255.

Chlupac, J., Filova, E., and Bacakova, L. 2009. Blood vessel replacement: 50 years of development and tissue engineering paradigms in vascular surgery. *Physiol Res*, 58(Suppl 2), S119–S139.

Creager, M. 2009. *Essential Atlas of Cardiovascular Disease.* New York: Springer.

Dabagh, M. and Al, E. 2005. Effects of polydimethylsiloxane grafting on the calcification, physical properties, and biocompatibility of polyurethane in a heart valve. *J Appl Polymer Sci*, 98, 758–766.

de Ruiter, G.C., Malessy, M.J., Yaszemski, M.J., Windebank, A.J., and Spinner, R.J. 2009. Designing ideal conduits for peripheral nerve repair. *Neurosurg Focus*, 26, E5.

Enderle, J., Blanchard, S., and Bronzino, J. 2005. *Introduction to Biomedical Engineering*, 2nd edn. Amsterdam, the Netherlands: Elsevier.

Erbel, R., Di Mario, C., Bartunek, J., Bonnier, J., De Bruyne, B., Eberli, F.R., Erne, P. et al. 2007. Temporary scaffolding of coronary arteries with bioabsorbable magnesium stents: A prospective, non-randomised multicentre trial. *Lancet*, 369, 1869–1875.

Farage, M.A., Miller, K.W., and Maibach, H.I. 2010. *Textbook of Aging Skin.* New York: Springer.

Faries, P.L., Logerfo, F.W., Arora, S., Hook, S., Pulling, M.C., Akbari, C.M., Campbell, D.R., and Pomposelli, F.B., Jr. 2000. A comparative study of alternative conduits for lower extremity revascularization: All-autogenous conduit versus prosthetic grafts. *J Vasc Surg*, 32, 1080–1090.

Farr, J., Cole, B., Dhawan, A., Kercher, J., and Sherman, S. 2011. Clinical cartilage restoration: Evolution and overview. *Clin Orthop Relat Res*, 469, 2696–2705.

Franklin, J.E., Marler, J.J., Byrne, M.T., Melvin, A.J., Clarson, S.J., and Melvin, D.B. 2009. Fiber technology for reliable repair of skeletal muscle. *J Biomed Mater Res B*, 90, 259–266.

Friedewald, V.E., Bonow, R.O., Borer, J.S., Carabello, B.A., Kleine, P.P., Akins, C.W., and Roberts, W.C. 2007. The Editor's Roundtable: Cardiac valve surgery. *Am J Cardiol*, 99, 1269–1278.

Fu, F.H., Bennett, C.H., Lattermann, C., and Ma, C.B. 1999. Current trends in anterior cruciate ligament reconstruction. Part 1: Biology and biomechanics of reconstruction. *Am J Sports Med*, 27, 821–830.

Gaziano, J.M. and Libby, P. 2009. *Essential Atlas of Cardiovascular Disease.* New York: Springer.

Ge, Z., Yang, F., Goh, J.C., Ramakrishna, S., and Lee, E.H. 2006. Biomaterials and scaffolds for ligament tissue engineering. *J Biomed Mater Res A*, 77, 639–652.

Georgiadis, G.S., Lazarides, M.K., Lambidis, C.D., Panagoutsos, S.A., Kostakis, A.G., Bastounis, E.A., and Vargemezis, V.A. 2005. Use of short PTFE segments (<6 cm) compares favorably with pure autologous repair in failing or thrombosed native arteriovenous fistulas. *J Vasc Surg*, 41, 76–81.

Ghanbari, H., Viatge, H., Kidane, A.G., Burriesci, G., Tavakoli, M., and Seifalian, A.M. 2009. Polymeric heart valves: New materials, emerging hopes. *Trends Biotechnol*, 27, 359–367.

Goda, T., Matsuno, R., Konno, T., Takai, M., and Ishihara, K. 2009. Protein adsorption resistance and oxygen permeability of chemically crosslinked phospholipid polymer hydrogel for ophthalmologic biomaterials. *J Biomed Mater Res B*, 89, 184–190.

Hanawa, T. 2009. Materials for metallic stents. *J Artif Organs*, 12, 73–79.

Harvitt, D.M. and Bonanno, J.A. 1999. Re-evaluation of the oxygen diffusion model for predicting minimum contact lens Dk/t values needed to avoid corneal anoxia. *Optom Vis Sci*, 76, 712–719.

Hausen, H. 2004. Benefits of topical fluorides firmly established. *Evid Based Dent*, 5, 36–37.

Heitz, R.F. and Enoch, J.M. 1987. Leonardo da Vinci: An assessment on his discourses on image formation in the eye. Fiorentini, A., Guyton, D.L., and Siegel, I.M., (ed.). In *Advances in Diagnostic Visual Optics*, Springer-verlag, Dusseldorf, pp. 19–26.

Hofbauer, P. and Smulders, F.J.M. 2011. The muscle biological background of meat quality including that of game species. Paulsen, P., Bauler, A., Vodnansky, M., Winkelmayer, R., and Smulders, F.J.M., (ed.). In *Game Meat Hygiene in Focus*. New York: Springer pp. 273–295.

Jepsen, S., Albers, H.K., Fleiner, B., Tucker, M., and Rueger, D. 1997. Recombinant human osteogenic protein-1 induces dentin formation: An experimental study in miniature swine. *J Endod*, 23, 378–382.

Johns Hopkins Medicine Health Alerts. 2009. Surgery for heart disease: Angioplasty vs. bypass surgery. http://www.johnshopkinshealthalerts.com/reports/heart_health/263-1.html?type=pf (accessed on April 12, 2012)

Kannan, R.Y. 2007. Silsesquioxane nanocomposites as tissue implants. *Plast Reconstr Surg*, 119, 1653–1662.

Kidane, A.G., Burriesci, G., Cornejo, P., Dooley, A., Sarkar, S., Bonhoeffer, P., Edirisinghe, M., and Seifalian, A.M., 2009. Current developments and future prospects for heart valve replacement therapy. *J Biomed Mater Res B*, 88, 290–303.

Klinkert, P., Post, P.N., Breslau, P.J., and Van Bockel, J.H. 2004. Saphenous vein versus PTFE for above-knee femoropopliteal bypass. A review of the literature. *Eur J Vasc Endovasc Surg*, 27, 357–362.

Lloyd, A.W., Faragher, R.G., and Denyer, S.P. 2001. Ocular biomaterials and implants. *Biomaterials*, 22, 769–785.

Lovegrove, J.M. 2004. Dental plaque revisited: Bacteria associated with periodontal disease. *J N Z Soc Periodontol*, 87, 7–21.

Mayo Clinic. 2010. Heart disease. http://www.mayoclinic.com/health/heart-disease/DS01120 (accessed on April 12, 2010)

Meek, M.F. and Coert, J.H. 2002. Clinical use of nerve conduits in peripheral-nerve repair: Review of the literature. *J Reconstr Microsurg*, 18, 97–109.

Morice, M.C., Serruys, P.W., Sousa, J.E., Fajadet, J., Ban Hayashi, E., Perin, M., Colombo, A. et al. 2002. A randomized comparison of a sirolimus-eluting stent with a standard stent for coronary revascularization. *N Engl J Med*, 346, 1773–1780.

Nakashima, M. 1994. Induction of dentine in amputated pulp of dogs by recombinant human bone morphogenetic proteins-2 and -4 with collagen matrix. *Arch Oral Biol*, 39, 1085–1089.

National Health Expenditure Projections 2009–2019. 2010. *Health & Human Services*, Washington, DC: Centers for Medicare & Medicaid Services.

Nicolson, P.C. and Vogt, J. 2001. Soft contact lens polymers: An evolution. *Biomaterials*, 22, 3273–3283.

Olah, A., Hillborg, H., and Vancso, G.J. 2005. Hydrophobic recovery of UV/ozone treated poly(dimethylsiloxane): Adhesion studies by contact mechanics and mechanism of surface modification. *Appl Surf Sci*, 239, 410–423.

Opdahl, A., Kim, S.H., Koffas, T.S., Marmo, C., and Somorjai, G.A. 2003. Surface mechanical properties of pHEMA contact lenses: Viscoelastic and adhesive property changes on exposure to controlled humidity. *J Biomed Mater Res A*, 67, 350–356.

Pennisi, E. 2002. Tending tender tendons. *Science*, 295, 1001.

Puskas, J.E., Munoz-Robledo, L.G., Hoerr, R.A., Foley, J., Schmidt, S.P., Evancho-Chapman, M., Dong, J., Frethem, C., and Haugstad, G. 2009. Drug-eluting stent coatings. *Wiley Interdiscip Rev Nanomed Nanobiotechnol*, 1, 451–462.

Refojo, M.F. 2004. Ophthalmological applications. In B.D. Ratner, A.S. Hoffman, F.J. Schoen, and J.E. Lemons (eds.), *Biomaterials Science*, 2nd edn. Amsterdam, the Netherlands: Elsevier, pp. 583–590.

Rey, C., Combes, C., Drouet, C., and Glimcher, M.J. 2009. Bone mineral: Update on chemical composition and structure. *Osteoporous Int*, 20, 1013–1021.

Riccotta, J.J. 2005. Vascular conduits: An overview. In R.B. Rutherford (ed.), *Vascular Surgery*. Philadelphia, PA: Elsevier-Saunders, pp. 688–695.

Ridley, H. 1951. Intra-ocular acrylic lenses. *Trans Ophthalmol Soc UK*, 71, 617–621.

Rush University Medical Center. 2012. Spinal cord trauma. http://health.rush.edu/healthinformation/hie%20multimedia/1/001066.aspx (accessed on December 19, 2012)

Sanan, A. and Haines, S.J. 1997. Repairing holes in the head: A history of cranioplasty. *Neurosurgery*, 40, 588–602.

Serruys, P.W., De Jaegere, P., Kiemeneij, F., Macaya, C., Rutsch, W., Heyndrickx, G., Emanuelsson, H. et al. 1994. A comparison of balloon-expandable-stent implantation with balloon angioplasty in patients with coronary artery disease. Benestent Study Group. *N Engl J Med*, 331, 489–495.

Sigwart, U., Puel, J., Mirkovitch, V., Joffre, F., and Kappenberger, L. 1987. Intravascular stents to prevent occlusion and restenosis after transluminal angioplasty. *N Engl J Med*, 316, 701–706.

Sloan, A.J. and Smith, A.J. 2007. Stem cells and the dental pulp: Potential roles in dentine regeneration and repair. *Oral Dis*, 13, 151–157.

Sloan, A.J. and Waddington, R.J. 2009. Dental pulp stem cells: What, where, how? *Int J Paediatr Dent*, 19, 61–70.

Soldani, G., Losi, P., Bernabei, M., Burchielli, S., Chiappino, D., Kull, S., Briganti, E., and Spiller, D. 2010. Long term performance of small-diameter vascular grafts made of a poly(ether) urethane–polydimethylsiloxane semi-interpenetrating polymeric network. *Biomaterials*, 31, 2592–2605.

Sommers, J.P. 2007. *Dental Expenditures in the 10 Largest States, 2004*. U.S. Department of Health and Human Services. Rockville, MD.

Stanec, S. and Stanec, Z. 1998. Reconstruction of upper-extremity peripheral-nerve injuries with ePTFE conduits. *J Reconstr Microsurg*, 14, 227–232.

Stehouwer, C.D., Clement, D., Davidson, C., Diehm, C., Elte, J.W., Lambert, M., and Sereni, D. 2009. Peripheral arterial disease: A growing problem for the internist. *Eur J Intern Med*, 20, 132–138.

Summitt, J.B., Robbins, J.W., Schwartz, R.S., and Santos, J. 2001. *Fundamentals of Operative Dentistry*, 2nd edn. Chicago, IL: Quintessence Publishing Co, Inc.

Theron, J.P., Knoetze, J.H., Sanderson, R.D., Hunter, R., Mequanint, K., Franz, T., Zilla, P., and Bezuidenhout, D. 2010. Modification, crosslinking and reactive electrospinning of a thermoplastic medical polyurethane for vascular graft applications. *Acta Biomater* (Online). www.elsevier.com/locate/actabiomat

Urist, M.R. and Mikulski, A.J. 1979. A soluble bone morphogenetic protein extracted from bone matrix with a mixed aqueous and nonaqueous solvent. *Proc Soc Exp Biol Med*, 162, 48–53.

Van Blitterswijk, C. 2008. *Tissue Engineering*. Amsterdam, the Netherlands: Elsevier.

Vunjak-Novakovic, G., Altman, G., Horan, R., and Kaplan, D.L. 2004. Tissue engineering of ligaments. *Annu Rev Biomed Eng*, 6, 131–156.

Wang, S., Yaszemski, M.J., Knight, A.M., Gruetzmacher, J.A., Windebank, A.J., and Lu, L. 2009. Photo-crosslinked poly(epsilon-caprolactone fumarate) networks for guided peripheral nerve regeneration: Material properties and preliminary biological evaluations. *Acta Biomater*, 5, 1531–1542.

Weber, F., Schneider, H., Schwarz, C., Holzhausen, C., Petzsch, M., and Nienaber, C.A. 2004. Sirolimus-eluting stents for percutaneous coronary intervention in acute myocardial infarction: Lesson from a case-controlled comparison of bare metal versus drug-eluting stents in thrombus-laden lesions. *Z Kardiol*, 93, 938–943.

Wichterle, O., Lim, D., and Dreifus, M. 1961. [On the problem of contact lenses]. *Cesk Oftalmol*, 17, 70–75.

World Health Organization. 2009. Visual impairment and blindness. http://www.who.int/mediacentre/factsheets/fs282/en/ (accessed on April 30, 2010).

CHAPTER 6

In Vitro Assessment of Cell–Biomaterial Interactions

Yong Wang, PhD

CONTENTS

6.1 INTRODUCTION

While the physicochemical and mechanical properties of biomaterials are important components to consider, the nature in which they interact with cells is equally important. A thorough understanding of how biomaterials interact with cells is critical, both *in vitro* and *in vivo*, to the proper design of implants for tissue regeneration. In this chapter, we focus on the interface between cells and biomaterials used in regenerative medicine and tissue engineering, with particular attention to methods of characterizing cell–biomaterial interactions and assessing cellular behavior on the surface of materials.

6.2 ASSESSMENT OF CELL–MATERIAL INTERACTIONS

Controlling cell–material interactions is critical to a variety of biological and biomedical applications such as regenerative engineering, surgical implantations, cell separation, and cell imaging (Kingshott and Griesser 1999; Shin et al. 2003; Ratner and Bryant 2004;

Cole et al. 2009). Thus, numerous approaches were developed in the past few decades to achieve cell adhesion or increase the resistance to cell adhesion on material surfaces. In general, the specific molecular recognition between ligands and cell receptors is used to enhance the interactions between cells and materials. Numerous affinity molecules have been derived from biological systems or chemically synthesized for this need (Shin et al. 2003). The most commonly used affinity molecules include gelatin, antibodies, and short peptides. These affinity molecules have been primarily used to functionalize materials to mimic the functionality of extracellular matrices for tissue engineering and regenerative medicine research and applications (Shin et al. 2003). Some of these applications require the prevention of cell adhesion, for the uncontrolled adhesion and accumulation of cells onto synthetic surfaces can adversely affect the functionality of various medical devices (Kingshott and Griesser 1999). At the molecular level, proteins and lipids can be rapidly adsorbed to the "naked" synthetic surface (i.e., bioadhesion), leading to subsequent adhesion of other molecules and cells (Kingshott and Griesser 1999). Therefore, research activities have been focused on modifying material surfaces to increase the resistance to bioadhesion. Various approaches and coating materials have been studied toward improving bioadhesion resistance. Of them, poly(ethylene glycol) (PEG)-based coatings have attracted the most attention (Ratner and Bryant 2004). The PEG polymers can be attached to a material surface through covalent conjugations, physical adsorption, or molecular interpenetration (Ratner and Bryant 2004). The use of optimized surface PEGylation can result in undetectable protein and cell adhesion for up to a month under normal cell culture conditions (Ma et al. 2006). Besides the studies aimed at promoting cell adhesion or increasing the resistance to cell adhesion, great efforts have also been made in developing materials and methods that can be used for capturing and releasing cells at specific time points (Cole et al. 2009). For instance, thermo- or photosensitive polymers or ligands can be immobilized on solid surfaces (Kushida et al. 1999; Akiyama et al. 2004; Auernheimer et al. 2005; Canavan et al. 2005; Yang et al. 2005; da Silva et al. 2007; Ohmuro-Matsuyama and Tatsu 2008). These polymers and ligands can be triggered by temperature or ultraviolet light and switch from an active to an inactive state. This feature can lead to the modulation of cell attachment on material surfaces. These reversible biointerfaces have been primarily investigated for monolayer cell cultures (Kushida et al. 1999; Akiyama et al. 2004; Auernheimer et al. 2005; Canavan et al. 2005; Yang et al. 2005; da Silva et al. 2007; Ohmuro-Matsuyama and Tatsu 2008), which have great potential for regenerative engineering applications. To limit the scope of discussion, this section does not elaborate on functionalizing material surfaces. The relevant information has been well described earlier. This section primarily focuses on the methodology for assessing cell–material interactions at the molecular and cellular level.

6.2.1 Evaluation of Ligand–Receptor Interactions at the Molecular Level

Materials developed for regenerative engineering are often functionalized with specific ligands that can communicate with cell receptors. The interactions between ligands and cell receptors can activate one or multiple intracellular signaling pathways. Eventually, the signals originating from the extracellular microenvironment are transmitted from the outside to the inside of a cell. The signal transduction will lead to the determination of the fate of a cell including differentiation, proliferation, migration, apoptosis, or other critical cellular functions. Additionally, the cell behavior in response to a material can also affect the functionality of the material such as material degradation or material encapsulation. Therefore, it is important to understand and quantify ligand–receptor interactions.

6.2.1.1 Kinetics and Thermodynamics of Molecular Recognition

When molecular recognition pairs are mixed together, the formation of ligand–receptor complexes is expected to occur. The molecular recognition process can be described with a simple equation:

$$L+R \Leftrightarrow LR \tag{6.1}$$

where L, R, and LR represent ligands, receptors, and ligand–receptor complexes, respectively. Because molecular recognition processes are determined by physical interactions, the formation of LR is a reversible, equilibrium reaction. The forward and reverse reactions are determined not only by their concentrations but also by two kinetic constants: the association rate constant (k_{on}) and the dissociation rate constant (k_{off}). The relationship between these parameters during the process of molecular recognition can be mathematically described with the following equation:

$$\frac{d[LR]}{dt} = k_{on}[L][R] - k_{off}[LR] \tag{6.2}$$

where [LR], [L], and [R] are used to describe the concentrations. At equilibrium, the time derivative on the left side of the equation is equal to zero. After the reorganization of this equation, it becomes

$$\frac{[L]_{eq}[R]_{eq}}{[LR]_{eq}} = \frac{k_{off}}{k_{on}} = K_d = \frac{1}{K_a} \tag{6.3}$$

where
  equilibrium is denoted with the subscript eq
  K_d is the dissociation constant
  K_a is the affinity constant

All of the parameters, including k_{on}, k_{off}, K_d, and K_a, can be determined by different experimental tools that will be introduced in later sections.

To better understand the molecular recognition between the ligands and the receptors, it is also necessary to discuss the thermodynamics of molecular recognition. We can use the Gibbs free energy, ideal gas constant, temperature, and concentrations to describe the thermodynamics by using the following equation:

$$\Delta G = \Delta G^0 + RT \ln \frac{[LR]}{[L][R]} \tag{6.4}$$

where

ΔG is the free energy at any moment
ΔG^0 is the standard-state free energy
R is the ideal gas constant
T is the temperature

The free energy, ΔG, is equal to zero at equilibrium. At equilibrium, Equation 6.4 can be written as

$$0 = \Delta G^0 + RT \ln \frac{[LR]_{eq}}{[L]_{eq}[R]_{eq}} \tag{6.5}$$

The combination of Equations 6.3 and 6.4 leads to

$$K_a = \exp\left(-\frac{\Delta G^0}{RT}\right) \tag{6.6}$$

6.2.1.2 Examination of Molecular Interactions of Free Molecules

The molecular interactions between ligands and cell receptors can be studied in terms of free molecules. There are quite a few methods that have been studied for this purpose. Of them, x-ray crystallography and nuclear magnetic resonance (NMR) have been widely used to understand molecular interactions (Bongrand 1999; Williamson 2009).

X-ray crystallography can be used to examine the contact area and the structure of the ligand, its receptor, and solvent molecules. Because antibodies have played a great role in various biological and biomedical applications including the development of novel biomaterials, crystallography has been used to study the molecular interactions between antibodies and antigens. For instance, the 3D structure of a lysozyme–antibody fragment complex was examined and refined by x-ray crystallographic techniques (Amit 1986). The results showed that the conformation of the tertiary structure of lysozyme did not change after being associated with the antibody fragment and revealed a high degree of complementarity between the lysozyme and the antibody fragment where the protrusions of the molecule well matched the depressions of the pairing molecule. In addition, 16 lysozyme residues tightly bound to 17 antibody residues to form the lysozyme–antibody interface characterized by 12 hydrogen bonds. The contact surface areas of the lysozyme and the antibody fragment were 748 and 690 Å^2, respectively. A later study further examined the 3D structures of the anti-lysozyme antibody fragment in its free and antigen-bound forms and revealed the critical role of water molecules in the molecular interactions between the ligand and the receptor (Bhat et al. 1994). Forty-eight water molecules were located at the lysozyme–antibody interface. Some of these water molecules formed a network to bridge the lysozyme and the antibody. The presence of the water molecules at the lysozyme–antibody interface weakened the hydrophobic interactions between the proteins that lead to a decrease in net entropy. The structural analysis was confirmed by the experimental measurements of change in enthalpy and entropy. These studies indicate that the main forces required for the formation of many ligand–receptor complexes arise from the hydrogen bonds between the ligand and the receptor, conformational stabilization, enthalpy of hydration, and van der Waals forces.

NMR spectroscopy is another tool available for understanding molecular interactions between ligands and receptors (Takeuchi and Wagner 2006). A distinguishing feature of NMR-based analysis is that this technique does not rely on the crystallization of ligand–receptor complexes. However, it is challenging to apply NMR to examine the molecular interactions of large biomolecules for three major reasons. First, complexes of large biomolecules have high molecular weights. Second, for a large system, it is difficult to directly measure the fast transverse relaxation. Third, it is difficult to assign NMR cross peaks due to the large number of resonances. To overcome these problems, much progress has been made in molecular labeling, deuteration, advanced pulse sequences, and exchange nuclear overhauser effect (NOE)/residual dipolar coupling (RDC) (Takeuchi and Wagner 2006). For instance, the isotope-edited NMR technique has been successfully applied to study the dynamics and conformation of the complexes formed by a peptide and antibody fragments (Tsang et al. 1992). Based on this technique, the specific resonances of an antigen bound to its antibody can be observed in a situation where its exchange rate is slow in comparison to the chemical shift time scale. In addition, local structural information can be acquired.

6.2.1.3 Examination of the Molecular Interactions between Ligands and Immobilized Receptors

The studies on free ligands and receptors can provide valuable information on molecular interactions. However, cell receptors or ligands exist in an immobilized form in real settings. Therefore, it is necessary to examine the molecular interactions between ligands and immobilized receptors. This goal can be achieved with various tools. Here, we will describe this goal by using surface plasmon resonance (SPR), atomic force microscopy (AFM), saturation transfer difference (STD) NMR, and flow cytometry.

6.2.1.3.1 Surface Plasmon Resonance SPR is a technique developed to examine the change of the refractive index of a sensor surface (McDonnell 2001). The change of the refractive index results from the binding of analytes to immobilized receptors on the sensor surface as the analytes in the solution flow on the surface. Because the refractive index can be examined in real time, the molecular interaction between ligands and receptors can be characterized in real time. Thus, the amount of analytes bound to the receptors can be measured. The real-time measurement of the change in the refractive index can be plotted as resonance units versus time, that is, a sensorgram, which can be used to calculate the association rate constant (k_{on}), the dissociation rate constant (k_{off}), and the equilibrium dissociation constant (K_d). The receptors can be immobilized onto the sensor surface with different methods. The commonly used sensor chips are functionalized with a carboxymethylated dextran matrix and a streptavidin-derivatized surface. Recently, dextran-free flat surfaces, nickel surfaces, and carboxymethylated surfaces with a reduced charge density have also been used to immobilize different types of molecules on the chip surface (McDonnell 2001). Because RGD peptides (R: arginine, G: glycine, D: aspartic acid) have been identified as key functional segments of fibronectin in promoting cell adhesion (Pierschbacher and Ruoslahti 1984), RGD has been used to functionalize various biomaterials in tissue engineering and regenerative medicine applications (Hersel et al. 2003). In addition, cell adhesive RGD sites have also been identified in other types of extracellular matrix proteins such as von Willebrand factor, collagen, laminin, osteopontin, vitronectin, and fibrinogen. Other RGD sequences have also been identified in membrane proteins on the surface of viruses and bacteria. One of the most well-studied cell receptors that bind to RGD peptides is the integrin. SPR has been used to understand the molecular interaction between RGD peptides and integrins (Liu et al. 2010). The SPR analysis revealed that the different cyclic RGD derivatives exhibited a different capability of binding to the immobilized integrin receptor, $\alpha_v\beta_3$ (Liu et al. 2010). The equilibrium dissociation constant (K_d) varied from 1×10^{-9} to 1×10^{-3} M. cRGDfK is a common peptide used for drug delivery and biomaterial functionalization. In fact, its K_d is only 1.3×10^{-6} M. The RGD derivative with the lowest K_d is cyclo[RGD-Ψ(triazole)-GK]. Its K_d is three orders of magnitude lower than that of cRGDfK. Clearly, SPR can be used to distinguish ligands with high or low affinity constants.

6.2.1.3.2 Atomic Force Microscopy   AFM is one of the most valuable tools for measuring matters at the nanoscale. The use of AFM has been found in many biological and biomedical applications, one of which is understanding the interactions of molecular pairs (Bongrand 1999). The operating principle is to move a ligand-coated surface toward a receptor-functionalized tip. The tip is mounted on a cantilever. When the surface is moving, the molecular interactions result in a continuous increase of the distractive force that can be examined by monitoring the deformation of the cantilever. With the increase in distance between the tip and the ligand-coated surface, the bonds formed between the ligand and the receptor are gradually ruptured. The rupture of the last bond will lead to a drastic change in the signal, which allows for the experimental determination of the unbinding force. The molecular pair of avidin/streptavidin and biotin has been well studied and used for various applications such as surface functionalization for enhancing cell adhesion (Anamelechi et al. 2007). Studies of this molecular pair through AFM have led to the acquisition of novel knowledge (Florin et al. 1994; Moy et al. 1994). It was found that the unbinding force was ~160 pN. This technique can also be used to determine the free energy, the reaction enthalpy, and the relationship between the unbinding force and the thermodynamic parameters (Moy et al. 1994). The AFM results showed that the effective rupture length was ~1 nm for the molecular pair (Moy et al. 1994).

6.2.1.3.3 Saturation Transfer Difference NMR   Though both SPR and AFM can provide useful information for understanding molecular interactions between ligands and receptors, the surface of solid materials is considerably different from the biophysical environment of a cell membrane and therefore does not faithfully recapitulate the functionality of cell surfaces. To solve such a problem, cell receptors can be intercalated into a biomimetic lipid membrane for studying ligand–receptor interactions (Meinecke and Meyer 2001). As previously mentioned, many NMR-based methods have been developed for understanding ligand–receptor interactions. The molecular interaction of a ligand and a bound receptor on the phospholipid bilayer has been studied by STD NMR (Meinecke and Meyer 2001). Because the receptor is inserted into the lipid bilayer, the slow tumbling of the lipid layer enables a very different saturation of the protein in the lipid bilayer. The saturation of the ligand is transferred from the lipid surface into the solution during the exchange between free and bound states. The application of different spectroscopy can eliminate signals resulting from free ligands. Thus, the STD NMR can be used to determine the binding strength of the ligands to the immobilized receptors. Based on this technique, the magnitude of the STD effect can be correlated to the concentration of the ligand. It was found that the equilibrium dissociation constant of cyclo(RGDfV) and $\alpha_{IIb}\beta_3$ was ~30–60 μM (Meinecke and Meyer 2001).

6.2.1.3.4 Flow Cytometry   Different from the methods mentioned earlier, flow cytometry can be used to directly analyze the interactions between a ligand and a receptor on the surface of a real cell (Sklar et al. 2002). Flow cytometry is a technique for measuring the fluorescence or light scatter of particles. Because flow cytometry can examine thousands of microparticles per second, this technique can sensitively and quantitatively measure complex binding kinetics and molecular interactions (Sklar et al. 2002). In the past, during the kinetic studies, a tube containing the sample was removed from the cytometer and then subjected to manual mixing. However, the manual operation can cause a dead time of ~10 s. Recent advances in optimizing the mixing procedure have decreased the dead time to subseconds, significantly improving the accuracy of the analysis. Thus, flow cytometry has been widely used to understand ligand–receptor interactions on cell surfaces and subsequently cell behavior in response to the ligand–receptor interactions. Experiments can be carried out to determine association or dissociation rate constants on the cell surface. For instance, the kinetic and equilibrium binding parameters of RGD in binding to glycoprotein IIb/IIIa on the surface of platelets have been quantified (Bednar et al. 1997). The RGD derivatives were labeled with a fluorescein moiety. The kinetic analysis indicated that the molecular interactions between RGD peptidomimetics and glycoprotein IIb/IIIa on the cell surface were a two-step binding reaction. In the first step, RGD derivatives bind to the glycoprotein IIb/IIIa with relatively low affinity to form a weak ligand–receptor complex. In the second step, after the binding, the low-molecular-weight RGD derivatives can induce conformational changes of the ligand–receptor complex. The rearrangement of the conformation is relatively slow with a rate in the tens of seconds (Bednar et al. 1997). The apparent equilibrium dissociation constant, K_d, is in the 10 nM range (Bednar et al. 1997).

6.3 EVALUATION OF CELL BEHAVIOR ON THE SURFACE OF MATERIALS

The fundamental understanding of the interactions between a ligand and its receptor can provide insightful information for the development of novel biomaterials in regenerative engineering applications. However, because the success of the applications depends on whether cells can behave as expected by communicating with the functionalized materials, it is undoubtedly necessary to directly evaluate cell behavior on the surface of a functionalized material surface. The use of *in vitro* cell culture approaches can facilitate the examination and screening of a large amount of material samples developed with different methods of surface functionalization before the use of animals for *in vivo* testing. Thus, this section will discuss the common approaches to characterizing cell behavior on the material surface.

6.3.1 Cell Source and Cell Culture

The simplest way to acquire cells for characterizing cell–material interactions is to purchase well-defined cell lines from a commercial source. For instance, the American Type Culture Collection (ATCC) is a biological resource center that has over 3500 cell lines from over 100 species (http://www.atcc.org/). A significant number of these cell lines were derived from human cells such as human aorta and human umbilical vein endothelial cells. Because these cell lines have been well established and characterized, they are reliable for pursuing reproducible studies in examining the biocompatibility of new biomaterials, new material surfaces, and the cell–material communications. However, in certain circumstances, some cell lines may not be stable in expressing critical biomarkers. Thus, an alternative method is to acquire cells directly from animals. The tissues of laboratory animals can be used to separate cells for primary or low-passaged cultures. For instance, vascular smooth muscle cells are very critical to the successful development of tissue-engineered blood vessels and therefore are important to the study of cell–material interactions. Vascular smooth muscle cells can be isolated from animals (e.g., mouse) with two common methods (Ray et al. 2001). One method is dependent on the culture of explanted vascular tissue and the migration of smooth muscle cells from the explanted tissues. The second method involves enzymatic digestion of vascular tissues followed by the plating of the dispersed smooth muscle cells. Stem cells have also been used to test the functionality of biomaterials for tissue regeneration. Adult stem cells can be isolated from bone marrow, and their differentiation into a desired cell type can be controlled by varying the properties (e.g., elasticity) of the materials (Engler et al. 2006). Cells can also be obtained from the biopsy of a human patient. Some human cells are commercially available from specialized companies (e.g., Provitro).

Cell culture for studying cell–material interactions can be carried out in two ways. One is static 2D cell culture, and the other is 3D dynamic cell culture. Static cell culture is much more commonly used because of its relative ease. In general, cell culture systems (e.g., Petri dishes) are covered by the materials to be studied. Cell suspension with the desired density is then incubated in the system at 37°C. Different parameters such as time, concentration of growth factors, and others can be varied during the culture to acquire the desired information (Yang et al. 2007). The advantages of static cell culture are its relative simplicity and reproducibility. However, to engineer a complex tissue and to understand 3D cell–material interaction, it is often necessary to carry out dynamic cell culture. For 3D dynamic cell culture, it is critical to realize the significance of nutrient/waste transports. The dynamic cell culture systems mainly include rotating bioreactors and perfusion systems (Shin 2007). In these systems, cell culture media can more efficiently penetrate the pore structures of materials and constructs to more accurately emulate the *in vivo* environment.

6.3.2 Evaluation of Cell Adhesion

The adhesion of specific cells to biomaterial surface is critical to the success of regenerative engineering. To achieve this success, specific ligands are usually used to functionalize biomaterials, as discussed in the initial portion of this chapter, to interact with target cell receptors and achieve the desired cell adhesion. During the studies of cell adhesion, it is important to bear in mind that cells need to be synchronized (Reinhart-King 2008). In general, cells are cultured until confluence, but not overgrown. In addition, it is also important to minimize adhesion-related background signals while culturing cells and in the preparation of a well-defined adhesive biomaterial. Cell adhesion is complex. It usually comprises a series of events, including cell binding to immobilized ligands on the material surface, cell spreading, actin polymerization and organization, and formation of focal adhesion (this step is usually mediated by integrins) (LeBaron and Athanasiou 2000). These events can be characterized by several common microscopy techniques such as phase contrast microscopy, fluorescence microscopy, and scanning electron microscopy (Hersel et al. 2003). Additionally, cell staining is sometimes required before cell examination.

The simplest way to evaluate cell adhesion is to use a microscope to count and examine cells. Here, the critical issue is to remove the cells that do not adhere to the material. The centrifugation assay has been developed to remove cells that do not strongly adhere to the material and to subsequently quantify the remaining cells (McClay et al. 1981). In general, cells are plated in a 96-well plate and allowed to attach to the substrate for a specified period of time. At a predetermined time point, the plate is inverted and centrifuged to detach loosely or unbound cells from the substrate. The parameters of centrifugation can be varied to satisfy different requirements. After centrifugation, the plate is removed from the centrifuge for cell counting and examination. The easiest way to count cells is to take the images of randomly chosen areas of each well and to evaluate the images with imaging software (e.g., ImageJ). The number of attached cells can also be treated with proteolytic enzymes for counting. The cells can be stained with trypan blue and counted manually by using a hemocytometer. Trypan blue is a reagent that penetrates dead cells, which allows one to discern and quantify dead and live cells. The number of cells can also be examined by testing the viability of cells (e.g., the MTT (3-(4,5-Dimethylthiazol-2-yl)-2, 5-diphenyltetrazolium bromide) assay) or the DNA content in cell lysates. Microscopic methods can also be used to characterize the cell area projected on the material surface.

Besides its usefulness in determining cell adhesion, the centrifugation assay is also useful for understanding the effect of forces on the detachment of a certain portion of cells. When ligand-mediated cell-specific binding and adhesion are studied, it is also important to use several controls to avoid artifact data. The controls include materials without ligands, materials with control ligands (i.e., inactive ligands), and cells that do not express specific receptors (Hersel et al. 2003). It is also desirable to perform a competition assay with the addition of competing free ligands into the cell culture medium. Based on these assays, it has been found that spacers, the surface distribution, and the surface density of ligands (e.g., RGD peptides) can significantly affect cell adhesion (Hersel et al. 2003).

6.3.3 Evaluation of Cell Migration

Cell migration is also a complex process. A number of signaling cascades occur during this process. Because the migration of cells on the material surface or into polymeric scaffolds is often desired for most regenerative engineering applications, it is necessary to perform an *in vitro* evaluation of this event. Cell migration can be studied in a uniform condition or a condition with chemical gradients. The latter is primarily used for the study of chemotaxis or haptotaxis. For instance, microfluidic flow has been used to produce gradient hydrogels to study cell migration (Burdick et al. 2004). However, the former one is relatively easier to perform. A commonly used method to examine cell migration is the wound-healing assay, which evaluates the behavior of cells in the state of confluence to migrate into a wounded area (Todaro et al. 1965; Reinhart-King 2008). When this assay is carried out, cells are allowed to adhere to the ligand-coated material surface and are grown to confluence. To create an artificial wound, a pipette tip can be dragged on the surface of the confluent cell monolayer. Thus, an area is scratched and represents the wounded area. Cells will then migrate to the wounded area as part of the healing process. At different time points, the healed area can be measured under a microscope with the aid of computer software. Thus, cell migration can be measured by correlating time with the quantity of cells residing in the wounded area. However, the wound-healing assay is an invasive assay because cells at the border of the wound are inevitably injured during the scratching. Additionally, the creation of cell debris affects the migration of cells. To address this question, an artificial barrier can be used to cover a portion of a material surface during the initial cell culture (Kumar et al. 2005). After the cells reach confluence, the barrier can be removed from the cell culture system. The operations involved in this method are mild and noninvasive.

6.3.4 Evaluation of Cell Proliferation

During cell growth, the number of cells increases. The increase in cell number is described as cell proliferation and can be examined by a number of methods. Cell counting is a relatively easy, straightforward method to study cell proliferation. The cell numbers can be quantified under a microscope with the aid of dye staining (e.g., trypan blue) or by the analysis of the activity of mitochondrial enzymes (e.g., MTT). Cell counting can be carried out at the predetermined time points for generating growth curves and calculating the doubling time (DT) of the cell population (Heiss et al. 2008). The DT can be calculated by the following equation:

$$DT = \frac{t}{3.32[\log N_t - \log N_0]} \qquad (6.7)$$

where

  t is the time between two measurements after cell seeding
  N_0 is the initial cell number
  N_t is the number of cells found in time t

Cell proliferation can also be characterized by the evaluation of a number of important parameters involved in the cell cycle. For instance, during cell proliferation, the DNA content and number of chromosomes increase. Thus, the increase of DNA can be correlated to cell proliferation. A traditional approach is to add ^{3}H-thymidine into the cell culture medium. During cell proliferation, ^{3}H-thymidine is incorporated into the DNA of a cell. Thus, higher levels of radioactivity will be measured where the proliferation rate is higher. Recently, new methods have been developed to avoid the use of radioactive reagents. For instance, a number of cell proliferation kits are commercially available based on the usage of bromodeoxyuridine (BrdU). BrdU is a synthetic nucleoside that can be incorporated into new DNA during DNA synthesis. The anti-BrdU antibodies can be added into the system for cell analysis based on immunocytochemical and cytometric approaches. The BrdU-based assay is as sensitive as ^{3}H-thymidine-based assay. Besides the studies on cell adhesion, cell migration, and cell proliferation, it is also valuable to study cell differentiation, cell viability, cell apoptosis, etc. These properties can be evaluated with the similar approaches as previously mentioned. For instance, the test for mitochondrial enzyme activity (e.g., MTT) that is used to analyze cell adhesion and cell proliferation is also often used for the examination of cell viability.

In summary, this chapter discusses the methodology and principles of evaluating the cell–material interactions at both the molecular and cell level. The ligand–receptor interactions can be examined in either soluble or immobilized states with the aid of various experimental tools. The cell–material interactions can be understood by the examination of cell adhesion, cell migration, cell proliferation, and many other critical cell functions.

ACKNOWLEDGMENT

The support from the National Science Foundation (DMR-0955358) is greatly acknowledged.

REFERENCES

Akiyama, Y., Kikuchi, A., Yamato, M., and Okano, T., Ultrathin poly(*N*-isopropylacrylamide) grafted layer on polystyrene surfaces for cell adhesion/detachment control. *Langmuir* 2004, 20(13), 5506–5511.

Amit, A. G., Mariuzza, R. A., Phillips, S. E., and Poljak, R. J., Three-dimensional structure of an antigen–antibody complex at 2.8 Å resolution. *Science* 1986, 233(4765), 747–753.

Anamelechi, C. C., Clermont, E. E., Brown, M. A., Truskey, G. A., and Reichert, W. M., Streptavidin binding and endothelial cell adhesion to biotinylated fibronectin. *Langmuir* 2007, 23(25), 12583–12588.

Auernheimer, J., Dahmen, C., Hersel, U., Bausch, A., and Kessler, H., Photoswitched cell adhesion on surfaces with RGD peptides. *J Am Chem Soc* 2005, 127(46), 16107–16110.

Bednar, B., Cunningham, M. E., McQueney, P. A., Egbertson, M. S., Askew, B. C., Bednar, R. A., Hartman, G. D., and Gould, R. J., Flow cytometric measurement of kinetic and equilibrium binding parameters of arginine–glycine–aspartic acid ligands in binding to glycoprotein IIb/IIIa on platelets. *Cytometry* 1997, 28(1), 58–65.

Bhat, T. N., Bentley, G. A., Boulot, G., Greene, M. I., Tello, D., Dall'Acqua, W., Souchon, H., Schwarz, F. P., Mariuzza, R. A., and Poljak, R. J., Bound water molecules and conformational stabilization help mediate an antigen–antibody association. *Proc Natl Acad Sci U S A* 1994, 91(3), 1089–1093.

Bongrand, P., Ligand–receptor interactions. *Rep Progr Phys* 1999, 62(6), 921–968.

Burdick, J. A., Khademhosseini, A., and Langer, R., Fabrication of gradient hydrogels using a micro-fluidics/photopolymerization process. *Langmuir* 2004, 20(13), 5153–5156.

Canavan, H. E., Cheng, X., Graham, D. J., Ratner, B. D., and Castner, D. G., Surface characterization of the extracellular matrix remaining after cell detachment from a thermoresponsive polymer. *Langmuir* 2005, 21(5), 1949–1955.

Cole, M. A., Voelcker, N. H., Thissen, H., and Griesser, H. J., Stimuli-responsive interfaces and systems for the control of protein–surface and cell–surface interactions. *Biomaterials* 2009, 30(9), 1827–1850.

da Silva, R. M., Mano, J. F., and Reis, R. L., Smart thermoresponsive coatings and surfaces for tissue engineering: Switching cell–material boundaries. *Trends Biotechnol* 2007, 25(12), 577–583.

Engler, A. J., Sen, S., Sweeney, H. L., and Discher, D. E., Matrix elasticity directs stem cell lineage specification. *Cell* 2006, 126(4), 677–689.

Florin, E. L., Moy, V. T., and Gaub, H. E., Adhesion forces between individual ligand–receptor pairs. *Science* 1994, 264(5157), 415–417.

Heiss, C., Wong, M. L., Block, V. I., Lao, D., Real, W. M., Yeghiazarians, Y., Lee, R. J., and Springer, M. L., Pleiotrophin induces nitric oxide dependent migration of endothelial progenitor cells. *J Cell Physiol* 2008, 215(2), 366–373.

Hersel, U., Dahmen, C., and Kessler, H., RGD modified polymers: Biomaterials for stimulated cell adhesion and beyond. *Biomaterials* 2003, 24(24), 4385–4415.

Kingshott, P. and Griesser, H. J., Surfaces that resist bioadhesion. *Curr Opin Solid State Mater Sci* 1999, 4(4), 403–412.

Kumar, G., Meng, J. J., Ip, W., Co, C. C., and Ho, C. C., Cell motility assays on tissue culture dishes via non-invasive confinement and release of cells. *Langmuir* 2005, 21(20), 9267–9273.

Kushida, A., Yamato, M., Konno, C., Kikuchi, A., Sakurai, Y., and Okano, T., Decrease in culture temperature releases monolayer endothelial cell sheets together with deposited fibronectin matrix from temperature-responsive culture surfaces. *J Biomed Mater Res* 1999, 45(4), 355–362.

LeBaron, R. G. and Athanasiou, K. A., Extracellular matrix cell adhesion peptides: Functional applications in orthopedic materials. *Tissue Eng* 2000, 6(2), 85–103.

Liu, Y., Pan, Y., and Xu, Y., Binding investigation of integrin alphavbeta3 with its inhibitors by SPR technology and molecular docking simulation. *J Biomol Screen* 2010, 15(2), 131–137.

Ma, H., Li, D., Sheng, X., Zhao, B., and Chilkoti, A., Protein-resistant polymer coatings on silicon oxide by surface-initiated atom transfer radical polymerization. *Langmuir* 2006, 22(8), 3751–3756.

McClay, D. R., Wessel, G. M., and Marchase, R. B., Intercellular recognition: Quantitation of initial binding events. *Proc Natl Acad Sci U S A* 1981, 78(8), 4975–4979.

McDonnell, J. M., Surface plasmon resonance: Towards an understanding of the mechanisms of biological molecular recognition. *Curr Opin Chem Biol* 2001, 5(5), 572–577.

Meinecke, R. and Meyer, B., Determination of the binding specificity of an integral membrane protein by saturation transfer difference NMR: RGD peptide ligands binding to integrin alphaIIbbeta3. *J Med Chem* 2001, 44(19), 3059–3065.

Moy, V. T., Florin, E. L., and Gaub, H. E., Intermolecular forces and energies between ligands and receptors. *Science* 1994, 266(5183), 257–259.

Ohmuro-Matsuyama, Y. and Tatsu, Y., Photocontrolled cell adhesion on a surface functionalized with a caged arginine–glycine–aspartate peptide. *Angew Chem Int Ed Engl* 2008, 47(39), 7527–7529.

Pierschbacher, M. D. and Ruoslahti, E., Cell attachment activity of fibronectin can be duplicated by small synthetic fragments of the molecule. *Nature* 1984, 309(5963), 30–33.

Ratner, B. D. and Bryant, S. J., Biomaterials: Where we have been and where we are going. *Annu Rev Biomed Eng* 2004, 6, 41–75.

Ray, J. L., Leach, R., Herbert, J. M., and Benson, M., Isolation of vascular smooth muscle cells from a single murine aorta. *Methods Cell Sci* 2001, 23(4), 185–188.

Reinhart-King, C. A., Endothelial cell adhesion and migration. *Methods Enzymol* 2008, 443, 45–64.

Shin, H., Fabrication methods of an engineered microenvironment for analysis of cell–biomaterial interactions. *Biomaterials* 2007, 28(2), 126–133.

Shin, H., Jo, S., and Mikos, A. G., Biomimetic materials for tissue engineering. *Biomaterials* 2003, 24(24), 4353–4364.

Sklar, L. A., Edwards, B. S., Graves, S. W., Nolan, J. P., and Prossnitz, E. R., Flow cytometric analysis of ligand–receptor interactions and molecular assemblies. *Annu Rev Biophys Biomol Struct* 2002, 31, 97–119.

Takeuchi, K. and Wagner, G., NMR studies of protein interactions. *Curr Opin Struct Biol* 2006, 16(1), 109–117.

Todaro, G. J., Lazar, G. K., and Green, H., The initiation of cell division in a contact-inhibited mammalian cell line. *J Cell Physiol* 1965, 66(3), 325–333.

Tsang, P., Rance, M., Fieser, T. M., Ostresh, J. M., Houghten, R. A., Lerner, R. A., and Wright, P. E., Conformation and dynamics of an Fab′-bound peptide by isotope-edited NMR spectroscopy. *Biochemistry* 1992, 31(15), 3862–3871.

Williamson, P. T. F., Solid-state NMR for the analysis of high-affinity ligand/receptor interactions. *Concepts Magn. Reson. A* 2009, 34A(3), 144–172.

Yang, J., Yamato, M., Kohno, C., Nishimoto, A., Sekine, H., Fukai, F., Okano, T., Cell sheet engineering: Recreating tissues without biodegradable scaffolds. *Biomaterials* 2005, 26(33), 6415–6422.

Yang, J., Yamato, M., Shimizu, T., Sekine, H., Ohashi, K., Kanzaki, M., Ohki, T., Nishida, K., and Okano, T., Reconstruction of functional tissues with cell sheet engineering. *Biomaterials* 2007, 28(34), 5033–5043.

CHAPTER 7

Host Response to Biomaterials and Its Implications in Regenerative Engineering

Lakshmi S. Nair, MPhil, PhD

CONTENTS

7.1 INTRODUCTION

The goal of regenerative engineering is to regenerate complex tissue, organ, and organ systems using advanced biomaterials, soluble and matrix-bound factors, and stem cell technology (Reichert et al. 2011). Advanced biomaterials and/or scaffolds that can mimic the physiological niche to modulate cell fate to support regeneration are one of the key elements in the regenerative engineering strategy. Several natural and synthetic polymers are currently used to develop scaffolds to support tissue regeneration either alone or as composites with cells and other biomolecules (Nair and Laurencin 2007). However, the clinical success of these technologies lies in the ability of these materials to function properly in the *in vivo* host environment. The innate and adaptive immune responses or host response to the implanted biomaterials and biomaterial–cell/growth factor composites therefore play a central role in determining their stability, biological functions, and the clinical outcome. The biological response to implanted materials is a complex series of events that involves many different cell types, bioactive molecules, and biochemical pathways. Implantation of a foreign material results in a foreign body response (FBR), the extent and nature of which depends on several factors such as the physicochemical aspects of the material and site of implantation. The goal of this chapter is to highlight the importance of FBR to biomaterials, to discuss ways to modulate the FBR, and to examine the impact this has on the success of regenerative engineering strategies. This chapter begins with a general discussion on wound healing and the different types of cells involved in the natural wound healing process followed by a discussion about the foreign body reaction to materials and the role of biomaterials in modulating the innate and adaptive immune systems.

7.2 EXAMPLES OF CLINICAL COMPLICATIONS DUE TO ADVERSE HOST RESPONSE TO BIOMATERIALS

Orthopedic implants (composed of metallic, polymeric, or ceramic biomaterials) play a major role in the clinical implant industry with the U.S. orthopedic implant market projected to rise to US\$23 billion by the year 2012 (Freedonia Group 2008). Despite the great advances in orthopedic biomaterials research during the past 75 years or so, the holy grail of a long-lasting orthopedic joint implant in a young active individual has yet to be achieved. One of the leading issues that adversely affects the longevity of current total joint arthroplasty (TJA) is aseptic loosening of an implant due to periprosthetic osteolysis (Hallab and Jacobs 2009; Wang 2011). Periprosthetic osteolysis arises from a local inflammatory reaction of the host immune system toward the wear particles and corrosion products from the implants. The host response to the wear particles, ranging in size from nanometers to millimeters, involves a local immune reaction that is predominantly mediated by macrophages. Figure 7.1 is a schematic showing the macrophage-mediated wear particle–induced inflammation around the implant leading to local tissue damage. Briefly, biomaterial wear particles induce monocyte–macrophage activation and secretion of proinflammatory cytokines such as interleukin (IL)-1β, IL-1α, tumor necrosis factor α (TNF-α), IL-6, IL-18, prostaglandin 2 (PGE2), and IL-8. Many of these cytokines are known to stimulate differentiation of osteoclast precursors to mature osteoclasts, which leads to increased bone resorption and decreased bone deposition, which results in bone loss at the tissue–implant interface and subsequent implant loosening (Hallab and Jacobs 2009; Beck et al. 2012).

Intracoronary stents present another example of clinical complications associated with adverse host response. Intracoronary stents are used increasingly for the treatment of atherosclerotic coronary disease (see Chapter 5; Farb et al. 1999). Recent studies indicate evidence of a chronic inflammatory reaction and endothelial dysfunction that could significantly affect the long-term patency of the stents. Several factors that have been identified to trigger the chronic inflammatory reaction include the host reaction to the foreign metallic material, vessel wall rupture during stent insertion, and the mechanical strain

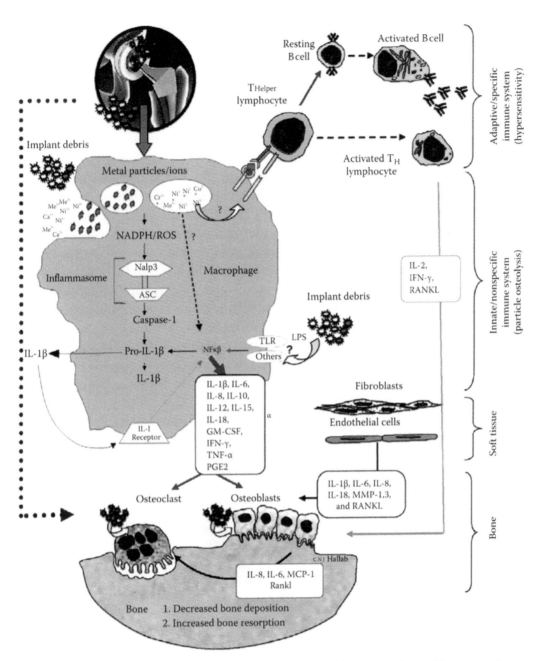

FIGURE 7.1 Wear particles induced inflammation mediated by macrophages. The macrophages ingest the debri and they in turn release proinflammatory cytokines leading to bone resorption and bone cell death. (Reproduced from Hallab, N.J. and Jacobs, J.J., *Bull. NYC Hosp. Jt. Dis.*, 67, 182, 2009.)

applied to the vessel wall by the material (Gomes and Buffolo 2006). The resulting endothelial dysfunction can also lead to post-angioplasty restenosis. Moreover, the adverse inflammatory and proliferative reactions most often will not localize to the injured vessel wall but will extend to the surrounding tissues and adjacent myocardium. This can lead to accelerated progression of the inflammatory process and atherosclerotic disease.

This warrants studies to understand the clinical significance of these complications and novel methods to control local and systemic inflammation. Coated or drug-eluting stents may be a major advance in addressing this challenge even though the long-term efficacy of these approaches is unknown and currently under study.

Another clinically relevant instance where the body's reaction to a foreign material merits study is biomaterial-induced fibrosis, which adversely affects the long-term use of neural prostheses (Szarowski et al. 2003). Neural prostheses are currently used clinically to address several peripheral and central nervous system conditions. Notable examples include cochlear implants and deep brain stimulation to alleviate symptoms due to Parkinson's disease (Bell et al. 1998; Caparros-Lefebyre et al. 2002). The long-term function of many of these devices is limited because of the resulting electrical and mechanical isolation of the prostheses from the brain with fibrous tissue encapsulation. Figure 7.2 shows the early and prolonged reactive host response to the implant upon insertion, the process that triggers the early reactive phase, which involves significant cellular rearrangement and cellular activation. During the prolonged reactive response, a compact sheath mostly composed of astrocytes and microglia will form around the electrode. The sheath will separate the neurons from the recording electrodes, which practically isolates the electrode from the brain tissue. This further highlights that a biomaterial-induced host response is a highly complex process, and understanding the cellular and biochemical pathways involved in it is a very important step in developing clinically viable approaches to improve implant performance.

Generally speaking, the activation of the innate and adaptive immune response can lead to a variety of localized and systemic clinical complications including inflammation, fibrosis, thrombosis, and infection. Moreover, the inflammatory response can also lead to accelerated degradation/corrosion of the biomaterial mainly via oxidative

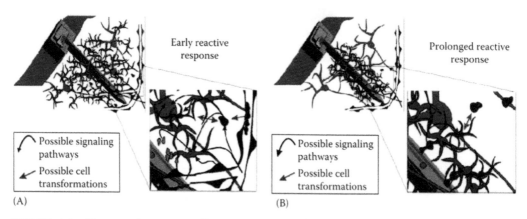

FIGURE 7.2 Cartoon depicting cellular responses following prostheses insertion. The early response (A) is characterized by a large region containing reactive astrocytes and microglia around inserted devices. The prolonged response (B) is characterized by a compact sheath of cells around insertion sites. Inserts depict potential cell–cell interactions and signaling pathways. Neurons (pink), astrocytes (red), monocyte-derived cells including microglia (blue), and vasculature (purple) are depicted. (Reproduced from Szarowski, D.H. et al., *Brain Res.*, 983, 23, 2003.)

products that are released by the activated inflammatory cells. These events will result in the development of a wound microenvironment that might or might not be conducive to the regenerative process, a process that requires tight spatial and temporal control of specific cells and biological factors. These points, demonstrated by the clinical examples earlier, indicate that an adverse host response to an implanted biomaterial is one of the critical barriers to achieving the vision of regenerative engineering, and need to be adequately addressed.

7.3 NATURAL WOUND HEALING RESPONSES TO INJURY/INFECTION

Tissue injury due to (1) trauma, (2) physical or chemical agents, or (3) bacterial, viral, or parasitic infection leads to a host response, which involves a plethora of events in an effort to restore the damaged area by either regeneration of native parenchymal cells, formation of fibroblastic scar tissue, or a combination of the two (Anderson et al. 2008). The natural wound healing process is composed of three main phases: (1) a coagulation/fibrinolysis phase during which a fibrin clot forms and is subsequently dissolved, (2) an inflammatory phase, which involves acute and chronic inflammation in a sequential fashion, and (3) a repair phase to reestablish tissue integrity and function (Tsirogianni et al. 2006).

Among these, the inflammatory phase plays a very important role in modulating the healing process and the degree of these responses is controlled by the nature of the tissue and the extent of injury/infection. A heterogeneous collection of blood cells called leukocytes, specialized to perform different functions in adaptive and innate immune responses, are involved in the different stages of the inflammatory process. Based on their appearance, the leukocytes are broadly classified into granulocytes and mononuclear cells. Granulocytes have prominent granules in their cytoplasm, vesicles containing a cocktail of different enzymes. Based on the histochemical properties of their granules, granulocytes are classified into neutrophils, basophils, and eosinophils. The mononuclear cells on the other hand do not have the multinucleate appearance of granular cells and are divided into monocytes, which are precursors for tissue, macrophages, and lymphocytes (Janeway et al. 2001).

Upon injury, acute inflammation sets in for a relatively short time. Inflammation is triggered by the degranulation of the mast cells and the subsequent release of preformed components such as histamine. Vascular phenomena play very important roles in acute inflammation, as vasodilation, or widening of the vessels, is one of the earliest occurring events, followed by increased vascular permeability that causes edema and inflammatory cell emigration. Polymorphonuclear leukocytes (PMNs) or neutrophils characterize the cellular component of acute inflammatory phase. Depending on the severity of the injury and/or the type of microbes, the inflammatory response can persist and become a chronic phase reaction. The chronic inflammatory phase is histologically less uniform compared to acute inflammation. There will be a gradual shift in the type of inflammatory cells from neutrophils to monocytes, macrophages, and lymphocytes. The resolution of inflammation, clearance of debris, and foreign agents initiates the reparative process that encompasses granulation tissue formation, angiogenesis, and recellularization. Sections 7.3.1 through 7.3.8 briefly discuss the different cells involved in the wound healing process.

7.3.1 Polymorphonuclear Phagocytic Cells

PMNs or neutrophils are estimated to form approximately 50%–70% of leukocytes in human blood (Klebanoff and Clark 1978). The neutrophil production and differentiation in the bone marrow is driven by the granulocyte colony-stimulating factor (GCSF) produced by monocytes. The neutrophils are phagocytic cells and they respond rapidly to chemotaxins and their major function is to migrate to sites of inflammation and ingest invading microorganisms by phagocytosis. These acute inflammatory cells are essential during the early stage of inflammation; however, if not cleared in time, they can damage healthy tissue through generation of free radicals and other mechanisms.

7.3.2 Mononuclear Phagocytic Cells

The mononuclear phagocytic system is composed of circulating monocytes, tissue macrophages, and dendritic cell (DC) lineage (Gordon et al. 1995). Apart from their phagocytic activity, these are multifunctional cells involved in many aspects of the immune system. These cells are responsible for the recognition of invading microbes and other foreign materials, reorganization of tissue during inflammation and wound healing, and the removal of tissue debris and apoptotic cells. The macrophage is the dominant cellular player in chronic inflammation and studies have indicated that they play a major role in biomaterial-induced host response. Not only do they function as phagocytic cells but they can also produce a wide range of biologically active products that are involved in matrix degradation and tissue remodeling. These include neutral proteases, chemotactic factors, arachidonic acid metabolites, complement components, coagulation factors, growth-promoting factors, and cytokines. The high plasticity of these cells is evident from recent studies indicating the potential to assume different phenotypes and functions in response to stimuli. Understanding macrophage–biomaterial interaction is therefore gaining significant interest in the research world and what is learned might contribute to the design of immunomodulatory biomaterials that support tissue regeneration. Figure 7.3 shows the different types of macrophages, their currently known inducers, phenotypes, and functions (Kou and Babensee 2011). The high plasticity of macrophages suggests the possibility of the primary phenotypes to blend into a variety of secondary phenotypes to perform different functions. Figure 7.3 also shows the ability of the cells to possibly modulate the adaptive immune system and determine the regenerative outcome.

DCs are hematopoietic in origin and, like macrophages, are an important class of antigen-presenting cells (APCs). DCs like macrophages have phagocytic ability and can produce a wide variety of complement proteins and cytokines, and therefore play a very important role in the innate immunity. Some of the recent studies indicate the potential of biomaterials, particularly composite materials with cells and biological factors, to modulate DC maturation and phenotypic polarization (Babensee 2008).

7.3.3 Lymphocytes

Lymphocytes are white blood cells and play a key role in the body's defense against foreign antigens. Three subsets of lymphocytes include (1) T lymphocytes, (2) B lymphocytes,

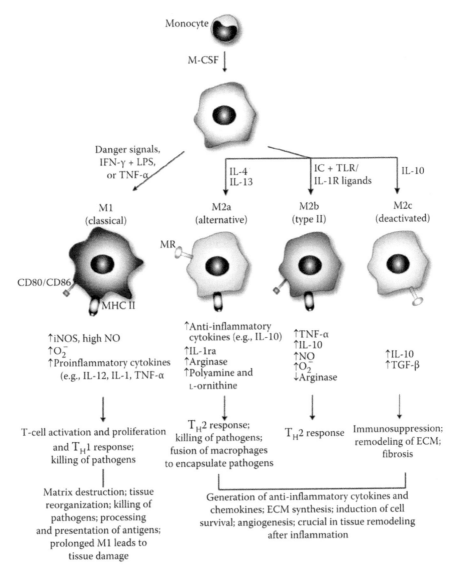

FIGURE 7.3 Illustration of different subsets of macrophages, their inducers, phenotype, and functions. The high plasticity of macrophages allows them to polarize into populations with different phenotypes and functions. In the presence of macrophage CSF (M-CSF), monocytes differentiate to form macrophages. Macrophages can acquire an M1 phenotype upon stimulation with IFN-γ, TNF-α, or LPS, which is characterized by high microbicidal and antitumor activity, production of proinflammatory cytokines, and activation of Th1 response. Similarly, macrophages can be alternatively activated into various M3 phenotypes such as M2a (induced by IL-4 and IL-13), M2b (induced by immune complex TLR or IL-1r ligands), and M2c (induced by IL-10). M2a and M2b are known to produce higher amounts of IL-10 and lower amounts of IL-12 and are associated with Th2 response. M2c produce higher levels of IL-10 and TGF-β and is associated with immune suppression and tissue remodeling. It is to be noted that these activation levels of macrophages are hypothetical ends of a spectrum of macrophage phenotypes, with actual macrophage phenotype should be viewed as within a continuum of functional states. (Reproduced from Kou, P.M. and Babensee, J.E., *J. Biomed. Mater. Res. A*, 96, 239, 2011.)

and (3) natural killer cells. Three major classes of T cells include (1) helper T cells, (2) cytotoxic T cells, and (3) suppresser T cells. The helper T cells (Th) with CD4+ markers are involved in multiple functions by virtue of their role in producing cytokines and chemokines. They can be either type 1 helper T cells (Th1 cells) or type 2 helper T cells (Th2 cells). The Th1 cells produce cytokines such as IL-1, interferon γ (IFN-γ), and TNF, which can activate complement-fixing Ab isotypes, macrophages, and cytotoxic T cells. The Th2 cells on the other hand are known to produce IL-4, IL-5, IL-6, and IL-10, cytokines that may not activate macrophages and therefore lead to production of non-complement-fixing Ab isotypes. The role of lymphocytes in host response to biomaterials is evident from their ability to adhere to biomaterial surfaces and activate macrophages and foreign body giant cells (Chang et al. 2009). B Lymphocytes are white blood cells involved in antibody production and are an integral part of the humoral immune system. Natural killer cells are cytotoxic cells involved in the programmed apoptosis of tumor cells and virus-infected cells.

7.3.4 Complement System

The complement system is composed of about 30 plasma proteins that play an important role in the innate immune defense system to clear foreign materials and microorganisms by direct lysis or phagocytosis via recruited leukocytes (Nilson et al. 2009). The complement proteins involved in this process remain inactive in the plasma until they are cleaved by proteases. It involves three distinct pathways: (1) the classical complement pathway that is triggered by the antigen–antibody complexes, (2) the lectin pathway, which is mediated by circulating soluble pattern-recognition receptors such as mannan-binding protein, and (3) the alternative complement pathway, which can be triggered without an antigen–antibody complex, such as by the presence of a foreign material leading to spontaneous activation of C3, a protein in the complement system (Ratner et al. 2004). The anaphylatoxins generated during the activation process can activate and recruit PMNs and monocytes to the target while the target-bound C3 fragments activate the recruited cells at the site. The activation pathways also lead to the formation of membrane attack complexes that can induce direct cell lysis by insertion into the cell lipid bilayer.

7.4 FOREIGN BODY RESPONSE TO BIOMATERIALS

The *in vivo* implantation of a biomaterial and the surgical trauma of implantation itself can induce an FBR (comprehensively reviewed by Anderson et al. 2008). Despite the similarity between the initial tissue response to an implanted biomaterial and the natural wound healing process, the nature and response of the infiltrated cells as well as a range of growth factors, cytokines, chemokines, matrix metalloproteinases (MMPs), and the inhibitors that mediate the FBR to a biomaterial depend considerably on the size, shape, surface chemistry, composition, contact duration, degradation, roughness, porosity, morphology, and sterility of the implanted material (Jones et al. 2008; Morais et al. 2010). The initial material-dependent response is mainly governed by the proteins or opsonins that adsorb onto the biomaterial shortly after implantation such as fibrinogen, complement proteins, and antibodies (Andrade and Hlady 1987). Neutrophils and macrophages have cell membrane receptors to recognize these opsonins. Denatured fibrinogen on a material surface could activate tissue phagocytes to release cytokines and chemokines, which in turn activate leukocytes and fibroblasts (Smiley et al. 2001). Immunoglobulin G (IgG) is another common opsonin. The biomaterial can also activate the alternative complement pathway due to the adsorption of complement protein C3b on the surface as well as the activation of the classical complement pathway due to the aspecific binding of antibodies on the surface. Similarly, the implantation process can cause an increase in endogenous damage-associated molecular patterns (DAMPs) that can adsorb on the biomaterial surface and in certain cases the biomaterial itself or additives in it can present molecular patterns that mimic pathogen-associated molecular patterns (PAMPs). All these can elicit a surface-associated innate activation of the mediated immune system leading to inflammatory cytokine production and subsequent chemokine recruitment of phagocytic cells. The phagocytic cells adhere to the biomaterial and if the size of the biomaterial is much larger than the cells, this can lead to frustrated phagocytosis wherein macrophages fuse to form foreign body giant cells. Frustrated phogocytosis may not always cause the engulfment of the biomaterial but can lead to increased secretion of inflammatory products in an attempt to degrade the material (Anderson et al. 2008). The foreign body reaction consists of foreign body giant cells and components of granulation tissue such as macrophages, fibroblasts, and capillaries. Studies have shown that the presence and extent of foreign body giant cells are greatly influenced by the form, topography, and properties of the biomaterial. Therefore, the same biomaterial in a particulate or powder form that can be phagocytosed may elicit a different degree of inflammatory response compared to the one in a form that cannot be phagocytosed. Figure 7.4 shows the size-dependent macrophage response to biomaterials (Kou and Babensee 2011). The macrophage and/or foreign body giant cells along with the granulation tissue surrounding the implant make up the foreign body reaction. A chronic inflammatory response mediated by macrophages, foreign body giant cells, lymphocytes, and plasma cells sets in if the implant elicits persistent inflammatory stimuli. Whether the biomaterial-mediated response will lead to tissue regeneration or scar tissue formation depends partially on the duration of the chronic inflammatory response that contributes to cytokine production and formation of granulation tissue (Boehler et al. 2011). The biomaterial–tissue microenvironment determines the immune phenotype of the macrophages, which in turn may determine the cytokines produced by the macrophages. It has been reported that macrophages can adopt a regenerative/anti-inflammatory (M2) phenotype after phagocytosis of debris (Brown et al. 2009). Similarly, a significant correlation has been noted between the progression of inflammatory macrophages (M1) to M2 and cytokine secretion profile of CD4+ helper T cells from Th1 to Th1 (which promotes the resolution of inflammation) (Figure 7.3). In summary, the physical, chemical, and biological properties of the biomaterial can modulate the host response. The intensity and the duration of the inflammatory response will determine the biocompatibility and regenerative outcome mediated by the material *in vivo*. Understanding the foreign body reaction to a biomaterial is therefore crucial while using them for regenerative purpose since FBR can favorably or adversely

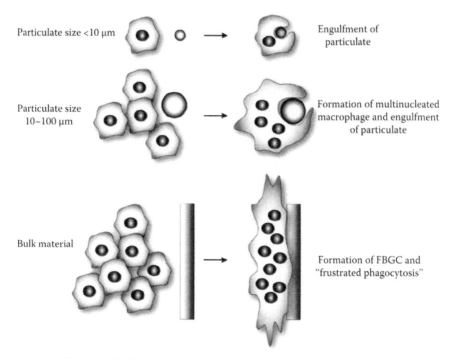

FIGURE 7.4 Differential behavior of macrophages toward biomaterials of different sizes. (Reproduced from Kou, P.M. and Babensee, J.E., *J. Biomed. Mater. Res. A*, 96, 239, 2011.)

affect the tissue repair process. Among the cells that react to a biomaterial implantation, macrophages play key roles in mediating the chronic inflammatory process associated with the FBR and are involved in modulating tissue repair and regeneration. Therefore, the past few years have seen significant interest in understanding macrophage behavior in response to biomaterial implantation. The following sections briefly describe the effect different biomaterial properties have on host response in terms of immune phenotype, cytokine release, biomaterial degradation, and fibrous capsule formation.

7.4.1 Effect of Biomaterial Surface Chemistry on Host Response

Some of the earlier studies that provided significant evidence of immune cell interactions with biomaterials were focused on the surface properties of the biomaterial. Smetana et al. (1993) demonstrated the direct correlation of surface chemistry on protein adsorption and macrophage adhesion and fusion. Using copolymers of 2-hydroxyethyl methacrylate and sodium methacrylate, surfaces with different carboxylic group contents were created to test the effect of surface chemistry on macrophage response. Increase in carboxylic acid content significantly decreased protein adsorption and macrophage adhesion and fusion. The significant reduction of macrophage adhesion and fusion *in vivo* supported the hypothesis that immune cells are able to detect very subtle differences in polymer surfaces. This was further verified by Barbosa et al. (2003) using self-assembled monolayers with well-defined surface chemistry. PMNs and mononuclear leukocytes isolated from human blood were used for the study and the surfaces were made on gold with alkane thiols having –COOH,

–OH, and –CH$_3$ terminal groups. The total number of cells adhered in the surfaces varied in the order of –CH$_3$ > –OH > –COOH > gold. The unique behavior of hydrophilic anionic polymeric surfaces was further confirmed by another study by Brodbeck et al. (2002a,b) indicating that these surfaces can induce increased apoptosis of macrophages compared to hydrophobic or cationic surfaces. Similarly, the surface chemistry can also modulate the cytokine release profile of the macrophages. Hydrophilic anionic surfaces were shown to significantly increase the expression of anti-inflammatory cytokine IL-10, and decreased the expression of the proinflammatory cytokine IL-8 by human monocytes (Brodbeck et al. 2002a,b). The hydrophilic, anionic surfaces also inhibited monocyte adhesion and IL-4-mediated macrophage fusion to form foreign body giant cells. Another related study investigated whether the leukocyte cytokine RNA profile *in vivo* depends on the surface chemistry of the implanted biomaterial (Brodbeck et al. 2003). That study showed the ability of hydrophilic surfaces to decrease the expression of inflammatory and wound healing cytokines, while cationic surfaces showed a strong early inflammatory response followed by a wound healing response. To maximize the influence of surface chemistry on cells to study the long-term fibrotic reaction, Kamath et al. created functionalized micrometer-sized particles to test their ability to modulate tissue response (Kamath et al. 2008). Polypropylene particles were functionalized with four different groups: –OH, –NH$_2$, CF$_x$, and –COOH using radiofrequency glow discharge plasma polymerization. A mouse subcutaneous implantation model was used to study their long-term tissue response. The study demonstrated that particles with –OH and –NH$_2$ functional groups elicit a strong fibrotic reaction with the formation of thick fibrous capsule and significant cellular infiltration into the implants. In contrast, the surfaces with –CF$_x$ and –COOH showed the least fibrotic reaction and cellular infiltration. Similarly, chemical modification to create hydrophilic surfaces on titanium dental implants with a microscale surface roughness was shown clinically to achieve better wound healing and osseointegration when compared to nonchemically modified implants with the same microscale surface roughness. In a similar study, Hamlet et al. (2012) investigated the cytokine profile of macrophages when cultured on hydrophilic microrough titanium implants and unmodified implants. After 24 h of culture on the hydrophilic surface, a murine leukemic monocyte cell line (RAW 264.7) showed a significant downregulation of key proinflammatory cytokines such as TNF-α, IL-1α, IL-1β, and the chemokine Ccl-2. These studies indicate the possibility of eliciting pro/anti-inflammatory immune response simply by modifying the biomaterial surfaces. Even though the exact mechanisms by which immune cells are recognizing and reacting to surfaces with different chemistries are not known yet, this is of significance from a tissue-engineering perspective since surface chemistries of porous scaffolds commonly used to support tissue regeneration can play a significant role in modulating the immune response and hence the regenerative process.

7.4.2 Effect of Biomaterial Topography and Architecture on Host Response

Similar to surface chemistry, the surface topography and architecture of the biomaterial scaffold have been shown to modulate immune cell response. Since macrophages play a key role in controlling normal wound healing and regenerative processes, several studies have investigated the effect of scaffold surface topography and architecture on macrophage response. A recent study by Chen et al. (2010) tested the hypothesis that topography on the biological scale (micrometer–nanometer range) provides a passive approach to modulate macrophage behavior in the absence of bioactive agents. Effect of topography on macrophage behavior was studied using parallel gratings of 250 nm–2 mm line widths imprinted on biocompatible polymers such as poly(caprolactone) (PCL), poly(lactic acid), and poly(dimethyl siloxane). Macrophage adhesion and elongation was found to increase as topography size decreased down to 500 nm while below that, cells appeared to be insensitive to the surface topography. In the first 6–48 h of the inflammation stage however, the macrophages showed functional differences with respect to the surface topography. Thus, reduced levels of TNF-α and VEGF secretion levels were found in samples with 1 μm gratings compared to nanoscale gratings and planar topography controls. While further studies are required to elucidate the mechanism behind the topographical cue–mediated responses as well as the *in vivo* response to these materials, the study confirmed the possibility of surface topography affecting macrophage behavior and subsequently perhaps the regenerative outcome.

An *in vivo* study by Sanders et al. (2000) showed interesting results in this context. The group investigated the effect of fiber diameter on the thickness of fibrous capsule formation and macrophage infiltration after subcutaneous implantation in a rat model over a range of fibers from 2–5 through 16–26 μm. The study demonstrated reduced fibrous capsule thickness as the diameter of fibers got smaller with the fiber diameters ranging from 2 to 5 μm showing the lowest macrophage density, comparable to that of the unoperated contralateral control skin. The macrophage density in fibers with diameters ranging from 6 to 26 μm was significantly higher than the smallest fiber diameter range. The authors have attributed the reduced fibrous capsule thickness and macrophage density for smaller fibers to the reduced cell–material contact surface area or to a curvature threshold effect that triggers cell signaling.

In natural tissue, the extracellular matrix (ECM) provides the structured microenvironment with mechanical, biochemical, and physical cues that facilitate cell–cell interactions and cell–ECM interactions for optimal cell function. The natural ECM is generally composed of a network of fibrous proteins and hydrated proteoglycans arranged in a unique tissue-specific three-dimensional architecture (collectively called structural/physical signals) in which other biomolecules (growth factors, chemokines, and cytokines) and various ions are bound (Nair et al. 2006). In short, the multifunctionality of the ECM is achieved via chemical/biological cues such as growth factors and biological molecules along with the unique tissue-specific hierarchical structural features. Therefore, it is apparent that ECM-mimicking synthetic biomaterials could significantly influence the response of tissue-specific cell types (Laurencin and Nair 2008). Some recent studies indicate that in addition to surface chemistry and surface properties of a biomaterial, the scaffold architecture can also influence immune cell response and can have significant impact on the foreign body reaction toward the scaffold. Studies show that porous structures tend to result in a moderate tissue response and promote faster healing with a thinner fibrous capsule compared to solid implants.

Cao et al. (2010) investigated the effect of scaffold architecture and topographical features on modulating *in vitro* and *in vivo* foreign body reaction using an ECM-mimicking electrospun nanofibrous scaffold. Random and aligned PCL nanofibrous scaffolds were developed using electrospinning with fiber diameters in the range of 313 ± 5 to 506 ± 24 nm, with PCL thin films serving as controls. Human monocytes were cultured on the scaffolds to follow cell density and morphology as a function of culture time (2 h, 3, 7, and 10 days). The study showed significant differences in initial monocyte adhesion on aligned and random fibers with aligned fibers showing significantly less number of cells. The *in vivo* host response to these scaffolds was evaluated by subcutaneous implantation in rats. The thickness of the fibrous capsule formed around the random and aligned nanofiber matrices was found to be significantly less than that formed around thin films. In addition, the aligned nanofiber matrices showed good cell infiltration whereas the random fiber matrices and thin film showed distinct fibrous capsule boundaries on the surface, supporting the notion that the architecture of the scaffold can significantly modulate host tissue response and play a key role in promoting or hindering tissue regeneration.

Ward et al. (2002) investigated the effect of scaffold porosity on host tissue response by following the thickness of the fibrous capsule and the extent of angiogenesis using a rat subcutaneous implantation model. The scaffolds investigated were solid polyurethane (PU), solid PU with silicone, and poly(ethylene oxide) (PU-S-PEO) with thickness of 300 and 2000 μm, porous poly(tetrafluoroethylene) (ePTFE), and porous poly(vinyl alcohol) (PVA) sponge. Compared to hydrophobic PU implants, the hydrophilic PU-S-PEO implants showed a significantly reduced fibrous capsule thickness. Within PU-S-PEO implants, the thinner implants showed lower fibrous capsule thickness compared to the thicker implants. The density of the fibrous capsule formed around the porous implants was found to be significantly lower than that formed around the solid implants. Moreover, the porous scaffolds showed a significant increase in new vessel formation around the porous implants compared to the solid implants. The study further supported a previous study by Hulbert et al. (1972) that compared the tissue response of porous and nonporous ceramic implants after intramuscular implantation in rabbits. That study showed that tissue around porous ceramic implants healed faster and exhibited a thinner fibrous capsule than nonporous implants. Moreover, the pore structure was filled with healthy vascularized connective tissue unlike the nonporous implants, which may have accounted for the more moderate tissue response to the porous implants.

A recent study by Madden et al. (2010) investigated the role of scaffold architecture in modulating the phenotypic polarization of macrophages and subsequent wound healing. Porous poly(2-hydroxyethyl methacrylate-*co*-methacrylic acid (pHEMA-*co*-MAA) hydrogels with an interconnected spherical pore network was created using a polymer fiber templating method. The channel size and spacing were controlled by varying the dimension of the template fibers from 45 to 150 μm to create pores ranging from 20 to 80 μm. Cardiac implantation of acellular scaffolds showed a significant increase in angiogenesis and reduced fibrotic response with scaffolds having pore size in the range of 30–40 μm. The increase in angiogenic activity of the scaffold coincided with the phenotypic polarization of the macrophages toward the M2 state. Even though the study has not determined where the scaffold-associated macrophages lie on the polarization continuum or how and to what extent they are modulating the neovascularization, it demonstrates the feasibility of varying macrophage phenotypes using scaffold architecture to support tissue regeneration by promoting neovascularization. The critical role of macrophage infiltration of tissue-engineered grafts in promoting neovascularization was confirmed by a recent study by Hibino et al. (2011).

7.4.3 Effect of Host Response on Biomaterial Degradation

Degradable biomaterials can be broadly classified into synthetic biomaterials and biological materials. Scaffolds made from biological materials are composed mainly of mammalian ECM components and undergo enzymatic degradation while scaffolds made from synthetic biomaterials mainly undergo hydrolytic degradation. This becomes relevant when considering the immune and inflammatory responses because the FBR is known to play a very important role in modulating biomaterial degradation.

Even though biological scaffolds generally exhibit an intense acute response, the long-term response, which may vary from chronic inflammation, fibrosis, and scarring or a site-appropriate, organized tissue remodeling, is determined by the nature of the material (Valentin et al. 2006). Ye et al. (2010) performed a study to understand the role of neutrophils in the foreign body reaction and how they modulate biomaterial degradation. Dermal sheep collagen disks cross-linked by glutaraldehyde (GDSC) and hexamethylene diisocyanate (HDSC) were studied as biomaterials using a subcutaneous implantation model in mice. The foreign body reaction toward the biomaterials was found to be significantly different. By day 28, 90% of GDSC was degraded whereas the HDSC remained unchanged throughout the time course. The molecular and cellular factors involved in the FBR indicated that GDSC showed much higher numbers of neutrophils at all time points compared to HDSC. Infiltration took place in two waves instead of one and appeared to be acting as a proinflammatory regulator by producing IL-6 and IFN-γ. Another interesting observation was the differences in the roles of macrophages in FBR of GDSC and HDSC even though similar numbers of macrophages were found in both the samples. In GDSC, macrophages degraded the biomaterial by means of MMPs and by phagocytosis. In contrast, in HDSC, the macrophages fused into giant cells that induced TIMP-1 expression via secretion of IL-10, resulting in a net decrease of MMP activity. In short, the absence of IFN-γ and phagocytic activity of macrophages, the high levels of TIMP-1 and consequent inhibition of collagenolytic activity may explain the absence of degradation of HDSC. These studies indicate the importance of biomaterial microenvironment in modulating inflammatory cell response and thereby the *in vivo* degradation of the material.

7.4.4 Effect of Host Response on Tissue Remodeling

The ability of biomaterials to modulate the FBR and support tissue remodeling was demonstrated by a study that evaluated commercially available ECM matrices: GraftJacket, Restore (procine small intestine submucosa [SIS]), and CuffPatch (cross-linked form of porcine SIS) (Valentin et al. 2006). The matrices showed profound differences in acute and chronic inflammatory responses and the downstream tissue remodeling process. Among the matrices, GraftJacket and Restore elicited the most intense acute inflammation. A persistent low-grade chronic inflammatory response was observed in GraftJacket and the implant was replaced with fibrous connective tissue. The Restore on the other hand was replaced with a mixture of muscle cells and organized connective tissue over time. The CuffPatch showed relatively slow remodeling compared to the Restore with a predominantly neutrophilic response initially followed by a persistent FBR.

The difference in immune response was partly attributed to the ability of biomaterials to induce phenotypic polarization of the immune cells. Badylak et al. (2008) investigated the difference in behavior of Restore and CuffPatch as a function of macrophage phenotype using a rat model. As discussed earlier, macrophage phenotypes are broadly classified into proinflammatory (M1), which is characterized by cells associated with classic signs of inflammation, and tissue remodeling (M2), which has been shown to promote immune regulation, tissue repair, and constructive tissue remodeling. At 1, 2, and 4 weeks, SIS showed an intense infiltration of mononuclear cells that were predominantly of an M2 type. By 16 weeks, the grafts were completely resorbed and the site was characterized by organized collagenous connective tissue. On the other hand, CuffPatch showed an intense mononuclear cell and polymorphonuclear cell response at 1 and 2 weeks surrounding the implant. At 4 weeks, a predominantly M1 profile was observed and at 16 weeks, mono and multinucleate giant cells were present and were associated with fibrosis around the scaffold. The study showed that even the chemical modification of the same material can lead to significant polarization of immune cells, thereby affecting biocompatibility.

Another related study investigated the effect of the presence of autologous or xenogeneic cells in ECM materials on macrophage phenotype and the subsequent tissue remodeling outcome (Brown et al. 2009). Partial-thickness defects in the abdominal wall musculature of rats were used to evaluate the tissue remodeling ability of autologous body wall tissue, acellular allogeneic body wall ECM, xenogeneic pig urinary bladder tissue, or acellular xenogeneic pig urinary bladder ECM. The study showed that the presence of cellular components in both autologous and xenogeneic tissue is capable of shifting the macrophage polarization predominantly to a proinflammatory phenotype (M1) and resulted in the formation of dense connective tissue and scarring. The acellular matrices on the other hand showed a predominantly M2 polarization and resulted in more constructive remodeling. Even though the underlying mechanism is not clear, the study suggests that the presence of cellular components can alter the host response to the biomaterial. The M1 polarization of the macrophages may be mediated by the cross talk between macrophages and activated DCs and the adaptive immune response (Kou and Babensee 2011).

Similarly, Allman et al. (2001) compared the immune response of xenogeneic and syngeneic muscle tissue to porcine SIS after subcutaneous implantation in mice. The xenogeneic tissue showed an intense immune response marked by the presence of PMNs in day 1. By day 10, a chronic inflammatory response was observed with a mixed population of neutrophils, T lymphocytes, and multinucleated giant cells. The tissue showed evidence of graft rejection by day 28 marked by necrosis, granuloma formation, and fibrous encapsulation. The syngeneic muscle tissue showed an initial acute inflammatory response. By day 10, however, there was minimal chronic inflammation and by day 28 tissue showed evidence of graft acceptance with the formation of organized tissue. The host response to the SIS was similar to that of syngeneic tissue with an acute inflammatory response followed by graft resorption and remodeling. The ability of biomaterials to modulate cell polarization is evident from the observation that the rejection of the xenografts was mediated by Th1 responses involving cytotoxic T cells, whereas the SIS elicited a Th2 response. Even though the relative roles of Th1 and Th2 cells in graft rejection are controversial, studies indicate that it is important to understand the immune cell polarization and the potential immunomodulatory activity of biomaterials.

7.5 CONCLUSIONS

Biomaterials either alone or combined with cells and biological factors will play a critical role in the functional regeneration of tissue and organs. The host immune response has increasingly been recognized as a key factor influencing regenerative outcomes. Even though the implications of immune cell phenotypes in repair and regeneration has not yet been conclusively established, studies so far have confirmed the ability of natural and synthetic biomaterials to modulate the host immune system via a myriad of mechanisms. Better understanding of the host immune response to biomaterials is needed to engineer novel immunomodulatory biomaterials that could sway the immune system to assist in the regenerative process.

REFERENCES

Allman AJ, McPherson TB, Badylak SF, Merrill LC, Kallakury B, Sheehan C, Raeder RH, Metzger DW. 2001. The xenogeneic extracellular matrix grafts elicit a TH-2 restricted immune response. *Transplantation* 71: 1631–1640.

Anderson JM, Rodriguez A, Chang DT. 2008. Foreign body reaction to biomaterials. *Semin Immunol* 20: 86–100.

Andrade JD, Hlady V. 1987. Plasma protein adsorption: The big twelve. *Ann N Y Acad Sci* 516: 158.

Babensee JE. 2008. Interaction of dendritic cells with biomaterials. *Semin Immunol* 20: 101–108.

Badylak SF, Valentin JE, Ravindra AK, McCabe GP, Stewart-Akers AM. 2008. Macrophage phenotype as a determinant of biologic scaffold remodeling. *Tissue Eng* 14: 1835–1842.

Barbosa JN, Barbosa MA, Aguas AP. 2003. Adhesion of human leukocytes to biomaterials: An in vitro study using alkanethiolate monolayers with different chemically functionalized surfaces. *J Biomed Mater Res A* 65: 429–434.

Beck RT, Illingworth KD, Saleh KJ. 2012. Review of periprosthetic osteolysis in total joint arthroplasty: An emphasis on host factors and future directions. *J Orthopaedic Res* 30: 541–6.

Bell TE, Wise KD, Andersen DJ. 1998. A flexible micromachined electrode array for a cochlear prosthesis. *Sens. Actuators A Phys* 66: 63–69.

Boehler RM, Graham JG, Shea LD. 2011. Tissue engineering tools for modulation of the immune response. *BioTechniques* 51: 239–254.

Brodbeck WG, Nakayama Y, Matsuda T, Calton E, Ziats NP, Anderson JM. 2002a. Biomaterial surface chemistry dictates adherent monocyte/macrophage cytokine expression in vitro. *Cytokine* 18: 311–319.

Brodbeck WG, Patel J, Voskerician G, Christenson E, Shive MS, Nakayama Y, Matsuda T, Ziats NP, Anderson JM. 2002b. Biomaterial adherent macrophage apoptosis is increased by hydrophilic and anionic substrates in vivo. *Proc Natl Acad Sci U S A* 99: 10287–10292.

Brodbeck WG, Voskerician G, Ziats NP, Nakayama Y, Matsuda T, Anderson JM. 2003. In vivo leukocyte cytokine mRNA responses to biomaterials are dependent on surface chemistry. *J Biomed Mater Res A* 64: 320–329.

Brown BN, Valentin JE, Stewart-Akers A, McCabe GP, Badylak SF. 2009. Macrophage phenotype and remodeling outcomes in response to biologic scaffolds with and without a cellular component. *Biomaterials* 30: 1482–1491.

Cao H, Mchugh K, Chew SY, Anderson JM. 2010. The topographical effect of electrospun nanofibrous scaffolds on the in vivo and in vitro foreign body reaction. *J Biomed Mater Res* 93A: 1151–1159.

Caparros-Lefebyre D, Blond S, Vermersch N, Pecheux J, Guieu HD, Petit H. 2002. Chronic thalamic stimulation improves tremor and levodopa induced dyskinesias in Parkinson's disease. *J Neurol Neurosurg Psychiatry* 56: 268–273.

Chang DT, Colton E, Matsuda T, Anderson JM. 2009. Lymphocyte adhesion and interactions with biomaterial adherent macrophages and foreign body giant cells. *J Biomed Mater Res A* 91: 1210–1220.

Chen S, Jones JA, Xu Y, Lo HY, Anderson JM, Leong KW. 2010. Characterization of topographical effects on macrophage behavior in a foreign body response model. *Biomaterials* 31: 3479–3491.

Farb A, Sangiorgi G, Carter AJ, Walley VM, Edwards WD, Schwartz RS, Virmani R. 1999. Pathology of acute and chronic coronary stenting in humans. *Circulation* 99: 44–52.

Gomes WJ, Buffolo E. 2006. Coronary stenting and inflammation: Implications for further surgical and medical treatment. *Ann Thorac Surg* 81: 1918–1925.

Gordon S, Clark D, Greaves D, Doyle A. 1995. Molecular immunobiology of macrophages: Recent progress. *Curr Opin Immunol* 7: 24–33.

Hallab NJ, Jacobs JJ. 2009. Biologic effects of implant debris. *Bull NYC Hosp Jt Dis* 67: 182–188.

Hamlet S, Alfarsi M, George R, Ivanovski S. 2012. The effect of hydrophilic titanium surface modification on macrophage inflammatory cytokine gene expression. *Clin Oral Implants Res* 23(5): 584–590.

Hibino N, Daniel TY, Duncan R, Rathore A, Dean E, Naito Y, Dardik A, Kyriakides T, Madri J, Pober S, Shinoka T, Breuer C. 2011. A critical role of macrophages in neovessel formation and the development of stenosis in tissue-engineered vascular grafts. *FASEB J* 25: 4253–4263.

Hulbert SF, Morrison SJ, Klawitter JJ. 1972. Tissue reaction to three ceramics of porous and non-porous structures. *J Biomed Mater Res* 6: 347–374.

Janeway CA, Travers P, Walport M, Shlomchik MJ. 2001. *Immunobiology: The Immune System in Health and Disease*, 5th edn. Garland Science, New York.

Jones JA, McNally AK, Chang DT, Qin LA, Meyerson H, Colton E et al. 2008. Matrix metalloproteinases and their inhibitors in the foreign body reaction on biomaterials. *J Biomed Mater Res A* 84: 158–166.

Kamath S, Bhattacharyya D, Padukudru C, Timmons RB, Tang LP. 2008. Surface chemistry influences implant-mediated host tissue responses. *J Biomed Mater Res A* 86: 617–626.

Klebanoff SJ, Clark RA. 1978. *The Neutrophil: Function and Clinical Disorders*. Oxford Press, New York.

Kou PM, Babensee JE. 2011. Macrophage and dendritic cell phenotypic diversity in the context of biomaterials. *J Biomed Mater Res A* 96: 239–260.

Laurencin CT, Nair LS (Eds.). 2008. *Nanotechnology and Tissue Engineering: The Scaffold*. CRC Press, Boca Raton, FL.

Madden LR, Mortisen DJ, Sussman EM, Dupras SK, Fugate JA, Cuy JL, Hauch KD, Laflamme MA, Murry CE, Ratner BD. 2010. Proangiogenic scaffolds as functional templates for cardiac tissue engineering. *PNAS* 107: 15211–15216.

Morais JM, Papadimitrakopoulos F, Burgess DJ. 2010. Biomaterials/tissue interactions: Possible solutions to overcome foreign body response. *AAPS J* 12: 188–196.

Nair LS, Bhattacharya S, Laurencin CT. 2006. Nanotechnology and tissue engineering: The scaffold based approach. In: Kumar OC (Ed.), *Tissue, Cell, and Organ Engineering. Nanotechnology for the Life Sciences Series.* Wiley-VCH Verlag GmBH & Co., Weinheim, Germany, pp. 1–56.

Nair LS, Laurencin CT. 2007. Biodegradable polymers as biomaterials. *Prog Polym Sci* 32: 762–798.

Nilson B, Korsgren O, Lambris JD, Ekdahl KN. 2009. Can cells and biomaterials in therapeutic medicine be shielded from innate immune recognition? *Trends Immunol* 31: 32–38.

Ratner BD, Hoffman AS, Schoen FJ, Lemons JE. 2004. *Biomaterials Science. An Introduction to Materials in Medicine,* 2nd edn. Elsevier, San Diego, CA.

Reichert WM, Ratner BD, Anderson J, Coury A, Hoffman AS, Laurencin CT, Tirrell D. 2011. Panel on the biomaterials grand challenges. *J Biomed Mater Res A* 96(2): 275–287.

Sanders JE, Stiles CE, Hayes CL. 2000. Tissue response to single-polymer fibers of varying diameters: Evaluation of fibrous encapsulation and macrophage density. *J Biomed Mater Res* 52: 231–237.

Smetana K, Vacik J, Houska M, Saouckova D, Lukas J. 1993. Macrophage recognition of polymers effect of carboxylate groups. *J Mater Sci Mater Med* 4: 526–529.

Smiley ST, King JA, Hancock WW. 2001. Fibrinogen stimulates macrophage chemokine secretion through toll-like receptor 4. *J Immunol* 167: 2887.

Szarowski DH, Andersen MD, Retterer S, Spence AJ, Isaacson M, Craighead HG, Turner JN, Shain W. 2003. Brain responses to micro-machined silicon devices. *Brain Res* 983: 23–35.

The Freedonia Group. 2008. *Orthopedic Implants: US Industry Forecasts for 2012 and 2017, USA.* Cleveland, OH. www.freedoniagroup.com

Tsirogianni AK, Moutsopoulos NM, Moutsopoulos HM. 2006. Wound healing: Immunological aspects. *Injury Int J Care Injured* 375: S5–S12.

Valentin JE, Badylak JS, McCabe GP, Badylak SF. 2006. Extracellular matrix bioscaffolds for orthopaedic applications. A comparative histologic study. *J Bone Joint Surg Am* 88: 2673–2686.

Wang W. 2011. Orthopaedic implant technology: Biomaterials from past to future. *Ann Acad Med Singapore* 40: 237–244.

Ward KW, Slobodzian EP, Tiekotter KL, Wood MD. 2002. The effect of microgeometry, implant thickness and polyurethane chemistry on the foreign body response to subcutaneous implants. *Biomaterials* 23: 4185–4192.

Ye Q, Harmsen MC, Luyn MJA, Bank RA. 2010. The relationship between collagen scaffold cross-linking agents and neutrophils in the foreign body reaction. *Biomaterials* 31: 9192–9201.

CHAPTER 8

Organ Regenerative Engineering

Cell Sources, Considerations, and Strategies

Anthony Atala, MD; Meng Deng, PhD; and Yusuf Khan, PhD

CONTENTS

8.1 INTRODUCTION

Patients suffering from diseased and injured organs may be treated with transplanted organs. However, there is a severe shortage of donor organs that is worsening yearly. As modern medicine increases the human lifespan, the aging population grows, and the need for organs grows with it, as aging organs are generally more prone to failure. Scientists in the field of regenerative medicine and tissue engineering apply the principles of cell transplantation, material science, and bioengineering to construct biological substitutes that can prolong life by reducing mortality from these diseases. Therapeutic cloning, where the nucleus from a donor cell is transferred into an enucleated oocyte in order to extract pluripotent embryonic stem cells, offers a potentially limitless source of cells for tissue engineering applications. The stem cell field is also advancing rapidly, opening new options for therapy. This chapter reviews recent advances that have occurred in regenerative medicine and describes applications of these new technologies that offer promise of a longer life to organ regenerative engineering.

The field of regenerative medicine encompasses various areas of technology, such as tissue engineering, stem cells, and cloning. Tissue engineering plays a major role in regenerative medicine and shows great promise toward the generation of biological substitutes for repair and restoration of damaged or diseased tissues/organs. Tissue engineering strategies generally involve the use of either acellular matrices or matrices with cells. Acellular matrices are characterized by the ability to serve as temporary cellular substrates that can be replaced by the extracellular matrix (ECM) proteins secreted by the in-growing cells. These matrices are often produced by a number of scaffold fabrication techniques or through decellularization of native tissues (Dahms et al. 1998, Piechota et al. 1998, Yoo et al. 1998, Chen et al. 1999). The efficacy of acellular tissue matrices lies in the body's own ability to regenerate for specific new tissue formation and ingrowth.

Cells constitute another important therapeutic component for tissue regeneration. Cells used for tissue engineering are isolated from a small biopsy of donor tissue that can be autologous (self), allogeneic (same species, different individual), or heterologous (such as bovine). Following *in vitro* expansion, these cells can be used either through injection (alone or with different carriers) or by implantation into the host with ECM-mimicking matrices. Compared to other cell donor sources, autologous cells from the host exhibit several advantages for tissue replacement including minimal complications and absence of host rejection (Cilento et al. 1994, Atala 1998, 1999, 2001, Yoo et al. 1998, 1999, Amiel and Atala 1999, Oberpenning et al. 1999, Amiel et al. 2006).

Most cell-based tissue engineering strategies involve the use of autologous cells from the diseased organ of the host. Aging itself is not a barrier to successful applications of engineered tissues, as cells can be expanded from young and old patients alike. However, there are a number of situations where expansion of primary autologous human cells is not feasible from a particular organ (e.g., the pancreas). In addition, a tissue biopsy obtained from patients suffering from extensive end-stage organ failure may not produce a sufficient number of normal cells for expansion and transplantation. Stem cells have thus emerged as an alternative source of cells for therapy, which are derived from discarded human embryos, fetal tissue, or adult sources such as bone marrow, fat, and skin.

Therapeutic cloning also contributes to the advances in the field of regenerative medicine. This type of cloning, which has also been called nuclear transplantation and nuclear transfer, involves the introduction of a nucleus from a donor cell into an enucleated oocyte to generate an embryo with a genetic makeup identical to that of the donor. Autologous stem cells can be derived from this source, which may have the future potential to be used therapeutically.

8.2 CELLS FOR USE IN TISSUE ENGINEERING

Please refer to Chapter 3 for an in-depth discussion of stem cells. In the following are many examples of various cell populations and their direct application to tissue regeneration.

8.2.1 Embryonic Stem Cells

Human embryonic stem cells are pluripotent stem cells derived from the inner cell mass of the embryo during the blastocyst stage (5 days post-fertilization). These cells display distinct characteristics in that they have the capacity to self-renew (proliferate in an undifferentiated but pluripotent state) indefinitely as well as retain the ability to differentiate into cells from all three embryonic germ layers (Brivanlou et al. 2003). Culture of human embryonic stem cells often requires the use of feeder layers consisting of mouse embryonic fibroblasts (MEFs) or human feeder cells (Richards et al. 2002). Recent advances have demonstrated the ability of growing these cells under feeder-free conditions (Amit et al. 2004), which can eliminate the potential influence of mouse viruses and proteins on these human cells. These cells have also been shown to be able to self-renew for more than 80 passages using established culture protocols (Thomson et al. 1998, Reubinoff et al. 2000).

The pluripotency of human embryonic stem cells has been demonstrated in a large number of *in vitro* studies showing that they can differentiate into cells from all three embryonic germ layers (ectoderm, mesoderm, and endoderm). In specific, ectodermal differentiation, mesodermal differentiation, and endodermal differentiation have been evidenced by the formation of skin and neurons (Schuldiner et al. 2000, 2001, Reubinoff et al. 2001, Zhang et al. 2001), blood, cardiac cells, cartilage, endothelial cells, and muscle (Kaufman et al. 2001, Kehat et al. 2001, Levenberg et al. 2002), and pancreatic cells (Assady et al. 2001), respectively. In addition, their capacity to form teratomas *in vivo* as well as embryoid bodies containing the three embryonic germ layers *in vitro* further exemplifies the pluripotency of human embryonic stem cells (Itskovitz-Eldor et al. 2000).

8.2.2 Laboratory-Generated Stem Cells

In addition, stem cells for tissue engineering could be generated through cloning procedures. In 1962, Gurdon reported the cloned frogs that were the first successfully cloned vertebrates derived from nuclear transfer, but the nuclei were derived from non-adult sources (Gurdon et al. 1958, Gurdon 1962a,b,c). In 1996, Campbell et al. (1996) produced live lambs that were the first-cloned mammals using nuclear transfer and differentiated epithelial cells derived from embryonic disks. It was not until a year later that Wilmut et al. (1997) reported the birth of Dolly, which was the first mammal derived from an adult somatic cell using nuclear transfer. Since then, there has been significant interest and tremendous progress in nuclear cloning technology. Animals from several species have been produced using nuclear transfer technology, including cattle (Cibelli et al. 1998), goats (Baguisi et al. 1999), mice (Wakayama et al. 1998), and pigs (Betthauser et al. 2000, De Sousa et al. 2002).

There are two different types of nuclear cloning: reproductive cloning and therapeutic cloning (Colman and Kind 2000, Vogelstein et al. 2002). Reproductive cloning involves creating an embryo that has the identical genetic material as its cell source by nuclear transfer and then implanting it into a uterus and allowing it to give rise to an infant that is a clone of the donor. This has been achieved for several mammalian species (e.g., sheep Dolly) and is banned in most countries for human applications. In contrast, therapeutic cloning that is also called somatic cell nuclear transfer (SCNT) is used to derive only embryonic stem cell lines that are genetically identical to the original donor. In this case, blastocysts are allowed to grow until a few hundred cell stages where embryonic stem cells can be obtained. These resulting autologous stem cells hold great therapeutic potential for tissue and organ replacement applications (Hochedlinger et al. 2004). According to data from the Centers for Disease Control, an estimated 3000 Americans die every day of diseases that could have been treated with stem cell-derived tissues (Lanza et al. 1999, 2001). Figure 8.1 illustrates the strategy of combining therapeutic cloning with tissue engineering to develop tissues and organs. The tissues and organs derived from therapeutic cloning could be transplanted into the original donor and would be recognized as "self" thereby circumventing the problems of rejection and immunosuppression that occur with transplantation of non-autologous tissues (Lanza et al. 1999).

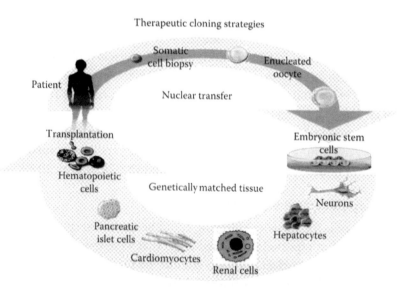

FIGURE 8.1 **Strategy for therapeutic cloning and tissue engineering.**

The application of therapeutic cloning in replacement therapy is currently hindered by several limitations associated with the SCNT technology, such as the low efficiency of the overall cloning process as well as poor survival rate for the majority of embryos derived from animal cloning after implantation (Solter 2000, Rideout et al. 2001, Hochedlinger and Jaenisch 2002). To achieve desirable cloning efficiency, further improvements are needed in the multiple complex steps of nuclear transfer involving enucleation and reconstruction, activation of oocytes, and cell cycle synchronization between donor cells and recipient oocytes (Dinnyes et al. 2002).

Recently, exciting reports of the successful transformation of adult cells into pluripotent stem cells through a type of genetic "reprogramming" have been published. Reprogramming is a technique that involves de-differentiation of adult somatic cells to produce patient-specific pluripotent stem cells, without the use of embryos. Cells generated by reprogramming would be genetically identical to the somatic cells (and thus, the patient who donated these cells) and would not be rejected. Yamanaka was the first to discover that MEFs and adult mouse fibroblasts could be reprogrammed into an "induced pluripotent state (iPS)" (Takahashi and Yamanaka 2006). This group used MEFs engineered to express a neomycin resistance gene from the *Fbx15* locus, a gene expressed only in ES cells. They examined 24 genes that were thought to be important for embryonic stem cells and identified four key genes that, when introduced into the reporter fibroblasts, resulted in drug-resistant cells. These were Oct3/4, Sox2, c-Myc, and Klf4. This experiment indicated that expression of the four genes in these transgenic MEFs led to the expression of a gene specific for ES cells. MEFs and adult fibroblasts were co-transduced with retroviral vectors, each carrying one of the four genes, and transduced cells were selected via drug resistance. The resultant iPS cells possessed the immortal growth characteristics of self-renewing ES cells, expressed genes specific for ES cells, and generated embryoid bodies *in vitro* and teratomas *in vivo*. When iPS cells were injected into mouse blastocysts, they contributed to a variety of cell types. However, although iPS cells selected in this way were pluripotent, they were not identical to ES cells. Unlike ES cells, chimeras made from iPS cells did not result in full-term pregnancies. Gene expression profiles of the iPS cells showed that they possessed a distinct gene expression signature that was different from that of ES cells. In addition, the epigenetic state of the iPS cells was somewhere between that found in somatic cells and that found in ES cells, suggesting that the reprogramming was incomplete.

These results were improved significantly by Wernig and Jaenisch in July 2007 (Wernig et al. 2007). Fibroblasts were infected with retroviral vectors and selected for the activation of endogenous *Oct4* or *Nanog* genes. Results from this study showed that DNA methylation, gene expression profiles, and the chromatin state of the reprogrammed cells were similar to those of ES cells. Teratomas induced by these cells contained differentiated cell types representing all three embryonic germ layers. Most importantly, the reprogrammed cells from this experiment were able to form viable chimeras and contribute to the germ line–like ES cells, suggesting that these iPS cells were completely reprogrammed. Wernig et al. observed that the number of reprogrammed colonies increased when drug selection was initiated later (day 20 rather than day 3 post-transduction). This suggests that reprogramming is a slow and gradual process and may explain why previous attempts resulted in incomplete reprogramming.

It has recently been shown that reprogramming of human cells is possible (Takahashi et al. 2007, Yu et al. 2007). Yamanaka showed that retrovirus-mediated transfection of *OCT3/4*, *SOX2*, *KLF4*, and *c-MYC* generates human iPS cells that are similar to hES cells in terms of morphology, proliferation, gene expression, surface markers, and teratoma formation. Thompson's group showed that retroviral transduction of *OCT4*, *SOX2*, *NANOG*, and *LIN28* could generate pluripotent stem cells without introducing any oncogenes (c-MYC). Both studies showed that human iPS were similar but not identical to hES cells.

Another concern is that these iPS cells contain three to six retroviral integrations (one for each factor) that may increase the risk of tumorigenesis. Yamanaka et al. studied the tumor formation in chimeric mice generated from Nanog-iPS cells and found 20% of the offspring developed tumors due to the retroviral expression of c-myc (Okita et al. 2007). An alternative approach would be to use a transient expression method, such as adenovirus-mediated system, since both Jaenisch and Yamanaka showed strong silencing of the viral-controlled transcripts in iPS cells (Meissner et al. 2007, Okita et al. 2007). This indicates that these viral genes are only required for the induction, not the maintenance, of pluripotency.

Another concern is the use of transgenic donor cells for reprogrammed cells in the mouse studies. Both studies used donor cells from transgenic mice harboring a drug resistance gene driven by *Fbx15*, *Oct3/4*, or *Nanog* promoters so that, if these ES cell-specific genes were activated, the resulting cells could be easily selected using neomycin. However, the use of genetically modified donors hinders clinical applicability for humans. To assess whether iPS cells can be derived from nontransgenic donor cells, wild-type MEF and adult skin cells were retrovirally transduced with Oct3/4, Sox2, c-Myc, and Klf4, and ES-like colonies were isolated by morphology alone, without the use of drug selection for *Oct4* or *Nanog* (Meissner et al. 2007). iPS cells from wild-type donor cells formed teratomas and generated live chimeras. This study suggests that transgenic donor cells are not necessary to generate IPS cells.

Although this is an exciting phenomenon, it is unclear why reprogramming adult fibroblasts and mesenchymal stromal cells have similar efficiencies (Takahashi and Yamanaka 2006). It would seem that cells that are already multipotent could be reprogrammed with greater efficiency, since the more undifferentiated donor nucleus, the better SCNT performs (Blelloch et al. 2006). This further emphasizes our limited understanding of the mechanism of reprogramming, yet the potential for this area of study is exciting.

8.2.3 Amniotic Fluid and Placental Stem Cells

Recent discovery of stem cells isolated from amniotic fluid and placenta provides an alternative source to the field of regenerative medicine. Amniotic fluid-derived stem (AFS) cells can be obtained from a small amount of fluid during amniocentesis, whereas placenta-derived stem cells can be obtained from a small biopsy of the chorionic villi. For example, Atala has reported the isolation of AFS cells that express embryonic and adult stem cell markers (De Coppi et al. 2007). It was found that these cells can be readily expanded without feeders in culture with a typical doubling time of about 36 h and do not form tumors *in vivo*. Lines showed the absence of senescence and maintenance of long telomeres and a normal karyotype for over 250 population doublings. AFS cells are pluripotent stem cells. Clonal human lines were able to yield differentiated cells corresponding to each of the three embryonic germ layers along adipogenic, osteogenic, myogenic, endothelial, neurogenic, and hepatic pathways. Furthermore, human AFS cells can give rise to differentiated cells, such as neuronal lineage cells, hepatic lineage cells, and osteogenic lineage cells with sufficient specialized function to have potential therapeutic utility. In the future, banking of these stem cells holds the promise for generating an attractive cell source for autologous therapy with a perfect genetic match in the treatment of newborns with congenital malformations as well as of adults (De Coppi et al. 2007).

8.2.4 Challenges with Cell-Based Organ Regeneration Strategies

One of the limitations of applying cell-based regenerative medicine techniques to organ replacement has been the inherent difficulty of growing specific cell types in large quantities. Even when some organs, such as the liver, have a high regenerative capacity *in vivo*, cell growth and expansion *in vitro* may be difficult. By studying the privileged sites for committed precursor cells in specific organs, as well as exploring the conditions that promote differentiation, one may be able to overcome the obstacles that limit cell expansion *in vitro*. For example, urothelial cells could be grown in the laboratory setting in the past, but only with limited expansion. Several protocols were developed over the past two decades that identified the undifferentiated cells and kept them undifferentiated during their growth phase (Liebert et al. 1991, 1997, Cilento et al. 1994, Scriven et al. 1997, Puthenveettil et al. 1999). Using these methods of cell culture, it is now possible to expand a urothelial strain from a single specimen that initially covered a surface area of 1 cm² to one covering a surface area of 4202 m² (the equivalent of one football field) within 8 weeks (Cilento et al. 1994). These studies indicated that it should be possible to collect autologous bladder cells from human patients, expand them in culture, and return them to the donor in sufficient quantities for reconstructive purposes (Liebert et al. 1991, 1997, Cilento et al. 1994, Harriss 1995, Freeman et al. 1997, Scriven et al. 1997, Nguyen et al. 1999, Puthenveettil et al. 1999). Major advances have been achieved within the past decade on the possible expansion of a variety of primary human cells, with specific techniques that make the use of autologous cells possible for clinical application.

8.3 TISSUE ENGINEERING OF SPECIFIC STRUCTURES

Collective efforts in the field of regenerative medicine have made significant progress in the development of tissues and organs for clinical application. Several specific bioengineered tissue structures are detailed in the following text.

8.3.1 Urethra

The urethra is the tube that carries urine from the bladder to the outside of the body. A number of disease states can cause strictures, or blockages, of the urethra, and many of these occur in response to pelvic injury in both men and women. Some strictures can be easily treated using urethral dilation or minor surgical procedures, but larger, more complex strictures often require the use of a tissue graft taken from another area of the body. Unfortunately, such a treatment requires several surgeries and can cause significant discomfort for the patient. Thus, the ability to regenerate or engineer urethral tissue would be advantageous. Various strategies have been proposed over the years for the regeneration of urethral tissue. Woven meshes of polyglycolic acid (PGA) without cells (Bazeed et al. 1983, Olsen et al. 1992) or with cells (Atala et al. 1992) were used to regenerate urethras in various animal models. Naturally derived collagen-based materials such as bladder-derived acellular submucosa (Chen et al. 1999), and an acellular urethral submucosa (Sievert et al. 2000), have also been tried experimentally in various animal models for urethral reconstruction.

The bladder submucosa matrix (Chen et al. 1999) proved to be a suitable graft for repair of urethral defects in rabbits. The neourethras demonstrated a normal urothelial luminal lining and organized muscle bundles. These results were confirmed clinically in a series of patients with a history of failed hypospadia reconstruction wherein the urethral defects were repaired with human bladder acellular collagen matrices (Figure 8.2) (Atala et al. 1999). The neourethras were created by anastomosing the matrix in an onlay fashion to the urethral plate. The size of the created neourethra ranged from 5 to 15 cm. After a 3-year follow-up, three of the four patients had a successful outcome in regard to cosmetic appearance and function. One patient who had a 15 cm neourethra created developed a subglanular fistula. The acellular collagen-based matrix eliminated the necessity of performing additional surgical procedures for graft harvesting, and both operative time and the potential morbidity from the harvest procedure were decreased. Similar results were obtained in pediatric and adult patients with primary urethral stricture disease using the same collagen matrices (El-Kassaby et al. 2003). Another study in 30 patients with recurrent stricture disease showed that a healthy urethral bed (two or fewer prior urethral surgeries) was needed for successful urethral reconstruction using the acellular collagen-based grafts (El-Kassaby et al. 2008). More than 200 pediatric and adult patients with urethral disease have been successfully treated in an onlay manner with a bladder-derived collagen-based matrix. One of its advantages over nongenital tissue grafts used for urethroplasty is that the material is "off the shelf." This eliminates the necessity of additional surgical procedures for graft harvesting, which may decrease operative time as well as the potential morbidity due to the harvest procedure.

The earlier techniques, using non-seeded acellular matrices, were applied experimentally and clinically in a successful manner for onlay urethral repairs. However, when tubularized urethral repairs were attempted experimentally, adequate urethral tissue regeneration was not achieved, and complications ensued, such as graft contracture and

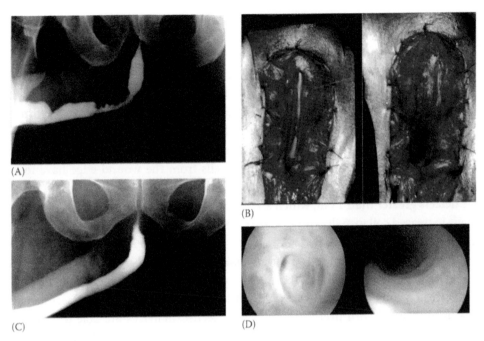

FIGURE 8.2   Tissue engineering of the urethra using a collagen matrix. (A) Representative case of a patient with a bulbar stricture. (B) During the urethral repair surgery, strictured tissue is excised, preserving the urethral plate on the left side, and matrix is anastamosed to the urethral plate in an onlay fashion on the right. The boxes in both photos indicate the area of interest, including the urethra, which appears white in the left photograph. In the left photograph, the arrow indicates the area of stricture in the urethra. On the right, the arrow indicates the repaired stricture. Note that the engineered tissue now obscures the native white urethral tissue in an onlay fashion in the right photograph. (C) Urethrogram 6 months after repair. (D) Cystoscopic view of urethra before surgery on the left side, and 4 months after repair on the right side.

stricture formation (De Filippo et al. 2002). Autologous rabbit bladder epithelial and smooth muscle cells were grown and seeded onto pre-configured tubular matrices. Entire urethra segments were resected, and urethroplasties were performed with tubularized collagen matrices either seeded with cells or without cells. The tubularized collagen matrices seeded with autologous cells formed new tissue that was histologically similar to native urethra. The tubularized collagen matrices without cells lead to poor tissue development, fibrosis, and stricture formation. These findings were confirmed clinically. A clinical trial using tubularized non-seeded small intestinal submucosa (SIS) for urethral stricture repair was performed in eight evaluable patients. Two patients with short inflammatory strictures maintained urethral patency. Stricture recurrence developed in the other six patients within 3 months of surgery (le Roux et al. 2005). Other cell types have also been tried experimentally in acellular bladder collagen matrices, including foreskin epidermal cells and oral keratinocytes (Fu et al. 2007, Li et al. 2008). Vascular endothelial growth factor gene-modified urothelial cells have also been used experimentally for urethral reconstruction (Guan et al. 2008).

The normal wound healing response to injury has been studied extensively, and this knowledge has been helpful in maximizing success for the engineering of tissues. At the time of tissue injury, cell ingrowth is initiated from the wound edges in order to cover the tissue defect. The cells from the edges of the native tissue are able to traverse short distances without any detrimental effects. If the wound is large, more than a few millimeters in distance or depth, increased collagen deposition, fibrosis, and scar formation ensue. Matrices implanted in wound beds are able to lengthen the distances that cells can traverse without initiating an adverse fibrotic response. However, these distances are also limited. The maximum distance that adjacent cells from the wound edge have to travel to create normal tissue over a biologic matrix is approximately 1 cm (Dorin et al. 2008). Tissue defects greater than 1 cm, which are treated with a matrix alone, without cells, usually have increased collagen deposition, increased fibrosis, and scar formation. Cell-seeded matrices implanted in wound beds are able to further lengthen the distance for normal tissue formation, without initiating an adverse fibrotic response. Studies in the field of regenerative medicine have shown that very large defects, greater than 30 cm, can be successfully treated using cell-seeded scaffolds. This explains the described experimental and clinical results noted with urethral repair. Non-seeded matrices are able to replace urethral segments when used in an onlay fashion because of the short distances required for tissue ingrowth. However, if a tubularized urethral repair is needed, the matrices need to be seeded with autologous cells in order to avoid the risk of stricture formation and poor tissue development.

Most recently, Raya-Rivera and colleagues were able to show that synthetic biomaterials can also be used in urethral reconstruction when they are tabularized and seeded with autologous cells (Raya-Rivera et al. 2011). This group used polyglycolic acid:poly(lactide-co-glycolic acid) scaffolds seeded with autologous cells derived from bladder biopsies taken from each patient. The seeded scaffolds were then used to repair urethral defects in five boys. Upon follow-up, it was found that most of the boys had excellent urinary flow rates post-operatively, and voiding cystourethrograms indicated that these patients maintained wide urethral calibers. Urethral biopsies revealed that the grafts had developed a normal-appearing architecture consisting of urothelial and muscular tissues.

8.3.2 Bladder

Currently, gastrointestinal segments are commonly used as tissues for bladder replacement or repair. However, gastrointestinal tissues are designed to absorb specific solutes, whereas bladder tissue is designed for the excretion of these same solutes. Because of this "mismatch," there can be serious consequences to using gastrointestinal tissue in the urinary tract, including infection, excess mucous production, formation of urinary stones, and even the development of malignancies. Due to the problems encountered with the use of gastrointestinal segments, numerous investigators have attempted alternative materials and tissues for bladder replacement or repair.

Over the last few decades, several bladder wall substitutes have been attempted with both synthetic and organic materials. Synthetic materials that have been tried in experimental and clinical settings include polyvinyl sponge, Teflon, collagen matrices, Vicryl

(PGA) matrices, and silicone. Most of these attempts have failed because of mechanical, structural, functional, or biocompatibility problems. Usually, permanent synthetic materials used for bladder reconstruction succumb to mechanical failure and urinary stone formation, and use of degradable materials leads to fibroblast deposition, scarring, graft contracture, and a reduced reservoir volume over time (Atala 1995, 1998). Because of this, there has been an increase in the use of various collagen-based matrices for tissue regeneration. Non-seeded allogeneic acellular bladder matrices have served as scaffolds for the ingrowth of host bladder wall components. The matrices are prepared by mechanically and chemically removing all cellular components from bladder tissue (Sutherland et al. 1996, Probst et al. 1997, Piechota et al. 1998, Yoo et al. 1998, Wefer et al. 2001). The matrices serve as vehicles for partial bladder regeneration, and relevant antigenicity is not evident. However, in multiple studies using various materials as non-seeded grafts for cystoplasty, the urothelial layer was able to regenerate normally, but the muscle layer, although present, was not fully developed (Kropp et al. 1996, Sutherland et al. 1996, Probst et al. 1997, Yoo et al. 1998, Jayo et al. 2008a,b, Zhang 2008). Studies involving acellular matrices that may provide the necessary environment to promote cell migration, growth, and differentiation are being conducted (Chun et al. 2007). With continued bladder research in this area, these matrices may have a clinical role in bladder replacement in the future.

Cell-seeded allogeneic acellular bladder matrices were used for bladder augmentation in dogs (Yoo et al. 1998). The regenerated bladder tissues contained a normal cellular organization consisting of urothelium and smooth muscle and exhibited a normal compliance. Biomaterials preloaded with cells before their implantation showed better tissue regeneration compared with biomaterials implanted with no cells, in which tissue regeneration depended on ingrowth of the surrounding tissue. The bladders showed a significant increase (100%) in capacity when augmented with scaffolds seeded with cells, compared to scaffolds without cells (30%). The acellular collagen matrices can be enhanced with growth factors to improve bladder regeneration (Kikuno et al. 2008).

It has been well established for decades that the bladder is able to regenerate generously over free grafts. Urothelium is associated with a high reparative capacity (de Boer et al. 1994). Bladder muscle tissue is less likely to regenerate in a normal fashion. Both urothelial and muscle ingrowth are believed to be initiated from the edges of the normal bladder toward the region of the free graft (Baker et al. 1958, Gorham et al. 1989). Usually, however, contracture or resorption of the graft has been evident. The inflammatory response toward the matrix may contribute to the resorption of the free graft. It was hypothesized that building the three-dimensional structure constructs *in vitro*, before implantation, would facilitate the eventual terminal differentiation of the cells after implantation *in vivo* and would minimize the inflammatory response toward the matrix, thus avoiding graft contracture and shrinkage. The dog study demonstrated a major difference between matrices used with autologous cells (tissue-engineered matrices) and those used without cells (Yoo et al. 1998). Matrices implanted with cells for bladder augmentation retained most of their implanted diameter, as opposed to matrices implanted without cells for bladder augmentation, in which graft contraction and shrinkage occurred. The histomorphology demonstrated a marked paucity of muscle cells and a more aggressive inflammatory reaction in the matrices implanted without cells. Epithelial–mesenchymal signaling is important for the differentiation of bladder smooth muscle (Master et al. 2003).

The results of initial studies showed that the creation of artificial bladders may be achieved *in vivo*; however, it could not be determined whether the functional parameters noted were caused by the augmented segment or by the intact native bladder tissue. To better address the functional parameters of tissue-engineered bladders, an animal model was designed in which a subtotal cystectomy was performed in dogs, with subsequent replacement of this bladder tissue with a tissue-engineered organ (Oberpenning et al. 1999). Cystectomy-only and non-seeded controls maintained average capacities of 20% and 46% of preoperative values, respectively. An average bladder capacity of 95% of the original precystectomy volume was achieved in the cell-seeded tissue-engineered bladder replacements. These findings were confirmed radiographically (Figure 8.3). The subtotal cystectomy reservoirs that were not reconstructed and the polymer-only reconstructed bladders showed a marked decrease in bladder compliance (10% and 42% total compliance). The compliance of the cell-seeded tissue-engineered bladders showed almost no difference from preoperative values that were measured when the native bladder was present (106%). Histologically, the non-seeded scaffold bladders presented a pattern of

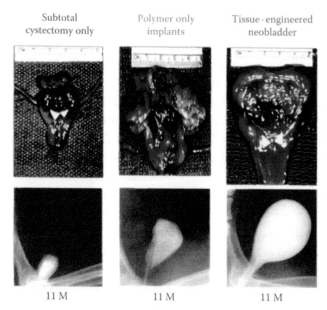

FIGURE 8.3 Gross specimens and cystograms at 11 months of the cystectomy-only, non-seeded controls, and cell-seeded tissue-engineered bladder replacements in dogs. The cystectomy-only bladder had a capacity of 22% of the preoperative value and a decrease in bladder compliance to 10% of the preoperative value. The non-seeded controls showed significant scarring with a capacity of 46% of the preoperative value and a decrease in bladder compliance to 42% of the preoperative value. An average bladder capacity of 95% of the original precystectomy volume was achieved in the cell-seeded tissue-engineered bladder replacements, and the compliance showed almost no difference from preoperative values that were measured when the native bladder was present (106%).

normal urothelial cells with a thickened fibrotic submucosa and a thin layer of muscle fibers. The retrieved tissue-engineered bladders showed a normal cellular organization, consisting of a trilayer of urothelium, submucosa, and muscle. Immunocytochemical analyses confirmed the muscle and urothelial phenotype. S-100 staining indicated the presence of neural structures (Oberpenning et al. 1999). These studies, performed with PGA-based scaffolds, have been repeated by other investigators, showing similar results in large numbers of animals in the long term (Jayo et al. 2008a,b). The strategy of using biodegradable scaffolds with cells can be pursued without concerns for local or systemic toxicity (Kwon et al. 2008). However, not all scaffolds perform well if a large portion of the bladder needs replacement. In a study using SIS for subtotal bladder replacement in dogs, both the unseeded and cell-seeded experimental groups showed graft shrinkage and poor results (Zhang et al. 2006). The type of scaffold used is critical for the success of these technologies. The use of bioreactors, in which mechanical stimulation is started at the time of organ production, has also been proposed as an important parameter for success (Farhat and Yeger 2008).

Atala's group has engineered human bladder tissues for patients requiring cystoplasty. In the pilot study of seven patients, autologous bladder urothelial and muscle cells were isolated and expanded *in vitro*, and seeded onto biodegradable bladder-shaped scaffold made of collagen, or a composite of collagen and PGA (Figure 8.4). The autologous engineered bladder constructs were implanted either with or without omental coverage. The composite engineered bladders with omental coverage resulted in improved functional parameters that were durable over a period of years (Figure 8.5) (Atala et al. 2006). It was also indicated from the study that the engineered bladders continued to develop with the increase in implantation time. This study represents a step forward to the development of anatomically functional engineered bladders. Nevertheless, this was a limited clinical experience, and the technology is not yet ready for wide dissemination, as further experimental and clinical studies are required. FDA Phase 2 studies have now been completed.

An area of concern in the field of tissue engineering in the past was the source of cells for regeneration. The concept of creating engineered constructs involves initially obtaining cells for expansion from the diseased organ. However, it was not known until recently whether the cell population obtained for later autologous implantation was normal and would lead to normal tissue formation. For example, would the cells obtained from a neuropathic bladder lead to the engineering of another neuropathic bladder? Cultured neuropathic bladder smooth muscle cells possess and maintain different characteristics than normal smooth muscle cells *in vitro*, as demonstrated by growth assays, contractility, adherence tests, and microarray analysis (Lin et al. 2004, Dozmorov et al. 2007, Hipp et al. 2008). However, when neuropathic smooth muscle cells were cultured *in vitro*, seeded onto matrices and implanted *in vivo*, the tissue-engineered constructs showed the same properties as the tissues engineered with normal cells (Lai et al. 2002). The progenitor cells, which reside within stem cell niches within each organ, are responsible for new cell differentiation and tissue formation during the normal process of tissue regeneration due to natural turnover, ageing, and tissue injury. It is known that genetically normal non-malignant progenitor cells, which are the reservoirs for new cell formation, are programmed to give

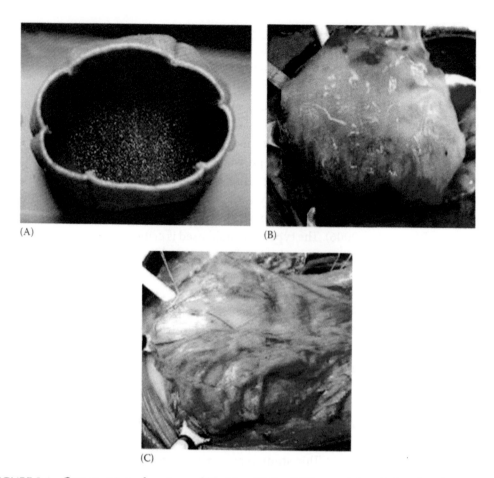

(A)

(B)

(C)

FIGURE 8.4   Construction of engineered bladder. (A) Scaffold material seeded with cells for use in bladder repair. (B) The seeded scaffold is anastamosed to native bladder with running 4–0 polyglycolic sutures. (C) Implant covered with fibrin glue and omentum.

rise to normal tissue, regardless of whether the niche resides in either normal or diseased tissues (Faris et al. 2001, Lai et al. 2002, Haller et al. 2005). Therefore, although the mechanisms for tissue self-assembly and regenerative medicine are not fully understood, it is known that the progenitor cells are able to "reset" their program for normal cell differentiation. The stem cell niche and its role in normal tissue regeneration remain a fertile area of ongoing investigation.

8.3.3 Kidney

The kidney is an organ consisting of multiple cell types and a complex functional anatomy that presents many challenges to reconstruct (Amiel and Atala 1999, Auchincloss and Bonventre 2002). While the metanephros is responsible for the development of the proximal section of the nephrons, the ureteric bud forms the collecting ducts and distal structures. The large vessels of the kidney are induced from extra renal tissues. Divergent embryologic origin converges to produce at least 26 distinct functional cells in the kidney (Al-Awqati and Oliver 2002). Earlier research in tissue engineering of the kidney has

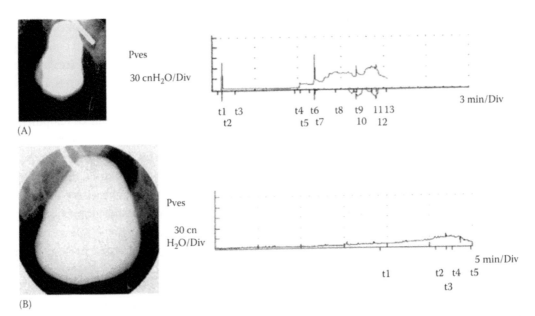

Pves

30 cnH₂O/Div

3 min/Div

t1 t3   t4 t6   t8 t9 1113
    t2   t5 t7   10 12

(A)

Pves

30 cn
H₂O/Div

5 min/Div

t1   t2 t4 t5
                t3

(B)

FIGURE 8.5 Cystograms and urodynamic studies of a patient before and after implantation of the tissue-engineered bladder. (A) Preoperative results indicate an irregular-shaped bladder in the cystogram (left) and abnormal bladder pressures as the bladder is filled during urodynamic studies (right). (B) Postoperatively, findings are significantly improved.

been focused on the development of extracorporeal renal support systems (Aebischer et al. 1987a,b, Ip et al. 1988, Lanza et al. 1996, MacKay et al. 1998, Humes et al. 1999a,b, Amiel et al. 2000, Joki et al. 2001). Still, there exists a need of a long-term transplantable device for patients with end-stage kidney disease, which can obviate the use of an extracorporeal perfusion circuit and immunosuppressive treatment.

Atala's group has explored the possibility of seeding an implantable biomaterial with a heterogeneous population of renal cells to evaluate function and viability. Atala et al. plated donor rabbit kidney cells, including distal tubules, glomeruli, and proximal tubules *in vitro*, and after expansion, these were seeded onto biodegradeable PGA scaffolds and implanted subcutaneously into athymic mice. The implants consisted of individual cell types and a mixture of all three. When examined histologically, progressive formation and organization of the nephron segments within the polymer fibers were noted. Additionally, BrdU incorporation into the renal cell DNA was confirmed (Atala et al. 1995). It was unclear if the tubular structures found on the scaffolds occurred *de novo* from the implanted cells or if they merely represented fragments of donor tubules that had survived the original dissociation and culture process intact. To further investigate this question, mouse renal cells were harvested and expanded in culture. Subsequently, a single cell suspension was created from the isolated cells, and these were seeded on biodegradable polymers and implanted into immune-competent synergic hosts. In this experiment, renal epithelial cells reconstituted tubular structures *in vivo*. The analyses of the retrieved implants indicated that the renal epithelial cells first organized into a structure with a solid center. Next, canalization into a hollow tube could be seen at 2 weeks.

Histological examination with nephron-specific lactins revealed successful reconstitution of proximal tubules, distal tubules, loops of Henle, collecting tubules, and collecting ducts. These results clearly showed that single cell suspensions grown *in vitro* are capable of reconstituting tubule structures. The tubules contained homogenous cell types within each tubule (Fung et al. 1996).

Further investigations by our group have demonstrated that renal tubular development from digested renal units is possible in the murine model as well. Joraku et al. (2009) developed an *in vitro* method for cultivation of renal cells that allowed for development of tubular structures. This technique involves digestion of the entire murine kidney followed by cultivation of the resulting cells in specific renal media. Immunohistochemistry revealed cells expressing proximal and distal tubule markers as well as markers for glomerular and endothelial cells. When these cells were allowed to grow on rat-tail type 1 collagen, cells from the thick ascending loop of Henle stained positive for Tamm–Horsfall protein in an architectural pattern reminiscent of natural tubules (Joraku et al. 2009).

Yoo et al. (1996) evaluated whether murine renal cells grown *in vitro* could produce functional results *in vivo*. They harvested the cells, expanded them in culture, and seeded them onto a tubular device constructed from polycarbonate. At one end of the tubular device was a Silastic catheter, which terminated into a reservoir. The device was subcutaneously implanted into athymic mice. The implanted device demonstrated extensive vascularization in addition to glomerular formation and highly organized tubular architecture. Immunohistochemistry for alkaline phosphatase showed positivity in the proximal tubule-like structures. Osteopontin, which is secreted by the proximal and distal tubular cells and the cells of the thin loop of Henle, was found on immunocytochemical staining of the tubular sections. In addition, the ECM of the newly formed tubules stained uniformly positive for fibronectin. Importantly, fluid collected in the reservoir of the device. This fluid was yellow, and the uric acid concentration was 66 mg/dL (as compared to 2 mg/dL in plasma). The creatinine concentration of the fluid (27.91 ± 7.56 mg/dL) was 8.2 times higher than that found in the serum (4.49 ± 0.08 mg/dL) (Yoo et al. 1996). These studies demonstrate that single cells can form multicellular structures, become organized into functional renal units, and are capable of unidirectional excretion of solutes through production of a urine-like fluid.

Next, Atala et al. explored the application of nuclear transplantation in the engineering of genetically identical renal tissue in a large-animal model, the cow (*Bos taurus*) (Lanza et al. 2002). In the study, renal cells were cloned from bovine fibroblasts of adult Holstein steers and seeded onto collagen-coated cylindrical polycarbonate membranes (Figure 8.6A). Renal devices with the capacity of collecting the excreted urinary fluid were created by connecting the ends of three membranes to catheters that terminated into a collecting reservoir (Figure 8.6B). These devices were transplanted subcutaneously and retrieved 12 weeks after implantation into the same donor animal. The implantation led to generation of functioning renal units that produced urine-like fluid and demonstrated unidirectional secretion and concentration of urea nitrogen and creatinine. Histological analysis of the explanted renal devices revealed extensive vascularization and formation of organized glomeruli- and tubule-like structures. There existed a clear

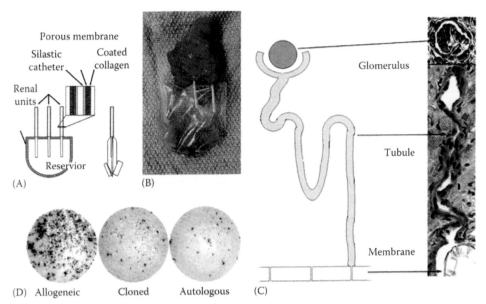

FIGURE 8.6   Combining therapeutic cloning and tissue engineering to produce kidney tissue. (A) Illustration of the tissue-engineered renal unit. (B) Renal unit seeded with cloned cells, 3 months after implantation, showing the accumulation of urine-like fluid. (C) Clear unidirectional continuity between the mature glomeruli, their tubules, and silastic catheter. (D) Elispot analyses of the frequencies of T cells that secrete IFNγ after stimulation with allogeneic renal cells, cloned renal cells, or nuclear donor fibroblasts. Cloned renal cells produce fewer IFNγ spots than the allogeneic cells, indicating that the rejection response to cloned cells is diminished. The presented wells are single representatives of duplicate wells.

continuity between the glomeruli, the tubules, and the Silastic catheter (Figure 8.6C). The expression of renal-specific mRNA and proteins was further confirmed in the retrieved tissues.

Several studies in the literature showed that bovine clones harbor the oocyte mitochondrial DNA (mtDNA), which might cause potential immunologic incompatibility resulting from the donor egg's mtDNA (Evans et al. 1999, Hiendleder et al. 1999, Steinborn et al. 2000). When cloned cells are transplanted back to the original nuclear donor, a T-cell response specific for mtDNA-encoded minor histocompatibility antigens (miHAs) may be stimulated owing to the differences in mtDNA-encoded proteins expressed by cloned cells (Fischer et al. 1991). This class of miHAs has been shown to stimulate both skin allograft rejection *in vivo* and expansion of cytotoxic T lymphocytes *in vitro* (Fischer et al. 1991), which could also be a barrier to successful clinical use of such cloned devices in patients with chronic rejection of major histocompatibility-matched human renal transplants (Hadley et al. 1992, Yard et al. 1993). Atala investigated a possible anti-miHA T-cell response to the cloned renal devices through both delayed-type hypersensitivity testing *in vivo* and Elispot analysis *in vitro*. The results suggested that there was no rejection response to the cloned renal cells, indicating that that rejection of cloned renal cells will not necessarily occur in the presence of oocyte-derived mtDNA (Figure 8.6D). This work has provided an important evidence in overcoming the histocompatibility problem of stem cell therapy (Yard et al. 1993).

These studies have demonstrated the efficacy of combining therapeutic cloning and tissue engineering for regeneration of tissues and organs. In general, autologous cells derived from nuclear transfer can be successfully harvested, expanded in culture, and transplanted back to the host with the use of engineered biodegradable scaffolds. Through the implantation, regeneration results from the single suspended cells organizing into desirable tissue structures that are genetically identical to those of the host.

Investigations into the possibility of using other cell types to produce renal tissue have also been promising. Perin et al. (2007) have been able to induce amniotic fluid/placental stem cells (AFPSCs) to differentiate into renal tissues. They labeled human AFPSC with a green fluorescent protein and microinjected the cells into developing murine embryonic kidneys. They found that the labeled cells assisted in forming both C- and S-shaped bodies, and the cells expressed RNA for early markers of renal development (Perin et al. 2007). This study demonstrates that AFPSC can differentiate into renal lineages when cultured *in vitro* with renal precursors. While promising, further *in vivo* studies and functional assays are required prior to clinical applications with AFPSC.

8.3.4 Male Reproductive Organs

A wide variety of pathologic penile conditions warrant the surgical intervention including penile carcinoma, trauma, severe erectile dysfunction, and congenital conditions such as ambiguous genitalia, hypospadias, and epispadias. The lack of sufficient autologous tissue is one of the major limitations of phallic reconstructive surgery. Nongenital autologous tissue sources have been used for decades. Phallic reconstruction was initially attempted in the late 1930s, with rib cartilage used as a stiffener for patients with traumatic penile loss (Frumpkin 1944, Goodwin and Scott 1952), but this process produced unsatisfactory functional and cosmetic results. Silicone rigid prostheses were popularized in the 1970s and have been used widely (Small et al. 1975, Bretan 1989). However, biocompatibility issues have been a problem in selected patients (Thomalla et al. 1987, Nukui et al. 1997). Tissue transfer techniques with flaps from various nongenital sources such as the groin and forearm have been used for genital reconstruction (Jordan 1999). However, operative complications such as infection, graft failure, and donor site morbidity are not negligible. Phallic reconstruction with autologous tissue, derived from the patient's own cells, may be preferable in selected cases.

One of the major components of the phallus is corporal smooth muscle. Initial experiments have shown that cultured human corporal smooth muscle cells may be used in conjunction with biodegradable polymers to create corpus cavernosum tissue *de novo* (Kershen et al. 2002). In a subsequent study, human corporal smooth muscle cells and endothelial cells seeded on biodegradable polymer scaffolds were able to form vascularized cavernosal muscle when implanted *in vivo* (Park et al. 1999). Later, in order to minimize any immune reactions that a synthetic biomaterial might cause, naturally derived acellular corporal tissue matrix with the same architecture as native corpora was developed. Acellular collagen matrices were derived from processed donor rabbit corpora using cell lysis techniques. Human corpus cavernosal muscle and endothelial cells were derived from donor penile tissue, and the cells were expanded *in vitro* and seeded on the acellular matrices. The matrices were covered with the appropriate cell architecture 4 weeks after implantation (Falke et al. 2003).

In order to look at the functional parameters of the engineered corpora, acellular corporal collagen matrices were obtained from donor rabbit penis, and autologous corpus cavernosal smooth muscle and endothelial cells were harvested, expanded, and seeded on the matrices. An entire cross-sectional segment of protruding rabbit phallus was excised, leaving the urethra intact. Cell-seeded matrices were interposed into the excised corporal space. Functional and structural parameters (cavernosography, cavernosometry, mating behavior, and sperm ejaculation) were followed, and histological, immunocytochemical, and Western blot analyses were performed up to 6 months after implantation. The engineered corpora cavernosa achieved adequate structural and functional parameters (Kwon et al. 2002). This technology was further confirmed when the entire rabbit corpora was removed and replaced with the engineered scaffolds. Most interestingly, mating activity in the animals with the engineered corpora appeared normal by 1 month after implantation. The presence of sperm was confirmed during mating and was present in all the rabbits with the engineered corpora. The female rabbits mated with the animals implanted with engineered corpora, and they conceived and delivered healthy pups. These studies demonstrate that penile corpora cavernosa tissue can be engineered. The engineered tissue is able to achieve adequate structural and functional parameters sufficient for erection, copulation, ejaculation, and conception in rabbits. Further studies will be needed to confirm the long-term functionality of these organs. In addition, further studies are needed to show that comparable human structures can also be engineered.

Patients with testicular dysfunction require androgen replacement for somatic development. Conventional treatment for testicular dysfunction consists of periodic intramuscular injections of chemically modified testosterone or, more recently, skin patch applications. However, long-term nonpulsatile testosterone therapy is not optimal and can cause multiple problems, including excessive erythropoiesis and bone density changes. To address the problem, a system was designed in which Leydig cells, which produce most of the testosterone in the male, were microencapsulated in an alginate-poly-L-lysine solution and injected into castrated animals. Serum testosterone was measured serially; the animals were able to maintain testosterone levels in the long term (Machluf and Atala 1998). These studies suggest that microencapsulated Leydig cells may be able to replace or supplement testosterone in situations where anorchia or testicular failure is present. Microencapsulated Leydig cells offer several advantages. For example, the encapsulation process creates a semipermeable barrier between the transplanted cells and the host's immune system, and it allows for the long-term physiologic release of testosterone.

Other studies have shown that testicular prostheses created with chondrocytes in bioreactors could be loaded with testosterone and that these prostheses could provide controlled testosterone release into the bloodstream when implanted. The prostheses were implanted in athymic mice with bilateral anorchia, and testosterone was released long term, maintaining the androgen level at a physiologic range (Raya-Rivera et al. 2008). One could envision combining the Leydig cell technology described earlier with engineered prostheses for the long-term functional replacement of androgen levels.

8.3.5 Female Reproductive Organs

Successful treatment of congenital malformations of the uterus is associated with profound clinical implications. For instance, patients with cloacal exstrophy and intersex disorders often suffer from the lack of sufficient uterine tissue for future reproduction. In that direction, Atala's group has explored the feasibility of developing engineered functional uterine tissue using autologous cells (Wang et al. 2003a). Using a rabbit model, they isolated autologous uterine smooth muscle and epithelial cells, expanded in culture, seeded onto designed uterine-shaped biodegradable polymer scaffolds, which were then implanted in the corresponding autologous animals for subtotal uterine tissue replacement. After 6 months of implantation, the implants were retrieved and subjected to a variety of compositional and functional analyses. The presence of normal uterine tissue components was confirmed by histological, immunocytochemical, and Western blot analyses, while the functional characteristics of these tissues were found to be comparable to those of normal uterine tissue through biomechanical analyses and organ bath studies. Ongoing work focuses on the breeding studies using these engineered uteri.

Similarly, several pathologic conditions, including congenital malformations and malignancy, can adversely affect normal vaginal development or anatomy. Vaginal reconstruction has traditionally been challenging due to the paucity of available native tissue. The feasibility of engineering vaginal tissue *in vivo* was investigated (De Filippo et al. 2003). Vaginal epithelial and smooth muscle cells of female rabbits were harvested, grown, and expanded in culture. These cells were seeded onto biodegradable polymer scaffolds, and the cell-seeded constructs were then implanted into nude mice for up to 6 weeks. Immunocytochemical, histological, and Western blot analyses confirmed the presence of vaginal tissue phenotypes. Electrical field stimulation studies in the tissue-engineered constructs showed similar functional properties to those of normal vaginal tissue. When these constructs were used for autologous total vaginal replacement, patent vaginal structures were noted in the tissue-engineered specimens, while the non-cell-seeded structures were noted to be stenotic (De Filippo et al. 2003).

8.3.6 Heart

In the United States, over 5 million people currently live with some form of heart disease, and many more are diagnosed each year. While many medications have been developed to assist the ailing heart, the treatment for end-stage heart failure still remains transplantation. Unfortunately, as with other organs, donor hearts are in short supply, and even when a transplant can be performed, the patient must endure the side effects created by lifelong immunosuppression. Thus, alternatives are desperately needed, and the development of novel methods to regenerate or replace damaged heart muscle using tissue engineering and regenerative medicine techniques is an attractive option.

Cell therapy for infracted areas of the heart is attractive, as these methods involve a rather simple injection into the damaged area of a patient's heart, rather than a rigorous surgical procedure, to complete. Various types of stem cells have been investigated for their potential to regenerate damaged or dead heart tissue in this manner. Skeletal muscle cells, bone marrow stem cells (both mesenchymal and hematopoietic), amniotic fluid stem cells, and embryonic stem cells have been used for this purpose. In this technique, cells are suspended in a biocompatible matrix that can range from simple normal saline to complex yet biocompatible hydrogels depending on the type of injection to be performed. The cells are either injected into the damaged area of the heart itself, or they are injected into the coronary circulation with the hope that they will home to the damaged area, take up residence there, and begin to repair the tissue. However, injectable therapies have been shown to be relatively inefficient, and cell loss is quite substantial. Newer methods of tissue engineering include the development of engineered "patches," which are comprised of cells adhered to a biomaterial that can theoretically be used to replace the damaged area of the heart. These techniques have promise, but require further research into the optimal cell types and biomaterials for this purpose before they can be used extensively in the clinic (see Jawad et al. 2007 for an excellent review of these methods).

However, the methods described earlier could only be used in cases where a relatively small section of heart muscle was damaged. In cases where a large area or even the whole heart has become nonfunctional, a more radical approach may be required. In these situations, the use of a bioartificial heart would be ideal, as rejection would be avoided and the problems associated with a mechanical heart (such as thromboembolus formation) would be abolished. To this end, Ott et al. (2008) recently developed a novel heart construct *in vitro* using decellularized cadaveric hearts. By reseeding the tissue scaffold that remained after a specialized decellularization process with various types of cells that make up a heart (cardiomyocytes, smooth muscle cells, endothelial cells, and fibrocytes) and culturing the resulting construct in a bioreactor system designed to mimic physiologic conditions, this group was able to produce a construct that could generate pump function on its own (Ott et al. 2008). This study suggests that production of bioartificial hearts may one day be possible.

8.3.7 Liver

The liver can sustain a variety of insults, including viral infection, alcohol abuse, surgical resection of tumors, and acute drug-induced hepatic failure. The current therapy for liver failure is liver transplantation. However, this therapy is limited by the shortage of donors and the need for lifelong immunosuppressive therapy. Cell transplantation has been proposed as a potential solution for liver failure. This is based on the fact that the liver has enormous regenerative potential *in vivo* suggests that in the right environment, it may be possible to expand liver cells *in vitro* in sufficient quantities for tissue engineering (Bhandari et al. 2001). Many approaches have been tried, including development of specialized media, co-culture with other cell types, identification of growth factors that have proliferative effects on these cells, and culture on three-dimensional scaffolds within bioreactors (Bhandari et al. 2001).

Extracorporeal bioartificial liver devices that use porcine hepatocytes have been designed and applied. These devices are designed to filter and purify the patient's blood as would the patient's own liver, and the blood is returned to the patient in a manner similar to kidney dialysis. Another cell-based approach is the injection of liver cell suspensions. This has been performed in animal models. Intraportal hepatocyte injection has also been used in patients with Crigler–Najjar Syndrome Type 1 (Fox et al. 1998); however, complications such as portal vein thrombosis and pulmonary embolism are major concerns, especially when large cell numbers are used (Nieto et al. 1989).

Finally, cells including stem cells, oval progenitor cells, and mature hepatocytes have been seeded onto liver-shaped biocompatible matrices to engineer artificial, implantable livers. These have been tested in various animal models (Gilbert et al. 1993, Kaufmann et al. 1999), but the transplantation efficiency as well as the functionality of these constructs was not optimal. Recently, however, Baptista and colleagues have reported a novel technique that may substantially advance the methods used to create tissue-engineered livers (Baptista et al. 2010). They describe the fabrication of three-dimensional naturally derived liver scaffolds with intact vasculature. To obtain these scaffolds, livers from donor animals of several different species were obtained and perfused with detergent solutions through the vascular network in order to remove all cellular components of the tissue while maintaining the ECM and the vasculature. They showed that the vasculature remained intact throughout the decellularization process and was subsequently able to handle fluid flow in a physiological manner. Thus, they were able to use this intact vascular tree to reseed the decellularized liver scaffold with endothelial cells and human fetal liver cells, and they showed that each cell type was able to engraft in its putative native location within the scaffold. Importantly, after cell engraftment within the scaffold, the cells were analyzed phenotypically, and it was shown that the cells displayed the appropriate endothelial, hepatic, and biliary epithelial markers, thus creating liver-like tissue *in vitro*. These results are a significant improvement in the bioengineering of whole organs and may provide the first fully functional bioengineered livers for use in organ transplantation and drug discovery.

8.3.8 Pancreas

Diabetes results from an insufficient mass of insulin-producing β-cells and affects more than 20 million people in the United States. Replacement or regeneration of functional β-cells allows physiological control of glycemia and is an attractive potential therapy for diabetes. Human islet transplantation is limited by the scarcity of donors and severe complication of immune suppression. Hence, research is directed toward the development of a cell-based approach that can generate sufficient numbers of transplantable β-cells or islets to meet the demands of patients with diabetes.

Efforts have utilized embryonic stem cells due to their potential to be differentiated to β-cells (Aguayo-Mazzucato and Bonner-Weir 2010, Mfopou et al. 2010). Many studies have demonstrated the ability to direct the differentiation of embryonic stem cells into pancreatic progenitors and insulin-secreting cells despite the lack of evidence in obtaining actual β-cells or islets (Soria et al. 2000, D'Amour et al. 2006, Kroon et al. 2008, Mao et al. 2009, Zhang et al. 2009, Shi 2010). Using a five-stage differentiation protocol mimicking *in vivo* pancreatic organogenesis, D'Amour et al. (2006) converted human embryonic stem cells to endocrine cells capable of producing the pancreatic hormones insulin, glucagon, somatostatin, pancreatic polypeptide, and ghrelin. Kroon et al. (2008) further showed that glucose-responsive endocrine cells can be generated from pancreatic endoderm derived from human embryonic stem cells after implantation into diabetic mice, which are functionally comparable to adult human islets. In addition to human embryonic stem cells, other stem cell types have also been shown to differentiate along the pancreatic lineage and normalize blood glucose levels through insulin secretion in the transplanted animals (Gabr et al. 2008, Chandra et al. 2009).

Given the benefit of reprogramming techniques to differentiate stem cells into terminally committed cell types, induced pluripotent stem cells constitute another attractive cell source for β-cell differentiation (Tateishi et al. 2008, Maehr et al. 2009, Zhang et al. 2009). Alipio et al. (2010) revealed the potential of induced pluripotent stem cells derived from fibroblasts to differentiate into insulin-secreting β-like cells *in vitro* and respond to glucose stimulation under physiological or pathological conditions. Direct reprogramming improves the efficiency of derivation of pancreatic-like cells from stem cells through introduction of pancreatic transcription factors that control β-cell-specific transcription of the insulin gene. For instance, Chiou et al. (2011) investigated the role of MafA in placenta-derived multipotent stem cells and found that MafA promoted the differentiation of placental-derived stem cells into insulin-producing cells that functionally restored the regulation of blood glucose levels in diabetic mice. In addition, reprogramming of AFS cells for differentiation into β-cells may also be achieved with the aid of appropriate genetic signaling. Current efforts focusing on the discovery and screening of small molecules to improve the reprogramming efficiency and avoid the safety concerns of transcription factors will accelerate the clinical translation of induced pluripotent stem cells (Feng et al. 2009, Zhu et al. 2010).

It has been suggested in the literature that appropriate differentiation and maintenance of functional phenotype may be fostered via three-dimensional organization of cell populations (Chung and Stainier 2008, Mao et al. 2009, Wang and Ye 2009). Van Hoof et al. (2011) created patterned size-controlled clusters for efficient production of pancreatic endocrine precursors from human embryonic stem cells. Thus, the efficacy of the earlier cell-based approaches for pancreas regeneration could be enhanced through the introduction of tissue engineering scaffolds providing a three-dimensional cellular environment. However, revascularization of a whole organ prior to implantation to ensure sufficient supply of oxygen in the core of three-dimensional structures is a challenge. In efforts to reconstruct vascularized pancreatic tissue *ex vivo*, Kaufman-Francis et al. (2012) developed a three-dimensional multi-culture model comprised of pancreatic islets, endothelial cells, and fibroblasts seeded on highly porous biocompatible polymeric scaffolds. It was demonstrated that prevascularized islets promoted survival, integration, and function of the engrafted engineered tissue in diabetic mice. Further studies remain to be conducted to evaluate the specific role of extracellular matrices on differentiation and cell-to-cell interactions as well as identify suitable scaffold and culture systems for implementation to clinical situations.

While encouraging results have been seen, there are hurdles concerning the clinical application of cell-based therapies such as the risk of tumor formation and destruction by the immune system via either allo- or autoimmunity. Future developments in cell differentiation, as well as encapsulation and immunomodulation techniques, may provide new advances in the area of pancreas regeneration.

8.3.9 Lung

Nearly 15 million individuals have been diagnosed with chronic obstructive pulmonary disease, and approximately 400,000 patients die from lung diseases annually in the United States. Human lungs have a poor ability to repair or regenerate, which makes the lung transplantation the primary therapy for replacement of lung tissue. However, this procedure is hindered by a severe shortage of donor lungs as well as low long-term survival rate resulting from chronic rejection and adverse effects of immunosuppressive treatment. A bioengineered transplantable lung that is structurally and functionally comparable to a donor lung could provide a viable solution to circumvent these problems. There are several key characteristics of a viable bioengineered lung. First, it supports the population and function of lung-specific cells. Second, it is characterized by hierarchical branching structures of airways and vasculature. Third, it provides alveolar barrier function so as to prevent any leakage of blood components into the airways. Fourth, it should have appropriate mechanical properties to enable ventilation at physiological pressures.

Considerable efforts have been made in engineering a functional lung tissue involving biomaterial scaffolds and *in vitro* culture systems. For example, pulmonary structures have been derived from stem cells both *in vitro* and *in vivo* (Pereira et al. 1995, Kotton et al. 2001, Giangreco et al. 2002, Kim et al. 2005, Cortiella et al. 2006, Loi et al. 2006, Reynolds et al. 2008). But these attempts do not generate a functional tissue that recapitulates the lung's complex architecture and participates in gas exchange (Nichols et al. 2009). In two recent reports, lung regeneration has been achieved through culture of pulmonary epithelium and vascular endothelium on the acellular lung matrix (Ott et al. 2010, Petersen et al. 2010). Petersen et al. (2010) performed lung decellularization to obtain a scaffold of ECM that retained the hierarchical branching structures of airways and vasculature. Acellular lung matrix was then cultured inside a biomimetic bioreactor that enabled seeding of vascular endothelium into the pulmonary artery and pulmonary epithelium into the trachea. Following *in vitro* culture, the engineered lung exhibited comparable microarchitecture and mechanical characteristics to those of native lung. The engineered lung was also capable of effecting gas exchange when implanted into rats. These encouraging results demonstrated the potential of a decellularization strategy in generating viable bioengineered lungs. Still, future work on the identification of autologous source of cells, differentiation, and maturation strategies remains to be done to facilitate clinical translation.

8.3.10 Intestine

Intestine is a complex organ with secretory and absorptive functions. Intestinal failure resulting from anatomical or functional loss of intestine impairs quality of life. Current treatment options for intestinal failure include total parenteral nutrition, intestinal elongation, and/or transplantation, which are associated with a number of limitations. For example, the intestinal transplant such as small bowel transplantation for pediatric small bowel syndrome is limited by the availability of donor organs, low success rate, and use of immunosuppression. Development of an artificial intestine by tissue engineering and stem cell-based therapies would provide an alternative option for the patients.

Since the first attempts in the 1980s (Vacanti et al. 1988), much progress has been made in the field of intestinal bioengineering. Many investigations have explored the use of intestinal epithelial organoid units for intestinal tissue generation, which allows partial restoration of gut function in a number of animal models (Choi and Vacanti 1997, Kim et al. 1999, Grikscheit et al. 2004, Sala et al. 2009). Sala et al. (2009) provided the first evidence in which tissue-engineered intestine was successfully generated in an autologous porcine model. In the study, organoid units, which are multicellular clusters with predominantly epithelial content, were generated through digestion of a resected jejunum from 6-week-old Yorkshire swine and loaded onto PGA-based tubes, which were subsequently implanted intraperitoneally in the autologous host. After 7 weeks of implantation, the tissue-engineered small intestine exactly recapitulated native intestine histology. The crypts in engineered intestine were also similar to those in native intestine. Control constructs with no organoid units implanted similarly did not result in engineered intestine tissue growth. Using an organoid units-on-scaffold approach, the same research group has recently demonstrated the growth of full thickness of engineered human intestine from postnatally derived organoid units in murine hosts (Levin et al. 2013). However, one of the major limitations of this approach is the difficulty to derive a sufficient number of organoid units for implantation, which may be overcome through the future advances in stem cell technology (Dunn 2008).

Stem cells are involved in the maintenance and function of intestine. For instance, the entire intestinal epithelium is regenerated every 3–7 days through the proliferation of intestinal epithelial stem/progenitor cells located at the base of the crypts. The number of stem cells per crypt is estimated to be between four and six. These cells are capable of differentiating into four different cell types, namely, goblet cells, Paneth cells, enteroendocrine cells, and enterocytes. Several proposed intestinal epithelium stem cell markers include Bmi1 (Sangiorgi and Capecchi 2008), Lgr5 (Barker et al. 2007), CD133 (Zhu et al. 2009), DCAMKL-1 (May et al. 2008), and Musashi-1 (Asai et al. 2005). Recent *in vitro* studies have demonstrated the capacity of isolated Lgr5-positive cells in building intestinal crypt–villus units without any mesenchymal niche as well as an epithelial tissue in which all four differentiated intestinal cell types are present (Sato et al. 2009). May et al. (2009) showed implantation of spheroids formed by DCAMKL-1-positive cells in the flanks of athymic nude mice generated glandular epithelial structures expressing multiple markers of gut epithelial lineage. In contrast to organoid units, these stem cells are readily expanded in culture, which makes them an attractive cell source for intestinal bioengineering. Several studies have been performed to investigate the potential of utilizing scaffolds to support cell growth and differentiation in three-dimensional environment both *in vitro* and *in vivo* (Wang et al. 2003b, Duxbury et al. 2004, Gupta et al. 2006, Sato et al. 2009). Totonelli et al. (2012) reported the creation of an acellular natural matrix from rat intestine through removal of cellular elements, which retains the intestinal architecture and connective tissue components as a base for developing functional intestinal tissue.

8.3.11 Brain

Brain consists of a highly organized network of interconnected cells (e.g., inhibitory and excitatory neurons as well as glial cells) and ECM imbued with biochemical and biophysical signals. The adult brain has limited healing capacity and thus represents a challenging management issue for the clinicians who treat patients with tissue insult resulting from diseases or traumatic brain injuries. Current treatment strategies include administration of pharmacological agents as well as maintenance of motility through rehabilitation. However, they have limited effectiveness and only result in alleviation of the symptoms such as cognitive, motor, and psychotic dysfunction. In that regard, a regenerative engineering strategy holds the promise to re-establish brain functionality and provide a potential solution to the patients. The intricate structure of the brain coupled with the complex signaling cascades associated with the neurological disorders present unique engineering and biological challenges. Scaffolds fabricated from various biomaterials in the form hydrogels, self-assembling peptides, and electrospun nanofibers have been explored for providing a microenvironment that promotes cell survival and connectivity, and re-establishment of a functional neural network (Pettikiriarachchi et al. 2010). Efforts have also been made to render scaffold bioactivity to enhance desirable cell–matrix and cell–cell interactions. In a recent report, Gurkan et al. (2012) utilized a digital tissue sculpting strategy to form a three-dimensional network of neurons recapitulating the spatial heterogeneity and mimic tissue architectural complexity of brain. In specific, digitally specified neural tissues were constructed from lithographically specified hydrogel containing neonatal rat primary cortical neurons. *In vitro* studies investigated the effect of three-dimensional spatial confinement on neural cell survival and neurite growth, which provides insights for the further development of bioengineered brain with a diversity of neuron types and connections. Future work to promote clinical translation of bioengineering efforts involves the combination of advances in stem cell science and advanced biomaterials to achieve tissue integration and functional recovery.

8.4 SUMMARY AND CONCLUSION

In summary, tremendous efforts in the field of regenerative medicine are currently underway experimentally for virtually every type of tissue and organ within the human body. Various tissues are at different stages of development, with some already being used clinically, a few in preclinical trials, and some in the discovery stage. Successful application of bioengineered tissues for tackling clinical challenges requires a convergence of stem cell science, advanced materials engineering, and developmental biology as well as close collaboration among scientists, engineers, and clinicians.

ACKNOWLEDGMENT

The authors wish to thank Jennifer L. Olson, Ph.D., for editorial assistance with this manuscript.

REFERENCES

Aebischer P, Ip TK, Miracoli L, Galletti PM. 1987a. Renal epithelial cells grown on semipermeable hollow fibers as a potential ultrafiltrate processor. *ASAIO Transactions* 33(3): 96–102.

Aebischer P, Ip TK, Panol G, Galletti PM. 1987b. The bioartificial kidney: Progress towards an ultrafiltration device with renal epithelial cells processing. *Life Support Systems* 5(2): 159–168.

Aguayo-Mazzucato C, Bonner-Weir S. 2010. Stem cell therapy for type 1 diabetes mellitus. *Nature Reviews Endocrinology* 6(3): 139–148.

Al-Awqati Q, Oliver JA. 2002. Stem cells in the kidney. *Kidney International* 61(2): 387–395.

Alipio Z, Liao W, Roemer EJ, Waner M, Fink LM, Ward DC et al. 2010. Reversal of hyperglycemia in diabetic mouse models using induced-pluripotent stem (iPS)-derived pancreatic beta-like cells. *Proceedings of the National Academy of Sciences of the United States of America* 107(30): 13426–13431.

Amiel GE, Atala A. 1999. Current and future modalities for functional renal replacement. *Urologic Clinics of North America* 26(1): 235–246.

Amiel GE, Komura M, Shapira O, Yoo JJ, Yazdani S, Berry J et al. 2006. Engineering of blood vessels from acellular collagen matrices coated with human endothelial cells. *Tissue Engineering* 12(8): 2355–2365.

Amiel GE, Yoo JJ, Atala A. 2000. Renal therapy using tissue-engineered constructs and gene delivery. *World Journal of Urology* 18(1): 71–79.

Amit M, Shariki C, Margulets V, Itskovitz-Eldor J. 2004. Feeder layer- and serum-free culture of human embryonic stem cells. *Biology of Reproduction* 70(3): 837–845.

Asai R. Okano H. Yasugi S. 2005. Correlation between Musashi-1 and c-hairy-1 expression and cell proliferation activity in the developing intestine and stomach of both chicken and mouse. *Development Growth and Differentiation* 47(8): 501–510.

Assady S, Maor G, Amit M, Itskovitz-Eldor J, Skorecki KL, Tzukerman M. 2001. Insulin production by human embryonic stem cells. *Diabetes* 50(8): 1691–1697.

Atala A. 1995. Commentary on the replacement of urologic associated mucosa. *Journal of Urology* 156: 338.

Atala A. 1998. Autologous cell transplantation for urologic reconstruction. *Journal of Urology* 159(1): 2–3.

Atala A. 1999. Creation of bladder tissue in vitro and in vivo. A system for organ replacement. *Advances in Experimental Medicine and Biology* 462: 31–42.

Atala A. 2001. Bladder regeneration by tissue engineering. *BJU International* 88(7): 765–770.

Atala A, Bauer SB, Soker S, Yoo JJ, Retik AB. 2006. Tissue-engineered autologous bladders for patients needing cystoplasty. *Lancet* 367(9518): 1241–1246.

Atala A, Guzman L, Retik AB. 1999. A novel inert collagen matrix for hypospadias repair. *Journal of Urology* 162(3 Pt 2): 1148–1151.

Atala A, Schlussel, R. N., Retik, A. B. 1995. Renal cell growth in vivo after attachment to biodegradable polymer scaffolds. *Journal of Urology* 153:4.

Atala A, Vacanti JP, Peters CA, Mandell J, Retik AB, Freeman MR. 1992. Formation of urothelial structures in vivo from dissociated cells attached to biodegradable polymer scaffolds in vitro. *Journal of Urology* 148(2 Pt 2): 658–662.

Auchincloss H, Bonventre JV. 2002. Transplanting cloned cells into therapeutic promise. *Nature Biotechnology* 20(7): 665–666.

Baguisi A, Behboodi E, Melican DT, Pollock JS, Destrempes MM, Cammuso C et al. 1999. Production of goats by somatic cell nuclear transfer. *Nature Biotechnology* 17(5): 456–461.

Baker R, Kelly T, Tehan T, Putnam C, Beaugard E. 1958. Subtotal cystectomy and total bladder regeneration in treatment of bladder cancer. *Journal of the American Medical Association* 168(9): 1178–1185.

Baptista PM, Siddiqui MM, Lozier G, Rodriguez SR, Atala A, Soker S. 2010. The use of whole organ decellularization for the generation of a vascularized liver organoid. *Hepatology* 53(2): 604–617.

Barker N, van Es JH, Kuipers J, Kujala P, van den Born M, Cozijnsen M et al. 2007. Identification of stem cells in small intestine and colon by marker gene Lgr5. *Nature* 449(7165): 1003–1007.

Bazeed MA, Thuroff JW, Schmidt RA, Tanagho EA. 1983. New treatment for urethral strictures. *Urology* 21(1): 53–57.

Betthauser J, Forsberg E, Augenstein M, Childs L, Eilertsen K, Enos J et al. 2000. Production of cloned pigs from in vitro systems. *Nature Biotechnology* 18(10): 1055–1059.

Bhandari RN, Riccalton LA, Lewis AL, Fry JR, Hammond AH, Tendler SJ et al. 2001. Liver tissue engineering: A role for co-culture systems in modifying hepatocyte function and viability. *Tissue Engineering* 7(3): 345–357.

Blelloch R, Wang Z, Meissner A, Pollard S, Smith A, Jaenisch R. 2006. Reprogramming efficiency following somatic cell nuclear transfer is influenced by the differentiation and methylation state of the donor nucleus 1. *Stem Cells* 24(9): 2007–2013.

Bretan PN. 1989. History of prosthetic treatment of impotence. In: Montague DK (ed.), *Genitourinary Prostheses*. Philadelphia, PA: WB Saunders, pp. 1–5.

Brivanlou AH, Gage FH, Jaenisch R, Jessell T, Melton D, Rossant J. 2003. Stem cells. Setting standards for human embryonic stem cells. *Science* 300(5621): 913–916.

Campbell KH, McWhir J, Ritchie WA, Wilmut I. 1996. Sheep cloned by nuclear transfer from a cultured cell line. *Nature* 380(6569): 64–66.

Chandra V, G S, Phadnis S, Nair PD, Bhonde RR. 2009. Generation of pancreatic hormone-expressing islet-like cell aggregates from murine adipose tissue-derived stem cells. *Stem Cells* 27(8): 1941–1953.

Chen F, Yoo JJ, Atala A. 1999. Acellular collagen matrix as a possible "off the shelf" biomaterial for urethral repair. *Urology* 54(3): 407–410.

Chiou SH, Chen SJ, Chang YL, Chen YC, Li HY, Chen DT et al. 2011. MafA promotes the reprogramming of placenta-derived multipotent stem cells into pancreatic islets-like and insulin+ cells. *Journal of Cellular and Molecular Medicine* 15(3): 612–624.

Choi RS, Vacanti JP. 1997. Preliminary studies of tissue-engineered intestine using isolated epithelial organoid units on tubular synthetic biodegradable scaffolds. *Transplantation Proceedings* 29(1–2): 848–851.

Chun SY, Lim GJ, Kwon TG, Kwak EK, Kim BW, Atala A et al. 2007. Identification and characterization of bioactive factors in bladder submucosa matrix. *Biomaterials* 28(29): 4251–4256.

Chung WS, Stainier DY. 2008. Intra-endodermal interactions are required for pancreatic beta cell induction. *Developmental Cell* 14(4): 582–593.

Cibelli JB, Stice SL, Golueke PJ, Kane JJ, Jerry J, Blackwell C et al. 1998. Cloned transgenic calves produced from nonquiescent fetal fibroblasts. *Science* 280(5367): 1256–1258.

Cilento BG, Freeman MR, Schneck FX, Retik AB, Atala A. 1994. Phenotypic and cytogenetic characterization of human bladder urothelia expanded in vitro. *Journal of Urology* 152(2 Pt 2): 665–670.

Colman A, Kind A. 2000. Therapeutic cloning: Concepts and practicalities. *Trends in Biotechnology* 18(5): 192–196.

Cortiella J, Nichols JE, Kojima K, Bonassar LJ, Dargon P, Roy AK et al. 2006. Tissue-engineered lung: An in vivo and in vitro comparison of polyglycolic acid and pluronic F-127 hydrogel/somatic lung progenitor cell constructs to support tissue growth. *Tissue Engineering* 12(5): 1213–1225.

Dahms SE, Piechota HJ, Dahiya R, Lue TF, Tanagho EA. 1998. Composition and biomechanical properties of the bladder acellular matrix graft: Comparative analysis in rat, pig and human. *British Journal of Urology* 82(3): 411–419.

D'Amour KA, Bang AG, Eliazer S, Kelly OG, Agulnick AD, Smart NG et al. 2006. Production of pancreatic hormone-expressing endocrine cells from human embryonic stem cells. *Nature Biotechnology* 24(11): 1392–1401.

de Boer WI, Schuller AG, Vermey M, van der Kwast TH. 1994. Expression of growth factors and receptors during specific phases in regenerating urothelium after acute injury in vivo. *American Journal of Pathology* 145(5):1199–1207.

De Coppi P, Bartsch G, Jr, Siddiqui MM, Xu T, Santos CC, Perin L et al. 2007. Isolation of amniotic stem cell lines with potential for therapy. *Nature Biotechnology* 25(1): 100–106.

De Filippo RE, Yoo JJ, Atala A. 2002. Urethral replacement using cell seeded tubularized collagen matrices. *Journal of Urology* 168(4 Pt 2): 1789–1792; discussion 1792–1783.

De Filippo RE, Yoo JJ, Atala A. 2003. Engineering of vaginal tissue in vivo. *Tissue Engineering* 9(2): 301–306.

De Sousa PA, Dobrinsky JR, Zhu J, Archibald AL, Ainslie A, Bosma W et al. 2002. Somatic cell nuclear transfer in the pig: Control of pronuclear formation and integration with improved methods for activation and maintenance of pregnancy. *Biology of Reproduction* 66(3): 642–650.

Dinnyes A, De Sousa P, King T, Wilmut I. 2002. Somatic cell nuclear transfer: Recent progress and challenges. *Cloning and Stem Cells* 4(1): 81–90.

Dorin RP, Pohl HG, De Filippo RE, Yoo JJ, Atala A. 2008. Tubularized urethral replacement with unseeded matrices: What is the maximum distance for normal tissue regeneration? *World Journal of Urology* 26(4): 323–326.

Dozmorov MG, Kropp BP, Hurst RE, Cheng EY, Lin HK. 2007. Differentially expressed gene networks in cultured smooth muscle cells from normal and neuropathic bladder. *Journal of Smooth Muscle Research* 43(2): 55–72.

Dunn JC. 2008. Is the tissue-engineered intestine clinically viable? *Nature Clinical Practice Gastroenterology and Hepatology* 5(7): 366–367.

Duxbury MS, Grikscheit TC, Gardner-Thorpe J, Rocha FG, Ito H, Perez A et al. 2004. Lymphangiogenesis in tissue-engineered small intestine. *Transplantation* 77(8): 1162–1166.

El-Kassaby A, Aboushwareb T, Atala A. 2008. Randomized comparative study between buccal mucosal and acellular bladder matrix grafts in complex anterior urethral strictures. *Journal of Urology* 179(4): 1432–1436.

El-Kassaby AW, Retik AB, Yoo JJ, Atala A. 2003. Urethral stricture repair with an off-the-shelf collagen matrix. *Journal of Urology* 169(1): 170–173; discussion 173.

Evans MJ, Gurer C, Loike JD, Wilmut I, Schnieke AE, Schon EA. 1999. Mitochondrial DNA genotypes in nuclear transfer-derived cloned sheep. *Nature Genetics* 23(1): 90–93.

Falke G, Yoo JJ, Kwon TG, Moreland R, Atala A. 2003. Formation of corporal tissue architecture in vivo using human cavernosal muscle and endothelial cells seeded on collagen matrices. *Tissue Engineering* 9(5): 871–879.

Farhat WA, Yeger H. 2008. Does mechanical stimulation have any role in urinary bladder tissue engineering? *World Journal of Urology* 26(4): 301–305.

Faris RA, Konkin T, Halpert G. 2001. Liver stem cells: A potential source of hepatocytes for the treatment of human liver disease. *Artificial Organs* 25(7): 513–521.

Feng B, Ng JH, Heng JC, Ng HH. 2009. Molecules that promote or enhance reprogramming of somatic cells to induced pluripotent stem cells. *Cell Stem Cell* 4(4): 301–312.

Fischer Lindahl K, Hermel E, Loveland BE, Wang CR. 1991. Maternally transmitted antigen of mice: A model transplantation antigen. *Annual Review of Immunology* 9: 351–372.

Fox IJ, Chowdhury JR, Kaufman SS, Goertzen TC, Chowdhury NR, Warkentin PI et al. 1998. Treatment of the Crigler-Najjar syndrome type I with hepatocyte transplantation. *New England Journal of Medicine* 338(20): 1422–1426.

Freeman MR, Yoo JJ, Raab G, Soker S, Adam RM, Schneck FX et al. 1997. Heparin-binding EGF-like growth factor is an autocrine growth factor for human urothelial cells and is synthesized by epithelial and smooth muscle cells in the human bladder. *Journal of Clinical Investigation* 99(5): 1028–1036.

Frumpkin AP. 1944. Reconstruction of male genitalia. *American Review of Soviet Medicine* 2: 14.

Fu Q, Deng CL, Liu W, Cao YL. 2007. Urethral replacement using epidermal cell-seeded tubular acellular bladder collagen matrix. *BJU International* 99(5): 1162–1165.

Fung LCT, Elenius, K., Freeman, M., Donovan, M. J., Atala, A. 1996. Reconstitution of poor EGFr-poor renal epithelial cells into tubular structures on biodegradable polymer scaffold. *Pediatrics* 98(Suppl): S631.

Gabr MM, Sobh MM, Zakaria MM, Refaie AF, Ghoneim MA. 2008. Transplantation of insulin-producing clusters derived from adult bone marrow stem cells to treat diabetes in rats. *Experimental and Clinical Transplantation* 6(3): 236–243.

Giangreco A, Reynolds SD, Stripp BR. 2002. Terminal bronchioles harbor a unique airway stem cell population that localizes to the bronchoalveolar duct junction. *American Journal of Pathology* 161(1): 173–182.

Gilbert JC, Takada T, Stein JE, Langer R, Vacanti JP. 1993. Cell transplantation of genetically altered cells on biodegradable polymer scaffolds in syngeneic rats. *Transplantation* 56(2): 423–427.

Goodwin WE, Scott WW. 1952. Phalloplasty. *Journal of Urology* 68(6): 903–908.

Gorham SD, French DA, Shivas AA, Scott R. 1989. Some observations on the regeneration of smooth muscle in the repaired urinary bladder of the rabbit. *European Urology* 16(6): 440–443.

Grikscheit TC, Siddique A, Ochoa ER, Srinivasan A, Alsberg E, Hodin RA et al. 2004. Tissue-engineered small intestine improves recovery after massive small bowel resection. *Annals of Surgery* 240(5): 748–754.

Guan Y, Ou L, Hu G, Wang H, Xu Y, Chen J et al. 2008. Tissue engineering of urethra using human vascular endothelial growth factor gene-modified bladder urothelial cells. *Artificial Organs* 32(2): 91–99.

Gupta A, Dixit A, Sales KM, Winslet MC, Seifalian AM. 2006. Tissue engineering of small intestine— Current status. *Biomacromolecules* 7(10): 2701–2709.

Gurdon JB. 1962a. Multiple genetically identical frogs. *Journal of Heredity* 53: 5–9.

Gurdon JB. 1962b. The developmental capacity of nuclei taken from intestinal epithelium cells of feeding tadpoles. *Journal of Embryology and Experimental Morphology* 10: 622–640.

Gurdon JB. 1962c. The transplantation of nuclei between two species of Xenopus. *Developmental Biology* 5: 68–83.

Gurdon JB, Elsdale TR, Fischberg M. 1958. Sexually mature individuals of *Xenopus laevis* from the transplantation of single somatic nuclei. *Nature* 182(4627): 64–65.

Gurkan UA, Fan Y, Xu F, Erkmen B, Urkac ES, Parlakgul G et al. 2012. Simple precision creation of digitally specified, spatially heterogeneous, engineered tissue architectures. *Advanced Materials*. doi: 10.1002/adma.201203261.

Hadley GA, Linders B, Mohanakumar T. 1992. Immunogenicity of MHC class I alloantigens expressed on parenchymal cells in the human kidney. *Transplantation* 54(3): 537–542.

Haller H, de Groot K, Bahlmann F, Elger M, Fliser D. 2005. Stem cells and progenitor cells in renal disease. *Kidney International* 68(5): 1932–1936.

Harriss DR. 1995. Smooth muscle cell culture: A new approach to the study of human detrusor physiology and pathophysiology. *British Journal of Urology* 75(Suppl 1): 18–26.

Hiendleder S, Schmutz SM, Erhardt G, Green RD, Plante Y. 1999. Transmitochondrial differences and varying levels of heteroplasmy in nuclear transfer cloned cattle. *Molecular Reproduction and Development* 54(1): 24–31.

Hipp J, Andersson KE, Kwon TG, Kwak EK, Yoo J, Atala A. 2008. Microarray analysis of exstrophic human bladder smooth muscle. *BJU International* 101(1): 100–105.

Hochedlinger K, Jaenisch R. 2002. Nuclear transplantation: Lessons from frogs and mice. *Current Opinion in Cell Biology* 14(6): 741–748.

Hochedlinger K, Rideout WM, Kyba M, Daley GQ, Blelloch R, Jaenisch R. 2004. Nuclear transplantation, embryonic stem cells and the potential for cell therapy. *Hematology Journal* 5(Suppl 3): S114–S117.

Humes HD, Buffington DA, MacKay SM, Funke AJ, Weitzel WF. 1999a. Replacement of renal function in uremic animals with a tissue-engineered kidney. *Nature Biotechnology* 17(5): 451–455.

Humes HD, MacKay SM, Funke AJ, Buffington DA. 1999b. Tissue engineering of a bioartificial renal tubule assist device: In vitro transport and metabolic characteristics. *Kidney International* 55(6): 2502–2514.

Hunter W. 1995. Of the structure and disease of articulating cartilages. 1743. *Clinical Orthopaedics and Related Research* 317: 3–6.

Ip TK, Aebischer P, Galletti PM. 1988. Cellular control of membrane permeability. Implications for a bioartificial renal tubule. *ASAIO Transactions* 34(3): 351–355.

Itskovitz-Eldor J, Schuldiner M, Karsenti D, Eden A, Yanuka O, Amit M et al. 2000. Differentiation of human embryonic stem cells into embryoid bodies compromising the three embryonic germ layers. *Molecular Medicine* 6(2): 88–95.

Jawad H, Ali NN, Lyon AR, Chen QZ, Harding SE, Boccaccini AR. 2007. Myocardial tissue engineering: A review. *Journal of Tissue Engineering and Regenerative Medicine* 1: 327–342.

Jayo MJ, Jain D, Ludlow JW, Payne R, Wagner BJ, McLorie G et al. 2008a. Long-term durability, tissue regeneration and neo-organ growth during skeletal maturation with a neo-bladder augmentation construct. *Regenerative Medicine* 3(5): 671–682.

Jayo MJ, Jain D, Wagner BJ, Bertram TA. 2008b. Early cellular and stromal responses in regeneration versus repair of a mammalian bladder using autologous cell and biodegradable scaffold technologies. *Journal of Urology* 180(1): 392–397.

Joki T, Machluf M, Atala A, Zhu J, Seyfried NT, Dunn IF et al. 2001. Continuous release of endostatin from microencapsulated engineered cells for tumor therapy. [See comment]. *Nature Biotechnology* 19(1): 35–39.

Joraku A, Stern KA, Atala A, Yoo JJ. 2009. In vitro generation of three-dimensional renal structures. *Methods* 47(2): 129–133.

Jordan GH. 1999. Penile reconstruction, phallic construction, and urethral reconstruction. *Urologic Clinics of North America* 26(1): 1–13.

Kaufman DS, Hanson ET, Lewis RL, Auerbach R, Thomson JA. 2001. Hematopoietic colony-forming cells derived from human embryonic stem cells. *Proceedings of the National Academy of Sciences of the United States of America* 98(19): 10716–10721.

Kaufman-Francis K, Koffler J, Weinberg N, Dor Y, Levenberg S. 2012. Engineered vascular beds provide key signals to pancreatic hormone-producing cells. *PLoS ONE* 7(7): e40741.

Kaufmann PM, Kneser U, Fiegel HC, Kluth D, Herbst H, Rogiers X. 1999. Long-term hepatocyte transplantation using three-dimensional matrices. *Transplantation Proceedings* 31(4): 1928–1929.

Kehat I, Kenyagin-Karsenti D, Snir M, Segev H, Amit M, Gepstein A et al. 2001. Human embryonic stem cells can differentiate into myocytes with structural and functional properties of cardiomyocytes. *Journal of Clinical Investigation* 108(3): 407–414.

Kershen RT, Yoo JJ, Moreland RB, Krane RJ, Atala A. 2002. Reconstitution of human corpus cavernosum smooth muscle in vitro and in vivo. *Tissue Engineering* 8(3): 515–524.

Kikuno N, Kawamoto K, Hirata H, Vejdani K, Kawakami K, Fandel T et al. 2008. Nerve growth factor combined with vascular endothelial growth factor enhances regeneration of bladder acellular matrix graft in spinal cord injury-induced neurogenic rat bladder. *BJU International* 103(10): 1424–1428.

Kim CF, Jackson EL, Woolfenden AE, Lawrence S, Babar I, Vogel S et al. 2005. Identification of bronchioalveolar stem cells in normal lung and lung cancer. *Cell* 121(6): 823–835.

Kim SS, Kaihara S, Benvenuto MS, Choi RS, Kim BS, Mooney DJ et al. 1999. Regenerative signals for intestinal epithelial organoid units transplanted on biodegradable polymer scaffolds for tissue engineering of small intestine. *Transplantation* 67(2): 227–233.

Kotton DN, Ma BY, Cardoso WV, Sanderson EA, Summer RS, Williams MC et al. 2001. Bone marrow-derived cells as progenitors of lung alveolar epithelium. *Development* 128(24): 5181–5188.

Kroon E, Martinson LA, Kadoya K, Bang AG, Kelly OG, Eliazer S et al. 2008. Pancreatic endoderm derived from human embryonic stem cells generates glucose-responsive insulin-secreting cells in vivo. *Nature Biotechnology* 26(4): 443–452

Kropp BP, Sawyer BD, Shannon HE, Rippy MK, Badylak SF, Adams MC et al. 1996. Characterization of small intestinal submucosa regenerated canine detrusor: Assessment of reinnervation, in vitro compliance and contractility. *Journal of Urology* 156(2 Pt 2): 599–607.

Kwon TG, Yoo JJ, Atala A. 2002. Autologous penile corpora cavernosa replacement using tissue engineering techniques. *Journal of Urology* 168(4 Pt 2): 1754–1758.

Kwon TG, Yoo JJ, Atala A. 2008. Local and systemic effects of a tissue engineered neobladder in a canine cystoplasty model. *Journal of Urology* 179(5): 2035–2041.

Lai JY, Yoon CY, Yoo JJ, Wulf T, Atala A. 2002. Phenotypic and functional characterization of in vivo tissue engineered smooth muscle from normal and pathological bladders. *Journal of Urology* 168(4 Pt 2): 1853–1857; discussion 1858.

Lanza RP, Chung HY, Yoo JJ, Wettstein PJ, Blackwell C, Borson N et al. 2002. Generation of histocompatible tissues using nuclear transplantation. *Nature Biotechnology* 20(7): 689–696.

Lanza RP, Cibelli JB, West MD. 1999. Prospects for the use of nuclear transfer in human transplantation. *Nature Biotechnology* 17(12): 1171–1174.

Lanza RP, Cibelli JB, West MD, Dorff E, Tauer C, Green RM. 2001. The ethical reasons for stem cell research. *Science* 292(5520): 1299.

Lanza RP, Hayes JL, Chick WL. 1996. Encapsulated cell technology. *Nature Biotechnology* 14(9): 1107–1111.

le Roux PJ. 2005. Endoscopic urethroplasty with unseeded small intestinal submucosa collagen matrix grafts: A pilot study. *Journal of Urology* 173(1): 140–143.

Levenberg S, Golub JS, Amit M, Itskovitz-Eldor J, Langer R. 2002. Endothelial cells derived from human embryonic stem cells. *Proceedings of the National Academy of Sciences of the United States of America* 99(7): 4391–4396.

Levin DE, Barthel ER, Speer AL, Sala FG, Hou X, Torashima Y et al. 2013. Human tissue-engineered small intestine forms from postnatal progenitor cells. *Journal of Pediatric Surgery* 48(1): 129–137.

Li C, Xu Y, Song L, Fu Q, Cui L, Yin S. 2008. Preliminary experimental study of tissue-engineered urethral reconstruction using oral keratinocytes seeded on BAMG. *Urologia Internationalis* 81(3): 290–295.

Liebert M, Hubbel A, Chung M, Wedemeyer G, Lomax MI, Hegeman A et al. 1997. Expression of mal is associated with urothelial differentiation in vitro: Identification by differential display reverse-transcriptase polymerase chain reaction. *Differentiation* 61(3): 177–185.

Liebert M, Wedemeyer G, Abruzzo LV, Kunkel SL, Hammerberg C, Cooper KD et al. 1991. Stimulated urothelial cells produce cytokines and express an activated cell surface antigenic phenotype. *Seminars in Urology* 9(2): 124–130.

Lin HK, Cowan R, Moore P, Zhang Y, Yang Q, Peterson JA, Jr. et al. 2004. Characterization of neuropathic bladder smooth muscle cells in culture. *Journal of Urology* 171(3): 1348–1352.

Loi R, Beckett T, Goncz KK, Suratt BT, Weiss DJ. 2006. Limited restoration of cystic fibrosis lung epithelium in vivo with adult bone marrow-derived cells. *American Journal of Respiratory and Critical Care Medicine* 173(2): 171–179.

Machluf M, Atala A. 1998. Emerging concepts for tissue and organ transplantation. *Graft* 1(1): 31–37.

MacKay SM, Funke AJ, Buffington DA, Humes HD. 1998. Tissue engineering of a bioartificial renal tubule. *ASAIO Journal* 44(3): 179–183.

Maehr R, Chen S, Snitow M, Ludwig T, Yagasaki L, Goland R et al. 2009. Generation of pluripotent stem cells from patients with type 1 diabetes. *Proceedings of the National Academy of Sciences of the United States of America* 106(37): 15768–15773.

Mao GH, Chen GA, Bai HY, Song TR, Wang YX. 2009. The reversal of hyperglycaemia in diabetic mice using PLGA scaffolds seeded with islet-like cells derived from human embryonic stem cells. *Biomaterials* 30(9): 1706–1714.

Master VA, Wei G, Liu W, Baskin LS. 2003. Urothlelium facilitates the recruitment and transdifferentiation of fibroblasts into smooth muscle in acellular matrix. *Journal of Urology* 170(4 Pt 2): 1628–1632.

May R, Riehl TE, Hunt C, Sureban SM, Anant S, Houchen CW. 2008. Identification of a novel putative gastrointestinal stem cell and adenoma stem cell marker, doublecortin and CaM kinase-like-1, following radiation injury and in adenomatous polyposis coli/multiple intestinal neoplasia mice. *Stem Cells* 26(3): 630–637.

May R, Sureban SM, Hoang N, Riehl TE, Lightfoot SA, Ramanujam R et al. 2009. Doublecortin and CaM kinase-like-1 and leucine-rich-repeat-containing G-protein-coupled receptor mark quiescent and cycling intestinal stem cells, respectively. *Stem Cells* 27(10): 2571–2579.

Meissner A, Wernig M, Jaenisch R. 2007. Direct reprogramming of genetically unmodified fibroblasts into pluripotent stem cells *Nature Biotechnology* 25(10): 1177–1181.

Mfopou JK, Chen B, Sui L, Sermon K, Bouwens L. 2010 Recent advances and prospects in the differentiation of pancreatic cells from human embryonic stem cells. *Diabetes* 59(9): 2094–2101.

Nguyen HT, Park JM, Peters CA, Adam RM, Orsola A, Atala A et al. 1999. Cell-specific activation of the HB-EGF and ErbB1 genes by stretch in primary human bladder cells. *In Vitro Cellular & Developmental Biology Animal* 35(7): 371–375.

Nichols JE, Niles JA, Cortiella J. 2009. Design and development of tissue engineered lung: Progress and challenges. *Organogenesis* 5(2): 57–61.

Nieto JA, Escandon J, Betancor C, Ramos J, Canton T, Cuervas-Mons V. 1989. Evidence that temporary complete occlusion of splenic vessels prevents massive embolization and sudden death associated with intrasplenic hepatocellular transplantation. *Transplantation* 47(3): 449–450.

Nukui F, Okamoto S, Nagata M, Kurokawa J, Fukui J. 1997. Complications and reimplantation of penile implants. *International Journal of Urology* 4(1): 52–54.

Oberpenning F, Meng J, Yoo JJ, Atala A. 1999. De novo reconstitution of a functional mammalian urinary bladder by tissue engineering. *Nature Biotechnology* 17(2): 149–155.

Okita K, Ichisaka T, Yamanaka S. 2007. Generation of germline-competent induced pluripotent stem cells 1. *Nature* 448(7151): 313–317.

Olsen L, Bowald S, Busch C, Carlsten J, Eriksson I. 1992. Urethral reconstruction with a new synthetic absorbable device. An experimental study. Scandinavian *Journal of Urology and Nephrology* 26(4): 323–326.

Ott HC, Clippinger B, Conrad C, Schuetz C, Pomerantseva I, Ikonomou L et al. 2010. Regeneration and orthotopic transplantation of a bioartificial lung. *Nature Medicine* 16(8): 927–933.

Ott HC, Matthiesen TS, Goh SK, Black LD, Kren SM, Netoff TI et al. 2008. Perfusion-decellularized matrix: Using nature's platform to engineer a bioartificial heart. *Nature Medicine* 14(2): 213–221.

Park HJ, Yoo JJ, Kershen RT, Moreland R, Atala A. 1999. Reconstitution of human corporal smooth muscle and endothelial cells in vivo. *Journal of Urology* 162(3 Pt 2): 1106–1109.

Pereira RF, Halford KW, O'Hara MD, Leeper DB, Sokolov BP, Pollard MD et al. 1995. Cultured adherent cells from marrow can serve as long-lasting precursor cells for bone, cartilage, and lung in irradiated mice. *Proceedings of the National Academy of Sciences of the United States of America* 92(11): 4857–4861.

Perin L, Giuliani S, Jin D, Sedrakyan S, Carraro G, Habibian R et al. 2007. Renal differentiation of amniotic fluid stem cells. *Cell Proliferation* 40(6): 936–948.

Petersen TH, Calle EA, Zhao L, Lee EJ, Gui L, Raredon MB et al. 2010. Tissue-engineered lungs for in vivo implantation. *Science* 329(5991): 538–541.

Pettikiriarachchi JTS, Parish CL, Shoichet MS, Forsythe JS, Nisbet DR. 2010. Biomaterials for brain tissue engineering. *Australian Journal of Chemistry* 63: 1143–1154.

Piechota HJ, Dahms SE, Nunes LS, Dahiya R, Lue TF, Tanagho EA. 1998. In vitro functional properties of the rat bladder regenerated by the bladder acellular matrix graft. *Journal of Urology* 159(5): 1717–1724.

Probst M, Dahiya R, Carrier S, Tanagho EA. 1997. Reproduction of functional smooth muscle tissue and partial bladder replacement. *British Journal of Urology* 79(4): 505–515.

Puthenveettil JA, Burger MS, Reznikoff CA. 1999. Replicative senescence in human uroepithelial cells. *Advances in Experimental Medicine and Biology* 462: 83–91.

Raya-Rivera AM, Baez C, Atala A, Yoo JJ. 2008. Tissue engineered testicular prostheses with prolonged testosterone release. *World Journal of Urology* 26(4): 307–314.

Raya-Rivera A, Esquiliano DR, Yoo JJ, Lopez-Bayghen E, Soker S, Atala A. 2011. Tissue-engineered autologous urethras for patients who need reconstruction: An observational study. 377(9772): 1175–1182.

Reubinoff BE, Itsykson P, Turetsky T, Pera MF, Reinhartz E, Itzik A et al. 2001. Neural progenitors from human embryonic stem cells. *Nature Biotechnology* 19(12): 1134–1140.

Reubinoff BE, Pera MF, Fong CY, Trounson A, Bongso A. 2000. Embryonic stem cell lines from human blastocysts: Somatic differentiation in vitro. [Erratum appears in *Nature Biotechnology* 2000 May 18(5): 559]. *Nature Biotechnology* 18(4): 399–404.

Reynolds SD, Zemke AC, Giangreco A, Brockway BL, Teisanu RM, Drake JA et al. 2008. Conditional stabilization of beta-catenin expands the pool of lung stem cells. *Stem Cells* 26(5): 1337–1346.

Richards M, Fong CY, Chan WK, Wong PC, Bongso A. 2002. Human feeders support prolonged undifferentiated growth of human inner cell masses and embryonic stem cells. *Nature Biotechnology* 20(9): 933–936.

Rideout WM, 3rd, Eggan K, Jaenisch R. 2001. Nuclear cloning and epigenetic reprogramming of the genome. *Science* 293(5532): 1093–1098.

Sala FG, Kunisaki SM, Ochoa ER, Vacanti J, Grikscheit TC. 2009. Tissue-engineered small intestine and stomach form from autologous tissue in a preclinical large animal model. *Journal of Surgical Research* 156(2): 205–212.

Sangiorgi E, Capecchi MR. 2008. Bmi1 is expressed in vivo in intestinal stem cells. *Nature Genetics* 40(7): 915–920.

Sato T, Vries RG, Snippert HJ, van de Wetering M, Barker N, Stange DE et al. 2009. Single Lgr5 stem cells build crypt-villus structures in vitro without a mesenchymal niche. *Nature* 459(7244): 262–265.

Schuldiner M, Eiges R, Eden A, Yanuka O, Itskovitz-Eldor J, Goldstein RS et al. 2001. Induced neuronal differentiation of human embryonic stem cells. *Brain Research* 913(2): 201–205.

Schuldiner M, Yanuka O, Itskovitz-Eldor J, Melton DA, Benvenisty N. 2000. Effects of eight growth factors on the differentiation of cells derived from human embryonic stem cells. *Proceedings of the National Academy of Sciences of the United States of America* 97(21): 11307–11312.

Scriven SD, Booth C, Thomas DF, Trejdosiewicz LK, Southgate J. 1997. Reconstitution of human urothelium from monolayer cultures. *Journal of Urology* 158(3 Pt 2): 1147–1152.

Shi Y. 2010. Generation of functional insulin-producing cells from human embryonic stem cells in vitro. *Methods in Molecular Biology* 636: 79–85.

Sievert KD, Bakircioglu ME, Nunes L, Tu R, Dahiya R, Tanagho EA. 2000. Homologous acellular matrix graft for urethral reconstruction in the rabbit: Histological and functional evaluation. *Journal of Urology* 163(6): 1958–1965.

Small MP, Carrion HM, Gordon JA. 1975. Small-Carrion penile prosthesis. New implant for management of impotence. *Urology* 5(4): 479–486.

Solter D. 2000. Mammalian cloning: Advances and limitations. *Nature Reviews Genetics* 1(3): 199–207.

Soria B, Roche E, Berna G, León-Quinto T, Reig JA, Martín F. 2000. Insulin-secreting cells derived from embryonic stem cells normalize glycemia in streptozotocin-induced diabetic mice. *Diabetes* 49(2): 157–162.

Steinborn R, Schinogl P, Zakhartchenko V, Achmann R, Schernthaner W, Stojkovic M et al. 2000. Mitochondrial DNA heteroplasmy in cloned cattle produced by fetal and adult cell cloning. *Nature Genetics* 25(3): 255–257.

Sutherland RS, Baskin LS, Hayward SW, Cunha GR. 1996. Regeneration of bladder urothelium, smooth muscle, blood vessels and nerves into an acellular tissue matrix. *Journal of Urology* 156(2 Pt 2): 571–577.

Takahashi K, Tanabe K, Ohnuki M, Narita M, Ichisaka T, Tomoda K et al. 2007. Induction of pluripotent stem cells from adult human fibroblasts by defined factors. *Cell* 131(5): 861–872.

Takahashi K, Yamanaka S. 2006. Induction of pluripotent stem cells from mouse embryonic and adult fibroblast cultures by defined factors. *Cell* 126(4): 663–676.

Tateishi K, He J, Taranova O, Liang G, D'Alessio AC, Zhang Y. 2008. Generation of insulin-secreting islet-like clusters from human skin fibroblasts. *Journal of Biological Chemistry* 283(46): 31601–31607.

Thomalla JV, Thompson ST, Rowland RG, Mulcahy JJ. 1987. Infectious complications of penile prosthetic implants. *Journal of Urology* 138(1): 65–67.

Thomson JA, Itskovitz-Eldor J, Shapiro SS, Waknitz MA, Swiergiel JJ, Marshall VS et al. 1998. Embryonic stem cell lines derived from human blastocysts. [Erratum appears in *Science* 1998 Dec 4; 282(5395): 1827]. *Science* 282(5391): 1145–1147.

Totonelli G, Maghsoudlou P, Garriboli M, Riegler J, Orlando G, Burns AJ et al. 2012. A rat decellularized small bowel scaffold that preserves villus-crypt architecture for intestinal regeneration. *Biomaterials* 33(12): 3401–3410.

Vacanti JP, Morse MA, Saltzman WM, Domb AJ, Perez-Atayde A, Langer R. 1988. Selective cell transplantation using bioabsorbable artificial polymers as matrices. *Journal of Pediatric Surgery* 23(1 Pt 2): 3–9.

Van Hoof D, Mendelsohn AD, Seerke R, Desai TA, German MS. 2011. Differentiation of human embryonic stem cells into pancreatic endoderm in patterned size-controlled clusters. *Stem Cell Research* 6(3): 276–285.

Vogelstein B, Alberts B, Shine K. 2002. Genetics. Please don't call it cloning! *Science* 295(5558): 1237.

Wakayama T, Perry AC, Zuccotti M, Johnson KR, Yanagimachi R. 1998. Full-term development of mice from enucleated oocytes injected with cumulus cell nuclei. *Nature* 394(6691): 369–374.

Wang T, Koh C, Yoo JJ. 2003a. *Creation of an Engineered Uterus for Surgical Reconstruction.* American Academy of Pediatrics Section on Urology, New Orleans, LA.

Wang X, Ye K. 2009. Three-dimensional differentiation of embryonic stem cells into islet-like insulin-producing clusters. *Tissue Engineering Part A* 15(8): 1941–1952.

Wang ZQ, Watanabe Y, Toki A. 2003b. Experimental assessment of small intestinal submucosa as a small bowel graft in a rat model. *Journal of Pediatric Surgery* 38(11): 1596–1601.

Wefer J, Sievert KD, Schlote N, Wefer AE, Nunes L, Dahiya R et al. 2001. Time dependent smooth muscle regeneration and maturation in a bladder acellular matrix graft: Histological studies and in vivo functional evaluation. *Journal of Urology* 165(5): 1755–1759.

Wernig M, Meissner A, Foreman R, Brambrink T, Ku M, Hochedlinger K et al. 2007. In vitro reprogramming of fibroblasts into a pluripotent ES-cell-like state. *Nature* 448(7151): 318–324.

Wilmut I, Schnieke AE, McWhir J, Kind AJ, Campbell KH. 1997. Viable offspring derived from fetal and adult mammalian cells. [Erratum appears in *Nature* 1997 Mar 13; 386(6621): 200]. *Nature* 385(6619): 810–813.

Yard BA, Kooymans-Couthino M, Reterink T, van den Elsen P, Paape ME, Bruyn JA et al. 1993. Analysis of T cell lines from rejecting renal allografts. *Kidney International* 39(Suppl): S133–S138.

Yoo J, Ashkar S, Atala A. 1996. Creation of functional kidney structures with excretion of kidney-like fluid in vivo. *Pediatrics* 98S: 605.

Yoo JJ, Meng J, Oberpenning F, Atala A. 1998. Bladder augmentation using allogenic bladder submucosa seeded with cells. *Urology* 51(2): 221–225.

Yoo JJ, Park HJ, Lee I, Atala A. 1999. Autologous engineered cartilage rods for penile reconstruction. *Journal of Urology* 162(3 Pt 2): 1119–1121.

Yu J, Vodyanik MA, Smuga-Otto K, Antosiewicz-Bourget J, Frane JL, Tian S et al. 2007. Induced pluripotent stem cell lines derived from human somatic cells. *Science* 38(5858): 1917–1920.

Zhang Y. 2008. Bladder reconstruction by tissue engineering—With or without cells? *Journal of Urology* 180(1): 10–11.

Zhang Y, Frimberger D, Cheng EY, Lin HK, Kropp BP. 2006. Challenges in a larger bladder replacement with cell-seeded and unseeded small intestinal submucosa grafts in a subtotal cystectomy model. *BJU International* 98(5): 1100–1105.

Zhang D, Jiang W, Liu M, Sui X, Yin X, Chen S et al. 2009. Highly efficient differentiation of human ES cells and iPS cells into mature pancreatic insulin-producing cells. *Cell Research* 19(4): 429–438.

Zhang SC, Wernig M, Duncan ID, Brustle O, Thomson JA. 2001. In vitro differentiation of transplantable neural precursors from human embryonic stem cells. *Nature Biotechnology* 19(12): 1129–1133.

Zhu L, Gibson P, Currle DS, Tong Y, Richardson RJ, Bayazitov IT et al. 2009. Prominin 1 marks intestinal stem cells that are susceptible to neoplastic transformation. *Nature* 457(7229): 603–607.

Zhu S, Li W, Zhou H, Wei W, Ambasudhan R, Lin T et al. 2010. Reprogramming of human primary somatic cells by OCT4 and chemical compounds. *Cell Stem Cell* 7(6): 651–655.

CHAPTER 9

Cardiovascular Regenerative Engineering

Rebekah A. Neal, PhD; Anusuya Das, PhD;
and Edward A. Botchwey, PhD

CONTENTS

9.1 INTRODUCTION

Pathologies of the cardiovascular system are becoming more pervasive as the world's population ages, highlighting the downfalls of current treatment practices and encouraging the search for regenerative medicine solutions. The World Health Organization's fact sheet (www.who.int) lists cardiovascular diseases as the number one cause of death globally, with 17.1 million people dying from cardiovascular diseases in 2004. Cardiovascular diseases are expected to remain the leading cause of death through at least 2030, underscoring the need for the development of new technologies and approaches to meet the global demand.

In the clinic, the most successful application of drug delivery for cardiovascular disease is drug-eluting stents (Garg and Serruys 2010). By 2005, over 80% of all stenting procedures used drug-eluting stent (Jeremias and Kirtane 2008), though concerns over safety have caused usage to drop slightly in the intervening years (Camenzind et al. 2007). In clinical trials to promote angiogenesis after myocardial infarction or other cardiovascular pathology, most clinical trials to date have sought to deliver growth factors in bolus, which led to angiogenesis *in vitro*, but have so far shown to be less than adequate for *in vivo* treatment (see Sefcik et al. 2008 for review). Clearly, new approaches are required to improve outcomes in cardiovascular pathologies, and regenerative medicine may be the ideal solution. Cardiovascular regenerative engineering encompasses the use of stem cells and other factors for both tissue-engineered solutions to cardiovascular deficits and recovery of function in disease states such as acute myocardial infarction. In attempts to overcome some of the traditional hurdles associated with cardiovascular disease treatment, therapeutic approaches have begun moving beyond an exclusive focus on orally delivered drugs and invasive surgeries toward controlled delivery of stem cells, proangiogenic and proinflammatory factors, and tissue-engineered solutions. These regenerative technologies exploit a greater understanding of molecular level pathways and stem cell biology to provide patient-specific solutions and encourage healing through stimulation of natural pathways.

9.2 ANATOMY OF THE CARDIOVASCULAR SYSTEM

The cardiovascular system consists of the heart and vasculature, where the heart functions as the mechanical pump to circulate blood, cells, and factors, and the vessels serve as channels for distribution to the tissues of the body. The heart is comprised of mainly cardiac muscle tissue and specialized contractile muscle cells, which provide the mechanical beat of the heart. Deoxygenated blood enters the right atrium through the superior vena cava and passes through the tricuspid valve to the right ventricle, which contracts to force the blood through the pulmonary artery into pulmonary circulation. In the lungs, gas exchange occurs to oxygenate the blood and remove carbon dioxide waste, and the newly oxygenated blood flows through the pulmonary vein into the left atrium. From the left atrium, the blood passes through the mitral valve and is pumped into circulation by the strongest chamber of the heart, the left ventricle. Heart valves prevent backflow between chambers of the heart and into the circulation. Both the aortic and pulmonary valves, which serve to prevent backflow into the ventricles from the circulation, are trileaflet valves. The mitral and tricuspid valves, which prevent backflow from the ventricles into the atria, are bileaflet valves. The valves are comprised mainly of endothelial cells (ECs) and interstitial cells. Valves have significant collagen content in their extracellular matrix (ECM) to provide strength, as well as elastin to provide elasticity, and glycosaminoglycans to aid in response to shear from blood flow.

The arterial system carries oxygenated blood from the heart to the body with high-pressure flow. Arteries divide into arterioles and then capillaries, the smallest vessels of the system. At the capillary level, diffusion into the tissue is possible, so oxygen and nutrients are removed from the blood and waste products are added as blood flows back to the heart through the veins with low-pressure flow. Based on their functionality and the need to withstand and respond to the pressure of blood flow, the arterial system and venous system exhibit structural differences.

The arterial system transports oxygenated blood from the left ventricle under high pressure and carries it throughout the body under pressure. Arteries have three main layers: the tunica intima, the tunica media, and the tunica adventitia.

The tunica intima lines the lumen of the vessel and consists of a single layer of ECs supported by a basement membrane of elastin with a sparse layer of branched vascular smooth muscle cells underneath. The ECs form a continuous interface between the vessel and blood and are selectively permeable. This layer is resistant to thrombosis, and the ECs secrete factors and cytokines, which mediate many vessel functions such as blood cell trafficking, vasomotor tone, cell growth, and vascular remodeling.

The middle layer, the tunica media, comprises several layers of vascular smooth muscle cells bundled into units bound by elastin, which are situated circumferentially around the vessel. These cells are responsible for the contractility of the vessel, maintain vasomotor tone, and regulate the dilation and contraction of the vessels in response to flow and other stimuli. Depending on the size of the vessel, multiple layers of smooth muscle cells may contribute to the thickness of the tunica media and contribute the most thickness to the vessel wall.

The outer layer, the tunica adventitia, is a loosely organized fibrous network containing elastin and fibroblasts. Also in this layer are blood vessels that supply cells in the larger vessel wall (called the vasa vasorum) and nerves that stimulate cells in the vessel wall (called the vasa nervosum).

The venous system transports deoxygenated blood back to the heart. This system is responsible for regulating blood distribution changes between central and peripheral circulation. The capillary system, where gas exchange occurs, maintains a tremendous surface area to allow for the movement of substances in and out of the circulation.

Due to the lower-pressure flow throughout the venous system when compared to the arterial system, the veins and venules exhibit thinner walls and larger overall diameters than comparable arteries and arterioles. In the veins, the tunica media contains fewer layers of smooth muscle cells and as a result is much weaker than the comparable layer in arteries. The capillaries themselves are small endothelial tubes that lack the organization of other layers of larger vessels. The endothelial layer is encapsulated by a basement membrane and a single layer of pericytes, and the tunica adventitia is merely a thin layer of connective tissue, which is integrated with surrounding tissue, providing the ideal environment for transport in and out of the bloodstream.

9.3 PHYSIOLOGY OF BLOOD VESSELS AND MICROVASCULAR REMODELING

The cardiovascular system is the first system to develop during embryogenesis as it is absolutely critical for the development of all other organs. Its function is to deliver oxygen and nutrients to the body and to remove cellular waste products. Sufficient vascularization and functioning circulation are requirements for all aspects of tissue growth, repair, and regeneration, from embryogenesis to wound healing. Embryogenesis will not be covered in depth in this chapter, except as the study of vascular growth and development in embryogenesis provides insights into microvascular remodeling in ischemia reperfusion injury and tissue engineering.

The process of vessel formation and remodeling is a continuum response to environmental stimuli such as hypoxia, paracrine signals, cell–matrix interactions, cell–cell interactions, and exogenous factors (Figure 9.1). This continuum, depicted in Figure 9.2, exists in both newly forming and regenerating tissues and helps to control assembly of the vasculature and formation of networks. A series of remodeling processes control complex cellular behaviors in a coordinated response to stimuli. The processes of neovascularization, angiogenesis, vasculogenesis, arteriogenesis, intussusception, and regression comprise this continuum reaction and are detailed later.

9.3.1 Vascular Growth and Remodeling

9.3.1.1 Neovascularization

The process of vasculogenesis was initially thought to only occur during embryogenesis, as it requires the formation of a vascular network *de novo* by stem or progenitor cells. Endothelial progenitor cells begin the process by forming into unstable, permeable tubes. Pericytes are then recruited and differentiated to line the vessel to produce a mature vessel phenotype, with structural integrity, basement membrane investment and production, and secretion of factors for the survival of the EC lining. These vessels are then incorporated into existing networks to establish blood flow.

In the adult, the presence of circulating endothelial progenitor cells as well as progenitor cells resident in the bone marrow suggests that vasculogenesis may be possible. For the remainder of this chapter, we will consider new vessel formation in an adult to be neovascularization, which will incorporate both the processes of adult vasculogenesis and sprouting angiogenesis.

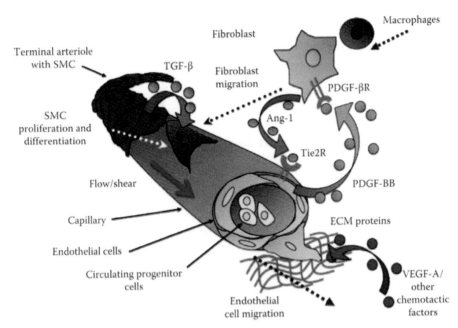

FIGURE 9.1 Different cellular populations, growth factors, and environmental signals that affect cell behaviors contribute to a coordinated remodeling response. (Adapted from Peirce, S.M. and Skalak, T.C., *Microcirculation*, 10(1), 99, 2003.)

9.3.1.2 Angiogenesis

Angiogenesis is the formation of new capillaries from existing capillary bed, and it involves complex coordination of multiple cell types and soluble and molecular signals. Stimulation of angiogenesis results from changes to the local tissue environment, typically inflammation or ischemia (hypoxia). It is crucial during development, healing, and for physiological processes such as menstrual cycles and reproduction. Two other cases are of particular interest. First, angiogenesis occurs during invasive tumor growth because of the additional nourishment required by the tumor. Second, it is essential for tissue-engineering purposes because it is necessary to be able to predict and control capillary development in scaffolds during *in vitro* and *in vivo* tissue development. The primary stages of angiogenesis can be categorized as (1) EC activation by chemotactic agents, (2) secretion of proteases into the matrix, (3) selection of ECs for sprouting, (4) capillary growth, (5) tubulogenesis, (6) nonangiogenic growth of blood vessels via capillary loop formation, and (7) formation of second-generation capillaries (Adams and Alitalo 2007). Two methods of angiogenesis exist, sprouting angiogenesis and intussusception, and these processes may occur independently or simultaneously in the tissue.

In sprouting angiogenesis, ECs resident on the vessel, typically a postcapillary venule, respond to an angiogenic stimulus by degrading the local basement membrane, migrating outward from the vessel toward the stimulus, and proliferating to form new capillary sprouts. Hypoxia typically drives sprouting angiogenesis, but other stimulatory signals such as high local expression of vascular endothelial growth factor (VEGF), stromal cell–derived factor 1 (SDF-1), or monocyte chemotactic protein 1 (MCP-1) can also encourage

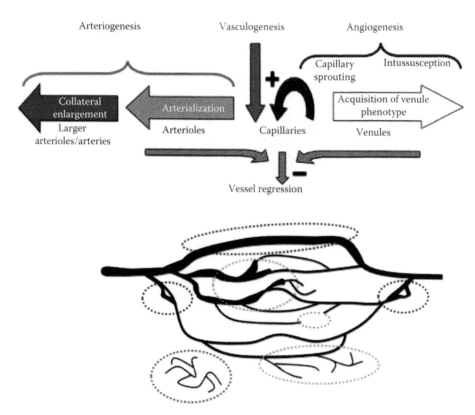

FIGURE 9.2 Vascular remodeling is a complex continuum of vascular adaptations invoked by a variety of environmental stimuli, which together determine the integrative control of vascular assembly and pattern formation. (Reproduced from Peirce, S.M. and Skalak, T.C., *Microcirculation*, 10(1), 99, 2003.)

angiogenesis. The progression begins with an increase in vessel permeability, which allows extravasation of plasma factors, which encourage EC migration. Matrix metalloproteinases (MMPs) secreted by these activated ECs break down the local basement membrane and allow the cells to migrate outward. ECs migrate and proliferate to form sprouts. The lumen forms through a process called canalization, and branches and loops in the new vessel are formed by anastomoses of sprouts with existing vessels to allow blood flow. Vascular smooth muscle cells wrap the vessel to stabilize and provide strength, and a new basement membrane is secreted around the vessel. Circulating endothelial progenitor cells may also play a role in the process, either by investing in the new vessels as differentiated ECs or by secreting growth factors, which stimulate sprouting. Local inflammatory responses by macrophages and mast cells may also release stimulatory factors to encourage angiogenesis. In tissue regeneration, several types of progenitor cells may play a role, pushing the process more toward vasculogenesis than the typical angiogenic response.

Angiogenesis by intussusception involves the splitting or partitioning of vessels into new vessels through the insertion of interstitial tissue. In this form of angiogenesis, interstitial tissue columns or pillars are inserted in the lumen of preexisting vessels. As the vessels grow and become stabilized and invested with smooth muscle cells, the ECs line the lumen partition to form two separate vessels and remodel the local vessel network. This response may be a transient phase where vessels are split with little new network expansion and allows for remodeling and integration of these new vessels into existing networks, reestablishing normal flow parameters for the tissue environment.

9.3.1.3 Arteriogenesis

The process of arteriogenesis encompasses arteriole and artery formation as well as collateral enlargement (Figure 9.3). Arteriolization is the process by which new arterioles are formed from existing capillaries in the network. Local inflammation or added hemodynamic stress can stimulate arteriolization. The vessel structure is modified by recruitment of perivascular cells, which then differentiate into the contractile smooth muscle cell phenotype required for high-pressure arteriolar flow. Smooth muscle cells residing on the vessel upstream of the event may also participate through proliferation, migration to the area, and investment in the remodeling capillary.

Collateral enlargement involves the enlargement of collateral vessels already in the network and may also include vessels in the vasa vasorum, the network that supplies the vessel wall. Hemodynamic stress causes EC activation, and ECs in turn degrade and reorganize the ECM to allow for vessel enlargement. Endothelial and vascular smooth muscle cells proliferate and enlarge the lumen and walls of the vessel to arteriole or artery functionality.

9.3.1.4 Regression

Vessel regression counterbalances angiogenesis to maintain a stable network. Regression often occurs in response to lessened flow or a hyperoxygenated environment. In hyperoxia, VEGF signaling is downregulated, decreasing cell–cell contact within the vessel wall and preventing vessel maintenance. By selectively paring down the vessel

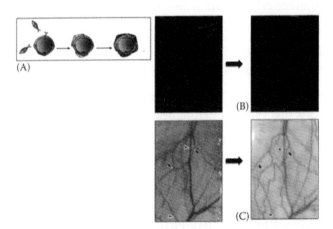

FIGURE 9.3   (A) Arteriogenesis is the process by which new arterioles form and existing arterioles structurally remodel. (B) Capillary arterialization: Recruitment of smooth muscle cells to capillaries in order to form new arteries. (C) Collateral enlargement: Enlargement of existing arterioles and arteries (following ischemia) in a mouse spinotrapezius model. (Courtesy of Peirce–Cottler Lab, Biomedical Engineering, University of Virginia, Charlottesville, VA.)

network in these regions, the cardiovascular system can maintain consistent function throughout the body.

9.3.2 Molecular Regulation of Angiogenesis

Angiogenesis and other processes in the continuum of vessel remodeling are regulated at a molecular level by a multitude of signaling molecules and growth factors. Many known participants are listed later, with a brief description of their role in the process. As this field is currently advancing rapidly, this list is not intended to be comprehensive, but rather an overview of many of the important molecules we understand to date (Krenning et al. 2009).

Angiopoietin 1 (Ang1): This molecule is required for the maturation and stabilization of blood vessels and plays a role in pericyte and vascular smooth muscle cell recruitment to immature vessels for stabilization.

Angiopoietin 2 (Ang2): This molecule is a natural antagonist of Ang1. It is expressed only at the site of vascular remodeling and is responsible for the destabilization of the vasculature.

Basic fibroblast growth factor (bFGF): Vessel formation during embryogenesis occurs through the differentiation of stem and progenitor cells into endothelial and blood cells. Blood island form, fuse, and create a vascular plexus, which is then remodeled and branched, blood flow begins, and the circulatory network is born. The differentiation of these early stem and progenitor cells into an endothelial lineage may be influenced by bFGF signaling.

Connexin 43 (Cx43): Connexin gap junction is found in several cell types and locations, including the heart. This junction controls communication between endothelial and mural cell progenitors. Deficiencies cause heart malformations and malfunction of blood flow from the heart.

Hepatocyte growth factor (HGF): This factor is secreted by mesenchymal cells and acts on ECs. It serves to stimulate cell migration and matrix degradation by ECs in microvascular remodeling.

Indian hedgehog (Ihh): This molecule is produced in the yolk sac ectoderm during embryogenesis. Inhibition of Ihh production disrupts EC differentiation and tube formation.

Interleukin 8 (IL-8): This molecule is produced by macrophages and ECs and is part of the inflammatory cascade that can lead to microvascular remodeling.

Platelet-derived growth factor B (PDGF-B): This molecule is secreted by proliferating ECs. It acts as a chemoattractant as well as a mitogen for pericytes and vascular smooth muscle cells and their precursors.

Placental growth factor (PlGF): This molecule is expressed in the placenta and part of the VEGF superfamily (binds to VEGF-R1). PlGF stimulates VEGF secretion by monocytes and recruits macrophages and monocytes to wound areas for healing.

Platelet tissue factor: This molecule is expressed by vascular smooth muscle cells and interstitial cells. It is required for the maturation of blood vessels and plays a role in pericyte and vascular smooth muscle cell recruitment to immature vessels for stabilization.

Quaking: This molecule is produced in yolk sac ectoderm during embryogenesis. Inhibition of quaking, or complete lack of the molecule, leads to disruption in vascular development.

Serum response factor (SRF): SRF is a transcription factor whose expression is upregulated by TGF-β in the induction of smooth muscle cell and pericyte differentiation. SRF is both necessary and sufficient to differentiate to smooth muscle cell phenotype.

Transforming growth factor β (TGF-β): This molecule induces the expression of vascular smooth muscle cell genes such as smooth muscle α-actin. It also induces vascular smooth muscle cell differentiation through SRF.

Vascular endothelial growth factor A (VEGF-A): This molecule is produced in yolk sac ectoderm during embryogenesis, and response is mediated by two receptor tyrosine kinases (VEGF-R2/Flk-1 and VEGF-R1/Flt-1). VEGF-A plays a role in modulating EC migration and tube formation. Without VEGF-A, healthy vessels are unable to form. In addition, VEGF-A contributes to vascular remodeling after exercise, injury, and collateral enlargement.

Identification of mature ECs and smooth vessel cells is critical during both *in vitro* and *in vivo* experiments. Genes that are indicative of mature ECs are Flt-1 (VEGF-R1), VE-cadherin, von Willebrand factor, and factor VIII, and those that represent smooth muscle cells are smooth muscle α-actin, calponin, and smooth muscle-22α.

9.3.3 Mechanisms of Structural Remodeling

Multiple mechanisms regulate structural remodeling. In the preceding section, growth factors and signaling mechanisms, which stimulate angiogenesis and vascular remodeling, were listed. In this section, we address other factors such as mechanical forces, cell responses, and ECM interactions that may drive structural remodeling.

9.3.3.1 Extracellular Matrix

ECs exist within an ECM environment bound to an array of ECM proteins. Multiple facets of that matrix play a role in EC behaviors such as the surface topography and soluble factors, which provide both biochemical and physical cues for the organization and fate of ECs. Cell–matrix interactions are established through integrins ($\alpha_v\beta_3$, $\alpha_5\beta_1$) and their receptors, mediated by focal adhesions, and allow signaling. The ECM contains collagen, fibronectin, laminin, and tenascin-c. These proteins may help regulate angiogenesis and neovascularization through cell adhesions, binding of growth factors, and providing stimuli for migration. Yamamura et al. (2007) studied the effect of substrate stiffness on bovine pulmonary microvascular ECs (BPMECs) and demonstrated that BPMECs cultured on flexible collagen gels form networks in 3 days and show extensive sprouting and formation of complex networks in 5 days, whereas the cells cultured on stiffer gels tend to form aggregates and thicker networks. Thus, matrix stiffness affects capillary formation. The presence of flow influences the directionality of capillaries. Helm et al. (2005) showed that interstitial flow on the order of 1 μm/s in combination with VEGF-induced directionality in capillary structures (in the direction of flow) and caused fibrin-bound VEGF to be released via proteolysis.

9.3.3.2 Hypoxia

A lack of oxygen in the local environment can drive angiogenesis. Within hypoxic regions, EC proliferation and sprouting are stimulated through hypoxia-inducible factor 1α (HIF-1α). HIF-1 is a nuclear factor, which is typically rapidly degraded in the cell in normoxia; however, in hypoxic conditions, the enzyme that breaks down HIF-1 is inhibited, and HIF-1α is stabilized. HIF-1α then upregulates VEGF to promote angiogenesis in the hypoxic region. In embryonic stem cells, hypoxia also upregulates VEGF and promotes angioblast specification. This occurs by the third week in development, when the oxygen needs of the embryo can no longer be met by diffusion alone. The production of VEGF causes endothelial progenitor cells to differentiate, proliferate, and form a network of tubules during vasculogenesis.

9.3.3.3 Hydrodynamic Shear

Blood flow produces shear forces within the lumen of the vessel on the layer of ECs. Changes in this shear force can affect the proliferation, differentiation, and active phenotype of these cells through modulation of gene expression and morphological changes to adapt to increased or decreased flow. The pumping of the heart produces cyclic strain in the tunica media, felt by the vascular smooth muscle cells. Changes in this strain can affect these cells in a similar manner.

9.4 CLINICALLY DRIVEN STRATEGIES FOR VASCULARIZATION

Given the complexity of the vascular system, it is no easy task to fix vascular problems. While current clinical approaches have proven functional, they are not without considerable limitations. However, with the considerable information becoming available to researchers, many novel strategies are now emerging. In the remainder of this chapter, we will consider two distinct but similar clinical problems, which drive efforts in cardiovascular regenerative medicine: (1) development of effective therapies to encourage neovascularization in tissue-engineered constructs and (2) recovery of function through revascularization after ischemic injury.

9.4.1 Tissue-Engineered Constructs

Tissue engineering is an interdisciplinary field that applies the principles of engineering and life sciences toward the development of biological substitutes that restore, maintain, or improve tissue function or a whole organ (Langer and Vacanti 1993).

Tissue-engineered constructs are developed to provide functional replacement for or encourage regeneration of injured, diseased, or dead tissues within the body. As such, these constructs must closely mimic the structures they seek to replace, with the microvasculature being a critical component for success. The vascular system supplies oxygen, nutrients, progenitor cells, and inflammatory cells to the tissue and removes metabolites and other waste to maintain a healthy environment. Diffusion can provide this function only within about 1 mm³ of the construct edge, limiting tissue-engineered solutions, which rely on diffusion to sizes that are not physiologically relevant for human disease treatment. In early tissue-engineered constructs, these diffusion limitations led to the formation of a necrotic

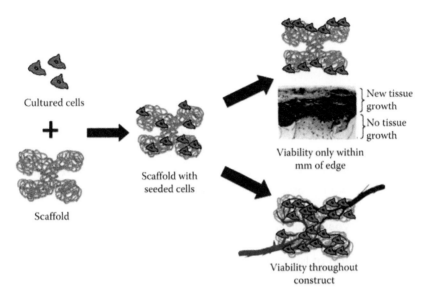

Cultured cells

Scaffold

Scaffold with
seeded cells

} New tissue growth

} No tissue growth

Viability only within
mm of edge

Viability throughout
construct

FIGURE 9.4 In recent years, tissue-specific scaffolds have been seeded with cells. However, upon implantation, cells in the center of the scaffold either die or migrate to the edges because of diffusion limitations (greater than a few cubic millimeter). Thus, the viability of every cell-seeded scaffold is only achieved when the construct is appropriately vascularized. (Adapted from Ishaug, S.L. et al., *J. Biomed. Mater. Res.*, 36(1), 17, 1997.)

core and, ultimately, failure of the implant (Figure 9.4; Ishaug et al. 1997). Endogenous neovascularization does not occur within an appropriately short time frame to prevent cell death within the construct, so alternative methods of stimulating neovascularization or generating a vessel network must be considered.

Current approaches to vascularization in tissue-engineered constructs include the following three main strategies (Lokmic and Mitchell 2008): (1) prevascularization of engineered tissues before implantation, (2) incorporation of proangiogenic factors into the matrix to encourage host vasculature to invest in the implant (Lee et al. 2002), and (3) seeding of ECs, vascular smooth muscle cells, progenitor cells, or stem cells within the construct to contribute to angiogenesis *in situ* (Schechner et al. 2000, Levenberg et al. 2005).

Some researchers seek to overcome the limitations of the host vasculature by generating prevascularized tissues. Constructs are prevascularized through an initial implantation to allow growth of vascular tissue, and tissue organization occurs around the forming vascular network. While this is a promising area of research, there is a concern over the time to treatment lost in the initial implantation stage, the potential for immune reactions if the initial implantation is done in a xenogenic model, and the inability to encourage this prevascularized network to merge with the host vasculature. Most applications to date rely on host vasculature to form connections and do not provide exogenous stimuli to encourage this merging.

Other researchers focus on delivering angiogenic factors or cytokines through the scaffolding used to form the tissue-engineered construct. With biodegradable scaffolds, concentration and release of the factor can be controlled to encourage capillary investment. To date, however, these studies have typically focused on single factor delivery with a single delivery profile, neglecting the complex scheme of cells and molecules involved in the angiogenesis cascade.

Many researchers evaluate various cell types for implantation, either preseeded and cultured on the construct or codelivered with the construct at the site of implantation. Mature ECs and smooth muscle cells can be added, but neither cell type is immune privileged and may ultimately cause graft versus host disease and graft rejection. Embryonic or adult stem cells left in their native undifferentiated state or predifferentiated toward an EC lineage are also used to populate constructs to form new vasculature. This area shows particular promise as these cells could be autologous and have the potential to differentiate into the various cell types involved in the angiogenic process.

9.4.2 Revascularization of Ischemic Tissue

Pathologies of the cardiovascular system, including chronic ischemic diseases and myocardial infarction, are the number one cause of death on a global scale. Most pathologies result from thrombotic events and vascular occlusions, which cause tissue ischemia. Current treatments focus on restoring perfusion to the ischemic tissue but do not typically include treatments to encourage tissue regeneration lost during ischemia. When perfusion is recovered, often the infarct size is reduced, cell death via apoptosis is prevented, and an entire organ may be saved from failure.

Most clinical trials to treat ischemia/reperfusion injury or acute myocardial infarction have focused on delivery of a single factor, such as a proangiogenic compound to encourage neovascularization, often released as a bolus to the site of injury. Studies like these have often failed to show efficacy at the clinical level, likely due to their simplicity. Single factor delivery overlooks the underlying complex physiology of angiogenesis and the coordinated response of multiple cell types, factors, and cytokines required to generate new vessels.

Other trials focus on delivering cell types such as predifferentiated stem cells or mobilizing circulating progenitor cells to the injury site to participate in tissue regeneration. While these therapies often show some level of efficacy over control treatments, limitations in cell tracking methods prohibit researchers from ascertaining whether the effects are due to cells actually participating in remodeling and regeneration efforts or secreting paracrine singles within the environment to encourage the endogenous healing response.

There is an overwhelming clinical need for greater understanding of the complex system of therapeutic neovascularization, both for tissue-engineered implants and for tissue regeneration after ischemic injury. Improvement in the ability to drive angiogenic stimulation and neovascularization of injury regions is critical if this technology is to become widely available as a therapy.

9.5 STEM CELLS IN CARDIOVASCULAR REGENERATIVE MEDICINE

One of the foremost obstacles in cardiovascular regenerative medicine, and in fact in all fields of regenerative medicine, is the current inability to induce vascularization in tissue, either ischemic tissue or engineered tissue constructs. We have discussed earlier the stimulators of these neovascularization or angiogenesis processes as including growth factors, ECM proteins, hypoxia, and hemodynamic shear forces. Without assistance, host vasculature cannot successfully revascularize an avascular tissue in time to prevent necrosis. To overcome this limitation, researchers have turned to stem cells, both embryonic and adult, as well as progenitor cells, which can either be precultured on tissue-engineered constructs or mobilized to the area of injury or disease.

9.5.1 Stem and Progenitor Cells

Embryonic stem cells are isolated from the early embryo, before cells have committed to a particular germ layer. These cells are considered to be pluripotent and can give rise to cells from any and all of the germ layers (Martin 1981, Thomson et al. 1998, Atala and Langer 2001).

Adult stem cells are tissue specific and isolated from the adult. Many tissues yield stem cells, such as bone marrow (hematopoietic and mesenchymal cells), adipose tissue, and others.

Progenitor cells exhibit clonality and a capacity for self-renewal. In addition, many progenitor cells also exhibit some level of multipotency, though less than most adult stem cells (Yi et al. 2010).

Embryonic stem cells have the most flexibility in differentiation. As such, embryonic stem cells can be used as a model system to interrogate issues associated with vascularizing tissue constructs, as well as aiding to elucidate the mechanisms involved in both vasculogenesis (typically in the embryo) and angiogenesis (Hanjaya-Putra and Gerecht 2009). Researchers have successfully grown embryonic stem cells within 3D scaffolds molded after a specific tissue (Gerecht et al. 2007, Huang et al. 2010, Liu et al. 2010). With the delivery of exogenous factors such as VEGF to promote angiogenesis or other factors to encourage differentiation down a specific tissue lineage, these cell-seeded constructs could ultimately be used to reconstruct entire organs. But before whole-organ regeneration is possible, embryonic stem cells can provide the platform by which microvascular network formation can be studied. With this platform, it may be possible to engineer the vascular supply *in vitro* before implantation into the host tissue or defect site and then induce the new vasculature to anastomose with the host system.

Embryonic stem cells can be cultured in suspension, which causes their spontaneous aggregation and the formation of embryoid bodies (Dang et al. 2004, Kurosawa 2007). These embryoid bodies then harbor populations of vascular progenitor cells, which can give rise to various vascular cell types including ECs and vascular smooth muscle cells (Levenberg et al. 2002, 2007). Researchers have shown that ECs differentiated *in vitro* from embryoid bodies have the capacity to form endothelial tubes on Matrigel (a 3D ECM equivalent available commercially). In addition, these differentiated ECs expressed endothelial markers discussed previously such as vascular endothelial cadherin (VE-cadherin), PECAM-1, CD-34, and VEGF-R2. These cells also display functional markers indicative of healthy ECs, such as von Willebrand factor, endothelial nitric oxide synthase (eNOS), and E-selectins, which allow for cell rolling and adhesion on the endothelial monolayer (Zhou and Gallicano 2006).

Vascular smooth muscle cells can also be differentiated from these embryoid bodies, which display the spindle-like morphology of smooth muscle cells and express markers indicative of a smooth muscle cell phenotype such as smooth muscle α-actin, calponin, smooth muscle 22, and smooth muscle myosin heavy chain (Ferreira et al. 2007, Levenberg et al. 2010).

There is a significant potential for embryonic stem cells differentiated into vascular cells such as endothelial and smooth muscle cells to contribute to neovascularization in a multitude of ways. Cells may contribute to mature blood vessels, which can then integrate into the host vasculature, may proliferate and contribute to the formation of new vessels, and may localize to the injury site and secrete factors, which encourage angiogenesis.

Biomaterial scaffolds may be the ideal structure with which to guide embryonic stem cell differentiation. Bioactive, biocompatible, and biodegradable scaffolds fabricated from natural materials (ECM proteins, plant material, agarose, alginate, dextrans, etc.) as well as synthetic materials (PLGA, PGSA) provide the appropriate geometry and structure to mimic the native tissue, and release of factors from these scaffolds can drive differentiation down a specific pathway.

9.5.1.1 Adult Stem Cells

Adult hematopoietic stem cells express CD-34 but not CD-38 and exhibit a small, spherical phenotype. They display a high nuclear to cytoplasm ratio and divide rarely. These stem cells give rise to blood cells (Griffin et al. 2010).

Adult mesenchymal stem cells are nonhematopoietic cells, which express CD-29, CD-44, CD-90, and CD-105 but do not express hematopoietic markers such as CD-14, CD-31, CD-34, and CD-45. As multipotent stem cells, they can differentiate into cell types, which arise from the mesoderm. For example, bone marrow (BMSCs) as well as adipose derived stem cells (ASCs) have been shown to give rise to adipocytes, osteoblasts, chondrocytes, tenocytes, and skeletal muscle cells. These cells have also been shown to modulate inflammation through the production of anti-inflammatory molecules that influence dendritic cells, inhibit T-cell proliferation, and modulate B-cell function (Rafei et al. 2009, Ohtaki 2008). Based on this immune-modulatory effect, when adult mesenchymal stem cells are injected or implanted allogeneically, they tend to lower the incidence of graft versus host disease (Lazarus et al. 2005).

Mesenchymal stem cells have been used to treat ischemic events as well as to seed tissue-engineered constructs. Intramyocardial injection of MSCs after myocardial infarction tends to aid in cell migration and retention at the site of injury and tissue recovery and survival (Mangi 2003).

While BMSCs received much of the early attention in the field of adult stem cells, ASCs are gaining favor for two main reasons. First, ASCs can be isolated from autologous adipose tissue through minimally invasive liposuction. Second, clinically relevant numbers can be obtained in just 1–2 h. These cells are typically located in the wall of the adipose vasculature. ASCs show particular promise for inclusion in tissue-engineered therapies due to this ready availability and expansion, secretion of factors, which promote angiogenesis and inhibit apoptosis, ability to differentiate into multiple relevant cell types, and capacity to modulate the immune system (Hong et al. 2010).

Currently, ASCs have been used to rescue and regrow vasculature in cardiac tissue after ischemic events (Cai et al. 2009). This rescue and regeneration may be due to paracrine secretion of angiogenic factors such as VEGF, HGF, bFGF, and Ang1; inflammatory factors such as IL-6, IL-8, IL-11, IL-17, and monocyte chemoattractant protein (MCP-1, -2); and mobilizing factors such as granulocyte–macrophage colony-stimulating factor (GM-CSF), macrophage CSF (M-CSF), and SDF-1. An alternative explanation is that instead of just secreting factors, which regulate the environment and encourage angiogenesis and immune protection, ASCs may contribute to new vessel formation by differentiating into ECs or vascular smooth muscle cells. Figure 9.5 shows the potential methods of cardiac regeneration.

Intravenous injection of ASCs shows improvement over BMSCs in restoring blood flow and revascularization after ischemic injury in rodent hind limb (Kim et al. 2007). In addition, injection of ASCs after acute myocardial infarction promotes angiogenesis, reduces cardiomyocyte apoptosis, and decreases inflammation. ASCs also aid in full-thickness wound healing, likely due to improved tissue vascularization (Lu et al. 2008).

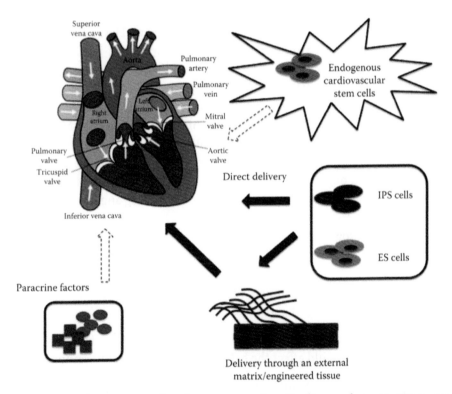

FIGURE 9.5 Potential routes to cardiac tissue regenerative. Cardiovascular progenitors, generated from human ES cells or iPS cells or isolated from the patients, could be directly implanted into the heart or used to seed an ECM in order to engineer muscle tissue. Alternatively, the endogenous regenerative capacity of the heart may be stimulated by extracellular factors such as neuregulin-1β, SDF-1. (Adapted from Yi, B.A. et al., *J. Clin. Invest.*, 120(1), 20, 2010.)

Despite these successes, several questions and concerns remain for clinical application of ASC therapy:

1. Are freshly isolated ASCs superior to culture-conditioned ASCs?

2. What changes occur after time in culture that affect ASCs phenotype and success rate *in vivo*?

3. Should autologous or allogeneic sources be used? Can off-the-shelf therapies with allogeneic sources be as good as autologous transplantation?

4. What are the ideal delivery approaches to maintain ASC viability and retain the maximum number at the injury site?

9.5.1.2 Progenitor Cells

Endothelial progenitor cells were first differentiated from peripheral blood mononuclear cells by Asahara et al. (1997). These cells express CD-34 and participate in vascular homeostasis and neovascularization. The most likely mechanism through which these cells induce neovascularization is paracrine signaling. In these cells, hypoxia induces production and secretion of proinflammatory and proangiogenic factors, which serve to alleviate the hypoxia through neovascularization (Hattori et al. 2001). More specifically, stabilized HIF-1α induces cellular transcription of VEGF, SDF-1, MCP-1, and angiopoietins in the local environment, which trigger the homing of circulating endothelial progenitor cells. VEGF signaling through its receptor VEGF-R2 causes an increase in local vascular permeability by breaking up adherens junctions and causing the internalization of VE-cadherin. Tight junctions are degrading by MCP-1, and local ECs increase their expression of cell adhesion molecules (E-selectin, ICAM-1, VCAM-1), which help to catch circulating endothelial progenitor cells. As the ECs extravasate, they secrete MMPs to degrade basement membrane into capillary-like tunnels, which become invested with ECs similar to the process of sprouting angiogenesis (Gavard and Gutkind 2006).

While endothelial progenitor cells show promise for revascularization, several questions and concerns remain for clinical application (Krenning et al. 2009):

1. How do these capillary-like tunnels become functional vessels, and what is the role of endothelial progenitors in that process?

2. Are there individual differences or tissue differences in ischemic or hypoxic environments that would affect the behavior of endothelial progenitor cells?

3. Are standard mechanisms of endothelial progenitor cell reaction and participation in endovascular remodeling affected by chronic disease environments? Does chronic disease affect the function and behavior of the local endothelium, which would affect progenitor cell recruitment?

9.5.1.3 Recovery of Heart Tissue after Ischemia with Stem and Progenitor Cells

Many current applications of stem and progenitor cells to cardiovascular medicine are applied to tissue-engineered constructs, which may ultimately lead to bioengineered heart muscle grafts, valves, vessels, and perhaps someday entire engineered hearts. To date, though, clinical trials typically seek to replenish lost cardiomyocytes in the heart.

Myocardial infarction can cause the loss of over a billion cardiomyocytes, resulting in ischemia and a loss of contractility in the region. Cardiomyocytes do not regenerate successfully in this situation, so other therapies are sought.

Two mechanisms of replacing cardiomyocytes with stem and progenitor cells are detailed in the following:

1. *Transplanted cells*: BMSCs transplanted into the defect area may differentiate into new cardiomyocytes to restore function; however, researchers have seen minimal positive benefits from supplying autologous stem cells to the infarct region (Korf-Klingebiel et al. 2008).

2. *Enhancing regenerative capacity of the heart*: In lower animals such as the newt, mature cells are able to dedifferentiate into progenitor cells, proliferate, and migrate through the injured region where they redifferentiate into mature cells. In other animals such as the zebra fish, signals from the injury recruit from the circulating and tissue-resident progenitor cells, which then differentiate to form mature cardiomyocytes and heal the infarct region (Poss et al. 2002, Bergmann et al. 2009).

Further research is under way to discover the appropriate panel and dosing of proangiogenic and proinflammatory signals to simulate the effects of stem and progenitor cells on neovascularization. Delivery of this panel of markers could encourage the regeneration of endogenous cells and enable the fabrication of biomaterial scaffolds with the appropriate stimuli to maintain or differentiate stem and progenitor cells to aid in microvascular remodeling at sites of injury and tissue-engineered implants. Most importantly, this type of scaffolding for regeneration has the potential for off-the-shelf availability in the clinic.

9.6 QUANTITATIVE ASSAYS OF ANGIOGENESIS

While both tissue engineering and tissue revascularization strategies are promising, assessing the efficacy of these approaches requires the use of quantitative and qualitative models of angiogenesis. To date, imaging limitations in cardiology have essentially prevented the imaging of smaller vessels, less than 100 μm in diameter. To study these vessels in tissue engineering and wound healing, researchers can use thin, transparent tissues to view and study small arterioles and capillaries. Direct intravital imaging allows for observation and quantitation of the behaviors of individual cells and their surrounding environments.

Current models of angiogenesis have been developed out of a desire for assays that are quantitative, inexpensive for the laboratory, quick to yield results, and require minimal special training. These models provide an insight into the anatomical, cellular, and functional aspects of microvascularization and the environments that encourage and inhibit angiogenesis.

Jain et al. (1997) described specific criteria for these angiogenesis assays:

1. Known quantities include R and C, which are used to generate dose–response curves:

   R = release rate of angiogenic factor/inhibitor

   C = spatial and temporal concentration distribution of angiogenic factor/inhibitor

2. If cells are used as source of angiogenic factor/inhibitor, they must be well-defined genetically.

3. Ability to quantify new vasculature and, thus, the need for a clear distinction between new vasculature and preexisting vasculature in the system

   a. *Structure* of new vasculature

      L = vascular length (may be vascular length density)

      A = vascular surface area

      V = volume of vessels

      N = number of vessels

      D = fractal dimensions

      BM = extent of basement membrane coverage in new vessels

   b. *Function* of new vasculature

      MR = EC migration rate

      PR = EC proliferation rate

      CR = canalization rate

      F = blood flow

      P = permeability

4. Effective and relatively harmless assay

   a. Avoid tissue damage as it causes inflammatory response and affects angiogenesis

   b. Ability to monitor noninvasively over long periods of time

   c. Cost-effective for laboratory use, quick to yield results

   d. Easy to use, reproducible model, reliable results

Intravital microscopy meets many of these requirements. This type of imaging is typically noninvasive or minimally invasive, provides a view of both temporal and spatial dynamics of the vascular system, and yields quantitative information on the physiological function of the system. Because clinically available imaging techniques lack the spatial resolution to observe processes on a cellular and subcellular level, intravital microscopy can provide insights into microvascular remodeling in the laboratory (Fukumura and Jain 2008).

To perform intravital microscopy, which has spatial resolution in the range of 1–10 μm, several requirements must be met. First, the tissue preparation must be optically transparent and accessible. Second, circulation must be visible using a molecular probe detected by the microscope. Some examples of these include the use of red blood cells as a contrast agent for transillumination or linearly polarized light, high-molecular-weight tracers for fluorescence microscopy, or optical coherence tomography. The microscope and detection system used are limited by resolution.

Light scattering by the tissue, as well as absorption of the light, limits both epifluorescence and confocal laser scanning microscopy to depths of around 100 μm into the tissue. If the tissue preparation is thin enough, these techniques, or even transillumination, may be sufficient. If depths of several hundred microns are required to satisfactorily view changes in the microvasculature, multiphoton laser scanning microscopy may be ideal, as the depth of resolution is greater and spatial resolution is retained. Finally, the researcher requires mathematical models, algorithms, or other method of quantification to extract information from images. Example measurements include vessel diameter, length, surface area, and volume, as well as characterization of branching patterns and quantification of intercapillary distances.

Intravital imaging is divided into three *in vivo* assays: chronic transparent windows, exteriorized tissue preparations, and *in situ* preparations. Other options include vascularization into polymer matrix implants (particularly relevant for tissue-engineering applications), excision of tissue, and several *in vitro* assays.

In vivo assays encompass microcirculatory preparations that can be viewed using light microscopy with red blood cells providing contrast to delineate the vasculature. Listed as follows are the advantages and disadvantages of each imaging system (Gavard and Gutkind 2006, Korf-Klingebiel et al. 2008):

1. *Chronic transparent chambers*

   Experimental systems: Rabbit ear chamber, dorsal skinfold in rodents (mouse, rat, hamster, rabbit), cranial windows in mouse or rat, and hamster cheek pouch window

   Advantages: These systems permit chronic and repeated observations over relatively long time periods.

   Disadvantages: These systems require recovery time after implantation for inflammatory response to lessen and vasculature to normalize before observations begin.

   a. Rabbit ear chamber

      i. Pros: Optically clearest preparation

      ii. Cons: 4–6 weeks before granulation tissue matures and factors can be added to the chamber, not immune-privileged site, too expensive

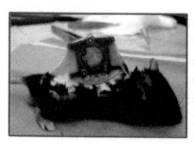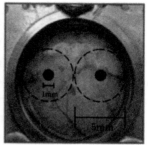

FIGURE 9.6   The dorsal skinfold window chamber model can be used to study the effects of growth factors on vascular remodeling *in vivo*. This backpack model allows polymers loaded with drugs to be implanted and assayed over time. Metrics such as total microvessel length or changes in vessel diameters can be easily quantified in this assay. (Courtesy of Botchwey Lab, Biomedical Engineering, Georgia Institute of Technology, Atlanta, GA.)

b. Dorsal skinfold window chamber model in rodents (Figure 9.6)

   i. Pros: Can use immune-deficient rodents (accept xenografts), less expensive

   ii. Cons: Optical quality not as good (thick tissue)

c. Hamster cheek pouch

   i. Pros: Immune-privileged site (accepts xenografts), less expensive than larger rodents

   ii. Cons: Optical quality not ideal (thick tissue)

d. Cranial window

   i. Pros: Lasts longer, better transplantability, elicits angiogenesis quickly, can investigate brain microenvironment

   ii. Cons: Mechanisms of enhanced angiogenesis unknown, visualization requires epi-illumination and injection of contrast agents

2. *Exterior tissue preparations (acute preparations)*

   Experimental systems: Hamster cheek pouch, rat or rabbit mesentery, mouse or rat liver, chick chorioallantoic membrane (CAM), mouse or rat air sac

   Advantages: These systems can be applied to virtually any tissue and can be inexpensive (chick CAM assay). A defined number of cells or construct with angiogenic agent can be injected via subcutaneous or intradermal route. Skin flap is then everted to measure and then sutured or stapled back in place, so tissue spends most of its time in native environment.

   Disadvantages: With these systems, the duration as well as frequency of observation is limited, and the preparation procedures may cause inflammation and affect the physiology of the local environment. Some trauma could result from frequently everting tissue, and difficulty may be encountered in viewing all new vessels.

3. *In situ preparations*

Example systems: Corneal pocket, iris implant

Corneal pocket more widely used

Advantages: These systems often require no invasive preparation and are natural sites for observing vessel growth.

Disadvantages: In these systems, vessel growth is in three dimensions and therefore more difficult to quantify after early stages. The rabbit model is ideal due to size of surgery site; however, smaller rodents have more difficult surgeries, but imaging in 3D is less important since tissue is thinner.

4. *Vascularization into biocompatible polymer matrix implants*

Experimental system: Polymer matrix, gel, or sponge containing known amount of angiogenic factor or cells is implanted on a vascular bed, and new vessels penetrating the matrix are measured.

Advantages: This type of system provides a realistic model for quantifying vessel ingrowth in response to angiogenic or antiangiogenic stimuli. Polymer implants can be combined with chronic window chamber models to offer noninvasive, real-time imaging and measurement of microvascular changes.

Disadvantages: Without combination with *in vivo* model, this type of system does not permit *in vivo* observation. A nonspecific immune response could be mounted by the host in response to the matrix implantation, so careful consideration of experimental controls is required.

5. *Excision of vascularized animal or human tissues*

Experimental system: Angiogenesis is characterized after tissue is excised by light or electron microscopy, histological examination, or other methods.

Advantages: This system is the only approach currently approved for human studies and permits subcellular and molecular level observation and analysis through histological techniques.

Disadvantages: This type of system is invasive and static, and no time course of changes is available, so kinetic and functional studies are impossible.

6. *In vitro assays*

Several *in vitro* platforms have been adapted for angiogenesis experiments in the last two decades. These can be broadly classified into proliferation, migration, differentiation, and microfluidic assays. Figure 9.7 is a diagrammatic representation of the factors in *in vitro* experimental design that affect assay outcomes.

a. *Proliferation assays.* The cell proliferation assays primarily rely on determining the net cell number. The increase in the cell number is measured by a cell counting device such as a hemocytometer, a coulter counter, or a Vi-CELL counter (Staton et al. 2009). DNA synthesis is an alternative measure of cell proliferation and is

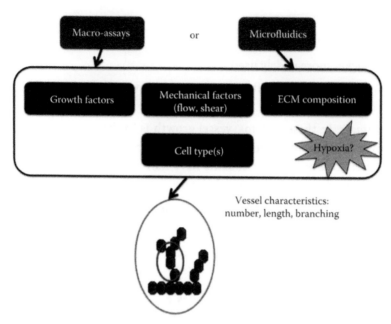

FIGURE 9.7 Factors in experimental design that affect assay outcomes like number, length, and branching of capillaries.

assayed by measuring the incorporation of [³H]thymidine into the DNA of the cell using scintillation counting, where the amount of radioactivity is proportional to the neosynthesis of DNA (Staton et al. 2009, Yu et al. 2004).

b. *Migration assays.* Migration assays are usually some form of a Boyden chamber assay. A summary of the different Boyden assays is provided by Staton et al. (2009) in their review of angiogenesis assays. These are 3D assays, which allow the passage of active cells toward an attractant (test angiogenic factor) placed in the lower chamber (Alessandri et al. 1983) with or without the filter being coated with single ECM proteins such as collagen or fibronectin or complex matrices, such as Matrigel (Albini et al. 2004). Transwells are a form of Boyden chamber assays that can be used to distinguish chemotaxis and chemokinesis. Though very useful, these assays have some drawbacks in that the assay needs a lot of optimization and using rare cells is difficult because of the need for high cell numbers. Additionally, imaging through the filter is difficult: the pores and cells cannot always be distinguished, the cell microenvironment is not always preserved, and the pore size tends to alter sprout formation characteristics.

c. *Differentiation assays.* Assays that simulate the formation of capillary-like tubules are regarded as representative of the later stages of angiogenesis known as differentiation. They are used extensively to assay novel compounds for pro- or antiangiogenic effects (Staton et al. 2009). Differentiation assays are useful in determining the tube formation behavior of ECs. They could be 3D assays where beads coated with ECs are dispersed in a matrix and allowed to form tubules or could be basic well assays where cells are seeded on a matrix and allowed to migrate and form tubes through it. Nakatsu et al. (2003) coated beads that were layered on top of the gel, where they provide necessary soluble factors that promote EC sprouting from the surface of the beads. In this assay, while the cells are exposed to a 3D environment, they do not have the same microenvironment, as the bead and the gel have different material characteristics. A spherical localization exposes the cells to a different concentration profile than what they would encounter *in vivo*. In other instances, cells are coated on a gel matrix (collagen, Matrigel, or fibronectin), exposed to various angiogenic agents, and allowed to form capillaries into the gel (Kanzawa et al. 1993, Lawley and Kubota (1989)). While this is very similar to the *in vivo* layout, cells usually see a different microenvironment as the precise environment around them cannot be controlled and most measurements are made based on bulk profiles. A further limitation common to all the 3D macroassays is that the gel has to be relatively thin to allow the diffusion of oxygen and nutrients (Staton et al. 2009).

d. *Microfluidic assays.* Over the last decade, microfluidic devices have been used extensively to study various biological processes. In addition to providing a cell microenvironment that replicates *in vivo* conditions better than macroassays, they may also enable 3D controlled experiments with a minimal number of agents and high temporal and spatial resolution. Unlike experiments conducted on the macroscale, like those in well plates, we can exert better control on the concentration and flow profiles in microfluidic devices. Moreover, we can have a better understanding of what the cell "sees." Thus, the results obtained can be correlated to the input conditions in a more precise manner. The amount of expensive reagents required for each experiment is reduced, and most devices also allow for better imaging of the experiments. While assays conducted in Boyden chambers cannot be easily imaged using a confocal microscope in 3D, experiments conducted in microfluidic devices can be. Many microfabricated devices have also been developed to induce and monitor cell migration in the channel in response to biochemical gradients or biomechanical forces (Gu et al. 2004, Chung et al. 2005, Tourovskaia et al. 2005, Gomez-Sjoberg et al. 2007). These methods have been used to apply well-defined biochemical gradients to cells either plated on a gel surface near the walls of a microfluidic channel (Jeon et al. 2002, Chung et al. 2005, Tourovskaia et al. 2005) or within gel scaffolds (Jeon et al. 2002, Frisk et al. 2007, Saadi et al. 2007). These techniques demonstrate the potential to be versatile tools for analyzing cellular responses under well-established gradients. The Kamm lab has used microfluidic devices that replicate a realistic 3D environment in combination with gradient and flow control to study cell migration and capillary morphogenesis (Figure 9.8; Chung et al. 2009). They studied responses of ECs when they were placed in coculture with physiologically relevant cell types such as cancer cell. Das et al. (2010a) characterized the effect of different concentrations of VEGF and Ang1 on various sprout characteristics.

Advantages: These systems permit control over experimental variables not available for *in vivo* assays. They are easy to monitor and permit examination of specific components of

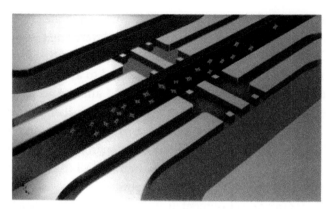

FIGURE 9.8 A microfluidic system for multicell culture in both 2D and 3D microenvironments can be used to examine the effects of different angiogenic factors on capillary formation. Each of the three channels (green, red, and blue) is separately addressable and can be seeded with cells or media alone, establishing concentration or pressure gradients. Gray regions are filled with 3D matrices of various compositions, with or without suspended cells. Overall dimension is of order 2 mm so all cells readily communicate with each other over physiological length scales. (Courtesy of Kamm Lab, Biological Engineering, Massachusetts Institute of Technology, Cambridge, MA.)

the system and have significantly lower costs than *in vivo* assays. They allow for the study of the effect of individual factors on the entire process, thus enabling a deeper understanding of driving mechanisms.

Disadvantages: These systems have not yet reached a level of standardization to permit quantitative comparisons across laboratory groups, and *in vitro* responses may not be indicative of *in vivo* outcomes.

9.7 COMPUTATIONAL MODELING OF NEOVASCULARIZATION

Cardiovascular regenerative medicine strives to recapitulate the complex process of neovascularization. Many of the obstacles faced in the field are due to the incredibly complex process of blood vessel formation and growth. Systems biology and computational modeling may provide tools to reach a greater understanding through the integration of complex biological data. These techniques can be applied to better understand and generate hypotheses about tissue-engineered constructs, revascularization after ischemic injury, and even pro- or antiangiogenic drug discovery.

This field of computational modeling in the cardiovascular system first arose with the theoretical modeling of transport and flow properties in the microcirculation in the Krogh cylinder model over 100 years ago (Krogh 1919). With the biomedical sciences and engineering, computational modeling has emerged as an interdisciplinary field drawing on the strengths of biologists, engineers, and computer modelers to develop mathematical and computational approaches, which permit the integration of significant amounts of data (Secomb et al. 2008). Particularly important is the integration of data across multiple levels such as spatial and temporal and scales from subcellular signaling processes to whole-tissue behavior.

A driving force behind systems biology and computational modeling is the lack of clinical success for angiogenic therapies. Many of these therapies involve single factor bolus delivery of a factor, which has been shown to promote angiogenesis *in vitro*. Unfortunately, this *in vitro* success does not consider the complexity of the *in vivo* system. Some studies take the first step toward addressing this complexity by examining delivery of combinations of factors; however, without specific knowledge as to which combinations will be success, this method can be prohibitively expensive as well as time-consuming for the researcher. Studies such as these, which seek to elucidate the ideal combination, delivery profile, and concentration of various factors, may be best suited to a computational approach, which may both generate and validate hypotheses before laboratory experiments are undertaken (Hirschi et al. 2002).

Systems biology and computational modeling provide the necessary tools to interrogate, characterize, and organize large groups of data. In addition, both spatial and temporal information can be combined into a single model to yield insights into vascular formation and remodeling. Scientists can generate biomechanical, biochemical, and biophysical data, and computational modeling can combine these data into a quantitative model. This time of computational modeling is ideal for a multiscale process such as angiogenesis (Sefcik et al. 2010).

Computational models are ideal methods to answer questions such as these (Peirce and Skalak 2003):

1. If a hypothesis exists, how can it be refined to a simpler set of experiments? If no hypothesis or multiple hypotheses exist, how can the most likely hypothesis be generated?

2. With the current knowledge gaps, which experiments would be the best to fill them?

3. With known parameters, which are the most important for system function? Which are unnecessary or redundant? Which are relevant for therapeutic intervention?

4. Which model (experimental) parameters are robust? To which parameters is the model most sensitive?

5. For the parameters that are difficult or impossible to quantify *in vivo*, what values does the model predict?

9.7.1 Types and Examples of Model Systems

Modeling is a useful tool for understanding the interplay between all the factors that affect a process and for the design of experiments of a predictive nature. Over the years, various models spanning different scales and focusing on different aspects of angiogenesis, an integral part of cardiovascular regeneration, have been developed. These can be classified as continuum models (Dallon and Othmer 1997, Anderson and Chaplain 1998, Levine et al. 2000, Chaplain and Anderson 2004, Chaturvedi et al. 2005, Chaplain et al. 2006) and discrete models (Stokes et al. 1991, Anderson and Chaplain 1998, Mantzaris et al. 2004, Chaplain et al. 2006).

Discrete models employ model units and behaviors, which are explicitly known or defined. Examples include agent-based modeling or cellular automata and systems of differential equations, which are solved at discrete points.

Continuous models describe processes, which are continuous in both time and space. These models are typically systems of differential equations solved continuously. One weakness is that cell-level details are ignored to maintain the continuum.

Stochastic models utilize probabilities to generate behaviors, taking into account the randomness of most biological processes. Examples include Markovian models where the model system retains no memory of past or present states or non-Markovian where all past, present, and future model states are considered.

Deterministic models define future states of the model based on the present and previous states. This type of model predicts a definite outcome, and when the same inputs are used, the same outcome will always result. These models can also be considered as predictive models and work best when the mechanism underlying the model is known, such as transport or hemodynamics.

The continuum models are based on conservation equations for chemotactic and haptotactic gradients. In one such continuum model, the Chaplain group models a "tissue response unit," which includes an EC, tumor angiogenic factor (TAF), and a generic matrix molecule. The numerical solution is obtained from a finite difference approximation subject to no flux boundary conditions and a specified initial condition. They have also developed a discretized version of the continuum model where the motion of the capillary in response to a tumor is governed by the EC at the tip (Anderson and Chaplain 1998).

A prime example of a discrete, stochastic model is the model developed by Stokes and Lauffenburger (Stokes et al. 1991) of EC migration. This particular model used differential equations to model the chemotactic activity and sensitivity of cells and illustrated the possibility of modeling these processes by observing population-level migration. This model helped pave the way for the use of dynamics based on system forces to simulate cells in migration (internal and external forces, matrix compliance, ECM stiffness). The main weakness of this model is its lack of complexity, cell types besides ECs, other factors, and ECM interactions.

The cellular Potts model (CPM) is a lattice-based model developed to describe the behavior of cellular structures and their interactions. It could be an agent-based model, which is a computational model that is based on one (or more) specific component(s) and its effect on the individual cells (agents) being modeled. The agents in these models are typically cells, capable of migration, proliferation, and other phenotypic changes in response to a defined set of rules. These rules represent known information about the local environment, endogenous and exogenous growth factor delivery, standard or applied mechanical stresses, and cell–cell and cell–matrix interactions. Rules can be established from published experimental data or empirically determined from simple calculations and assumptions, and each agent (cell) responds independently to these rules, generating a population behavior, which may guide hypotheses or experimental design. A 2D agent-based model of angiogenesis based on CPM has been developed by Pierce et al. (2004), where they identify multiple cell types and growth factors.

Their cell-level rule-based model of network growth in mesenteric tissue predicts emergent behavior like new vessel formation, vessel length extensions, and recruitment of contractile perivascular cells in response to localized pressure, circumferential strain, and focal application of growth factor. The Sherratt group has used an extension of the Potts model to simulate malignant cells and quantified invasion morphology as a function of cell–cell adhesion (Turner and Sherratt 2002). In a recent approach, the Popel group has developed a multiscale integrative model with specific modules for various growth factor receptor pairs and ECM proteolysis (Qutub 2009). Their model considers the cellular response to oxygen in skeletal muscles (Ji et al. 2005), oxygen delivery by hemoglobin-based oxygen carriers (Tsoukias et al. 2007), and a cell-based model that incorporated the microvascular network, skeletal muscle fibers, and kinetics of VEGF binding, which results in angiogenesis via reorganization of existing capillaries (Qutub and Popel 2009). Das et al. (2010b) have developed a 3D hybrid continuum model that combines deterministic response of the ECM and the stochastic cellular behavior that can predict emergent patterns in *in vitro* microfluidic devices. Other models include a random walk model (Plank and Sleeman 2004), which is distinguished by the fact that it places no restrictions on the direction of capillary growth, an individual cell-based 2D mathematical model of tumor angiogenesis in response to a diffusible angiogenic factor, and a fractal-based model in which the smaller pieces of the system show "statistical self-similarity" to the whole and the anatomical entities are given a fractal dimension. Random walk models that incorporate biochemical cascades when VEGF binding occurs have also been developed (Levine et al. 2002). Physiological models, for instance a model of corneal angiogenesis, have also been developed. Jackson and Zheng have developed one such model that integrates a mechanical model of cell elongation with a biochemical model of cell phenotype variation (Jackson and Zheng 2010).

9.7.2 VEGF as a Candidate for Computational Modeling

VEGF is perhaps the most popularly studied and well-known angiogenic agent; however, its complexity and that of its signaling pathways are often underestimated. There are at least 17 known homodimeric forms of VEGF, as well as an unknown number of heterodimeric forms, and all have distinct binding characteristics. The receptors for VEGF are also complicated and allow multiple signaling pathways per ligand. VEGF is expressed by multiple cell types across a range of tissues and can be regulated by a multitude of factors (mechanical, environmental, inflammatory). Experiments utilizing VEGF, and even models built to describe VEGF signaling or cellular response to exogenous VEGF, typically consider only one or several components, losing tremendous amounts of information about the whole system. While models such as these may lead to the attainment of incomplete information, they are still useful. However, a computational model containing all known information about VEGF signaling would permit researchers to make better inferences (Mac Gabhann and Popel 2008).

Since VEGF signaling plays a significant role in neovascularization in both recovery after ischemic injury and in tissue-engineered constructs, a greater understanding of the pathways and mechanisms underlying this activity could lead to more efficacious therapies.

Additionally, VEGF cross talk with other growth factors like Ang1, and PDGF is also important in understanding the cue-signal-response mechanism of capillary formation and development. Thus, a computational model that incorporates various biochemical and biomechanical factors will prove to be very useful. An integrated model such as this could save billions of dollars in drug development and lead to improved angiogenic (vascularization in ischemic tissues, tissue-engineered implants) and antiangiogenic (decrease tumor growth) therapies.

9.7.3 Value of Modeling

Computational models add value to many applications, especially when complex processes or expensive experiments are required. They provide us with invaluable tools that can increase basic science knowledge through compilation and interpretation of data; support biomedical development of devices, materials, and solutions for which cellular interactions and behaviors must be understood; perform genetic and proteomic experiments, which are difficult or impossible to do *in vivo* to verify activity or mechanisms of a factor; provide high-throughput, low-cost analysis for drug, device, or material development; and observe and track the behavior of multiple (thousands) of cells in response to injury, repair, and exogenously delivered factors.

To that end, many programs have been developed for the use of researchers who seek to add computational modeling to their experimental toolbox. A selection is outlined in the following, with current web links for further information.

9.7.4 Computational Programs and Tools

Cardiome Project and Microcirculation Physiome Project

Launched in response to Physiome Project (http://www.physiome.org/)

To archive and disseminate quantitative data and models of function and behavior of molecules, cells, tissues, organs, and organisms

To create a World Wide Web–accessible database of the microcirculation—library of architectural and hemodynamic data to facilitate research in transport and regulation of blood flow and build knowledge of comparative physiology of microcirculation

Ingenuity Pathways Analysis (http://www.ingenuity.com/)

Founded in 1998 by Stanford graduate students, Ingenuity Systems is a company that is taking on the challenge of next-generation knowledge management for the life sciences community. Our long-term focus on innovation in semantic search, ontology, and software development has allowed us to create groundbreaking technologies that help life science researchers more effectively search, explore, visualize, and analyze biological and chemical findings related to genes, proteins, and small molecules (e.g., drugs).

Connectivity Map (http://www.broadinstitute.org/cmap/)

The Connectivity Map (also known as cmap) is a collection of genome-wide transcriptional expression data from cultured human cells treated with bioactive small molecules and simple pattern-matching algorithms that together enable the discovery of functional connections between drugs, genes, and diseases through the transitory feature of common gene-expression changes. You can learn more about cmap from our papers in Science and Nature Reviews Cancer.

Pathway Interaction Database (http://pid.nci.nih.gov/)

Biomolecular interactions and cellular processes assembled into authoritative human signaling pathways

CellML (http://www.cellml.org/)

The purpose of CellML is to store and exchange computer-based mathematical models. CellML allows scientists to share models even if they are using different modeling tools. It also enables them to reuse components from one model:

Sefcik review (*Tissue Engineering* 2010)

Secomb review (*Microcirculation* 2008)

Mac Gabhann review (*Microcirculation* 2008)

Peirce review (*Microcirculation* 2008)

Hirschi (Little) review (*Annals of New York Academy of Sciences* 2002)

9.8 SUMMARY

There are many facets to cardiovascular tissue engineering, and we have summarized the advances made in the experimental (*in vivo* and *in vitro*), analytical (imaging), and computational (modeling) fronts in the recent years. The current progress has been made possible because of the collaborative efforts in medicine, biomaterials, and computational and systems biology. While the use of tissue-engineered constructs to replace or regenerate cardiovascular tissues in a clinical setting is possible, such collaborations and intelligent design of experiments are imperative to achieve those goals. Development of better techniques that enable live *in vivo* imaging, more reproducible *in vitro* assays, methods to discern the temporal effects of pro- and antiangiogenic factors, and comprehensive computational models are some directions for the focus of future efforts. It is conceivable that a therapy that is combinatorial such that it uses more than one of the approaches mentioned in this chapter becomes successful in the near future.

REFERENCES

Adams RH, Alitalo K. 2007. Molecular regulation of angiogenesis and lymphangiogenesis. *Nat Rev Mol Cell Biol.* 8:464–478.

Albini A, Benelli R, Noonan DM, Brigati C. 2004. The "chemoinvasion assay": A tool to study tumor and endothelial cell invasion of basement membranes. *Int J Dev Biol.* 48:563–571.

Alessandri G, Raju F, Gullino PM. 1983. Mobilization of capillary endothelium *in vitro* induced by effectors of angiogenesis *in vivo*. *Cancer Res.* 43:1790–1797.

Anderson AR, Chaplain MA. 1998. Continuous and discrete mathematical models of tumor induced angiogenesis. *Bull Math Biol.* 60:857–899.

Asahara T, Murohara T, Sullivan A, Silver M, van der Zee R, Li T, Witzenbichler B, Schatteman G, Isner JM. 1997. Isolation of putative progenitor endothelial cells for angiogenesis. *Science.* 275(5302):964–967.

Atala and Langer. October 26, 2001. *Methods of Tissue Engineering,* 1st edn. Academic Press.

Bergmann O, Bhardwaj RD, Bernard S, Zdunek S, Barnabé-Heider F, Walsh S, Zupicich J et al. 2009. Mesenchymal stromal cells ameliorate experimental autoimmune encephalomyelitis by inhibiting CD4 Th17 T cells in a CC chemokine ligand 2-dependent manner. *J Immunol.* 182:5994–6002.

Cai L, Johnstone BH, Cook TG, Tan J, Fishbein MC, Chen PS, March KL. 2009. IFATS collection: Human adipose tissue-derived stem cells induce angiogenesis and nerve sprouting following myocardial infarction, in conjunction with potent preservation of cardiac function. *Stem Cells.* 27(1):230–237.

Camenzind E, Steg PG, Wijns W. 2007. Stent thrombosis late after implantation of first-generation drug-eluting stents: A cause for concern. *Circulation.* 115(11):1440–1455.

Chaplain M, Anderson A. 2004. Mathematical modelling of tumour-induced angiogenesis: Network growth and structure. *Cancer Treat Res.* 117:51–75.

Chaplain MA, McDougall SR, Anderson AR. 2006. Mathematical modeling of tumor induced angiogenesis. *Annu Rev Biomed Eng.* 8:233–257.

Chaturvedi RHC, Kazmierczak B, Schneider T, Izaguirre JA, Glimm T, Hentschel HG, Glazier JA, Newman SA, Alber MS. 2005. On multiscale approaches to three-dimensional modeling of morphogenesis. *J R Soc Interf.* 2:237–253.

Chung L, Flanagan, Rhee S, Schwarz P, Lee A, Monuki E, Jeon N. 2005. Human neural stem cell growth and differentiation in a gradient-generating microfluidic device. *Lab Chip.* 5(4):401–406.

Chung S, Sudo R, Mack PJ, Wan CR, Vickerman V, Kamm RD. 2009. Cell migration into scaffolds under co-culture conditions in a microfluidic platform. *Lab Chip.* 9(2):269–275.

Dallon JC, Othmer HG. 1997. A discrete cell model with adaptive signaling for aggregation of *Dictyostelium discoideum. Philos Trans R Soc Lond B Biol Sci.* 352(1351):391–417.

Dang SM, Gerecht-Nir S, Chen J, Itskovitz-Eldor J, Zandstra PW. 2004. Controlled, scalable embryonic stem cell differentiation culture. *Stem Cells.* 22(3):275–282.

Das A, Asada H, Lauffenburger D, Kamm RD. 2010a. A hybrid continuum-discrete modeling approach to predict and control angiogenesis: Analysis of combinatorial growth factor and matrix effects on vessel sprouting morphology. *Phil Trans R Soc A.* 368:2937–2960.

Das A, Lauffenburger D, Asada H, Kamm R. 2010b. Determining cell fate transition probabilities to VEGF/Ang 1 levels: Relating computational modeling to microfluidic angiogenesis studies [Quick Edit]. *Cell Mol Bioeng.* 3(4):1–16.

Ferreira LS, Gerecht S, Fuller J, Shieh HF, Vunjak-Novakovic G, Langer R. 2007. Bioactive hydrogel scaffolds for controllable vascular differentiation of human embryonic stem cells. *Biomaterials.* 28:2706–2717.

Frisk T, Rydholm S, Liebmann T, Svahn HA, Stemme G, Brismar H. 2007. A microfluidic device for parallel 3-D cell cultures in asymmetric environments. *Electrophoresis.* 28:4705–4712.

Fukumura D, Jain RK. 2008. Imaging angiogenesis and the microenvironment. *APMIS.* 116(7–8):695–715 [Review].

Garg S, Serruys PW. 2010. Coronary stents: Current status. *J Am Coll Cardiol.* 56(10 Suppl):S1–S42.

Gavard J, Gutkind JS. 2006. VEGF controls endothelial-cell permeability by promoting the beta-arrestin-dependent endocytosis of VE-cadherin. *Nat Cell Biol.* 8(11):1223–1234.

Gerecht S, Burdick JA, Ferreira LS, Townsend SA, Langer R, Vunjak-Novakovic G. 2007. Hyaluronic acid hydrogel for controlled self-renewal and differentiation of human embryonic stem cells. *Proc Natl Acad Sci U S A.* 104:11298–11303.

Gomez-Sjoberg R, Leyrat AA, Pirone DM, Chen CS, Quake SR. 2007. Versatile, fully automated, microfluidic cell culture system. *Anal Chem.* 79:8557–8563.

Griffin M, Greiser U, Barry F, O'Brien T, Ritter T. 2010. Genetically modified mesenchymal stem cells and their clinical potential in acute cardiovascular disease. *Discov Med.* 9(46):219–223.

Gu, X. Zhu, N. Futai, B. Cho, S. Takayama. 2004. Computerized microfluidic cell culture using elastomeric channels and Braille displays. *Proc Natl Acad Sci U S A.* 101(45):15861–15866.

Hanjaya-Putra D, Gerecht S. 2009. Vascular engineering using human embryonic stem cells. *Biotechnol Prog.* 25(1):2–9 [Review].

Hattori K, Heissig B, Tashiro K, Honjo T, Tateno M, Shieh JH, Hackett NR, Quitoriano MS, Crystal RG, Rafii S, Moore MA. 2001. Plasma elevation of stromal cell-derived factor-1 induces mobilization of mature and immature hematopoietic progenitor and stem cells. *Blood.* 97(11):3354–3360.

Helm CL, Fleury ME, Zisch AH, Boschetti F, Swartz MA. 2005. Synergy between interstitial flow and VEGF directs capillary morphogenesis *in vitro* through a gradient amplification mechanism. *Proc Natl Acad Sci U S A.* 102(44):15779–15784.

Hirschi KK, Skalak TC, Peirce SM, Little CD. 2002. Vascular assembly in natural and engineered tissues. *Ann N Y Acad Sci.* 961:223–242 [Review].

Hong SJ, Traktuev DO, March KL. 2010. Therapeutic potential of adipose-derived stem cells in vascular growth and tissue repair. *Curr Opin Organ Transplant.* 15(1):86–91.

Huang CC, Liao CK, Yang MJ, Chen CH, Hwang SM, Hung YW, Chang Y, Sung HW. 2010. A strategy for fabrication of a three-dimensional tissue construct containing uniformly distributed embryoid body-derived cells as a cardiac patch. *Biomaterials.* 31(24):6218–6227.

Ishaug SL, Crane GM, Miller MJ, Yasko AW, Yaszemski MJ, Mikos AG. 1997. Bone formation by three-dimensional stromal osteoblast culture in biodegradable polymer scaffolds. *J Biomed Mater Res.* 36(1):17–28.

Jackson T, Zheng X. 2010. A cell-based model of endothelial cell migration, proliferation and maturation during corneal angiogenesis. *Bull Math Biol.* 72(4):830–868.

Jain RK, Schlenger K, Höckel M, Yuan F. 1997. Quantitative angiogenesis assays: Progress and problems. *Nat Med.* 3(11):1203–1208 [Review].

Jeon, H. Baskaran, S. Dertinger, G. Whitesides, L. Van De Water, M. Toner. 2002. *Nat Biotechnol.* 9(5):627–635.

Jeremias A, Kirtane A. 2008. Balancing efficacy and safety of drug-eluting stents in patients undergoing percutaneous coronary intervention. *Ann Intern Med.* 148(3):234–238.

Ji JW, Tsoukias NM, Goldman D, Popel AS. 2005. A computational model of oxygen transport in skeletal muscle for sprouting and splitting modes of angiogenesis. *J Theor Biol.* 241(1):94–108.

Kanzawa S, Endo H, Shioya N. 1993. Improved *in vitro* angiogenesis model by collagen density reduction and the use of type III collagen. *Ann Plast Surg.* 30:244–251.

Kim Y, Kim H, Cho H, Bae Y, Suh K, Jung J. 2007. Direct comparison of human mesenchymal stem cells derived from adipose tissues and bone marrow in mediating neovascularization in response to vascular ischemia. *Cell Physiol Biochem.* 20(6):867–876.

Korf-Klingebiel M, Kempf T, Sauer T, Brinkmann E, Fischer P, Meyer GP, Ganser A, Drexler H, Wollert KC. 2008. Bone marrow cells are a rich source of growth factors and cytokines: Implications for cell therapy trials after myocardial infarction. *Eur Heart J.* 29(23):2851–2858.

Krenning G, van Luyn MJ, Harmsen MC. 2009. Endothelial progenitor cell-based neovascularization: Implications for therapy. *Trends Mol Med.* 15(4):180–189 [Review].

Krogh A. 1919. The supply of oxygen to the tissues and the regulation of the capillary circulation. *J Physiol.* 152(6):457–474.

Kurosawa H. 2007. Methods for inducing embryoid body formation: *In vitro* differentiation system of embryonic stem cells. *J Biosci Bioeng.* 103(5):389–398.

Langer R, Vacanti JP. 1993. Tissue engineering. *Science.* 260(5110):920–926.

Lawley TJ, Kubota Y. 1989. Induction of morphologic differentiation of endothelial cells in culture. *J Invest Dermatol.* 93:59S–61S.

Lazarus HM, Koc ON, Devine SM, Curtin P, Maziarz RT, Holland HK, Shpall EJ, McCarthy P, Atkinson K, Cooper BW, Gerson SL, Laughlin MJ, Loberiza FR, Jr. Moseley AB, Bacigalupo A. 2005. Cotransplantation of HLA-identical sibling culture-expanded mesenchymal stem cells and hematopoietic stem cells in hematologic malignancy patients. *Biol Blood Marrow Transplant* 11:389–398.

Lee H, Cusick RA, Browne F, Ho Kim T, Ma PX, Utsunomiya H, Langer R, Vacanti JP. 2002. Local delivery of basic fibroblast growth factor increases both angiogenesis and engraftment of hepatocytes in tissue-engineered polymer devices. *Transplantation.* 73:1589.

Levenberg S, Ferreira LS, Chen-Konak L, Kraehenbuehl TP, Langer R. 2010. Isolation, differentiation and characterization of vascular cells derived from human embryonic stem cells. *Nat Protoc.* 5(6):1115–1126.

Levenberg S, Golub JS, Amit M, Itskovitz-Eldor J, Langer R. 2002. Endothelial cells derived from human embryonic stem cells. *Proc Natl Acad Sci U S A.* 99:4391–4396.

Levenberg S, Rouwkema J, Macdonald M, Garfein ES, Kohane DS, Darland DC, Marini R, Van Blitterswijk CA, Mulligan RC, D'Amore PA, Langer R. 2005. Engineering vascularized skeletal muscle tissue. *Nat Biotechnol.* 23:879–884.

Levenberg S, Zoldan J, Basevitch Y, Langer R. 2007. Endothelial potential of human embryonic stem cells. *Blood.* 110:806–814.

Levine HA, Sleeman BD, Nilsen-Hamilton M. 2000. A mathematical model for the roles of pericytes and macrophages in the initiation of angiogenesis. I. The role of protease inhibitors in preventing angiogenesis. *Math Biosci.* 168(1):77–115.

Levine HA, Tucker AL, Nilsen-Hamilton M. 2002. A mathematical model for the role of cell signal transduction in the initiation and inhibition of angiogenesis. *Growth Factors.* 20(4):155–175.

Liu T, Zhang S, Chen X, Li G, Wang Y. 2010. Hepatic differentiation of mouse embryonic stem cells in three-dimensional polymer scaffolds. *Tissue Eng Part A.* 16(4):1115–1122.

Lokmic Z, Mitchell GM. 2008. Engineering the microcirculation. *Tissue Eng Part B Rev.* 14(1):87–103 [Review].

Lu F, Mizuno H, Uysal CA, Cai X, Ogawa R, Hyakusoku H. 2008. Improved viability of random pattern skin flaps through the use of adipose-derived stem cells. *Plast Reconstr Surg.* 121(1):50–58.

Mac Gabhann F, Popel AS. 2008. Systems biology of vascular endothelial growth factors. *Microcirculation.* 15(8):715–738 [Review].

Mangi AA, Noiseux N, Kong D, He H, Rezvani M, Ingwall JS, Dzau VJ. 2003. Mesenchymal stem cells modified with Akt prevent remodeling and restore performance of infarcted hearts. *Nat Med* 9:1195–1201.

Mantzaris NV, Webb S, Othmer HG. 2004. Mathematical modeling of tumor-induced angiogenesis. *J Math Biol.* 49(2):111–187.

Martin GR. 1981. Isolation of a pluripotent cell line from early mouse embryos cultured in medium conditioned by teratocarcinoma stem cells. *Proc Natl Acad Sci U S A.* 78(12):7634–7638.

Nakatsu M, Richard CA, Sainson, Jason N, Aoto Kevin L Taylor, Mark Aitkenhead, Sofía Pérez-del-Pulgar, Philp M Carpenter and Christopher CW Hughesa. 2003. Angiogenic sprouting and capillary lumen formation modeled by human umbilical vein endothelial cells (HUVEC) in fibrin gels: The role of fibroblasts and Angiopoietin-1. *Microvascular Research* 66:102–112.

Ohtaki H, Ylostalo JH, Foraker JE, Robinson AP, Reger RL, Shioda S, Prockop DJ. 2008. Stem/progenitor cells from bone marrow decrease neuronal death in global ischemia by modulation of inflammatory/immune responses. *Proc Natl Acad Sci USA* 105:14638–14643.

Peirce SM, Skalak TC. 2003. Microvascular remodeling: A complex continuum spanning angiogenesis to arteriogenesis. *Microcirculation.* 10(1):99–111 [Review].

Peirce SM, Van Gieson EJ, Skalak TC. 2004. Multicellular simulation predicts microvascular patterning and *in silico* tissue assembly. *FASEB J.* 18(6):731–733.

Plank MJ, Sleeman BD. 2004. A reinforced random walk model of tumour angiogenesis and anti-angiogenic strategies. *Math Med Biol.* 20(2):135–181.

Poss KD, Wilson LG, Keating MT. 2002. Heart regeneration in zebrafish. *Science.* 298(5601): 2188–2190.

Qutub A, Gabhann F, Karagiannis E, Vempati P, Popel A. 2009. Multiscale models of angiogenesis. *IEEE Eng Med Biol Mag.* 28(2):14–31.

Qutub AA, Popel AS. 2009. Elongation, proliferation & migration differentiate endothelial cell phenotypes and determine capillary sprouting. *BMC Syst Biol.* 3:13.

Rafei M, Campeau PM, Aguilar-Mahecha A, Buchanan M, Williams P, Birman E, Yuan S et al. 2009. Mesenchymal stromal cells ameliorate experimental autoimmune encephalomyelitis by inhibiting CD4 Th17 T cells in a CC chemokine ligand 2-dependent manner. *J Immunol* 182:5994–6002.

Saadi, S. Rhee, F. Lin, B. Vahidi, B. Chung and N. Jeon. 2007. Generation of stable concentration gradients in 2D and 3D environments using a microfluidic ladder chamber. *Biomed Microdevices.* 9(5):627–635.

Schechner JS, Nath AK, Zheng L, Kluger MS, Hughes CC, Sierra-Honigmann MR, Lorber MI, Tellides G, Kashgarian M, Bothwell AL, Pober JS. 2000. *In vivo* formation of complex microvessels lined by human endothelial cells in an immunodeficient mouse. *Proc Natl Acad Sci U S A.* 97(16):9191–9196.

Secomb TW, Beard DA, Frisbee JC, Smith NP, Pries AR. 2008. The role of theoretical modeling in microcirculation research. *Microcirculation.* 15(8):693–698 [Review].

Sefcik LS, Petrie Aronin CE, Botchwey EA. 2008. Engineering vascularized tissues using natural and synthetic small molecules. *Organogenesis.* 4(4):215–227.

Sefcik LS, Wilson JL, Papin JA, Botchwey EA. 2010. Harnessing systems biology approaches to engineer functional microvascular networks. *Tissue Eng Part B Rev.* 16(3):361–370 [Review].

Staton CA, Reed MW, Brown NJ. 2009. A critical analysis of current *in vitro* and *in vivo* angiogenesis assays. *Int J Exp Pathol.* 90(3):195–221.

Stokes CL, Lauffenburger DA, Williams SK. 1991. Migration of individual microvessel endothelial cells: Stochastic model and parameter measurement. *J Cell Sci.* 99(Pt 2):419–430.

Thomson JA, Itskovitz-Eldor J, Shapiro SS, Waknitz MA, Swiergiel JJ, Marshall VS, Jones JM. 1998. Embryonic stem cell lines derived from human blastocysts. *Science.* 282(5391):1145–1147. [Erratum in *Science.* 1998;282(5395):1827.]

Tourovskaia A, Figueroa-Masot X, Folch A. 2005. Differentiation-on-a-chip: A microfluidic platform for long-term cell culture studies. *Lab Chip.* 5(1):14–19.

Tsoukias NM, Goldman D, Vadapalli A, Pittman RN, Popel AS. 2007. As computational model of oxygen delivery by hemoglobin-based oxygen carriers in three-dimensional microvascular networks. *J Theor Biol.* 248(4):657–674.

Turner S, Sherratt JA. 2002. Intercellular adhesion and cancer invasion: A discrete simulation using the extended Potts model. *J Theor Biol.* 216(1):85–100.

Yamamura N, Sudo R, Ikeda M, Tanishita K. 2007. Effects of the mechanical properties of collagen gel on the *in vitro* formation of microvessel networks by endothelial cells. *Tissue Eng.* 13(7):1443–1453.

Yi BA, Wernet O, Chien KR. 2010. Pregenerative medicine: Developmental paradigms in the biology of cardiovascular regeneration. *J Clin Invest.* 120(1):20–28 [Review].

Yu CH, Wu J, Su YF, H. PY, Liang YC, Sheu MT, Lee WS. 2004. Anti-proliferation effect of 3-amino-2-imino-3,4-dihydro-2*H*-1,3-benzothiazin-4-one (BJ-601) on human vascular endothelial cells: G0/G1 p21-associated cell cycle arrest. *Biochem Pharmacol.* 67:1907–1916.

Zhou X, Gallicano GI. 2006. Microvascular tubes derived from embryonic stem cells sustain blood flow. *Stem Cells Dev.* 15(3):335–347.

CHAPTER 10

Bone Regenerative Engineering

Yusuf Khan, PhD; Anil Magge, BS;
and Cato T. Laurencin, MD, PhD

CONTENTS

10.1 INTRODUCTION

Bone is one of the several types of connective tissue found in the body, along with cartilage, ligament, tendon, and muscle. Bone serves three primary functions in the body: it provides (a) mechanically stable points for muscle attachment, (b) protection to internal organs, and (c) stores of ions necessary for normal bodily function (Sarkar et al. 2001). Mechanically sound bone can fail, however, from excessive physical loading, disease, or bone density decrease as a function of aging. In fact, as the average age of the U.S. population rises the number of bone injuries requiring some sort of orthopedic intervention continues to rise as well. This need sustains a large commercial industry in which ~3 million musculoskeletal procedures are performed annually in the United States grossing more than $2.5 billion annually. Worldwide, the orthopedic biomaterials market is considerably higher, approximately $14 billion, with a large percentage of this coming from joint replacements and a smaller percentage from fracture management (Ratner et al. 2004). The nature of these procedures varies considerably with the nature of the injury.

10.2 CLINICAL CHALLENGES WITH BONE REPAIR

Typically, a simple fracture of a long bone will heal with nothing more than rigid external fixation from a cast to allow the normal healing mechanisms to occur (see Section 10.4 for details about healing bone). More extreme bone injuries, where the bone has multiple fractures that cannot be easily set or where there is excessive bone loss from trauma or tumor resection, may require treatment beyond simple external fixation. These bone defects often mandate surgical intervention. On rare occasions, even simple fractures may require treatment beyond rigid external fixation. In approximately 5%–10% of all fractures, there is no sign of healing after several weeks. If the fracture remains unhealed for at least 12 weeks, the bony defect is now considered a fracture nonunion (Khan et al. 2008). While there are some recognized causes of nonunions such as excessive motion between fractured ends after fixation, a gap between fractured ends after fixation, or remanipulation of the fracture site (Caputo 1999), there are a subpopulation of nonunions that still occur in the absence of such causes. In these instances, surgical intervention in mandated.

In certain disease states such as osteoarthritis, it may not be the bone itself that is injured but the overlying cartilage that lines the ends of the long bones. Osteoarthritis can occur as a normal function of aging or in instances of excessive wear and tear in a joint. Unlike a focal cartilage injury, the injured cartilage in osteoarthritis spans a large portion of the articulating surface. While many researchers are attempting to find strategies to engineer new cartilage, the most predominant way of treating osteoarthritis is to replace the entire joint. This surgical intervention may require some sort of bony supplement to complete the surgical repair since replacing an entire joint (typically a hip or knee) requires the substantial removal of bone. While much of the removed bone is replaced by the implant material, it may be necessary to include supplementary bony implants.

Each of these real clinical scenarios requires some sort of surgical procedure in which a bony supplement, natural or synthetic, is implanted to facilitate healing. This bony supplement minimally should be biocompatible and encourage bone ingrowth and repair. There are a number of bone-healing strategies that span from materials like metals, ceramics, and polymers, to biological approaches such as cell implantation and protein delivery from degradable materials. To fully understand and appreciate the advantages and shortcomings of current strategies and to begin to consider new designs and approaches, a good understanding of bone biology is necessary.

10.3 BONE BIOLOGY

Bone itself is composed of an extracellular matrix and several different cell types each with its own specific function. The matrix is composed of 95% type I collagen and 5% proteoglycans and noncollagenous proteins (Einhorn 1996). Proteoglycans are high-molecular-weight complexes of proteins and polysaccharides typically found in structural and connective tissues. One example of a proteoglycan is a glycosaminoglycan, commonly found in both bone and cartilage. Partially what makes bone a unique tissue type is its ability to form and deposit crystalline salts. These salts form a mineralized coating around cells embedded within the extracellular matrix providing strength and rigidity to the tissue, but the bone still has some inherent mechanical flexibility. The mineralized coating is composed primarily of calcium and phosphate in a ratio that forms a calcium-deficient carbonated hydroxyapatite (CHA) (see Table 10.2 later in chapter). It is this matrix that also provides the body with necessary ions such as calcium and phosphate.

10.3.1 Cells of Bone

A discussion about bone repair must include bone cells, beginning with the stem cell. A comprehensive discussion of stem cells is given in Section 10.3 so details given in this chapter will pertain more specifically to bone. Stem cells are generally divided into three categories: embryonic stem cells, hematopoietic stem cells, and mesenchymal stem cells (MSCs). Hematopoietic stem cells give rise to neutrophils, lymphocytes, natural killer cells, dendritic cells, macrophages, and monocytes. Bone marrow (BM)-resident MSCs give rise to chondrocytes, adipocytes, reticular stroma, and osteoblasts (Nombela-Arrieta et al. 2011). Criteria to classify stem cells as such are based in part on their function compared to other cell types (Potten and Loeffler 1990). A stem cell of a particular tissue type would be a cell

- Lacking certain tissue-specific differentiation markers

- Capable of proliferation

- Able to self-maintain the population of cells

- Able to produce many differentiated, functional daughter cells

- Able to regenerate the appropriate tissue after injury

The earlier definition best describes stem cells derived from human embryos, which are capable of assuming any cell type given the appropriate surroundings and conditions.

10.3.1.1 Mesenchymal Stem Cells

During embryonic development, the embryo consists of three germ or cell layers: the ectoderm, the endoderm, and the mesoderm (Alberts et al. 1994). The endoderm develops into the liver, lungs, pancreas, and alimentary canal. The ectoderm develops into the epidermis, nerves, skin of the mouth, nasal cavity, bladder, etc. The cells of the mesodermal layer eventually develop into several connective tissue types including muscle, blood, lymph tissue, bone, cartilage, tendon, ligament, and fat. The cells of the mesoderm are called MSCs and are also found in the marrow of postnatal organisms, although only about 1 in 100,000 nucleated marrow cells is a MSC. Using various *in vitro* culture techniques, the MSCs can be differentiated into bone, cartilage, tendon, ligament, muscle, fat, skin, and marrow stroma (Alberts et al. 1994).

10.3.1.2 Differentiation of Mesenchymal Stem Cells toward the Osteoblast Lineage

The development of a bone cell from initial to terminal differentiation is marked by both cellular morphological characteristics and the appearance and disappearance of biochemical markers, each of which may vary depending on the cell type studied (primary cell vs. cell line) as well as the surroundings (*in vivo* vs. *in vitro*). It is important to appreciate the fact that the progression from stem cell to osteocyte does not follow a well-defined pattern with clearly delineated stages. However, for the sake of clarity, the development of a bone cell has been divided into three stages: proliferation, extracellular matrix development and maturation, and mineralization. These stages are roughly correlated with five phases of cell differentiation: osteoprogenitor cell, preosteoblast, osteoblast, osteocyte, and bone lining cell (Bruder et al. 1998).

10.3.1.3 Osteoprogenitor Cell

The osteoprogenitor cell has poorly defined morphological and molecular characteristics (Bruder et al. 1998) but appears spindle-like, similar to a fibroblast, and is located adjacent to the preosteoblast at the site of newly forming bone. Osteoprogenitors are considered to be in the proliferative phase of bone development. Of the most common bone markers, only osteopontin is evident at the later stages of the osteoprogenitor cell. The osteoprogenitor is a highly proliferative cell type that is capable of reproducing other osteoprogenitor cells as well as daughter cells.

10.3.1.4 Preosteoblasts

The daughter cells are preosteoblasts and are identifiable *in vivo* by both location and ultrastructure (Aubin and Liu 1996, Aubin 2008). The preosteoblast is found along the borders of newly forming bone and appears cuboidal in shape. Preosteoblasts produce type I collagen, alkaline phosphatase, and osteopontin in limited amounts and possess a limited ability to divide. Thus, preosteoblasts mark the end of the proliferative phase and the beginning of the extracellular matrix development and maturation phase. Differentiation of preosteoblasts gives rise to osteoblasts (Aubin and Liu 1996).

10.3.1.5 Osteoblasts

Osteoblasts, like preosteoblasts, also appear cuboidal in shape and occupy a slightly more interior position on the boundary of newly forming bone than osteoblasts. Osteoblasts secrete the matrix that eventually envelopes them within the new bone and so are located that much deeper into the bone layer. Osteoblasts produce abundant alkaline phosphatase, osteopontin, and bone sialoprotein, and lesser amounts of osteocalcin early on but begin producing more abundant amounts of osteocalcin as they mature. Osteoblasts also begin producing collagenase at this point, marking the beginning of remodeling. Osteoblasts are considered post proliferative and encompass the end of the matrix maturation phase and the beginning of the mineralization phase. The mature osteoblast is capable of producing type I collagen for matrix development, proteoglycans, hormones, and growth factors for further matrix maturation and mineralization. Differentiation of the osteoblast gives rise to the osteocyte (Aubin and Liu 1996).

10.3.1.6 Osteocytes

The osteocyte is responsible for maintaining the mineralized tissue through limited abilities of both synthesis and resorption of the matrix. Further, the osteocyte initiates the intramatrix diffusion network for nutrients by extending filopodial processes from its place in a lacuna to adjacent cells within the matrix. New bone is formed in concentric sheets, or lamellae, that surround tubes called Haversian canals, through which blood vessels pass to provide nutrients. As osteoblasts form new bone along the inner edge of these concentric circles, subsequent lamellae are migrated outward from the center. The canaliculi provide the transfer of nutrients from newly formed lamellae to older layers of bone (see Figure 10.1). This method of bone formation is typical of cortical, or compact bone (see Figure 10.2). The osteocyte is considered postproliferative and becomes embedded in the matrix that it produced during its osteoblastic phase. Osteocytes are smaller than osteoblasts, have decreased or no alkaline phosphatase production, and are considered to be metabolically inactive. They continue, however, to produce osteocalcin, bone sialoprotein, and osteopontin (Nijweide et al. 1996, Klein-Nulend and Bonewald 2008).

Compact bone and spongy (cancellous bone)

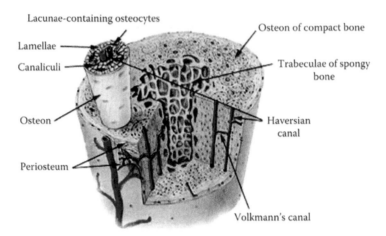

FIGURE 10.1 **Cross section of a long bone showing compact bone, trabecular bone, osteons, canaliculi, and Haversian canal system. (From http://training.seer.cancer.gov/anatomy/skeletal/tissue.html; http://en.wikipedia.org/wiki/File:Illu_compact_spongy_bone.jpg)**

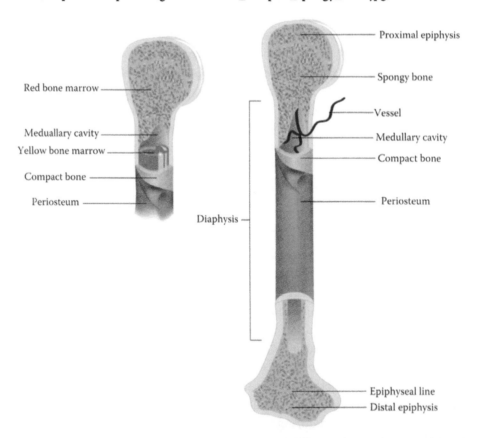

FIGURE 10.2   Anatomy of a long bone showing cortical and trabecular bone. (From mykhan/123RF stock photo; http://www.123rf.com/photo_9233645_human-bone-anatomy-illustration-showing-detailed-anatomy-of-human-bone-isolated-white-background-har.html)

10.3.1.7 Bone Lining Cells

In the mature adult where formation of new bone occurs outside of bone borders, the bone is lined with flat cells that are considered mature osteoblasts. That is, they are located at the bone margins but are no longer producing matrix. These cells have little known function, but some speculation states that they may be osteoblast precursors (Einhorn 1996).

10.3.1.8 Osteoclasts

Osteoclasts are differentiated from hematopoietic stem cells found in the circulating blood. Osteoclasts are the cells responsible for the resorption of bone and are characterized by two distinct plasma membrane types: a ruffled border and a clear or sealing zone (Einhorn 1996, Sims and Baron 2002). The clear or sealing zone forms a barrier (resorption lacuna) around the ruffled border, which is responsible for bone resorption. The osteoclast synthesizes hydrochloric acid (Mulari et al. 2003) and collagenase that are excreted at the ruffled border at high extracellular concentrations. This highly acidic secretion dissolves the hydroxyapatite crystals forming the mineralized extracellular bone matrix. Then several enzymes and collagenase are released that destroy the collagen matrix that secures the hydroxyapatite crystals to the bone. With the matrix degraded and dislodged, the degradation products are then removed from the resorption lacuna, or resorption pits, and released into the extracellular space.

10.3.2 Bone Types

Cortical bone, one of the two types of bone, is typical of the outer layers of most bones and occupies the majority of the long bones (see Figure 10.2). Cortical bone is 80%–90% mineralized with very few pores and void spaces, making it very strong and capable of maintaining the mechanical and protective requirements of the skeleton. The second type of bone is trabecular, or cancellous bone, and is much less dense than cortical, is found on the interior of most bones (see Figure 10.2). Only about 15%–25% of its content is mineralized, but it is rich in BM, blood vessels, and connective tissue, making the primary role of trabecular bone metabolic as opposed to structural.

10.4 FRACTURE HEALING

When a bone has sustained an injury, there are several stages that characterize the healing process (Carano and Filvaroff 2003). With a structural failure of bone, there are many aspects beyond the actual bone break that must be understood. Imperative to the health of the bone prior to breaking is an adequate nutrient supply, which is partially maintained by blood. In the event of a break, this blood supply may be compromised. Further, there are numerous tissues including ligament, tendon, and muscle that may or may not have been affected by the break. The process of healing all these elements is a multidimensional event with an overlapping timeline, but can be divided into three broad stages: inflammation, repair, and remodeling (Claes et al. 2012).

10.4.1 Stage I: Inflammation

The initial response to fracture is largely cellular, with a hematoma occurring and platelets, macrophages, monocytes, and polymorphonuclear neutrophils collecting at the injury site and beginning the clean-up and repair process. Cell death occurs where there has been an interruption of blood flow due to the break, with necrotic bone evident at the point of fracture. Within 8 h after the injury and continuing for the first 24 h post-injury, there is an elevated level of cell division not only adjacent to the injury site but, in the case of long bone fractures, throughout the entire bone (McKibbon 1978). This elevated cell division rate subsides within a few days throughout the majority of the bone, but continues at the injury site weeks into the healing process. At this point, MSCs, osteoprogenitor cells, fibroblasts, and endothelial cells arrive at the fracture site from the marrow within the medullary canal, from the periosteum, and from soft tissue that may be adjacent to the injury site. These cells in combination with endogenous growth factors and proteins begin the rebuilding process. New blood vessels begin to form and the repair process begins to form new bone (Carano and Filvaroff 2003).

10.4.2 Stage II: Soft and Hard Callus Formation

As the inflammation slowly subsides, a fibrous tissue layer called a callus forms around the fracture (Carano and Filvaroff 2003). Within this callus, the bone is remodeled over the course of several weeks. The initial callus formed is a soft callus that is a cartilaginous/bony tissue with cartilage forming at the edges of the callus and bone forming within the fracture site. This soft callus provides limited stability to the fracture site in compression but is not rigid enough to prevent flexure of the fracture. As time passes, however, the cartilage is converted to woven bone through endochondral ossification and bone is also formed directly from MSCs and preosteoblasts within the callus (Ostrum 2000). Both of these healing processes result in an increase of the mechanical rigidity of the site.

10.4.3 Stage III: Bone Remodeling

In the final stage of healing, the woven bone formed within the callus is slowly remodeled as lamellar bone (Carano and Filvaroff 2003). Further, the mineralized callus is slowly remodeled via osteoclast resorption to return the bone to its original diameter in response to the stresses seen by the bone, and the medullary canal is remodeled as well. This remodeling stage may take years to complete and in the case of adults may only remodel to a limited degree but not completely. The bone will, however, remodel completely in children. This may be partially due to the relatively thicker, and therefore more cellular, periosteum in children than adults (Caputo 1999).

10.5 CURRENT STRATEGIES FOR BONE REPAIR

The aforementioned process describes typical healing for a bony fracture, but as mentioned earlier this can be hindered either due to the nature or severity of an injury or due to an underlying pathology. In those instances where additional intervention is required, surgeons have a small armamentarium from which to choose that includes (1) "natural" implant materials like autografts and allografts, (2) synthetic materials like implantable plastics, metals, and ceramics that have been fashioned into screws, rods, pins, plates, and entire joints and are intended to provide mechanical fixation and support with little to no bioactivity with surrounding bone, and (3) natural and synthetic materials that are engineered to be bioactive, that is to interact with cells and tissues after implantation to facilitate healing. This latter category often includes biodegradable materials capable of delivering cells and therapeutic molecules like growth factors and capable of being formed into two-dimensional and three-dimensional structures that encourage healing and host bone ingrowth. Following is an overview of tools available to help regenerate bone, starting with the current gold standard for bone repair, the autograft.

10.5.1 Autograft

An autograft is tissue that has been harvested from one region of the patient's body and reimplanted into another region of that same patient. In these instances, the patient serves as his/her own donor, which has considerable advantages over tissue transplanted from another individual. Tissue taken from and reimplanted into the same patient will not contain any risk of immunogenic response or disease transfer since tissue is native to the patient (Laurencin et al. 2006). Further, in the case of bone autografts, the tissue also possesses many of the cells, proteins, growth factors, and mechanical/structural elements necessary for complete bone healing, repair, and/or regeneration. While the autograft is an ideal tool for bone repair, it also has its shortcomings. Autograft tissue is typically harvested from the iliac crest of the pelvis because of the trabecular, or porous, bone found there and because the iliac crest is not directly load bearing, rather it is a site of muscle attachment. The trabecular bone harvested from the iliac crest is more porous than cortical bone, typically found in the center portion, or diaphyseal region, of the long bones in the arms and legs (see Figure 10.2). The porous nature of trabecular bone makes the tissue osteoconductive, or capable of supporting osteoblast attachment, migration throughout its three-dimensional structure, and proliferation (Khan et al. 2008). The osteoconductivity of trabecular bone is better suited for bony defects because its pore structure allows neighboring bone at the defect site to grow into and incorporate the implanted tissue more readily, leading to more rapid healing. The trabecular bone harvested from the iliac crest is rich in marrow, blood, stem, and progenitor cells, proteins, and growth factors ideally suited for further assisting neighboring bone at the defect site to incorporate the transplanted tissue and speed healing. This combination of cells, proteins, and growth factors give autografts the ability not only to allow cells to migrate and proliferate but also to drive undifferentiated stem and progenitor cells down the osteoblastic lineage (Khan et al. 2008). This capability, termed osteoinductivity, is an essential part of the clinical success seen with autografts, and is integral in the healing capabilities autografts have in defects, such as the nonunions described earlier, that would not otherwise be capable of healing. One can imagine, though, that the amount of bone that can be harvested from the iliac crest would be limited since harvesting the bone is in fact creating a new injury site, and harvesting too much bone would result in the new injury potentially being as bad or worse than the original defect. This new injury that is being created along the iliac crest typically heals itself over time but is now susceptible to the same complications likely for any injury like excessive pain, infection, poor healing outcome, etc. In total, this creation of additional injury sites and the potential complications associated with them is commonly termed donor-site morbidity. The potential for donor-site morbidity and the limitations of available donor tissue are two of the more substantial drawbacks of autografts. So, while autografts have a number of positive attributes their drawbacks necessitate alternative strategies. One of the more common alternatives to the autograft is the allograft.

10.5.2 Allograft

In general, the term allograft refers to tissue harvested from a member of the same species and implanted into a donor (or, person to person). Bone allografts are harvested from donor patients, typically cadavers, and either treated through a freeze-drying process, stored as fresh frozen grafts, or demineralized to form demineralized bone matrix (DBM). Freeze-dried and fresh frozen allografts maintain their microstructure and general structural integrity while DBM becomes a powder-like substance that does not have any mechanical integrity on its own (Costain and Crawford 2009). With fresh frozen allografts, there is a small but present risk of disease transmission from the donor to the recipient. In fact, there have been cases of disease transmission from donor to recipient in the early 2000s (Laurencin et al. 2006). While freeze-dried tissue is treated to eliminate these possibilities, the treatment in turn eliminates the potential osteoinductivity of the graft, reducing its overall healing potential (Laurencin et al. 2006). DBM powder is commonly mixed with solutions to form a putty-like substance that can be shaped and molded (Laurencin et al. 2006). DBM still contains many of the proteins that facilitate healing so these putties are quite effective in promoting bone formation, but the putties have little to no mechanical strength and lack a pore structure, limiting their osteoconductivity and thus suitability for certain defects. Not all defects can be treated solely with an autograft or allograft though. Some injuries may require more rigid hardware like metallic rods, pins, or screws, or in the case of more invasive surgical procedures like joint replacement, an implant formed from a combination of metals, ceramics, and polymers.

10.5.3 Orthopedic Implant Materials

Metals are used as screws to fuse one or more bones or bone parts together, as rods to stabilize long bones, and as plates and pins to hold pieces of bone together. Ceramics are used as articulating surfaces in artificial joints and as bone void fillers and in these capacities are largely nonresorbable. Polymers, generally nondegradable polymers, are used as articulating surfaces in artificial joints and also as cements to affix implants to surrounding bone after implantation. While these fixation devices and nondegradable implants do aid in bone repair, they rely to a large extent on mechanical fixation, load bearing, and durability and less so on bioactive integration with and regeneration of surrounding tissue. A subset of tools for bone repair, the bone graft substitutes, includes degradable polymers, ceramics, and composites of the two (Laurencin et al. 2006). While metals, ceramics, and nondegradable polymers have dominated orthopedic repair for some time, advances in materials science have brought both degradable polymers and novel ceramics to the forefront of orthopedic device research, both in conjunction with implant materials and as bone graft substitutes designed for bone regeneration. Following is a brief summary of metals, ceramics, and polymers as orthopedic fixation devices and implants and a more in-depth discussion of degradable polymers, ceramics, and composites of the two as materials designed for regenerative engineering of bone.

10.5.3.1 Metals

Metals as biomaterials are broadly organized into three categories: stainless steel, cobalt-based alloys, and titanium and titanium alloys. Each category has had a significant presence in orthopedics as rods, screws, plates, and rigid components of knee and hip replacements. They differ from one another in their material content, mechanical properties, weight, and resistance to corrosion. Stainless steel contains a number of metals including iron, nickel, chromium, and carbon. There have been modifications to the content of stainless steel for orthopedic implants over time to enhance its biocompatibility; for instance, molybdenum has been added to reduce corrosion in salty aqueous environments (like the human body), while the carbon content has been reduced for the same reason. The latest version of stainless steel, commonly referred to as 316L, is currently used for orthopedic devices. Despite efforts to reduce corrosion (added molybdenum and reduced carbon content), it is still more appropriate for temporary implants like screws, plates, and nails due to its poor corrosion resistance relative to other metals available for implants (Park and Lakes 2007). The cobalt-based alloys include cobalt–chromium–molybdenum alloys, with varying trace amounts of other metals such as tungsten, nickel, and iron. They are typically stronger and with higher nickel content more corrosion-resistant than stainless steel but may subsequently have lower wear resistance than other metals so are less suited for articulating surfaces. Concerns existed with the higher nickel content alloys of potential toxicity from wear particles so despite the better resistance to corrosion the alloys with higher nickel content are not widely used for articulating surfaces. Titanium and titanium alloys are used for both dental and orthopedic applications. They tend to have higher corrosion resistance than both stainless steel and cobalt-based alloys but lower wear resistance and mechanical properties. While the mechanical properties of the titanium alloys are more susceptible to wear and crack propagation, the reduced properties, closer to those of the bone surrounding the material after implantation than other metals, may serve to reduce the likelihood of a phenomenon called stress shielding, which can negatively impact healing.

When a material is used as either a support or replacement for bone, it is important to have the mechanical strength of the implant be similar to that of the surrounding bone. If not, the bone around the implant is seen by the body as superfluous (since the physical loading is sustained by the implanted metals of greater strength) and is resorbed. This creates problems because the surrounding bone is necessary to secure hip or knee implant stems, and resorption of this bone can lead to implant loosening. For this reason, one basic design criteria of orthopedic implants and scaffolds is to match as closely as possible the mechanical properties of surrounding bone. A quick look at the mechanical properties of metals used in orthopedics (see Table 10.1) shows the disparity between certain metals and human bone. This, among other factors, has motivated the development of new materials for orthopedics, some of which are discussed later (see Section 10.6).

Another caveat in the utility of metals as orthopedic implants is corrosion. When a metal is placed in an aqueous environment (like the human body) that contains ions, oxygen,

TABLE 10.1   Mechanical Properties of Metals Commonly Used as Orthopedic
Devices and Human Bone

Material	Elastic Modulus	Yield Strength (MPa)	Tensile Strength (MPa)
Stainless Steel 316L	190 GPa	190–690	490–1350
Cobalt–chromium alloys	210–250 GPa	448–1500	650–1800
Titanium and Ti-based alloys	110–116 GPa	170–1000	240–1100
Cortical bone	4–17 GPa	7–180	—
Trabecular bone	12–900 MPa	0.15–13	—

Sources: *Biomaterials Science*, 2nd edn., Ratner, B.D., Hoffman, A.S., Schoen, F.J., and
Lemons, J.E., Copyright 2004, Elsevier; from Springer Science + Business
Media: *Biomaterials: An Introduction*, 2007, Park, J. and Lakes, R.S.; Athanasiou,
K.A. et al., *Tissue Eng.*, 6(4), 361, 2000.

Note the large discrepancy in cortical and trabecular bone and the metals used to
repair it.

and other dissolved compounds, an electrochemical reaction takes place. This reaction, called corrosion, can erode a metal. This corrosion liberates ions from the metal to the surrounding milieu that, on its own, can be hazardous to the individual, but also leads to physical and mechanical compromise of the implant itself. Corrosion can be minimized by passivation, the spontaneous formation of a thin oxide layer along the metal surface when the metal comes in contact with oxygen, which hinders (but does not completely prevent) the transfer of ions from the metal to the surrounding fluid. Damage to this oxide layer by scratching the surface of the metal can accelerate corrosion. While the oxide layer can spontaneously reform on the metal to resist corrosion, repeated scratches, through cyclic motion for instance, can re-damage it over time. Corrosion can also occur between metallic components that are designed to fit snugly with no gaps, like a screw in a screw hole, but have been poorly machined or engineered. The resulting crack or crevice between two poor-fitting components can become oxygen-poor and the passivation layer can be compromised, leaving a vulnerable spot for corrosive degradation. Repeated loading of an implant can cause microcracks that, while not necessarily catastrophic to the mechanical strength of the implant, may break the passivation layer and initiate corrosion. The corrosion will wear away at the metal at that point and ultimately increase the crack and lead to implant failure. Finally, since corrosion is based on the electrochemical potential of the metal, if two dissimilar metals are placed next to each other, say a screw of one metal type placed in a screw hole of another metal type, they can create their own electric potential and initiate the exchange of ions locally, leaving one as the ion donor and the other as the ion sink, initiating corrosion. The concept of corrosion is explained in detail in Chapter 4.

10.5.3.2 Bioinert Ceramics

Ceramic materials are solid, inorganic compounds consisting of metallic and nonmetallic elements that are held together by ionic and covalent bonding (see Chapter 4 for details). Ceramics for bony repair have been used as one of the components of total joint replacements, as stand-alone implant materials, and as one of several materials

TABLE 10.2 Various Types of Calcium Phosphates, Their Molecular Formula, and Ca/P Ratios

Calcium Phosphates Type	Molecular Formula	Ca/P Ratio
Tricalcium phosphate (TCP)	$Ca_3(PO_4)_2$	1.5
Hydroxyapatite (HA)	$Ca_{10}(PO_4)_6(OH)_2$	1.67
Calcium-deficient hydroxyapatite (CDHA)	$Ca_9(HPO_4)(PO_4)_5(OH)$	1.5
Tetracalcium phosphate (TTCP)	$Ca_4(PO_4)_2O$	2
Octacalcium phosphate (OCP)	$Ca_8(HPO_4)_2(PO_4)_4 \cdot 5H_2O$	1.33
Carbonated hydroxyapatite	$Ca_{10-x}(PO_4)_{6-x}(CO_3)_x(OH)_2$	1.7–1.8

blended together to make composites. As components of total joint replacements, the bioinert ceramics alumina (Al_2O_3) and zirconia (ZrO_2) have been chosen for their overall biocompatibility and high wear resistance (compared to metals or nondegradable polymers). Alumina has been used for over 40 years as a choice for the articulating surface in joint replacements, but zirconia was introduced in the mid-1980s as an alternative to alumina for the femoral head component given its superior mechanical properties and wear resistance. While successful as articulating surfaces, zirconia and alumina are less suited as synthetic bone grafting material given their nonresorbability and susceptibility to fracturing in failure (vs. elastically or plastically deforming). Other ceramics, notwithstanding, are very well suited for bone repair stemming in part from the mineral content of bone itself, a form of calcium phosphate known as calcium-deficient CHA. Like other apatites, it has a calcium and phosphate component in a specific proportion (Ca/P ratio) but is associated with a hydroxyl group and thus is referred to as hydroxyapatite. The stoichiometrically stable form of hydroxyapatite is that with a Ca/P ratio of 1.67 as can be seen by its molecular formula $Ca_{10}(PO_4)_6(OH)_2$. There are several other non apatitic calcium phosphates that are distinguished from one another by their molecular formulae, Ca/P ratios (see Table 10.2), crystal structures as seen by x-ray diffraction patterns, and solubilities. The Ca/P ratios of other calcium phosphates that differ from 1.67 tend to have higher dissolution rates than stoichiometric hydroxyapatite, which is an important point when considering the design of bone graft substitutes capable of being resorbed and remodeled by the host environment because hydroxyapatite, in its most stable, crystalline form is very slow to degrade. In fact, very often it is either nondegradable or incapable of being resorbed and subsequently remodeled by osteoclasts during healing (Van Landuyt et al. 1995). This can lead to hydroxyapatite particles associated with implant materials remaining long after the implant has either been degraded or resorbed or with nondegradable implants long after the surrounding bone has grown into the implant material. Although these particles may lie dormant for several years without incident, the nondegradable hydroxyapatite particles do not lend themselves to tissue regenerative applications as they do not participate in bone remodeling and may even prevent it over time (Sarkar et al. 2001). So when considering viable materials for bone repair, alternatives with more resorbability should be considered. For instance, tricalcium phosphate (TCP) differs from hydroxyapatite in both molecular formula and Ca/P ratio (see Table 10.2), as do calcium-deficient hydroxyapatite (CDHA) and CHA in which a carbonate ion (CO_3) is incorporated into the ceramic. All three are less stable than stoichiometric hydroxyapatite so they can be more readily resorbed by osteoclasts. They also dissolve more rapidly than stoichiometric HA, allowing for bone remodeling and complete scaffold replacement over time. These calcium phosphates tend to interact with their environment in a more active way than those used as articulating surfaces for joints. These bioactive calcium phosphates are discussed in greater depth later.

10.5.3.3 Nondegradable Polymers

Polymers are large molecules made from combinations of smaller molecules consisting of primarily carbon, hydrogen, oxygen, and nitrogen. These structures have been utilized and designed for several orthopedic applications. Many of the properties of these molecules are dictated by their chemical structures, the molecular weight, the physical structure, isomerism, and crystallinity. Polyethylene and polymethylmethacrylate (PMMA) are two examples of nondegradable polymers currently used as orthopedic implant materials.

10.5.3.3.1 Polyethylene   Polyethylene consists entirely of ethylene monomer units linked together to form long polymer chains (see Chapter 4 for general information about polymers). There are several kinds of polyethylene (low-density polyethylene [LDPE], high-density polyethylene [HDPE], ultrahigh-molecular-weight polyethylene [UHMWPE]) that are synthesized with different relative molecular masses and chain architectures. LDPE refers to low-density polyethylene with a relative molecular mass of less than 50,000 g/mol. HDPE is a linear polymer with a relative molecular mass up to 200,000 g/mol. In comparison, UHMWPE has a relative molecular mass ranging from 2 to 6×10^6 g/mol. The typical modern UHMWPE used in implants has a relative molecular mass of >4 to 6×10^6 g/mol. UHMWPE has a higher ultimate strength and impact strength than HDPE, and UHMWPE is significantly more abrasion and wear resistant than HDPE, making it desirable from a clinical perspective. With its high abrasion and wear resistance, UHMWPE has been one of a few materials used as the articulating surface for both hips and knees in combination with metallic counterparts. Sterilizing UHMWPE with γ- or electron beam irradiation tends to increase this wear resistance and decrease crack propagation when done in carefully controlled conditions by cross-linking the polymer (see Chapter 4 for more details). More recently, annealing and incorporating vitamin E into the polymer have been evaluated for even better wear properties (Sobieraj and Rimnac 2009). While advances in materials processing continue to reduce the effects of wear on UHMWPE, the side effects of wear, resulting particles, and debris can pose a risk to the health of a joint. In bulk form and prior to the formation of wear particles, polyethylene is relatively inert and exhibits little or no degradation or biological incompatibility. However, polyethylene wear particles that break free from the bulk can elicit an osteolytic host response. Polyethylene wear particles induce a macrophage response, which leads to osteolysis and aseptic loosening in total joint arthroplasties. In the 1990s, wear of polyethylene components and osteolysis after total knee arthroplasties were reported with increased frequency and motivated the advances discussed earlier in wear resistance technology (Kurtz et al. 2011).

10.5.3.3.2 Polymethylmethacrylate   Another commonly used nondegradable polymer for orthopedic repair is PMMA. Unlike UHMWPE, which is used primarily for articulating surfaces, PMMA is used as a cement to secure implant materials to surrounding bone, such as a hip stem that has been implanted into a femur. PMMA is a nondegradable polymer that secures implants into bone by forming a mechanical interlock between the implant and host bone rather than through adhesive properties. It comes as a powder and a liquid that, when mixed together, polymerize and harden over 5–15 min. When the liquid phase of the cement (the monomer) is mixed with the powder phase of the cement (the polymer and initiator), the result is an exothermic reaction that raises the local temperature from 40°C to 90°C, depending on the testing location (at the core of the cement vs. at the bone–cement interface) and thickness of the cement (Leeson and Lippitt 1993, Poitout 2004), which can result in some necrosis of the bone around the cement as it cures. While this quality of PMMA as bone cement would seem to disqualify it from use, it nevertheless is still widely used, and to be sure continues to show utility. Given the role of PMMA, certain mechanical properties are mandated like appropriate resistance to creep, good wear resistance, and suitable yield stress (Ratner et al. 2004). Its mechanical properties are similar to strong trabecular bone but the fact that it is not resorbable, and therefore is never renewed or replaced by newly forming bone, leaves PMMA vulnerable to normal wear and tear of any nondegradable material under constant loading. Over time, PMMA can fracture from high levels of mechanical loading, incomplete polymerization upon initial mixing, or poor bone–cement implant bonding due to eccentrically shaped bone or air voids in the cement after implantation (Poitout 2004). Over time, these irregularities can lead to implant loosening, which can lead to further instabilities in the joint and irregular wear or failure of the joint as a whole. While commonly used and certainly effective, these clear limitations do suggest that alternative strategies would be worth investigating. While the nondegradable materials like UHMWPE and PMMA are effective, they exemplify an approach to bone repair that is based on bioinert materials *designed not to* interact with surrounding tissue. It may, however, be valuable to consider the design and use of bioactive materials that are *designed to* interact with surrounding tissue. This is a fundamental tenet of a regenerative engineering strategy for bone repair.

10.6 REGENERATIVE ENGINEERING OF BONE

Approaches to repairing bone have evolved over the last several decades as documented by the chronological advancement in the tools available to the orthopedic surgeon. Implants have evolved from relatively simple metals, ceramics, and polymers that were initially chosen for their intrinsic properties like mechanical strength, corrosion resistance, wear resistance, chemical stability, and inertness, to materials that were designed to function specifically as biological implants and interact with the body to facilitate and even enhance bone repair. The field is continuing to evolve from one facilitating the repair of tissues to one now considering the regeneration of tissues. This is the core of regenerative engineering to utilize materials science, developmental biology, and stem cell technology toward the regeneration of tissues. Regenerative engineering, like tissue engineering, relies on degradable materials, mostly polymers and ceramics, as substrates for cell attachment, proliferation, and differentiation. These materials can be capable of withstanding mechanical loading, are easily formed and shaped, and to some degree can serve as cues to guide progenitor cells in cell migration, proliferation, or differentiation. Substrate-guided cell behavior is an important tool that has emerged with advances in materials science, imaging, and substrate synthesis technology. The ability to guide cell behavior by modifying the surface of materials with nanoscale precision has opened up a new dimension of scaffold synthesis in which a surface architecture that may only measure a fraction of the size of the cell it supports can influence the behavior of that cell. As with conventional tissue engineering, it is important to provide an osteoconductive scaffold structure onto which cells can attach, proliferate, and migrate. It is also important that a scaffold be osteoinductive and have the capacity to guide undifferentiated progenitor cells toward the osteoblastic lineage. Generally speaking, a three-dimensional structure can be designed to be osteoconductive by engineering an interconnected pore structure, but adding osteoinductivity to that scaffold usually requires the incorporation and subsequent delivery of specific growth factors. Recent studies, however, have shown how blending polymers and ceramics may impart osteoinductivity without the use of growth factors. With the advances in nanoscale materials science, it is now foreseeable that this capability may be engineered into the surface architecture of the scaffold. Later is a discussion of degradable polymers that are suitable candidates for scaffold development, bioactive ceramics that are a step beyond the bioinert ceramics discussed earlier, and composites of the two that have been investigated in the research lab. Finally, a brief overview of scaffolds interacting with progenitor and stem cells is given.

10.6.1 Degradable Polymers

There are a number of degradable polymers available to the orthopedic regenerative engineer. They differ by their modes of synthesis, degradation time, degradation mechanism, and physicochemical nature. The vast majority of polymers used for regenerating tissue degrade through hydrolysis, or the breakdown of the polymer backbone in the presence of water, which makes intuitive sense given the aqueous milieu of the body. Within hydrolytically degradable polymers, there are two general modes of degradation: surface erosion and bulk degradation. This is explained in detail in Chapter 4 but briefly, surface eroding polymers are generally more hydrophobic than bulk-degrading polymers because their overall hydrophobicity limits the penetration of water into the material and leaves it confined to the periphery. Polymers that are less hydrophobic may permit the penetration of water into the bulk of the material so the degradation can begin at the center of the material. The polymer begins to degrade from the inside out but maintains its overall structure. Over time, the degradation continuously breaks the polymer down until it is unable to maintain its physical shape and physically breaks down. While many polymers exhibit one of these modes of degradation, it is possible to exhibit both as well. As a general rule, surface eroding polymers offer advantages for drug delivery since the release of polymer, and subsequently any drug payload, can take place more gradually. In practice, however, both types of polymers are used for both engineered scaffold synthesis for tissue regeneration and drug delivery applications. Another mode of degradation is through enzymatic activity. Enzymatically degrading polymers generally have hydrolytically sensitive bonds but do not appreciably degrade without some physiological enzymatic activity. When considering polymers for bone regeneration, it is important to have a material that has the mechanical integrity required for the bony site, but also a degradation time that will allow for healing before resorption and remodeling. Some capacity to deliver factors is important, but the overriding consideration may be one of mechanical integrity. The choice of polymers includes a number of synthetic materials, but also a shorter list of naturally derived polymers.

10.6.1.1 Collagen

Collagen is a natural polymer that is ubiquitous in the human body. Collagen is the primary component of a number of musculoskeletal tissues like ligament, cartilage, tendon, and bone and thus has found favor as a material for musculoskeletal regeneration. While it lacks the compressive strength of bone, it has been paired with other materials like calcium phosphates that impart mechanical stability. This is a well-reasoned approach given that native bone is made up of a collagen network that has been mineralized by osteoblasts for strength and collagen is degraded enzymatically by the body. Some commercially available products have used this premise to form bone graft substitutes. Collagraft® (Zimmer Inc.), for instance, is a commercially available scaffold for bone repair composed of calcium phosphate and collagen. It is available as thin sponge-like strips that are placed within a defect site. Healos® (Depuy Inc.) is another example of a collagen sponge that has been blended with calcium phosphate for bone repair applications. While collagen scaffolds do have utility for bone repair, the nature of collagen limits its utility as a load-bearing scaffold so there are limits to its stand-alone utility.

10.6.1.2 Chitosan

Another natural polymer that has found favor as a bone repair substrate is chitosan. Chitosan is derived from chitin, a polysaccharide that is the main constituent in the exoskeletons of arthropods (Ulery et al. 2011). Chitin alone is relatively insoluble and therefore difficult to work with as a biomaterial so it is chemically deacetylated to form chitosan that is enzymatically degradable. The degree of deacetylation dictates in part how readily the material is resorbed (the lower the deacetylation, the longer the degradation), so degradation kinetics can be partially controlled by controlling this process.

10.6.1.3 Poly(α-Hydroxy Esters)

Several synthetic degradable polymers have been used as scaffolds for bone regeneration as well. The first, and most commonly used, are the poly(α-hydroxy esters). They include polylactide (PLA), polyglycolide (PGA), and their copolymer poly(lactide-*co*-glycolide) (PLGA). These polymers degrade through hydrolysis to their constituent parts, lactic acid and glycolic acid, which are further broken down by the body and harmlessly excreted as H_2O and CO_2. The lactic acid and glycolic acid are, as expected, acidic in nature and can cause some minor degree of inflammation but by and large PLA, PGA, and PLGA are considered biocompatible. They are perhaps the most widely studied polymers as a bone regeneration scaffold material in part because their physicochemical properties make them relatively easy to form, melt, mold, and shape. They are also one of the few degradable polymers that have been cleared or approved by the FDA for medical applications. Specifically, PLA has been formed into pins, screws, and plates for orthopedic fixation. PGA alone has been used as degradable suture material in the past, but more recently has been combined with PLA when used for suture materials to give the quickly degrading PGA a bit more stability. The copolymer PLGA has been used extensively for a number of clinical materials including sutures. The utility of PLGA from a research perspective comes in the variable degradation time depending on the ratio of lactic acid:glycolic acid in the copolymer. For instance, 50:50 PLGA degrades in about 1–2 months while 85:15 PLGA degrades in about 5–6 months (Ulery et al. 2011). Vicryl, a commercially available PLGA polymer, has a LA:GA ratio of 10:90 and loses all its strength in about a month but may remain for several more months (Middleton and Tipton 2000). While the ratio of LA:GA does influence the degradation time, the three-dimensional structure of a scaffold and its location within the body can also impact the degradation time. As discussed earlier, a more porous structure will degrade more rapidly than a solid material, and a material subject to greater fluid transfer will degrade faster than one in static environment. PLA, PGA, and PLGA are bulk degrading polymers making them good candidates for bone regeneration scaffolds, but also have utility as drug and factor delivery vehicles given the variability of degradation times.

10.6.1.4 Polyphosphazenes

Polyphosphazenes are a family of degradable polymers that are defined by alternating phosphorus and nitrogen along the backbone. PPHOS, as they are more commonly referred to, can be made to have a wide variety of mechanical, physicochemical, and degradative properties by varying the constituent molecules that form the side groups to the P–N backbone. This inherent flexibility and the large library of side group molecules available make PPHOS a good candidate material for drug and growth factor delivery (Zhang et al. 2006, Oredein-McCoy et al. 2009, Park et al. 2010) in part because they can be fabricated as particles (Jun et al. 2007, Yang et al. 2008, 2010), fibers (Nair et al. 2004), thin films (Deng et al. 2008), and sintered microspheres (Nukavarapu et al. 2008). Similarly, the flexibility of synthesis, overall robust mechanical properties, and tunable, predictable degradation times have made PPHOS a desirable platform for orthopedic-related materials research alone and as a composite (Nair et al. 2004, Deng et al. 2008, 2010, Nukavarapu et al. 2008).

10.6.1.5 Polyhydroxyalkanoates

Polyhydroxyalkanoates are degradable polymers formed either synthetically or as a waste product of bacteria. Poly(3-hydroxybutyrate) is the most common polymer in this family. It degrades through surface erosion due to its inherent hydrophobicity and tends to degrade slowly, but has been combined with 3-hydroxyvalerate to form (3-hydroxybutyrate-co-3-valerate) (PHBV) as a way to control degradation. As the valeric acid component increases, the degradation time decreases (Liu et al. 2010).

10.6.1.6 Polycaprolactone

Polycaprolactone (PCL) is a degradable polymer that has had limited usage as a bone regeneration scaffold in part due to its very long degradation time (~2 years *in vivo*) and its elastic nature at body temperature. The long degradation time makes it more suitable for drug delivery applications though, and its overall high degree of solubility has encouraged others to form blends between it and other degradable polymers (Hutmacher et al. 1996). When formed as a copolymer with PLA, the degradation time can be shortened to just a few months (Hutmacher et al. 1996).

10.6.2 Bioactive Calcium Phosphates

Calcium phosphates are an obvious choice as a biomaterial for bone repair and regeneration given that it is the primary inorganic component of normal healthy human bone. There are, however, subsets of calcium phosphates that differ from those that have been traditionally used as bone graft substitutes. As mentioned earlier, deviating from stoichiometrically stable calcium phosphates like hydroxyapatite enhances resorbability of the ceramic, and this resorbability leads to greater dissolution after implantation. Upon dissolution of calcium phosphate, the liberated ions will be available for new bone formation. This may happen because the dissolution of calcium phosphate results in an increased concentration of calcium and phosphate ions locally forcing apatite crystals to precipitate out of solution and incorporate other locally available ions like carbonate to form new bone mineral (Daculsi et al. 1989). This dissolution/reprecipitation process has been described in detail by Ducheyne et al. (1992). Initially, ions are liberated from the ceramic to the surrounding fluid via dissolution. These dissolution rates are determined by (1) the stoichiometric stability of the ceramic, with those differing from the thermodynamically stable 1.67 having higher dissolution rates and (2) the crystallinity of the ceramic, with those of smaller crystal size and thus more surface area having higher dissolution rates. Then the ions undergo reprecipitation from the surrounding solution onto the surface of the material. With this precipitation, calcium phosphate crystals form while present osteoblasts mineralize the collagen fibrils of the extracellular matrix. These combine to facilitate the attachment of the implant, be it a ceramic, a polymer, or a composite of the two, to neighboring bone at the implant site. The presence of calcium phosphate in an implanted material may also initiate further calcium phosphate development by preexisting osteoblasts, either through the liberation of calcium or through the stimulation of calcium phosphate crystal formation. Once new mineral crystals are formed, they may stimulate additional crystals to form (Daculsi et al. 1990). Studies examining the effect of dissolution rate on overall healing have shown that increased rates of dissolution result in enhanced healing and mineral formation (Ducheyne et al. 1990, de Bruijn et al. 1994, Morgan et al. 1996). Further, calcium phosphates have been shown to be osteoconductive when implanted next to preexisting bone and, in some cases, osteoinductive as evidenced by the ectopic bone formation within porous hydroxyapatite blocks implanted into abdominal muscles of baboons (Ripamonti 1996). For all these reasons, it has become of interest to encourage the formation of an apatitic layer onto a material rather than rely solely on the preimplantation content of the

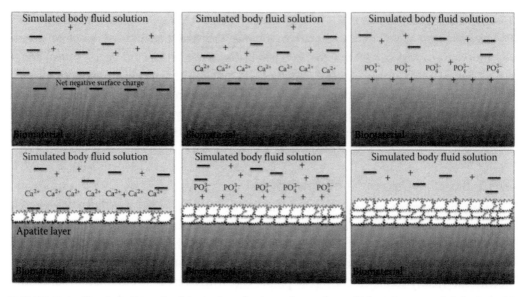

FIGURE 10.3 Precipitation of calcium phosphate on the surface of bioactive materials in ion-rich simulated body fluid. As the ions adhere to the surface of the material, the resulting change in surface charge encourages the deposition of oppositely charged ions, leading to the precipitation of calcium phosphate.

biomaterial. Initiating apatite deposition may also improve mechanical properties of an implant by providing a ceramic coating on a non ceramic, say polymeric, material. With this, several researchers have embraced the notion of dissolution and reprecipitation but have bypassed the dissolution step. To mimic the ion-rich milieu seen after ceramic dissolution, some or all ions commonly seen in the body (Na^+, Ca^{2+}, K^+, Mg^{2+}, Cl^-, HPO_4^{2-}, HCO^{3-}, SO_4^{2-}) are mixed to form a simulated body solution (Kokubo et al. 1990). The ions present in this solution precipitate out and form a ceramic coating on the polymeric material (Kim et al. 2005) much like it occurs from ion dissolution described earlier (see Figure 10.3). So a biomaterial can be pre mineralized *in vitro* and then implanted *in vivo*, having a jump-start to the mineral deposition stage of healing.

10.6.3 Polymer–Ceramic Composites

Combining polymers and ceramics together into one structure can capitalize on the benefits of each material while in some instances minimizing the drawbacks of each material as well. For instance, the brittle nature of ceramics can be minimized by forming composites with polymers that have greater ductility and may undergo plastic deformation without losing mechanical integrity better than ceramics, while at the same time the osteogenic capacity of ceramics can be imparted to non osteogenic polymers. Several composites have been studied with calcium phosphates and an array of polymers including PLAs, PLGA, PMMAs, chitosan, collagen, and others. Some composites have been designed to be suitable for bone attachment and ingrowth, others have included calcium phosphates to impart certain mechanical properties, and others have examined the influence of the calcium phosphate on both *in vitro* cell growth and *in vivo* healing.

Several groups have investigated the benefits of adding hydroxyapatite to a scaffold to increase mechanical properties. Deng et al. added nanocrystalline hydroxyapatite to a PLA solution to form solvent–cast composite matrices and found a steady increase in tensile modulus as hydroxyapatite loading increased from a low of 1.66 GPa for polymer without hydroxyapatite up to 2.47 GPa for a 10.5% hydroxyapatite content (Deng et al. 2001). It was theorized that the increase in tensile modulus was due to (1) an increase in rigidity over the polymer alone when the hydroxyapatite was added and (2) the resulting strong adhesion between the two materials. Wang et al. combined polyamide, a bioinert polymer, with both microcrystalline and nanocrystalline hydroxyapatite and compared resulting bending strength and tensile strength. As the ceramic content of each composite increased, so did the bending strength. For both bending and tensile strength, the addition of nanocrystalline hydroxyapatite increased the properties over those with microcrystalline hydroxyapatite (Wang et al. 2002). It was theorized that the smaller crystals of the nanocrystalline HA resulted in higher surface areas and thus greater surface energy, surface activity, and thus bonding between the polymer and the HA. Finally, Abu Bakar et al. examined the effect of varying amounts of hydroxyapatite added to polyetheretherketone, a polymer used in orthopedic devices, as an injection-molded composite by varying hydroxyapatite content between 0% and 40% by volume. Results indicate that Young's modulus increased from ~3 to 15 GPa as hydroxyapatite content increased from 0% to 40% but tensile strength decreased from 80 to 44 MPa along the same increase in HA content (Abu Bakar et al. 2003). Examination of the load–displacement curves indicates that as the HA content decreased the brittle nature of the composite also decreased. This agrees well with the common complaint of ceramics failing in a brittle fashion in load-bearing situations, and also supports the theory behind forming composites between polymers and ceramics; the polymers become stronger with the addition of the ceramic, and the brittle nature of the ceramic is reduced with the addition of the polymer. Balac et al. (2002) attempted to understand the effect of hydroxyapatite particle shape and volume fraction in a PLA/collagen/hydroxyapatite composite scaffold using finite element analysis and found fewer stress concentrations throughout the matrix with an increased hydroxyapatite volume fraction but a reduced dependence on this as the hydroxyapatite particles were modeled as spherical, suggesting yet another design consideration for the composite scaffold.

The advantages of ceramics in composites are not limited to hydroxyapatite. Lin et al. combined PLA with TCP to make composite rods for orthopedic internal fixation by dissolving the polymer and creating a suspension of TCP particles within the polymer solution (Lin et al. 1999). The suspension was added to rod-shaped molds and heated to harden the polymer. It was determined that the elastic modulus of the rods increased with increasing TCP content, indicating that TCP shares the same reinforcing capabilities as hydroxyapatite. It was also found that the addition of TCP slowed the rate of degradation of the rods. It was theorized that this may have been due to the TCP dissolving in solution and causing hydroxyapatite to precipitate on its surface, which was less susceptible to dissolution and thus protected the composite from a more rapid dissolution/degradation. Further, with the TCP protected from dissolution, it formed a protective seal between the aqueous environment and the PLA, thus reducing the rate of hydrolytic degradation that PLA typically undergoes in an aqueous environment. A similar study by Imai et al. examined the effect of blending TCP with a PLA blend on degradation and found results similar to Lin et al. (Imai et al. 1999). However, they attributed the delayed degradation of the polymer in the presence of TCP to the ability of the TCP to neutralize the acidic oligomers from the degradation of the PLA, which if left unchecked will result in the autocatalytic degradation of the polymer. This theory of the calcium phosphate regulating the acidic degradation products is further supported by Schiller and Epple (2003). It is reasonable to suppose that the presence of the resorbable TCP may not only improve mechanical properties but also decrease both degradation rate and possibly harmful acidic degradation products.

While hydroxyapatite is commonly referred to as the mineral content of bone, it is actually a subset of hydroxyapatite, CDHA that is the true ceramic found in bone (Posner 1969, Durucan and Brown 2000a,b). With this in mind, Durucan et al. have synthesized a CDHA through hydrolysis of TCP at 37°C and combined it with PLA and PLGA to form composites (Durucan and Brown 2000a,b). X-ray diffraction patterns of the CDHA show an amorphous or nanocrystalline ceramic formed that strongly resembles HA with traces of α-TCP (Durucan and Brown 2000a,b), while composites formed with PLGA showed a range of mechanical properties between 13 and 24 MPa tensile strengths depending on the CDHA content. The hydrolysis of TCP at body temperature is an important parameter as it may predict the *in vivo* behavior of certain ceramics into CDHA. Laurencin et al. has developed a composite microsphere-based scaffold in which composite microspheres are formed with a nanocrystalline hydroxyapatite within each microsphere (Khan et al. 2005, 2007, Cushnie et al. 2008). This was accomplished by synthesizing the calcium phosphate within each microsphere as the microsphere was formed in a water/oil/water emulsion system. Through this approach, it was possible to form a composite scaffold with well-dispersed hydroxyapatite in a form that would be easily resorbed and lend itself to calcium phosphate reprecipitation *in vitro* and *in vivo* (see Figure 10.4). This reprecipitation of dissolution products onto a negatively charged scaffold surface has been seen elsewhere (Kim et al. 2005) and is illustrated in Figure 10.3. This has stimulated studies where the precipitation of calcium phosphate is not a by-product, but the goal.

For instance, Murphy et al. has shown that a calcium phosphate coating can be precipitated onto a PLGA surface by incubating the polymer in an ion-rich simulated body fluid (SBF) solution (Murphy et al. 2000). After a 16 day incubation in the SBF at room temperature, a continuous, carbonated apatite coating was seen throughout the scaffold. The compressive modulus of the scaffold increased fivefold over the incubation as the apatite coating increased, all with no modification to the polymer itself. Other groups have sought to modify the polymeric surface to encourage a more rapid deposition of ceramic. Song et al. (2003) modified a poly(2-hydroxyethyl methacrylate) (pHEMA) polymeric scaffold to form a carboxylate-rich outer layer that would encourage the attachment and deposition of a ceramic layer by exposing carboxyl groups for ceramic deposition, leading to a better bond between the polymer and ceramic. The liberated ions from the dissolved hydroxyapatite precipitated on the surface of the treated pHEMA. X-ray diffraction confirmed that a nanocrystalline layer of hydroxyapatite had formed

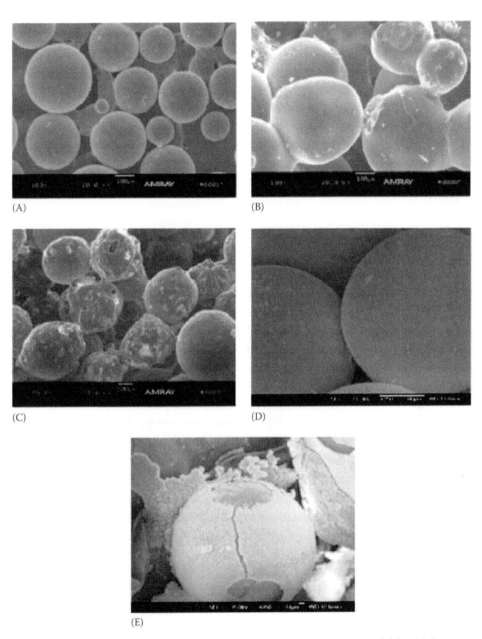

FIGURE 10.4 Scanning electron micrographs of (A) pure polymeric scaffolds, (B) low ceramic content scaffolds, and (C) high ceramic content scaffolds prior to SBF incubation. SEM micrographs of (D) pure polymeric scaffolds and (E) low ceramic content scaffolds after 6 weeks of incubation showing robust CaP precipitation on composite scaffolds but no evidence of precipitation with pure polymeric scaffolds. (With kind permission from Springer Science + Business Media: *J. Mater. Sci.*, In situ synthesized ceramic–polymer composites for bone tissue engineering: Bioactivity and degradation studies, 42(12), 2007, pp. 4183–4190, Khan, Y., Kelleher, J., Cushnie, E., Laurencin, C.T.)

on the surface of the polymer. Varma et al. (1999) incubated phosphorylated chitosan films in SBF for 20 days to induce a porous, poorly crystalline hydroxyapatite coating on top of the calcium phosphate layer. Lawson and Czernuszka (1999) performed a similar experiment with collagen films that were incubated in reservoirs of calcium and phosphate ions. This study demonstrated the ability to control the ceramic precipitate by varying the pH of the solution, with higher pH producing a calcium phosphate similar to poorly crystalline hydroxyapatite. It was also noted that both the amount of ceramic that precipitated on the surface and the compressive modulus of the composite increased as the concentration of ions in the solution increased as well. These ceramic surfaces were characterized and determined to possess a nanocrystalline phase, which has been shown to enhance both osteoblast adhesion and osteoclast functionality (Webster et al. 2000, 2001).

10.6.4 Stem Cells and Biomaterials in Regenerative Engineering

Central to the goals of regenerative engineering is the use of undifferentiated stem cells in combination with scaffolds designed to influence the fate of stem cells. Many researchers have sought the use of human MSCs in combination with scaffolds like porous ceramics to stimulate bone growth at the sites of fractures. It has been shown that MSCs in combination with a suitable scaffold possess a significant osteogenic potential and therefore lend themselves to being use to promote bone growth. Within the past 5 years, many studies performed by researchers around the world have utilized MSCs in conjunction with polymeric, ceramic, and metallic biomaterials to enhance bone repair but these studies are often difficult to assess against other published studies due to the lack of established standards of protocol. For instance, the ceramic-based studies often differ by the type of ceramic used and their osteoinductive abilities. While numerous successful *in vivo* animal studies (Caplan 2007) and *in vitro* cellular evaluations (Goldthwaite 2006) have been reported, variations in MSC isolation and culture techniques and the lack of consistent methodologies for MSC transplantation have made the use of MSCs as a clinical alternative still ahead of its time (Siddappa et al. 2007). Nevertheless, much work is being done toward better understanding how MSCs function in conjunction with biomaterials for orthopedic regeneration.

In a study performed in 2010, Janicki et al. attempted to solve this issue of clinical transplantation of MSCs. The group showed it is possible to induce *in vivo* endochondral ossification by chondrogenic pre induction of constructs composed of human MSC seeded on β-TCP granules and subsequently transplanted into immunodeficient mice, resulting in fully developed ossicles consisting of bone and marrow tissue (Janicki et al. 2010). In another study performed by Xu et al., *in vivo* bone-regenerative potential of a novel bioactive composite scaffold of glass–collagen–hyaluronic acid–phosphatidylserine (BG-COL-HYA-PS) hybridized with MSCs was investigated in a rat bone defect model. MSCs were cultured for 2 weeks *in vitro* on the scaffold before implantation into the defect. A cell-free scaffold and an untreated defect were used as controls. The results from histology, x-ray, and mechanical testing experiments revealed that the scaffold exhibited a low inflammatory response and foreign body response up to 3 weeks. At week 6, those responses disappeared after the resorption of scaffolds and the formation of new bone. Compared with the unseeded scaffold or empty defect group, MSCs seeded into the porous scaffold dramatically enhanced the efficiency of new bone formation and biomechanical integrity of the femur (Xu et al. 2010).

Another group studied posterolateral spinal fusion used in the treatment of patients with degenerative spinal disorders. In this study, they investigated the effectiveness of a MSC/hydroxyapatite/type I collagen hybrid graft for posterolateral spinal fusion in a rabbit model. The results suggested that the MSCs differentiated into osteoblasts and produced extracellular matrix in the hybrid graft. Increased alkaline phosphatase activity, indicative of stem cell differentiation toward the osteoblastic lineage, was noted as was mRNA of Cbfa-1 and osteopontin, also markers of the osteoblastic lineage. Radiographs and computed tomography images showed a continuous bone bridge and a satisfactory fusion mass incorporated into the transverse processes (Huang et al. 2011).

Other groups, including Zhao et al., have sought ways to form a mechanically strong injectable paste to help deliver stem cells to the defect site to engender bony growth. The group attempted to combine calcium phosphate cement (CPC) paste with injectable hydrogel microbeads that contained encapsulated human umbilical cord MSCs (hUCMSCs). The CPC–cell–hydrogel composite paste was fully injectable under small injection forces at no detriment to cells as cell viability matched that in hydrogel without CPC after injection. Mechanical properties of the construct matched reported values of cancellous bone, and were much higher than previous injectable polymeric and hydrogel carriers. hUCMSCs in the injectable constructs differentiated into osteoblasts, yielding high alkaline phosphatase, osteocalcin, collagen type I, and osterix gene expressions at 7 days (which were 50–70-fold higher than those at 1 day). Mineralization was seen after 14 days and was 100-fold than at 1 day. The encapsulated hUCMSCs remained viable, osteodifferentiated, and synthesized bone mineral supporting the conclusion that the new injectable stem cell construct with load-bearing capability may enhance bone regeneration in minimally invasive and other orthopedic surgeries (Zhao et al. 2010).

Guo et al. investigated the delivery of marrow MSCs both with and without transforming growth factor-β1 (TFG-β1), a well-characterized growth factor for bone formation, from biodegradable hydrogel composites on the repair of osteochondral defects in a rabbit model. This work investigated the delivery of marrow MSCs, with or without the growth factor (TGF-β1), from biodegradable hydrogel composites on the repair of osteochondral defects in a rabbit model (Guo et al. 2010).

Another animal model study performed by Peng et al. aimed to develop a novel approach for treatment of large bone defect in the femoral head in patients in which osteonecrosis has occurred. In this study, biphasic calcium phosphate (BCP) ceramic scaffolds were fabricated by a 3D gel lamination technique based on micro-computed tomography images of the cancellous bone microarchitecture of femoral heads and then seeded with autologous BM-derived MSCs *in vitro*. The cell–scaffold composite was implanted into a bone defect surgically induced in canine femoral head. The osteointegration and new bone formation was significantly greater with BCP scaffold implantation with than without BMSC seeding and showed greater strength and compressive modulus in the repair site.

Micro-CT-based bone ceramic scaffolds seeding with BMSC might be a promising way to repair bone defects in the femoral head (Peng et al. 2011). Many additional animal models have been used and many have shown the benefits of combining biomaterials like ceramics (Nair et al. 2009).

10.7 CONCLUSION

The field of orthopedic biomaterials has a long and successful history. A number of different implant materials spanning metals, polymers, and ceramics have been used and improved through continuous modification over the years, leaving us with highly specialized materials ideally suited to their particular tasks. Despite the significant advances in biomaterials for orthopedic applications, there are still identifiable deficits in their performance and considering a new approach is well supported. Toward this, researchers have been developing degradable polymers and resorbable ceramics that, rather than designed to be bioinert, are designed specifically to interact with the healing tissue and at a minimum support healing, and at a maximum enhance it. Regenerative engineering of bone seeks to capitalize on this approach toward bioactive materials by concentrating on the importance of the material itself and how these materials interact with undifferentiated cells to further enhance healing. While relatively new in its concept, bioactive materials for bone regeneration have been very successful thus far and their continued study and development is well supported, if not essential.

REFERENCES

Abu Bakar MS, Cheng MHW, Tang SM, Yu SC, Liao K, Tan CT, Khor KA, Cheang P. Tensile properties, tension–tension fatigue and biological response of polyetherketone–hydroxyapatite composites for load-bearing orthopedic implants. *Biomaterials.* 24:2245–2250, 2003.

Alberts B, Bray D, Lewis J, Raff M, Roberts K, Watson JD. *Molecular Biology of the Cell*, 3rd edn. Garland Publishing, Inc., New York, 1994.

Athanasiou KA, Zhu C, Lanctot DR, Agrawal CM, Wang X. Fundamentals of biomechanics in tissue engineering of bone. *Tissue Eng.* 6(4):361–381, 2000.

Aubin JE. Mesenchymal stem cells and osteoblast differentiation. In: *Principles of Bone Biology*, JP Bilezikian, LG Raisz, GA Rodan, eds. Academic Press, San Diego, CA, Chapter 4, pp. 85–107, 2008.

Aubin JE, Liu F. The osteoblast lineage. In: *Principles of Bone Biology*, JP Bilezikian, LG Raisz, GA Rodan, eds. Academic Press, San Diego, CA, Chapter 2, pp. 51–67, 1996.

Balac I, Uskokovic PS, Aleksic R, Uskokovic D. Predictive modeling of the mechanical properties of particulate hydroxyapatite reinforced polymer composites. *J Biomed Mater Res.* 63(6):793–799, 2002.

Bruder SP, Jaiswal N, Ricalton NS, Mosca JD, Kraus KH, Kadiyala S. Mesenchymal stem cells in osteobiology and applied bone regeneration. *Clin Orthop.* 355 Suppl:S247–S256, 1998.

Caplan AI. Adult mesenchymal stem cells for tissue engineering versus regenerative medicine. *J Cell Physiol.* 213(2):341–347, 2007.

Caputo E. Healing of bone and connective tissues. In: *Orthopaedics: Principles of Basic and Clinical Science*, F Bronner, RV Worrell, eds. CRC Press, Boca Raton, FL, pp. 201–216, 1999.

Carano RAD, Filvaroff EH. Angiogenesis and bone repair. *Drug Discov Today.* 8(21):980–989, 2003.

Claes L, Recknagel S, Ignatius A. Fracture healing under healthy and inflammatory conditions. *Nat Rev Rheumatol.* 8(3):133–43, 2012.

Costain DJ, Crawford RW. Fresh-frozen vs. irradiated allograft bone in orthopaedic reconstructive surgery. *Injury*. 40(12):1260–1264, 2009.

Cushnie E, Khan Y, Laurencin CT. Amorphous hydroxyapatite-sintered polymeric scaffolds for bone tissue regeneration: Physical characterization studies. *J Biomed Mater Res*. 84(1):54–62, 2008.

Daculsi G, LeGeros RZ, Heughebaert M, Barbieux I. Formation of carbonate–apatite crystals after implantation of calcium phosphate ceramics. *Calcif Tissue Int*. 46:20–27, 1990.

Daculsi G, LeGeros RZ, Nery E, Lynch K, Kerebel B. Transformation of biphasic calcium phosphate ceramics in vivo: Ultrastructural and physicochemical characterization. *J Biomed Mater Res*. 23:883–894, 1989.

de Bruijn JD, Bovell YP, van Blitterswijk CA. Structural arrangements at the interface between plasma sprayed calcium phosphates and bone. *Biomaterials*. 15(7):543–550, 1994.

Deng X, Hao J, Wang C. Preparation and mechanical properties of nanocomposites of poly(D,L-lactide) with Ca-deficient hydroxyapatite nanocrystals. *Biomaterials*. 22(21):2867–2873, 2001.

Deng M, Nair, LS, Nukavarapu SP, Kumbar SG, Jiang T, Krogman NR, Singh A, Allcock HR, Laurencin CT. Miscibility and in vitro osteocompatibility of biodegradable blends of poly[(ethyl alanato) (p-phenyl phenoxy) phosphazene] and poly(lactic acid–glycolic acid). *Biomaterials*. 29(3):337–349, 2008.

Deng M, Nair LS, Nukavarapu SP, Kumbar SG, Jiang T, Weikel AL, Krogman NR, Allcock HR, Laurencin CT. In situ porous structures: A unique polymer erosion mechanism in biodegradable dipeptide-based polyphosphazene and polyester blends producing matrices for regenerative engineering. *Adv Funct Mater*. 20(17):2794–2806, 2010.

Ducheyne P, Beight J, Cuckler J, Evans B, Radin S. Effect of calcium phosphate coating characteristics on early post-operative bone tissue growth. *Biomaterials*. 11(8):531–540, 1990.

Ducheyne P, Bianco P, Radin S, Schepers E. Bioactive materials: Mechanisms and bioengineering considerations. In: *Bone-Bonding*, P Ducheyne, T Kokubo, CA van Blitterswijk, eds. Reed Healthcare Communications, heiderdorp, Netherlands, pp. 1–12, 1992.

Durucan C, Brown PW. Calcium-deficient hydroxyapatite–PLGA composites: Mechanical and microstructural investigation. *J Biomed Mater Res*. 51(4):726–734, 2000a.

Durucan C, Brown PW. Low temperature formation of calcium-deficient hydroxyapatite–PLA/PLGA composites. *J Biomed Mater Res*. 51(4):717–725, 2000b.

Einhorn T. Biomechanics of bone. In: *Principles of Bone Biology*, JP Bilezikian, LG Raisz, GA Rodan, eds. Academic Press, San Diego, CA, Chapter 3, pp. 25–38, 1996.

Goldthwaite C. Using stem cells to build new bones: A tissue engineering frontier. In: *Regenerative Medicine*. Department of Health and Human Services, 2006.

Guo X, Park H, Young, S. Repair of osteochondral defects with biodegradable hydrogel composites encapsulating marrow mesenchymal stem cells in a rabbit model. *Acta Biomater*. 6(1):39–47, 2010.

Huang J, Lin S, Chen, L. The use of fluorescence-labeled mesenchymal stem cells in poly(lactide-co-glycolide)/hydroxyapatite/collagen hybrid graft as a bone substitute for posterolateral spinal fusion. *J Trauma*. 1495–1502, 2011.

Hutmacher D, Hürzeler MB, Schliephake H. A review of material properties of biodegradable and bioresorbable polymers and devices for GTR and GBR applications. *Int J Oral Maxillofac Implants*. 11(5):667–678, 1996.

Imai Y, Fukuzawa A, Watanabe M. Effect of blending tricalcium phosphate on hydrolytic degradation of a block polyester containing poly(L-lactic acid) segment. *J Biomater Sci Polym Edn*. 10(7):773–786, 1999.

Janicki P, Kasten P, Kleinschmidht K. Chondrogenic pre-induction of human mesenchymal stem cells on β-TCP: Enhanced bone quality by endochondral heterotopic bone formation. *Acta Biomater*. 6(8):3292–3301, 2010.

Jun YJ, Kim JH, Choi SJ, Lee HJ, Jun MJ, Sohn YS. A tetra(L-lysine)-grafted poly(organophosphazene) for gene delivery. *Bioorg Med Chem Lett*. 17(11):2975–2978, 2007.

Khan Y, Katti DS, Laurencin CT. A novel polymer-synthesized ceramic composite based system for bone repair: Osteoblast growth on scaffolds with varied calcium phosphate content. In: *Nanoscale Materials Science in Biology and Medicine*, CT Laurencin, E Botchwey, eds. *MRS Proceedings*, Materials Research Society, Warrendale, PA, Volume 845, pp. 63–67, 2005.

Khan Y, Kelleher J, Cushnie E, Laurencin CT. In situ synthesized ceramic–polymer composites for bone tissue engineering: Bioactivity and degradation studies. *J Mater Sci.* 42(12):4183–4190, 2007.

Khan Y, Laurencin CT. Fracture repair with ultrasound: Clinical and cell-based evaluation. *J Bone Joint Surg.* 90:138–144, 2008.

Khan Y, Yaszemski MJ, Mikos AG, Laurencin CT. Tissue engineering of bone: Material and matrix considerations. *J Bone Joint Surg.* 90:36–42, 2008.

Kim HM, Himeno T, Kokubo T, Nakamura T. Process and kinetics of bonelike apatite formation on sintered hydroxyapatite in a simulated body fluid. *Biomaterials.* 26(21):4366–4373, 2005.

Klein-Nulend J, Bonewald LF. The osteocyte. In: *Principles of Bone Biology*, JP Bilezikian, LG Raisz, GA Rodan, eds. Academic Press, San Diego, CA, Chapter 8, pp. 153–174, 2008.

Kokubo T, Kushitani H, Sakka S, Kitsugi T, Yamamuro T. Solutions able to reproduce in vivo surface-structure changes in bioactive glass-ceramic A-W. *J Biomed Mater Res.* 24(6):721–734, 1990.

Kurtz SM, Gawel HA, Patel JD. History and systematic review of wear and osteolysis outcomes for first-generation highly crosslinked polyethylene. *Clin Orthop Relat Res.* 469(8):2262–2277, 2011.

Laurencin C, Khan Y, El-Amin SF. Bone graft substitutes. *Expert Rev Med Dev.* 3(1):49–57, 2006.

Lawson AC, Czernuszka JT. Production and characterization of a collagen calcium phosphate composite for use as a bone substitute. *Mater Res Soc Symp Proc.* 550:273–278, 1999.

Leeson MC, Lippitt SB. Thermal aspects of the use of polymethylmethacrylate in large metaphyseal defects in bone. A clinical review and laboratory study. *Clin Orthop Relat Res.* (295):239–245, 1993.

Lin FH, Chen TM, Lin CP, Lee CJ. The merit of sintered PDLLA/TCP composites in management of bone fracture internal fixation. *Artif Organs.* 23(2):186–194, 1999.

Liu H, Pancholi M, Stubbs J III, Raghavan D. Influence of hydroxyvalerate composition of polyhydroxy butyrate valerate (PHBV) copolymer on bone cell viability and in vitro degradation. *J Appl Polymer Sci.* 116(6):3225–3231, 2010.

McKibbon B. The biology of fracture healing in long bones. *J Bone Joint Surg Br.* 60(2):150–162, 1978.

Middleton JC, Tipton AJ. Synthetic biodegradable polymers as orthopedic devices. *Biomaterials.* 21:2335–2346, 2000.

Morgan J, Holtman KR, Keller JC, Stanford CM. In vitro mineralization and implant calcium phosphate–hydroxyapatite crystallinity. *Implant Dent.* 5(4):264–271, 1996.

Mulari MT, Zhao H, Lakkakorpi PT, Vaananen HK. Osteoclast ruffled border has distinct subdomains for secretion and degraded matrix uptake. *Traffic.* 4(2):113–125, 2003.

Murphy WL, Kohn DH, Mooney DJ. Growth of continuous bonelike mineral within porous poly(lactide-co-glycolide) scaffolds in vitro. *J Biomed Mater Res.* 50(1):50–58, 2000.

Nair LS, Bhattacharyya S, Bender JD, Greish YE, Brown PW, Allcock HR, Laurencin CT. Fabrication and optimization of methylphenoxy substituted polyphosphazene nanofibers for biomedical applications. *Biomacromolecules.* 5(6):2212–2220, 2004.

Nair M, Varma H, Menon K. Reconstruction of goat femur segmental defects using triphasic ceramic-coated hydroxyapatite in combination with autologous cells and platelet-rich plasma. *Acta Biomater.* 5(5):1742–1755, 2009.

Nijweide PJ, Burger EH, Klein Nulend J, Van der Plas A. The osteocyte. In: *Principles of Bone Biology*, JP Bilezikian, LG Raisz, GA Rodan, eds. Academic Press, San Diego, CA, Chapter 9, pp. 115–126, 1996.

Nombela-Arrieta C, Ritz J, Silberstein LE. The elusive nature and function of mesenchymal stem cells. *Nat Rev Mol Cell Biol.* 12:126–131, 2011.

Nukavarapu SP, Kumbar SG, Brown JL, Krogman NR, Weikel AL, Hindenlang MD, Nair LS, Allcock HR, Laurencin CT. Polyphosphazene/nano-hydroxyapatite composite microsphere scaffolds for bone tissue engineering. *Biomacromolecules.* 9(7):1818–1825, 2008.

Oredein-McCoy O, Krogman NR, Weikel AL, Hindenlang MD, Allcock HR, Laurencin CT. Novel factor-loaded polyphosphazene matrices: Potential for driving angiogenesis. *J Microencapsul.* 26(6):544–555, 2009.

Park M-R, Chun C, Ahn S-W, Ki M-H, Cho C-S, Song S-C. Sustained delivery of human growth hormone using a polyelectrolyte complex-loaded thermosensitive polyphosphazene hydrogel. *J Control Release.* 147(3):359–367, 2010.

Park J, Lakes RS. *Biomaterials: An Introduction.* Springer, New York, 2007.

Peng J, Wen C, Wang A. Micro-CT-based bone ceramic scaffolding and its performance after seeding with mesenchymal stem cells for repair of load-bearing bone defect in canine femoral head. *J Biomed Mater Res B Appl Biomater.* 96(2):316–325, 2011.

Poitout D. *Biomechanics and Biomaterials in Orthopaedics.* Springer, Basel, Switzerland, 2004.

Potten CS, Loeffler M. Stem cells: attributes, cycles, spirals, pitfalls and uncertainties. Lessons for and from the crypt. *Development.* 110(4):1001–1020, 1990.

Posner AS. Crystal chemistry of bone mineral. *Physiol Rev.* 49:760–792, 1969.

Ratner BD, Hoffman AS, Schoen FJ, Lemons JE. *Biomaterials Science*, 2nd edn. Elsevier, San Diego, CA, 2004.

Ripamonti U. Osteoinduction in porous hydroxyapatite implanted in heterotopic sites of different animal models. *Biomaterials.* 17(1):31–35, 1996.

Sarkar MR, Wachter N, Patka P, Kinzl L. First histological observations on the incorporation of a novel calcium phosphate bone substitute material in human cancellous bone. *J Biomed Mater Res (Appl Biomater).* 58:329–334, 2001.

Schiller C, Epple M. Carbonated calcium phosphates are suitable pH-stabilizing fillers for biodegradable polyesters. *Biomaterials.* 24(12):2037–2043, 2003.

Siddappa R, Licht C, van Blitterswijk J. Donor variation and loss of multipotency during in vitro expansion of human mesenchymal stem cells for bone tissue engineering. *J Orthop Res.* 25(8):1029–1041, 2007.

Sims, NA, Baron R. Bone: Structure, function, growth and remodeling. In: *Orthopaedics*, R Fitzgerald, H Kaufer, AL Malkani, eds. Mosby, Inc., Philadelphia, PA, Section 2, Chapter 2, pp. 147–159, 2002.

Sobieraj MC, Rimnac CM. Ultra high molecular weight polyethylene: Mechanics, morphology, and clinical behavior. *J Mech Behav Biomed Mater.* 2(5):433–443, 2009.

Song J, Saiz E, Bertozzi CR. A new approach to mineralization of biocompatible hydrogel scaffolds: An efficient process toward 3-dimensional bonelike composites. *JACS.* 125:1236–1243, 2003.

Ulery BD, Nair LS, Laurencin CT. Biomedical applications of biodegradable polymers. *J Polym Sci B Polym Phys.* 49(12):832–864, 2011.

Van Landuyt P, Li F, Keustermans JP, Streydio JM, Delannay F, Munting E. The influence of high sintering temperatures on the mechanical properties of hydroxyapatite. *J Mater Sci Mater Med.* 6:8–13, 1995.

Varma HK, Yokogawa Y, Espinosa FF, Kawamoto Y, Nishizawa K, Nagata F, Kameyama T. Porous calcium phosphate coating over phosphorylated chitosan film by a biomimetic method. *Biomaterials.* 20(9):879–884, 1999.

Wang X, Li Y, Wei J, de Groot K. Development of biomimetic nanohydroxyapatite/poly(hexamethylene adipamide) composites. *Biomaterials.* 23:4787–4791, 2002.

Webster TJ, Ergun C, Doremus RH, Siegel RW, Bizios R. Specific proteins mediate enhanced osteoblast adhesion on nanophase ceramics. *J Biomed Mater Res.* 51(3):475–483, 2000.

Webster TJ, Ergun C, Doremus RH, Siegel RW, Bizios R. Enhanced osteoclast like cell functions on nanophase ceramics. *Biomaterials.* 22(11):1327–1333, 2001.

Xu C, Su P, Weng Y. A novel biomimetic composite scaffold hybridized with mesenchymal stem cells in repair of rat bone defects models. *J Biomed Mater Res A.* 95(2):495–503, 2010.

Yang Y, Xu Z, Chen S, Gao Y, Gu Y, Chen L, Pei Y, Li Y. Histidylated cationic polyorganophosphazene/DNA self-assembled nanoparticles for gene delivery. *Int J Pharm.* 353(1–2), 277–282, 2008.

Yang Y, Zhang Z, Chen L, Gu W, Li Y. Urocanic acid improves transfection efficiency of polyphosphazene with primary amino groups for gene delivery. *Bioconjug Chem.* 21, 419–426, 2010.

Zhang JX, Li XJ, Qiu LY, Li XH, Yan MQ, Jin Y, Zhu KJ. Indomethacin-loaded polymeric nanocarriers based on amphiphilic polyphosphazenes with poly(*N*-isopropylacrylamide) and ethyl tryptophan as side groups: Preparation, in vitro and in vivo evaluation. *J Control Release.* 116(3), 322–329, 2006.

Zhao L, Weir M, Xu H. An injectable calcium phosphate-alginate hydrogel–umbilical cord mesenchymal stem cell paste for bone tissue engineering. *Biomaterials.* 6502–6510, 2010.

CHAPTER 11

Engineering Tissue-to-Tissue Interfaces

Nancy M. Lee, MEng; Nora T. Khanarian, PhD;

Jung Hyun Park, PhD; and Helen H. Lu, PhD

CONTENTS

11.1 INTRODUCTION

Orthopedic injuries and diseases commonly affect soft tissues such as ligaments and tendons, which connect bone to bone and muscle to bone, respectively. While recent developments in tissue engineering have led to advancements in the regeneration of these tissues, much less attention has been paid to the interfaces or insertion sites that connect these soft tissues to bone. Orthopedic interfaces exhibit a gradient of structural and mechanical properties. The integrity of these regions are essential to facilitating synchronized joint motion, mediating load transfer between distinct tissue types and sustaining heterotypic cellular communication necessary for interface function and homeostasis (Benjamin et al. 1986; Lu and Jiang 2006; Woo et al. 1988). However, these critical junctions are also prone to injury, and healing is typically incomplete after surgical repair. The need for interface regeneration is underscored by the fact that the failure to restore the intricate tissue-to-tissue interface has been reported to compromise graft stability and long-term clinical outcome (Friedman et al. 1985; Robertson et al. 1986).

This chapter reviews the current biological fixation strategies aimed at engineering the junction between soft tissue and bone. The interface tissue engineering challenge is rooted in the complexity of the musculoskeletal system and the structural intricacy of both hard and soft tissues. Although these tissues are comprised of distinct cellular populations, both must operate in unison to facilitate physiological function and maintain homeostasis. Interfaces often exhibit a unique biochemical composition, which is distinct from the tissues they connect. Furthermore, the transition between various tissue types is characterized by a high level of heterogeneous structural organization. In light of this complexity, functional tissue engineering involves utilizing cells, growth factors, and biomaterial scaffolds in a variety of ways to engineer tissues *in vitro* and *in vivo*. This chapter focuses on complex scaffold design currently used to regenerate soft tissue-to-bone interfaces, in particular the ligament-to-bone and tendon-to-bone interface. Each section will begin with a brief description of the current understanding of the requirements for biomimetic and functional interface scaffold design, which have been distilled through characterization of the structure–function understandings of the native interface. This is followed by a brief review of scaffold design currently researched for soft tissue-to-bone interface tissue engineering. Lastly, potential challenges and future directions in this rapidly expanding area of functional tissue engineering will be discussed.

11.2 SCAFFOLD DESIGN FOR LIGAMENT-TO-BONE INTERFACE TISSUE ENGINEERING

Ligaments connect bone to bone and are composed primarily of collagenous fibers. The Anterior cruciate ligament (ACL) is one of the four primary ligaments in the human knee and is the most commonly injured knee ligament with ~100,000 reconstruction surgeries reported annually in the United States (Gotlin and Huie 2000). Current treatment solutions for ACL reconstruction include biological (allografts, autografts) and synthetic grafts. However when the interface is involved in ACL injuries, it is crucial to achieve functional integration of these grafts with the existing host environment. Various approaches for 3D scaffold design have been recently studied for ACL regeneration, and those which mimic the native interface with gradual changes of mechanical, structural, and biological properties are highly desirable (Table 11.1).

Elucidation of the structure–function relationship at this ligament-to-bone junction is essential for ACL regeneration. Given that the ACL insertion site is representative of other soft tissue-to-bone interfaces (Spalazzi et al. 2006c), these understandings also have a broader impact to the field of orthopedic tissue engineering. The ligament-to-bone junction is characterized by the transition from three distinct tissues (ligament, fibrocartilage, and bone); fibrocartilage tissue is further divided into mineralized and non mineralized regions. The ligament region is composed of fibroblasts embedded in a collagenous matrix. The non mineralized fibrocartilage consists of chondrocytes in a proteoglycan-rich matrix containing collagen I and II. The mineralized fibrocartilage zone includes chondrocytes surrounded by a calcified matrix containing collagen X. Finally, subchondral bone is made up of osteoblasts, osteoclasts, and osteocytes in a mineralized collagen matrix. The existence of the fibrocartilage transition reduces the accumulation of stress concentrations and enables the transfer of complex loads between soft and hard tissues.

Early efforts to design and fabricate 3D scaffolds for the ligament-to-bone interface focused on improving the fixation of ligament grafts with bone. For example, ceramic materials such as calcium phosphate cements help to improve bone tissue growth and organization in animal ACL reconstruction procedures (Huangfu and Zhao 2007; Tien et al. 2004). Tendons have been coated with a calcium phosphate layer prior to surgery

TABLE 11.1   Scaffolds for Ligament-to-Bone Tissue Engineering

Study	Scaffold Design	Study Model	Outcomes
Dunn et al. (1992)	Collagen fibers with PMMA bone fixation plugs	*In vivo*/Rabbit model	Supported development of functional neoligament tissue
Bitar et al. (2005)	Phosphate-based fibers	*In vitro*/Human osteoblasts and fibroblasts	Cell differentiation maintained by both cell types and strongly related to fiber composition
1. Lu et al. (2005) 2. Cooper et al. (2007)	Multi-region knitted PLLA fiber scaffold	1. *In vitro*/Rabbit ACL cells 2. *In vivo*/Rabbit model with primary ACL cells	1. Supported long-term matrix deposition 2. Demonstrated scaffold healing and mechanical strength *in vivo*
Spalazzi et al. (2006a)	Triphasic Phase A: PLGA mesh Phase B: PLGA (85:15) microspheres Phase C: PLGA–bioglass composite	*In vitro*/Bovine fibroblast (phase A), osteoblast (phase C) coculture	Supported cell proliferation and matrix production while maintaining distinct cellular regions
Phillips et al. (2008)	3D poly(L-lysine) retrovirus gradient	*In vitro*/Rat dermal fibroblasts	Cells displayed spatial patterns of transcription factor expression, differentiation. and matrix deposition
Spalazzi et al. (2008a)	Triphasic Phase A: PLGA mesh Phase B: PLGA (85:15) microspheres Phase C: PLGA–bioglass composite	*In vivo*/Rat model with bovine, fibroblasts, chondrocytes, osteoblasts	Interface-like matrix heterogeneity maintained
Spalazzi et al. (2008b)	PLGA (85:15) nanofibers PLGA (85:15) microspheres	*In vitro*/Bovine patellar tendon graft	Upregulation of fibrocartilage markers after 7 days of tendon compression
Ma et al. (2009)	Ligament–bone constructs from rat BMSC	*In vivo*/Rat model	Tissues grew and remodeled quickly with partial restoration of knee function
Paxton et al. (2009)	Poly(ethylene glycol) hydrogel with HA	*In vitro*/Rat Achilles tendon fibroblasts	Inclusion of HA in PEG hydrogel enhanced mechanical strength and cell attachment
1. Paxton et al. (2010a) 2. Paxton et al. (2010b)	Brushite cement anchors with cell-seeded fibrin gels	*In vitro*/Rat Achilles tendon fibroblasts	1. Anchor shape altered longevity and strength of the bone–ligament interface 2. SEM and Raman microscopy suggested regeneration of tidemark between brushite and cell-seeded gel
Lee et al. (2011)	PLCL (60:40 mol%) scaffold with (1) fibrochondrocyte and BMP2 delivered via heparin hydrogel and (2) fibroblast regions	*In vitro*/Rabbit patellar ligament fibroblasts and meniscal fibrochondrocytes *In vivo*/Murine model with rabbit fibroblasts and fibrochondrocytes	*In vitro* and *in vivo* studies confirm increased calcium and GAG production and increased mechanical properties of hydrogel-containing scaffold

intended to foster integration with bone (Mutsuzaki et al. 2004). In another example, periosteum grafts in conjunction with growth factors have been shown to enhance bone tunnel osteointegration (Chen et al. 2003; Kyung et al. 2003; Rodeo et al. 1999). However, these efforts centered on developing single-phased scaffolds have limited potential for regenerating the multi region ligament-to-bone interface. Consequently, the resultant graft–bone junction continues to exhibit poor mechanical stability, which remains one of the primary causes of graft failure. Therefore, biomimetic scaffolds that recapitulate the complexity of the multilayered ligament-to-bone interface are needed.

The ideal scaffold design for regenerating the ligament-to-bone interface is a stratified scaffold that mimics the three distinct tissue regions found in native tissue. The scaffold should support the growth and differentiation of the relevant cell populations, directing cellular interactions, as well as promoting the formation and maintenance of extracellular matrix heterogeneity. The scaffold must also exhibit a gradation in mechanical properties that mimics the native insertion site, with magnitudes comparable to those of the ligament-to-bone interface. An additional consideration is that the scaffold must be biodegradable at a relevant timescale in order to be gradually replaced by the host tissue. Finally, in order to be clinically relevant, the engineered graft must be easily adaptable with current ACL reconstruction grafts, or pre incorporated into the design of ligament replacement grafts.

Inspired by these design criteria, Spalazzi et al. (2006a) reported on a triphasic scaffold for ligament-to-bone interface tissue engineering. Each phase of the scaffold—phase A (ligament), phase B (fibrocartilage), and phase C (bone)—is fabricated from poly(lactide-*co*-glycolide) (PLGA), each with varying ratios of PGA and PLA. Phases A, B, and C consist of PLGA (10:90) mesh, PLGA (85:15) microspheres, and sintered PLGA (85:15) and bioactive glass composite microspheres, respectively. This innovative approach centers on a single integrated scaffold with three distinct but continuous phases. Using this stratified scaffold, the interactions between the three interface-relevant cell populations, fibroblasts, chondrocytes, and osteoblasts, were evaluated both *in vitro* and *in vivo*. *In vitro* assessment revealed that fibroblasts and osteoblasts were selectively distributed on phases A and C, respectively, whereas both cell types were co localized on phase B (Spalazzi et al. 2006a). Furthermore, *in vivo* tri culture of fibroblasts (phase A), chondrocytes (phase B), and osteoblasts (phase C) resulted in abundant matrix production and tissue infiltration (Spalazzi et al. 2008a; Figure 11.1).

These pioneering studies the potential that multiphase biomimetic scaffolds coupled with the spatial control of interface-relevant cell types have in the regeneration of multiple tissue types using a single scaffold system. In terms of clinical application, the triphasic scaffold can be used to guide the re establishment of an anatomic fibrocartilage interfacial region directly on soft tissue grafts. Specifically, the scaffold can be utilized as a graft collar during ACL reconstruction. The feasibility of such an approach was recently demonstrated with a mechanoactive scaffold based on a composite of PLGA 85:15 nanofibers and sintered microspheres (Spalazzi et al. 2008b). It was observed that scaffold-induced compression of tendon grafts resulted in significant matrix remodeling and the upregulation of fibrocartilage interface-related markers such as type II collagen, aggrecan, and transforming

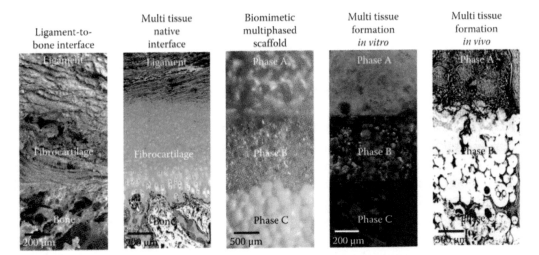

| Ligament-to-bone interface | Multi tissue native interface | Biomimetic multiphased scaffold | Multi tissue formation *in vitro* | Multi tissue formation *in vivo* |

FIGURE 11.1 Soft tissue-to-bone repair. The native ligament-to-bone interface exhibits distinct yet continuous tissue regions, including ligament, fibrocartilage, and bone (Neonatal Bovine: SEM 5 kV, 30×; Histology-Modified Goldner Masson Trichrome Stain). A triphasic stratified scaffold mimics multiphase tissues. *In vitro* co-culture of fibroblasts and osteoblasts on the triphasic scaffold induced a segregation of specific cell types and matrix deposition on phases. Fibroblasts and osteoblasts were selectively localized on phases A and C, respectively. Both cell types were co-localized on phase B. Distinct tissue regions were formed on the triphasic scaffold *in vivo*.

growth factor β3 (TGF-β3). These results suggest that the stratified scaffold can be used to induce the formation of an anatomic fibrocartilage interface directly onto biological ACL reconstruction grafts.

In summary, a promising strategy to achieving ligament-to-bone interface regeneration is to first address the difficult problem of soft tissue-to-bone integration *ex vivo* by pre-engineering the multi tissue interface through a stratified scaffold design, and then focusing on the relatively less challenging task of bone-to-bone integration *in vivo*. In the design of such scaffolds, one must consider that each region of the scaffold must be engineered with physiologically relevant mechanical properties. Building upon this scaffold-based approach, interface-relevant cell types, and bioactive molecules, such as growth factors and cytokines, can also be integrated into the stratified scaffold as efforts to recapitulate the complex nanoscale to microscale organization of the native ligament-to-bone interface.

11.3 SCAFFOLD DESIGN FOR TENDON-TO-BONE INTERFACE TISSUE ENGINEERING

The tendon-to-bone interface displays a zonal distribution of cells and extracellular matrix components, similar to that of the ligament-to-bone interface (Benjamin et al. 1986; Blevins et al. 1997). While the tendon-to-bone and ligament-to-bone interfaces are physiological and biochemically similar, differences arise in the loading environment, mineral distribution, and surgical repair methods. Thus it is expected that the tissue engineering strategies applied should also differ. To date, current efforts in tendon-to-bone interface tissue engineering have centered on rotator cuff repair. There is a clear clinical need for functional solutions to integrative tendon-to-bone repair, as existing surgical strategies and mechanical fixation methods for rotator cuff repair often result in the incomplete healing of these complex tissues and are associated with a high incidence of failure (Coons and Alan 2006; Derwin et al. 2006; Galatz et al. 2004; Iannotti et al. 2006). Grafting solutions, designed to target interface formation and biological fixation, are thus necessary to address this challenge. Several groups have evaluated the feasibility of integrating tendon with bone or biomaterials through the formation of an anatomic insertion site. By surgically reattaching tendon to bone using a rat Achilles tendon avulsion model, Fujioka et al. (1998) reported cellular reorganization at the reattachment site, along with the formation of calcified and noncalcified fibrocartilage-like regions. Additionally, periosteum (Chang et al. 2009) and demineralized bone matrix (Sundar et al. 2009) have been explored for tendon-to-bone interface regeneration. The periosteum is known to be a source of multipotent stem cells that have the potential to differentiate into osteogenic and chondrogenic lineages. Chang et al. (2009) sutured a periosteal flap between the torn end of a rabbit infraspinatus tendon and bone. At 4 weeks, fibrous tissue was observed at the interface between the rotator cuff tendon and bone, which later remodeled into a fibrocartilage-like matrix after 12 weeks. A significant increase in failure load over time indicated a progressive increase in tendon-to-bone integration with healing. Demineralized bone matrix (DBM), which has also demonstrated osteogenic and chondrogenic properties, was explored by Sundar et al. (2009) in a patellar tendon ovine model. DBM was interposed between patellar tendon and osteotomized bone and resulted in significantly improved function weight bearing as well as the deposition of fibrocartilage and mineralized fibrocartilage at the tendon-to-bone interface (Table 11.2).

The delivery of osteoinductive growth factors (Rodeo et al. 2007) and the inhibition of matrix metalloproteinases (MMP) during the healing process (Bedi et al. 2010; Gulotta et al. 2010) have also been explored to improve tendon-to-bone integration. Rodeo et al. (2007) utilized a type I collagen sponge to deliver a mixture of osteoinductive growth factors, harvested from platelet-rich plasma, to the infraspinatus tendon-to-bone interface in an ovine model. Enhanced bone, soft tissue, and fibrocartilage formation, as well as an increase in tendon attachment strength were noted in the growth factor treated groups. Bedi et al. (2010) explored the effect of MMP inhibition on tendon-to-bone healing and insertion site regeneration in a rat rotator cuff model. Recombinant α-2 macroglobulin (A2M) protein, a universal MMP inhibitor, was applied at the tendon-to-bone interface, resulting in enhanced fibrocartilage formation, greater collagen organization, and a reduction in collagen degradation.

In addition to biological grafts and cytokines, synthetic biomaterials have been investigated for tendon-to-bone integration. Implantation of a polyglycolide fiber mesh in a rat model was shown to lead to the formation of an organized fibrovascular matrix at the infraspinatus tendon-to-bone junction (Yokoya et al. 2008). Recently, nanofiber scaffolds have been explored for tendon-to-bone interface tissue engineering, largely due to their biomimetic potential and physiological relevance. Through modification of fabrication methods, these scaffolds can be fabricated to match the native tendon matrix,

TABLE 11.2   Scaffolds for Tendon-to-Bone Tissue Engineering

Study	Scaffold Design	Study Model	Outcomes
Chang et al. (2009)	Periosteum attached to end of transected end of tendon	*In vivo*/Infraspinatus tendon–bone repair in rabbit model	1. Extensive fibrocartilage and bone formation at interface 2. Significant increase in failure load at interface region over time
Li et al. (2009)	PLGA and PCL nanofibers (unaligned) with a gradient of calcium phosphate across scaffold	*In vitro*/MC3T3 cells (mouse preosteoblasts)	1. Gradation in mineral across scaffold produced a gradient in stiffness 2. Gradient in cell density observed, higher in regions of increased mineral concentration
Sundar et al. (2009)	Demineralized bone matrix (DBM) interposed between tendon and bone	*In vivo*/Patellar–patellar tendon–bone repair in ovine model	Augmentation with DBM increased area of fibrocartilage and mineralized fibrocartilage found at interface
Moffat et al. (2009a,b)	PLGA (85:15) nanofiber scaffolds (aligned and unaligned)	*In vitro*/human rotator cuff tendon fibroblasts	1. Tendon fibroblasts organized and produced matrix oriented according to the underlying nanofiber organization 2. Matrix deposition and scaffold mechanical properties mimicked that of human rotator cuff tendons
Moffat et al. (2010, 2011)	Biphasic nanofiber-based scaffold (aligned): Phase A: PLGA (85:15) Phase B: PLGA + HA	*In vitro*/bovine full thickness chondrocytes and *In vivo*/rat mesenchymal stem cells in an athymic rat model	1. Scaffold mineral distribution mimics that of native insertion sites 2. Synthesis of fibrocartilage-like matrix on phases A and B 3. Regional mineral distribution maintained 4. Increase in mineral density and osteointegration over time
Xie et al. (2010)	PLGA nanofiber scaffold with an aligned-to-random gradient in structure	*In vitro*/rat tendon fibroblasts	Both scaffold regions supported cell proliferation and collagen type I deposition. Cell morphology and matrix deposition oriented according to nanofiber organization

with controlled alignment, high surface area-to-volume ratio, permeability, and porosity (Li et al. 2002, 2007; Ma et al. 2005; Pham et al. 2006). Moffat et al. (2009a) evaluated the effects of PLGA nanofiber organization (aligned vs. unaligned) on human tendon fibroblast attachment and matrix deposition. Nanofiber alignment was found to be the primary factor guiding tendon fibroblast morphology, alignment, and integrin expression. Types I and III collagen, the dominant collagen types of the supraspinatus tendon, were synthesized on the nanofiber scaffolds and it was shown that their deposition was also controlled by the underlying fiber orientation. Furthermore, scaffold mechanical properties, which were directly related to fiber alignment, decreased as the polymer degraded but remained within range of those reported for the native supraspinatus tendon (Itoi et al. 1995).

Building upon these promising results, Moffat et al. (2008) designed a stratified, composite nanofiber system consisting of distinct yet continuous noncalcified and calcified regions intended to mimic the organization of native tendon-to-bone insertion. The biphasic scaffold was produced by electrospinning, with phase A comprised of aligned PLGA nanofibers to support the regeneration of the non mineralized fibrocartilage region, and phase B, which is based on aligned PLGA nanofibers embedded with nanoparticles of hydroxyapatite (PLGA-HA) to support the regeneration of the mineralized fibrocartilage region. The biphasic scaffold design has been evaluated both *in vitro* and *in vivo* (Moffat et al. 2010). A chondrocyte-mediated fibrocartilage-like extracellular matrix was found on each scaffold phase mineral distribution was also maintained, with a calcified fibrocartilage formed on phase B through which the biphasic scaffold can integrate with the surrounding bone tissue.

These studies collectively demonstrate the importance of regenerating the tendon-to-bone interface and the promise of different tissue-engineering methodologies for achieving tendon-to-bone healing and integration. Functional tendon-to-bone interface tissue engineering focuses on the design of biomimetic scaffolds that are pre engineered to recapitulate the inherent structural, mechanical, and biochemical heterogeneity of the native interface. To this end, biomaterials, combined with physiologically relevant growth factors and cytokines to guide cellular differentiation, have shown immense potential in enhancing tendon-to-bone integration.

11.4 SUMMARY AND FUTURE DIRECTIONS

This chapter provides an overview of current concepts in interface tissue engineering, focusing on strategies for the design of biomimetic scaffolds fabricated that exhibit a gradation of mechanical and structural properties. Specifically, stratified scaffolds have been designed to mimic the structure and function of the native soft tissue-to-bone interface while exercising spatial control over heterotypic cell interactions and supporting the formation of integrated multi tissue systems. The vast potential of multiphased scaffold systems is evident from the *in vitro* and *in vivo* evaluations described here for the integrative repair of ligament and tendon injuries. Moreover, these novel scaffolds can be further refined by incorporating well controlled compositional and growth factor gradients, as well as through the use of biochemical and biomechanical stimulation to encourage tissue growth and maturation. It is anticipated that functional and integrative soft tissue repair will be realized through the coupling of cell-based and scaffold-based approaches. Clinically, stratified scaffolds would significantly improve current soft tissue repair strategies by encouraging functional integration with host tissue and stimulating interface formation while also enabling biological fixation.

While it is apparent that interface tissue engineering will be instrumental for the *ex vivo* development and *in vivo* regeneration of integrated musculoskeletal tissue systems with biomimetic functionality, there remains a number of challenges in this exciting area. These include the need for a greater understanding of the structure–function relationship existing at the native tissue-to-tissue interface, as well as the precise biological mechanisms governing interface development and regeneration. Furthermore, the *in vivo* host environment, in addition to the precise effects of biological, chemical, and physical stimulation on interface regeneration must be thoroughly evaluated to enable the formation and homeostasis of the neo interface. Physiologically relevant *in vivo* models are also needed to determine the clinical potential of the designed scaffolds. In summary, regeneration of tissue-to-tissue junctions through interface tissue engineering using either biological or tissue-engineered grafts represents a promising strategy for achieving biological fixation and integrative soft tissue repair. It is anticipated that these efforts will lead to the development of a new generation of functional fixation devices for soft tissue repair as well as augmenting the clinical translation potential of tissue-engineered grafts. Moreover, by bridging distinct types of tissue, interface tissue engineering will be instrumental for the development of integrated musculoskeletal tissue systems or total joint systems with biomimetic complexity and functionality.

REFERENCES

Bedi, A., Kovacevic, D., Hettrich, C., Gulotta, L. V., Ehteshami, J. R., Warren, R. F., and Rodeo, S. A. 2010. The effect of matrix metalloproteinase inhibition on tendon-to-bone healing in a rotator cuff repair model. *J. Shoulder. Elbow. Surg.* 19:384–391.

Benjamin, M., Evans, E. J., and Copp, L. 1986. The histology of tendon attachments to bone in man. *J. Anat.* 149:89–100.

Bitar, M., Knowles, C., Lewis, M. P., and Salih, V. 2005. Soluble phosphate glass fibres for repair of bone-ligament interface. *J. Mater. Sci. Mater. Med.* 16:1131–1136.

Blevins, F. T., Djurasovic, M., Flatow, E. L., and Vogel, K. G. 1997. Biology of the rotator cuff tendon. *Orthop. Clin. North Am.* 28:1–16.

Chang, C. H., Chen, C. H., Su, C. Y., Liu, H. T., and Yu, C. M. 2009. Rotator cuff repair with periosteum for enhancing tendon–bone healing: A biomechanical and histological study in rabbits. *Knee Surg. Sports Traumatol. Arthrosc* 17:1447–1453.

Chen, C. H., Chen, W. J., Shih, C. H., Yang, C. Y., Liu, S. J., and Lin, P. Y. 2003. Enveloping the tendon graft with periosteum to enhance tendon–bone healing in a bone tunnel: A biomechanical and histologic study in rabbits. *Arthroscopy* 19:290–296.

Coons, D. A. and Alan, B. F. 2006. Tendon graft substitutes–rotator cuff patches. *Sports Med. Arthrosc.* 14:185–190.

Cooper, J. A., Jr., Sahota, J. S., Gorum, W. J., Carter, J., Doty, S. B., and Laurencin, C. T. 2007. Biomimetic tissue-engineered anterior cruciate ligament replacement. *Proc. Natl. Acad. Sci. USA* 104:3049–3054.

Derwin, K. A., Baker, A. R., Spragg, R. K., Leigh, D. R., and Iannotti, J. P. 2006. Commercial extracellular matrix scaffolds for rotator cuff tendon repair. Biomechanical, biochemical, and cellular properties. *J. Bone Joint Surg. Am.* 88:2665–2672.

Dunn, M. G., Tria, A. J., Kato, Y. P., Bechler, J. R., Ochner, R. S., Zawadsky, J. P., and Silver, F. H. 1992. Anterior cruciate ligament reconstruction using a composite collagenous prosthesis. A biomechanical and histologic study in rabbits. *Am. J. Sports Med.* 20:507–515.

Friedman, M. J., Sherman, O. H., Fox, J. M., Del Pizzo, W., Snyder, S. J., and Ferkel, R. J. 1985. Autogeneic anterior cruciate ligament (ACL) anterior reconstruction of the knee. A review. *Clin. Orthop.* 196:9–14.

Fujioka, H., Thakur, R., Wang, G. J., Mizuno, K., Balian, G., and Hurwitz, S. R. 1998. Comparison of surgically attached and non-attached repair of the rat Achilles tendon–bone interface. Cellular organization and type X collagen expression. *Connect. Tissue Res.* 37:205–218.

Galatz, L. M., Ball, C. M., Teefey, S. A., Middleton, W. D., and Yamaguchi, K. 2004. The outcome and repair integrity of completely arthroscopically repaired large and massive rotator cuff tears. *J. Bone Joint Surg. Am.* 86-A:219–224.

Gotlin, R. S. and Huie, G. 2000. Anterior cruciate ligament injuries. Operative and rehabilitative options. *Phys. Med. Rehabil. Clin. N. Am.* 11:895–928.

Gulotta, L. V., Kovacevic, D., Montgomery, S., Ehteshami, J. R., Packer, J. D., and Rodeo, S. A. 2010. Stem cells genetically modified with the developmental gene *MT1–MMP* improve regeneration of the supraspinatus tendon-to-bone insertion site. *Am. J. Sports Med.* 38:1429–1437.

Huangfu, X. and Zhao, J. 2007. Tendon–bone healing enhancement using injectable tricalcium phosphate in a dog anterior cruciate ligament reconstruction model. *Arthroscopy* 23:455–462.

Iannotti, J. P., Codsi, M. J., Kwon, Y. W., Derwin, K., Ciccone, J., and Brems, J. J. 2006. Porcine small intestine submucosa augmentation of surgical repair of chronic two-tendon rotator cuff tears. A randomized, controlled trial. *J. Bone Joint Surg. Am.* 88:1238–1244.

Itoi, E., Berglund, L. J., Grabowski, J. J., Schultz, F. M., Growney, E. S., Morrey, B. F., and An, K. N. 1995. Tensile properties of the supraspinatus tendon. *J. Orthop. Res.* 13:578–584.

Kyung, H. S., Kim, S. Y., Oh, C. W., and Kim, S. J. 2003. Tendon-to-bone tunnel healing in a rabbit model: The effect of periosteum augmentation at the tendon-to-bone interface. *Knee Surg. Sports Traumatol. Arthrosc.* 11:9–15.

Lee, J., Il Choi, W., Tae, G., Kim, Y. H., Kang, S. S., Kim, S. E., Kim, S. H., Jung, Y., and Kim, S. H. 2011. Enhanced regeneration of the ligament-bone interface using a poly(L-lactide-co-epsilon-caprolactone) scaffold with local delivery of cells/BMP-2 using a heparin-based hydrogel. *Acta Biomater.* 7:244–257.

Li, W. J., Laurencin, C. T., Caterson, E. J., Tuan, R. S., and Ko, F. K. 2002. Electrospun nanofibrous structure: A novel scaffold for tissue engineering. *J. Biomed. Mater. Res.* 60:613–621.

Li, W. J., Mauck, R. L., Cooper, J. A., Yuan, X., and Tuan, R. S. 2007. Engineering controllable anisotropy in electrospun biodegradable nanofibrous scaffolds for musculoskeletal tissue engineering. *J. Biomech.* 40:1686–1693.

Li, X. R., Xie, J. W., Lipner, J., Yuan, X. Y., Thomopoulos, S., and Xia, Y. N. 2009. Nanofiber scaffolds with gradations in mineral content for mimicking the tendon-to-bone insertion site. *Nano Letters* 9:2763–2768.

Lu, H. H., Cooper, J. A., Jr., Manuel, S., Freeman, J. W., Attawia, M. A., Ko, F. K., and Laurencin, C. T. 2005. Anterior cruciate ligament regeneration using braided biodegradable scaffolds: In vitro optimization studies. *Biomaterials* 26:4805–4816.

Lu, H. H. and Jiang, J. 2006. Interface tissue engineering and the formulation of multiple-tissue systems. *Adv. Biochem. Eng. Biotechnol.* 102:91–111.

Ma, J., Goble, K., Smietana, M., Kostrominova, T., Larkin, L., and Arruda, E. M. 2009. Morphological and functional characteristics of three-dimensional engineered bone-ligament-bone constructs following implantation. *J. Biomech. Eng.* 131:101017.

Ma, Z., Kotaki, M., Inai, R., and Ramakrishna, S. 2005. Potential of nanofiber matrix as tissue-engineering scaffolds. *Tissue Eng.* 11:101–109.

Moffat, K. L. 2010. Biomimetic nanofiber scaffold design for tendon-to-bone interface tissue engineering, PhD thesis, Columbia University, New York.

Moffat, K. L., Kwei, A. S., Spalazzi, J. P., Doty, S. B., Levine, W. N., and Lu, H. H. 2009a. Novel nanofiber-based scaffold for rotator cuff repair and augmentation. *Tissue Eng. Part A* 15:115–126.

Moffat, K. L., Levine, W. N., and Lu, H. H. 2008. *In vitro* evaluation of rotator cuff tendon fibroblasts on aligned composite scaffold of polymer nanofibers and hydroxyapatite nanoparticles. *Transactions of the 54th Orthopaedic Research Society.*

Moffat, K. L., Wang, I. N., Rodeo, S. A., and Lu, H. H. 2009b. Orthopedic interface tissue engineering for the biological fixation of soft tissue grafts. *Clin. Sports Med.* 28:157–176.

Moffat, K. L., Zhang, X., Greco, S., Boushell, M. K., Guo, X. E., Doty, S. B., Soslowsky, L. J., Levine, W. N., and Lu H. H. 2011. In vitro and in vivo evaluation of a bi-phasic nanofiber scaffold for integrative rotator cuff repair. *Trans. Orthop. Res. Soc.* 36:482.

Mutsuzaki, H., Sakane, M., Nakajima, H., Ito, A., Hattori, S., Miyanaga, Y., Ochiai, N., and Tanaka, J. 2004. Calcium-phosphate-hybridized tendon directly promotes regeneration of tendon–bone insertion. *J. Biomed. Mater. Res. A.* 70:319–327.

Paxton, J. Z., Donnelly, K., Keatch, R. P., and Baar, K. 2009. Engineering the bone-ligament interface using polyethylene glycol diacrylate incorporated with hydroxyapatite. *Tissue Eng. Part A* 15:1201–1209.

Paxton, J. Z., Donnelly, K., Keatch, R. P., Baar, K., and Grover, L. M. 2010a. Factors affecting the longevity and strength in an in vitro model of the bone-ligament interface. *Ann. Biomed. Eng.* 38:2155–2166.

Paxton, J. Z., Grover, L. M., and Baar, K. 2010b. Engineering an in vitro model of a functional ligament from bone to bone. *Tissue Eng. Part A* 16(11):3515–3525.

Pham, Q. P., Sharma, U., and Mikos, A. G. 2006. Electrospinning of polymeric nanofibers for tissue engineering applications: A review. *Tissue Eng.* 12:1197–1211.

Phillips, J. E., Burns, K. L., Le Doux, J. M., Guldberg, R. E., and Garcia, A. J. 2008. Engineering graded tissue interfaces. *Proc. Natl. Acad. Sci. USA* 105:12170–12175.

Robertson, D. B., Daniel, D. M., and Biden, E. 1986. Soft tissue fixation to bone. *Am. J. Sports Med.* 14:398–403.

Rodeo, S. A., Potter, H. G., Kawamura, S., Turner, A. S., Kim, H. J., and Atkinson, B. L. 2007. Biologic augmentation of rotator cuff tendon-healing with use of a mixture of osteoinductive growth factors. *J. Bone Joint Surg. Am.* 89:2485–2497.

Rodeo, S. A., Suzuki, K., Deng, X. H., Wozney, J., and Warren, R. F. 1999. Use of recombinant human bone morphogenetic protein-2 to enhance tendon healing in a bone tunnel. *Am. J. Sports Med.* 27:476–488.

Spalazzi, J. P., Dagher, E., Doty, S. B., Guo, X. E., Rodeo, S. A., Lu, H. H. 2008a. In vivo evaluation of a multiphased scaffold designed for orthopaedic interface tissue engineering and soft tissue-to-bone integration. *J. Biomed. Mater. Res. A* 86:1–12.

Spalazzi, J. P., Doty, S. B., Moffat, K. L., Levine, W. N., and Lu, H. H. 2006a. Development of controlled matrix heterogeneity on a triphasic scaffold for orthopedic interface tissue engineering. *Tissue Eng.* 12:3497–3508.

Spalazzi, J. P., Gallina, J., Fung-Kee-Fung, S. D., Konofagou, E. E., and Lu, H. H. 2006b. Elastographic imaging of strain distribution in the anterior cruciate ligament and at the ligament–bone insertions. *J. Orthop. Res.* 24:2001–2010.

Spalazzi, J. P., Vyner, M. C., Jacobs, M. T., Moffat, K. L., and Lu, H. H. 2008b. Mechanoactive scaffold induces tendon remodeling and expression of fibrocartilage markers. *Clin. Orthopaed. Relat. Res.* 466:1938–1948.

Sundar, S., Pendegrass, C. J., and Blunn, G. W. 2009. Tendon bone healing can be enhanced by demineralized bone matrix: A functional and histological study. *J. Biomed. Mater. Res. B Appl. Biomater.* 88:115–122.

Tien, Y. C., Chih, T. T., Lin, J. H., Ju, C. P., and Lin, S. D. 2004. Augmentation of tendon–bone healing by the use of calcium-phosphate cement. *J. Bone Joint Surg. Br.* 86:1072–1076.

Woo, S. L., Maynard, J., Butler, D. L., Lyon, R. M., Torzilli, P. A., Akeson, W. H., Cooper, R. R., and Oakes, B. 1988. Ligament, tendon, and joint capsule insertions to bone. In *Injury and Repair of the Musculoskeletal Soft Tissues*, S. L. Woo and J. A. Bulkwater, eds., pp. 133–166. Savannah, GA: American Academy of Orthopaedic Surgeons.

Xie, J., Li, X., Lipner, J., Manning, C. N., Schwartz, A. G., Thomopoulos, S., and Xia, Y. 2010. "Aligned-to-random" nanofiber scaffolds for mimicking the structure of the tendon-to-bone insertion site. *Nanoscale.* 2:923–926.

Yokoya, S., Mochizuki, Y., Nagata, Y., Deie, M., and Ochi, M. 2008. Tendon–bone insertion repair and regeneration using polyglycolic acid sheet in the rabbit rotator cuff injury model. *Am. J. Sports Med.* 36:1298–1309.

CHAPTER 12

Neural Regenerative Engineering

Shyam Aravamudhan, PhD and Ravi V. Bellamkonda, PhD

CONTENTS

12.1 INTRODUCTION

Neural regeneration following a disorder or injury to an adult mammalian nervous system is a complex biological phenomenon. During the last two decades, strategies for neural repair, functional replacement, and regeneration have included neuroprosthetic devices (Wickelgren 2004, Abbott 2006, Scott 2008), pharmacological treatments (Chau et al. 1998, Antri et al. 2003, Landry et al. 2006), stem cell–based therapies (Bareyre 2008, Coutts and Keirstead 2008), tissue-engineering approaches (Bellamkonda 2006, Kim et al. 2008, Clements et al. 2009, Orive et al. 2009), advanced neurorehabilitation (Chau et al. 1998, De Leon et al. 1999, Tillakaratne et al. 2002, Ichiyama et al. 2008), and neurobiological interventions that modulate plasticity and potentially promote neuroprotection. However, in spite of profound advances in the bioengineering strategies and in molecular-scale understanding of neural pathologies, currently no effective long-term treatment is available to restore complete function for a host of neural pathologies including spinal cord injury (SCI), peripheral nerve injury (PNI), stroke, traumatic brain injury (TBI), Parkinson's disease, Huntington's disease, amyotrophic lateral sclerosis (ALS), Alzheimer's disease, and multiple sclerosis (MS). Even though no single strategy has yet restored complete function after a neural pathology, neurobiologists, tissue engineers, and neuroprosthetists are optimistic that effective clinical therapies are within reach, if combinatorial therapies aimed at targeting multiple factors are implemented synergistically. This chapter represents an exploration of the hypotheses that a specific combination of biomaterial, pharmacological, cell replacement, drug delivery, and electrical stimulation, together with plasticity-promoting and neurorehabilitation-locomotor training, may interact synergistically to activate and enable functional circuits. While these disciplines have very different approaches to tackle the problem, the critical issue is—how can these diverse solutions be implemented in a manner that they are convergent, synergistic, and complementary rather than antagonistic? In this chapter, we will try to highlight convergent themes among currently parallel fields of *Rehabilitation*, *Regenerative Medicine*, and *Neural Prosthetics* so that they can synergistically achieve the common goal of restoring function after neural damage.

A neurological deficit is caused due to either loss of cells, or interruption of connections between cells or due to a loss of networks that include cells and their interconnections. For example, in the case of a severe SCI, supraspinal inputs to lumbosacral circuits are lost, leading to dramatic loss of function (Courtine et al. 2008, Ichiyama et al. 2008, Kubasak et al. 2008). Although spontaneous recovery after SCI occurs occasionally, in most instances significant damage results in permanent disability (Schwab and Bartholdi 1996). Current clinical approaches for SCI include use of high dose of methylprednisolone (MP) to help limit secondary injury, surgery to stabilize and decompress the spinal cord, and intensive medical or rehabilitative care. Although these treatments provide some benefits, no long-term restoration of function has been observed. Therefore, it reasonably follows that there is a critical and unmet clinical need to develop bioengineering intervention strategies that account for the complex pathophysiology of CNS or PNS and to optimize functional recovery. In this chapter, we review the clinical consequences of traumatic neural injuries, followed by current regenerative strategies and their deficiencies and finally discuss the need for better solutions to existing clinical problems. This chapter begins with a general discussion on physiology of the nervous system, followed by a discussion of the epidemiology and pathogenesis of traumatic peripheral, spinal, and brain injuries, and finally presents challenges associated with promoting repair and regeneration.

12.2 ANATOMY AND PHYSIOLOGY OF THE NERVOUS SYSTEM

The nervous system is divided into central and peripheral sections, along with the separate autonomic system. The central nervous system (CNS) consists of the brain, spinal cord, optic, olfactory, and auditory systems, while the peripheral nervous system (PNS) broadly consists of the nerves to the trunk and extremities. Specifically, the PNS consists of the cranial nerves arising from the brain, the spinal nerves arising from the spinal cord, and sensory nerve cell bodies (such as dorsal root ganglia) and their processes.

12.2.1 Cellular Components of the Nervous System

Two cell types are primarily found in the nervous system—neurons and glia. Neurons, which consist of a cell body (soma) and its extensions (axons and dendrites), are the basic structural and functional elements of the nervous system (Figure 12.1). Ganglia (clusters of sensory nerve soma) are located just outside the spinal column. While dendrites transmit electrical signals to the neuron cell body, the axon conducts impulses away. Glial cells (Schwann cells—PNS and astrocytes and oligodendrocytes—CNS) are support cells that aid the function of neurons. Another type of glial cell in the brain and spinal cord are the microglia, the resident macrophages and thus act as the main form of active immune defense in the CNS. Astrocytes perform many functions, including biochemical support of endothelial cells (blood–brain barrier [BBB]), provision of nutrients to the nervous tissue, maintenance of extracellular ion balance, and a principal role in the repair and scarring process following traumatic brain or SPIs. Glial cells are more abundant than neurons, and unlike neurons, which cannot undergo mitosis, glial cells possess some capacity for cell division. However, neurons can regenerate a severed portion or sprout new processes

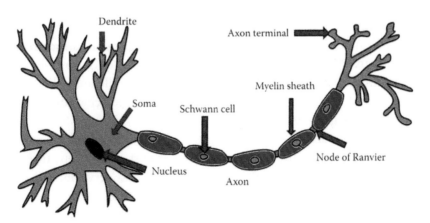

FIGURE 12.1   **Anatomy of a typical neuron.**

under certain conditions. In the PNS, sheaths of living Schwann cells surround all axons and myelinate them. The Schwann cells, in response to injury, attain a "regenerative" phenotype by producing extracellular matrix and trophic factor proteins that largely aid regeneration.

12.2.2 Central Nervous System

The brain and spinal cord make up the CNS, with the brain coordinating higher-level functions and the spinal cord serving mainly as the communication pathway between the brain and the periphery. The spinal cord is composed of dendrites, axons, and cell bodies. The spinal gray matter, which is located more centrally within the cord, contains the cell bodies of excitatory neurons, as well as glial cells and blood vessels. The gray matter is surrounded by a white matter, which helps to protect and insulate the spinal cord. White matter consists of axons and glial cells, including oligodendrocytes, astrocytes, and microglia (immune cells). Oligodendrocytes serve to myelinate the axons in the CNS, whereas astrocytes contribute to the blood–nerve barrier, separating the CNS from blood proteins and cells. In contrast to axons in the PNS, axons in CNS do not possess the continuous basement membrane and sheath of Schwann cells. Instead, axons are surrounded by an insulating myelin sheath, which are wrappings of the cell membrane of oligodendrocytes. The myelin serves to increase the nerve impulse propagation velocity, an important factor for axons that extend long distances (up to 1 m). Furthermore, axons project from the white matter into bundles, called as fascicles, which then exit the spinal column, travel through PNS–CNS transition zone to enter the PNS region.

12.2.3 Peripheral Nervous System

A peripheral nerve (PN) is composed of connective tissue and neural components. These are responsible for the innervations of the skin and skeletal muscles and contain electrically conductive fibers called axons, whose cell bodies reside in or near the spinal cord (Kerns 2008). There are three types of nerve fibers in PNS: (1) motor fibers, where axons originate in the anterior horn of the spinal cord and terminate in the neuromuscular ending of skeletal muscle; (2) sensory fibers, the peripheral projections of dorsal root ganglion neurons and terminate at the periphery; and (3) sympathetic fibers, the postganglionic processes of neurons innervating blood vessels or the skin's glandular structures (Valentini 2000). All axons are wrapped by support cells called Schwann cells. However, nerve fibers can be either unmyelinated or myelinated (Landon 1975). While unmyelinated fibers are composed of several axons, enveloped as a group by a single Schwann cell, myelinated fibers consist of a single axon, enveloped individually by a single Schwann cell. The connective tissue structures of the PN consist of three distinct sheaths: endoneurium, perineurium, and epineurium, from innermost to outermost, respectively. These structures form a framework that organizes and protects the axons and nerve fibers (Landon 1975, Kerns 2008). The perineurium and its endoneurial contents constitute a fascicle, which is the basic structural unit of a peripheral nerve. Most peripheral nerves, as stated earlier, contain several fascicles with many myelinated and unmyelinated axons. In a normal PNS development, the morphological structures (axon, Schwann cell, and components of epineurium, perineurium, and endoneurium) are of crucial importance for the integrity of various body functions, as they control tissues, organs, and systems (Landon 1975, Valentini 2000).

12.3 NEURAL INJURIES

Next, we describe the pathophysiology of both CNS and PNS trauma, so that readers can achieve a better understanding of the mechanisms of TBI, SCI, and PNI and the basis for current and future treatment approaches.

12.3.1 CNS Trauma

TBI and traumatic SCI result when an external physical insult causes damage or trauma. Although a direct mechanical insult with contusion secondary to a fracture accompanied with the dislocation of adjacent bony structures is a common feature and the initiating factor in the pathophysiology of CNS trauma, the force distribution and the resulting cellular responses are currently not well understood. As stated earlier, both the brain and spinal cord are composed of gray matter, consisting of neuronal cell bodies and white matter, consisting of myelinated axons. A blunt traumatic impact to the brain's outer gray matter results in large degree of cell body damage, while a high-speed impact, in addition also includes axonal damage to deeper regions of the brain. In contrast, the spinal cord's outer layer consists of axonal tracts, and primary damage from either compression or blunt trauma includes damage to both gray and white matter, especially given the relatively smaller thickness of the spinal cord compared to the brain. Within the injured core, nerve cells, axons, and blood vessels are damaged at the moment of injury. Normal blood flow is disrupted leading to ischemia, oxygen deprivation at the injury site, and instantaneous cell death and necrosis. The axonal membranes are damaged, causing electrolytic shifts at the site of injury. Regardless of the initial location of the insult to the CNS, injury is an ongoing process, with primary damage leading to a cascade of devastating events leading to secondary injury. Ischemia, electrolytic shifts, and edema continue to affect the cell body and axonal function, resulting in continued dysfunction and prolonged degeneration.

As stated earlier, the heterogeneity of TBI pathology remains poorly understood. TBI caused by a physical insult that surpasses structural and functional thresholds (Jennett et al. 2001) results in cerebral compression, laceration, contusion, edema, hemorrhage, and ischemia (Graham et al. 2005). On the cellular level, the primary injury triggers a number of pathogenic cascades, which then destroy cellular cytoarchitecture (Yatsiv et al. 2005). These cascades are responsible for secondary cellular injury, which can lead to neurodegeneration for over a year post-TBI (McIntosh et al. 1998a,b). These cellular level effects from TBI often lead to motor (loss of ambulation, balance, coordination, fine motor skills, strength, and endurance) and cognitive (loss of communication, information processing, memory, and perceptual skills) impairment (Levin et al. 1990, Raghupathi 2004, Hall et al. 2005, Povlishock and Katz 2005). Clinically, TBI severity is rated using the Glasgow coma score, which includes assessment of eye, verbal, and motor responses to give a combined score ranging from 3 (deep coma or dead) to 15 (fully alert). A Glasgow coma score ≤8 is considered severe, 9–12 is moderate, and ≥13 is minor (Stalhammar and Starmark 1986).

Based upon the understanding of pathophysiology, the most clinically relevant intervention is the detection, avoidance, and treatment of secondary insults. The presence of a secondary insult is the single most important treatable factor in improving TBI outcome, although this has only a modest effect on decreasing the propagation of cell and tissue damage and does not promote or improve clinical outcomes—repair or regeneration. Although several therapies have shown benefit in preclinical models, there have been notable failures in clinical translation, with trials failing to confirm functional benefits in human subjects (McIntosh et al. 1998a,b, Mammis et al. 2009). Thus, current treatment for TBI remains largely supportive, directed toward management of cerebral edema and intracranial hypertension using temporizing measures (McAllister 2009). None of these interventions have been definitively demonstrated to improve long-term functional outcome (Galvin and Mandalis 2009, Giles 2009, Zasler 2009).

SCI can be broadly classified into (1) dislocation, (2) lateral bending, (3) axial loading, (4) rotation, and (5) hyperflexion or hyperextension, although severe injuries often result from a combination of more than one of these types (Lisak 2009). There are other ways to classify SCI. One could categorize SCI according to whether the patient is para- (thoracic, lumbar, or sacral spinal segment involved) or tetraplegic (cervical segment involved) (Harkey et al. 2003), whether it is primary or secondary SCI, an upper or lower motoneuron lesion, traumatic (direct) or nontraumatic (indirect), an open or a closed lesion. The severity of injury is ranked on the American Spinal Injury Association (ASIA) scale of A to E, where A is a complete SCI with no motor or sensory function in the perineal region and B through E reflect improving motor function below the site of injury (Ackery et al. 2004). The annual incidence rate of SCI varies considerably from country to country (2.5–57.8 per million populations). SCI is most frequent in young adults, a grim statistic compounded by the lifelong disability. The main causes of injuries in the economically developed countries are vehicular accidents and sporting accidents, whereas falling from a height is the most common cause in less-developed regions. The combined negative health, sociological implications, and the economic impact are enormous (Carlson and Gorden 2002, Corso et al. 2006), which prompt for urgent clinically effective treatments. The complexity of the CNS and variability in clinical presentation make such efforts to repair damaged CNS and to restore complete function extremely challenging.

The regrowth of axons is not possible because CNS has multiple factors at the cellular as well as molecular level which act as barriers for regeneration and make the environment hostile for endogenous regeneration (Schwab et al. 1993, Tatagiba et al. 1997, Fawcett and Asher 1999, Hagg and Oudega 2006). In particular, astroglial scar consists of reactive astrocytes and invades meningeal fibroblasts, expressing inhibitory molecules such as CSPGs (Silver and Miller 2004). In addition, the injured spinal cord contains inhibitory molecules from myelin debris, such as Nogo (Caroni et al. 1988, Schwab and Caroni 1988, Chen et al. 2000) and myelin-associated proteoglycan (Mukhopadhyay et al. 1994, Wang et al. 2002). However, recent strategies aimed at overcoming these inhibitory cues have resulted in encouraging regeneration of lesioned SCI axons. These strategies include the neutralization of myelin inhibitors (Bregman et al. 1995, GrandPre et al. 2002), and degradation of inhibitory CSPGs in the glial scar (Bradbury et al. 2002, Yick et al. 2003). Furthermore, limited axonal regrowth and sprouting has also been demonstrated following administration of growth-promoting molecules and pathways such as exogenous neurotrophic factors (Oudega and Hagg 1996, Grill et al. 1997, Bradbury et al. 1999), cell transplantation strategies—Schwann cell bridges (Bunge 1994), genetically modified fibroblasts (Liu et al. 1999), olfactory ensheathing cells (OECs) (Li et al. 1997), stem cells (Lu et al. 2003), and modulation of pro-regenerative neuronal signaling pathways (Neumann and Woolf 1999, Qiu et al. 2002). There is, however, no known definitive combinatorial strategy that can target the multiple domains, alter the pathophysiology of injury site, and bring a significant functional change to the patient's condition. Although complete recovery of function in an injured spinal cord is still not possible in a clinical setting, numerous efforts to promote repair and regeneration after SCI are actively being pursued. Bradburg and McMohan (2006) postulated the following main goals in order to overcome failure of SCI axonal regeneration: (1) initiate and maintain axonal growth; (2) direct regenerating axons to reconnect with their target neurons; and (3) reconstitute the original spinal cord circuitry, which would potentially lead to complete functional recovery. Although many interventions have now been reported to promote functional recovery after experimental SCI, none has fulfilled all three of these aims together (Bradbury and McMahon 2006). However, recent progress in regenerative medicine and combinatorial approaches has led to new approaches for the treatment of CNS injuries and thus renewed hope for complete recovery of function.

12.3.2 Peripheral Nerve Injury

PNIs present a significant clinical challenge, as more than 300,000 PNS trauma cases are reported every year in the United States (Noble et al. 1998). Injuries to the PNS are a major source of disability, impairing the ability to move muscles and/or feel normal sensations, or resulting in painful neuropathies. The most severe PNI is a complete nerve transection. Severe PNI results in complex pathophysiological changes at the injury site, including morphological and metabolic changes. These complex changes occur almost immediately in the proximal and distal segments, and in the distal endings of both muscle end plates and sensory receptors. In the proximal end, axons degenerate for some distance back from the site of injury, leaving the corresponding endoneurial tubes (basal laminae of Schwann cell) behind as empty cylinders. This retrograde degeneration may extend over one or several internodal segments, the length depending on the severity of the lesion. The distal portions begin to degenerate as a result of protease activity and separation from the metabolic resources of the nerve cell bodies (Schmidt and Leach 2003). The degeneration is a slow process of known as Wallerian degeneration. This process starts immediately after injury and involves myelin breakdown and proliferation of Schwann cells. Schwann cells and macrophages are recruited to the injury site, and over a period of 3–6 weeks they phagocytize (clear) all the myelin and cellular debris (Stoll et al. 1989). In addition to clearing debris, macrophages and Schwann cells also produce cytokines, which will enhance axon growth (Chaudhry et al. 1992). Following this clearance, regeneration begins at the proximal end and continues toward the distal stump. New axonal sprouts usually emanate within hours of injury from the nodes of Ranvier, the nonmyelinated areas of axons located between Schwann cells.

Functional reinnervation requires the advancing sprouts to pass a critical area between the proximal and distal stumps of the cut nerve: the interstump zone. The success of the nerve regeneration is, to a great extent, dependent on what happens in this critical area and in what way local chemical and cellular reaction can influence the growth of sprouts toward their peripheral pathways. In humans, axon regeneration occurs at a rate of about 2–5 mm/day; thus, significant PN injuries can take many months to heal (Jacobson and Guth 1965).

The clinical solution is to appose the two nerve ends and suture them together without generating tension where possible. If the gap is large, such that tensionless apposition is not possible, a nerve autograft—typically patient's own sural nerve—is used as a bridge. While autografts represent the best clinical option today with several advantages: (1) biocompatible, (2) nontoxic, and (3) provide a support structure to promote axonal adhesion, extension, and ECM formation, there are also many drawbacks including their availability, donor site morbidity, and loss of function (Lee and Wolfe 2000). Therefore, there is a clear and urgent clinical need to find alternative approaches that match or exceed the performance of autografts. However, a serious drawback to the use of autografts is that the availability of disposable nerve segments is limited, and multiple lengths of nerve graft might be often needed to bridge the gap between the injured nerve stumps (Ansselin and Davey 1988). In addition, autografts contain inhibitory CSPGs, which may reduce their performance (Groves et al. 2005). Another serious drawback is that there may be a dependence on the type of autograft used for the modality of nerve regenerated. Using sural nerve grafts (which are the most commonly used autograft in humans) may exclude regenerating motor nerves (Nichols et al. 2004). Therefore, there is an opportunity for alternative bioengineering strategies to bridge nerve gaps. Driven by this need, several strategies are being pursued, primarily involving the use of hollow polymeric "guidance channels" (NeuroGen and Integra Life Sciences) alone or using guidance channels as carriers for hydrogel-based scaffolds for nerve repair (Dodla and Bellamkonda 2008). However, these have attained limited success, and present an opportunity for prostheses, regenerative medicine, and tissue engineering to fill this void. Figure 12.2 shows the desired characteristics for the bioengineered scaffold for peripheral nerve regeneration.

12.4 CLINICAL CHALLENGES AND OPPORTUNITIES

Spontaneous regeneration and regrowth of the proximal segment of the injured spinal cord or peripheral nerve has been an important target for regenerative medicine as well as neuroscientific research. As stated earlier, several key elements such as glial cells and their products, in the case of SCI, contribute to the lack of regeneration or the inhibitory environment. Various models of complete spinal cord transection have played an important role in identifying these underlying mechanisms, although such models may not accurately represent the events after traumatic SCI (Table 12.1). Later, we discuss some of the key mechanisms and challenges that hinder the current approaches for regeneration after both CNS and PNS trauma. Several reviews have addressed this aspect of neuroengineering research (Shoichet et al. 2008). As stated earlier, the physical insults to brain or spinal cord

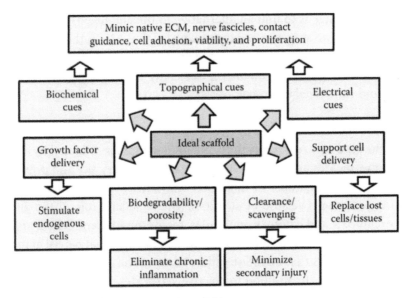

FIGURE 12.2 **Properties of the ideal neural scaffold.**

TABLE 12.1 Key Events (Physical, Cellular, and Molecular) after Traumatic CNS Injuries and
Potential Regenerative Approaches

Key Events after CNS Injury	Underlying Mechanism	Repair Strategies
Primary damage		
Cell death—necrosis (minutes to hours)	Oxidative stress	Antioxidant therapy
BBB/BSCB breakdown	Infiltration of macrophages, fibroblasts, inflammatory molecules into the site of injury	Neuroprotective and reparative molecules
Secondary damage		
Cell death—apoptosis (hours to days/weeks)	Limited endogenous progenitor cells to replace the damaged glia and neurons	Cell replacement; neurotrophin administration; modulation of cell signaling; rehabilitation
Demyelination (days to months)	Oligodendrocyte loss; loss/block of function	Cell replacement; neurotrophin administration
Glial scar formation (days to weeks)	Reactive gliosis; ECM remodeling	Degradation of ECM molecules; modulation of inflammation
Axon degeneration and retraction (days to months)	Inhibitory/repulsive environment—Nogo, OMG, MAG, CSPG	Modulation of intracellular signaling; physical guidance channels with chemical cues

initially cause necrotic cell death and damage to the underlying tissue, followed by multiple
secondary events, for example, opening of the BBB or blood–spinal cord barrier (BSCB),
inflammation, edema, ischemia, excitotoxicity, increase in free radicals, and altered cell
signaling and gene expression (Gaetz 2004). This cascade of secondary events leads to
more cell death, demyelination, axonal degeneration, and glial scar (Fawcett 2006). In the

case of PNI, the challenge is to find an alternative to the autologous nerve graft and thus eliminate the need for two surgeries and the removal of tissue from the patient. Thus neural engineering strategies for the PNS have focused on developing alternative treatments to the nerve graft (e.g., nerve guidance channels), especially for larger defects, and improving recovery rates and functional outcomes.

12.4.1 Glial Scar

Formation of the glial scar represents the acute injury response initiated by activated glial cells (including astrocytes and microglia) to contain the injury site and promote healing. Recent evidence shows a number of molecular similarities between the SCI and dermal wound healing processes (Velardo et al. 2004). The beneficial role of the glial response helps buffer excitotoxic and cytotoxic molecules, repair the BBB and BSCB, and isolate the site of injury (Eddleston and Mucke 1993). However, glial cells that persist at the injury site produce inhibitory factors that manifest within hours of the original trauma and severely limit axonal regeneration. In addition to reactive astrocytes, scar formation also involves oligodendrocyte precursor cells, microglia, and macrophages. After injury, up-regulation of chondroitin sulfate proteoglycans (CSPGs) (Fawcett and Asher 1999), which are associated with astrocytes and oligodendrocyte precursors, is a major contributor to the inhibitory properties of the CNS glial scar (Properzi et al. 2003). As part of a nascent regenerative response, severed CNS axons can develop new axonal sprouts that extend very short distances and then will recede because of the inhibitory environment to regeneration (Schwab and Bartholdi 1996).

12.4.2 Myelin/Oligodendrocyte Inhibitory Molecules

The glial scar also includes myelin/oligodendrocyte inhibitory molecules and their inhibitory effects have been studied extensively (Schwab 2004). The Nogo family (Nogo-A, -B, and -C) of oligodendrocyte membrane proteins is a well-known inhibitory signal for neurite outgrowth. Myelin-associated glycoprotein, oligodendrocyte myelin glycoprotein, semaphorin 4D, and ephrin B3 are other identified inhibitory molecules in the oligodendrocyte membrane. To achieve axonal regeneration, which is particularly crucial following SCI, the physical and chemical inhibitory environment of the glial scar must be overcome. For example, Fawcett et al. found that the CSPG in the glial scar can be degraded by using an enzyme chondroitinase ABC, resulting in limited regeneration success (Rhodes and Fawcett 2004). Fournier et al. reported neutralization of inhibitory myelin environment following injury by targeting the Rho-kinase receptor (Fournier et al. 2003).

12.4.3 Blood–Brain Barrier and Blood–Spinal Cord Barrier

The damage or opening created to the BBB and BSCB is the hallmark of CNS injury. In general, these barriers protect the brain and spinal cord from biochemical fluctuations in the periphery. A breach in the BBB or BSCB permits infiltration of macrophages, fibroblasts, and inflammatory molecules into the site of injury. This further activates astrocytes, contributing to the inhibitory environment, which as stated earlier will physically and chemically obstruct axonal regeneration.

12.4.4 Inflammation

While some inflammation is clearly needed to limit degeneration and address the cell debris resulting from CNS injury, there is active discussion on whether the inflammatory response should be further enhanced (Lenzlinger et al. 2001, Correale and Villa 2004). The proinflammatory cytokines are released within minutes following TBI/SCI, with acutely harmful effects—BBB and BSCB disruption, and cell death. However, they are beneficial at later time points by inducing synthesis of anti-inflammatory cytokines, by inducing neurotrophic factor secretion, and by promoting proliferation of oligodendrocyte precursor cells that may help in remyelination (Morganti-Kossmann et al. 2002). Because of the dual nature of the inflammatory response, treatments for TBI and SCI that target specific cells or proteins involved in the inflammatory response must be approached with caution. Schwartz and Yoles (2005) found that the injection of macrophages to the injured spinal cord can be beneficial, yet clinical trials have not continued. As Schwann cells rather than macrophages and microglia seem to provide most of the debris clean-up after injury, other groups have questioned the utility of inflammatory response (Bao et al. 2004, Gomes-Leal et al. 2004). In general, Schwann cells have shown some functional benefits on their own (Fouad et al. 2005).

In summary, the complex environment after TBI/SCI exhibit different aspects of inhibition and cell death, together with endogenous attempts at repair and regeneration. While significant efforts have been made to reduce inhibitory molecules following CNS injury, much less attention has been given to the role of endogenous repair proteins, such as fibronectin and laminin (Tate et al. 2007). Therefore, the key challenges and opportunities for CNS and PNS nerve repair and regeneration are to (1) direct regenerating axons to reconnect with their target neurons in a potentially hostile milieu with appropriate cues, including scaffolds, matrices, and substrates; (2) correct and/or strengthen connections formed by axonal sprouting; (3) activate "residual" neural circuitry and CNS plasticity that has survived the neural injury; and (4) "condition" the innervating muscle. However, one significant difference between the PNS and CNS is the capacity for the peripheral nerves to regenerate, while the CNS axons do not regenerate appreciably in their native environment because of the presence of inherent inhibitory molecules (Eftekharpour et al. 2008). Currently, the goal of various bioengineering efforts in the CNS domain is mainly geared toward creating a permissive "axonal regeneration" environment. This environment will, in future, involve a combination of physical and biochemical cues, cellular components, along with plasticity-promoting and neuroprosthetic strategies to target multiple inhibitory factors and challenges. In addition to regenerative strategies, neuroprotective strategies will seek to limit secondary injury (or the cascade of degenerative events) as a way to limit the loss of function following injury.

12.5 NEURAL REGENERATION APPROACHES

In 1911, Tello first demonstrated the ability of CNS fibers to regenerate into a PN graft (Tello 1911). Ramón y Cajal in 1928 noticed the scar formation, following SCI, postulating a role in axonal regeneration. He implied that the deficit in CNS axonal regeneration was not an inability of the axons themselves to regrow but that it was due to an environment lacking in nutritive substances and a scar barrier (Cajal 1928). David and Aguayo (1982) showed evidence for long PN bridges circumventing the spinal cord carrying CNS axonal processes for remarkable distances, for example, from the lower medulla to the thoracic cord. In a follow-up study, Richardson et al. (1984) demonstrated that the distance of injury to the cell body was a crucial determinant for regeneration. In all these experiments, no fibers were observed to leave the graft to reenter the distal spinal cord. In contrast to the PNS, regeneration in the CNS was still deficient. Recent reports have indicated that the injured brain or spinal cord may attempt to repair through developmental processes, as evidenced by increases in neurogenesis and angiogenesis that occur following TBI (Dash et al. 2001). These significant findings have guided a new generation of regenerative strategies. While these recent breakthroughs offer promise in restoring complete function, a number of challenges still remain because of the complex and dynamic CNS milieu.

It is clear from the earlier discussion that restoration of complete function will require multiple interventions (or combinatorial interventions) that result in targeting multiple regenerative domains (secondary injury, regenerative medicine, electrical stimulation, and plasticity) rather than finding a single "magic bullet" regenerative factor or therapeutic strategy. The nervous system, after an injury, constantly changes as a function of time. Consequently, different therapeutic strategies can be designed to work at different points of time to achieve maximum recovery of function (Figure 12.3). For example, in the case of traumatic SCI, early surgery (within the first 24 h) and pharmacological treatments may be used in the acute phase to prevent secondary complications (Bracken 1990, 2001), and then in the sub-chronic phase, treatments for prevention of delayed apoptotic degeneration of oligodendrocyte may be used (Totoiu and Keirstead 2005). Finally, in the chronic phase, treatments such as cell transplantation, locomotor training, and neuroprosthetic strategies may be employed. Efforts to treat traumatic CNS injures can be broadly divided into two categories: (1) neuroprotection, minimization of cell damage, death, and axonal degeneration caused by the cascade

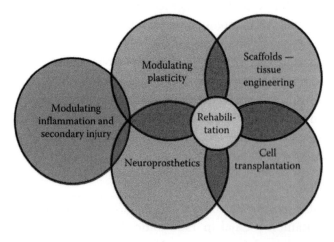

FIGURE 12.3 Convergent themes among various therapeutic strategies to restore complete function.

TABLE 12.2 Current Therapeutic Strategies to Stimulate Nerve Repair/Regeneration after Traumatic Injury

Current Therapeutic Strategies after Neural Injury		References
1	Rehabilitation	Management of pain and secondary complications Preventive care Training of neural circuits	Freehafer (1998), Protas et al. (2001), Weidner et al. (2001)
2	Modification of neural environment	Pharmacological interventions Neurotrophic factors Antibodies to inhibitory molecules (CNS)	Bracken (1990), Patist et al. (2004), Bradbury et al. (2002)
3	Modulation of plasticity	Pharmacological interventions Biomolecular therapeutics Exogenous electrical activity	Garcia-Alias et al. (2008), Silver and Miller (2004), Musienko et al. (2009)
4	Cell and gene therapy	Neural and mesenchymal stem cells Olfactory ensheathing cells Schwann cells Genetically modified cells Macrophages Regeneration-associated genes	Coutts and Keirstead (2008), Fovad et al. (2005), Li et al. (2006)
5	Biomaterials/tissue engineering	Guidance channels Cell-seeded and acellular scaffolds Growth factor delivery ECM molecule delivery	Ngo et al. (2003), Kim et al. (2008), Koshimune et al. (2003), Jain et al. (2006), Dodla and Bellamkonda (2008)
6	Neural prostheses	Functional electrical stimulation Axonal regeneration Neuromotor prostheses Non invasive and invasive electrodes	Mensinger et al. (2000), Hamid and Hayek (2008), Gazula et al. (2004), Sadowsky (2001)

of secondary events and (2) neural regeneration, promotion of plasticity and axonal growth. For neural regeneration following traumatic SCI, axonal growth is required across the injury site, through the glial scar, and to the appropriate target. Because of the progressive nature of cell death, a sustained neuroprotective therapy may be required to alleviate or reduce neurological disability and render the damaged CNS more receptive to regenerative strategies. An ideal treatment strategy(ies) will have to exploit and complement endogenous repair mechanisms while suppressing inhibitory mechanisms. In summary, the three main research avenues to promote complete regeneration and repair are summarized in Table 12.2: (1) minimizing initial and secondary injury; (2) modifying regenerative environment; and (3) electrical stimulation (Hamid and Hayek 2008). Next, we discuss some promising therapeutic interventions currently being explored in the fields of neurorehabilitation, regenerative medicine, and neuroprosthesis.

12.5.1 Regenerative Medicine

The aim of regenerative medicine is to repair, replace, or regenerate cells, tissues, or organs to restore impaired function (Langer and Vacanti 1993, Daar and Greenwood 2007). Specifically, neuroprotection and neural regeneration using (1) growth factor/drug delivery vehicle, (2) support matrix for cell transplantation, (3) tissue-engineering/ biomaterial strategies, and (4) combinatorial methods are discussed here.

12.5.1.1 Drug Delivery

Drug delivery strategies have been investigated to both limit degeneration and promote regeneration following traumatic injury. In the case of TBI, current treatment methods in clinical practice primarily aim to reduce intracranial pressure in an effort to minimize brain damage caused by swelling. However, these therapies have resulted only in modest functional outcomes (Roberts et al. 1998). Furthermore, these treatments do not provide sustained efforts that promote repair or regeneration. Similar results occurred with other drugs including free radical scavengers and steroids (Narayan et al. 2002). An important reason for these failures is due to the treatment targeting only a single mechanism, which may be insufficient in light of the multifaceted pathology. In the future, therapies that address multiple pathological events will be developed.

To limit degeneration after SCI, the goal has been to preserve functional behavior through axonal sparing and reduced lesion volumes. While the extent of primary injury is determined by the initial trauma, which is beyond control, the severity of secondary injury can be potentially modulated through the use of pharmacological agents such as MP, an anti-inflammatory steroid. MP is a synthetic corticosteroid that is clinically used for the treatment of acute SCI. The National Acute Spinal Cord Injury Study II (NASCIS II) demonstrated that MP given within 8 h following SCI can improve neural recovery in humans (Bracken 1990). Typically, MP is administered in high doses systemically (30 mg/kg bolus injection followed by a 5.4 mg/kg/h infusion over 23 h). Even though the underlying therapeutic mechanisms are unclear, MP-mediated inhibition of lipid peroxidation and inflammatory response are thought to offer important therapeutic benefits after SCI (Hall 1992, 1993). The effect of systemic MP delivery into the injured SC have been demonstrated in various studies and discussed in detail (Kim et al. 2009). However, the use of systemic high dose of MP causes adverse side effects including wound infections, pneumonia, and acute corticosteroid myopathy accompanied by only modest improvements in neural recovery (Gerndt et al. 1997, Qian et al. 2005). Bellamkonda group suggested that most of the side effects of MP-based therapy are related to the high systemic dosage and its associated toxicity, and that the relatively modest neural effects are a reflection of inefficient dosing to the injury site (Kim et al. 2009). Therefore, while MP has huge promise, its delivery to the injury site is likely to be the major impediment for effective and widespread clinical use. Other molecules that have been investigated by systemic delivery include GM-1 gangliosides, minocycline (Wells et al. 2003), and cAMP moderators (Pearse et al. 2004). The intervention time course with neuroprotective strategies has typically been within 24–72 h of traumatic injury, but pharmacological intervention is transient.

An important consideration is the route of drug delivery. Molecules have been delivered systemically and injected locally via epidural, intrathecal, and intramedullary routes. While the majority of pharmacological efforts for TBI have used systemic delivery, potential treatments for SCI have explored various local delivery options. Bellamkonda group reported on a novel localized MP drug delivery system using biodegradable PLGA-based nanoparticles (NP).

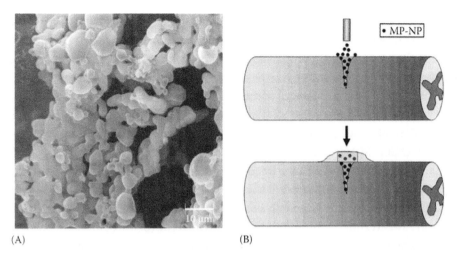

FIGURE 12.4   Methylprednisolone-encapsulating PLGA nanoparticles (MP-NP). (A) An SEM image of the lyophilized MP-NPs. Scale bar = 1 μm. (B) Schematic of topical and local delivery of the MP-NPs onto dorsal over-hemisection lesioned spinal cord. (Reproduced from *Biomaterials*, 30(13), Kim, Y.T., Caldwell, J.M., and Bellamkonda, R.V., Nanoparticle-mediated local delivery of methylprednisolone after spinal cord injury, 2582–2590, Copyright 2009, with permission from Elsevier.)

When delivered via the hydrogel–nanoparticle system, MP entered the injured SC and diffused up to 1.5 mm deep and up to 3 mm laterally into the injured spinal cord within 2 days (Figure 12.4). Furthermore, the topically delivered MP significantly decreased the early inflammation inside the contusion injured spinal cord. This was evidenced by a significant reduction in the number of ED-1[+] macrophages/activated microglia, along with significantly diminished expression of proinflammatory proteins including Calpain and iNOS. Also, a significantly reduced lesion volume 7 days after contusion injury was observed (Chvatal et al. 2008). In a following study, using a rat model of SCI compared the efficacy of controlled, nanoparticle (NP)-enabled local delivery of MP to the injured spinal cord with systemic delivery of MP, and a single local injection of MP without nanoparticles. The data clearly demonstrated that sustained local delivery of MP-NPs soon after SCI significantly decreased the reactivity of the early markers of injury/secondary injury, reduced lesion volume, and improved functional outcomes (Kim et al. 2009). These results were obtained using a remarkably low dose of MP (400 mg/animal). The dosage used was approximately 1/20th of the systemically administered dose (7–8 mg/animal). The benefits of MP-NP sustained, local delivery onto the lesion site were apparent within the first 24 h after injury (i.e., significantly increased expression of anti-apoptotic protein along with decreased expression of proapoptotic-related proteins).

12.5.1.2 Plasticity Modulation

Following CNS damage, some degree of spontaneous recovery does occur in both humans and rodents, in part due to the rearrangements of spared neural networks (denoted as "plasticity"). Here, plasticity refers to the growth and sprouting of axons leading to anatomical rewiring of CNS circuits. Plasticity of connections in the spinal cord also provides some capacity for adaptation to injury (Weidner et al. 2001, Raineteau et al. 2002) and represents a target for therapeutic intervention (Thallmair et al. 1998, Chuah et al. 2004). Enhancing the CNS plasticity has in recent times become a major research area for functional recovery after complete SCI. The basis for this regeneration is thought to be promotion of localized axonal sprouting facilitated by plasticity modulation, which creates bypass routes when projected tracts are interrupted (Raineteau et al. 2001, Bareyre et al. 2004, Vavrek et al. 2006). In general, many molecules including myelin-associated inhibitors NOGO, MAG, and Omgp as well as family of matrix molecules—CSPGs— inhibit axonal growth and plasticity. Recent experimental treatments have found that adult CNS plasticity can return to levels seen in childhood by either blocking inhibitory effects of Nogo-A or digesting CSPGs in PNNs or by other mechanisms (Buchli and Schwab 2005, Galtrey and Fawcett 2007, Dunlop 2008). Garcia-Alias et al. (2008) demonstrated anatomical plasticity of corticospinal tract (CST) as well as modest improvement of forelimb function after only injecting chondroitinase ABC (ChABC) immediately after almost complete CST axon severing. So the current question in SCI rehabilitation is whether it can be made more effective by temporarily creating a plastic CNS environment. Recent studies have explored this current opinion, using a combination of plasticity-modulating treatment and rehabilitation to promote locomotor recovery (Garcia-Alias et al. 2009). However, the results so far have raised more questions in regard to whether the different strategies tend to compete with each other or by emphasizing a specific rehabilitation or behavior, other behaviors will be damaged.

12.5.1.3 Cell Transplantation

Exploiting cell transplantation offers a great potential to produce specific beneficial factors or to replace lost cells and tissue. Advantages of transplanting cells include the ability to target multiple neuroprotective and neuroregenerative mechanisms and the ability to provide a sustained treatment. An important strategy in this domain is the replenishment of lost cell types by stem cell–based therapies (Lindvall and Kokaia 2006, Eftekharpour et al. 2008, Kim and de Vellis 2009). Cells, particularly stem cells, can adapt to their environment and are thus able to evolve with the pathology of the brain and spinal cord. Even though endogenous stem cells are present in the spinal cord with the inherent capacity to regenerate, recovery of function with just endogenous cells is difficult and limited after traumatic SCI. However in recent years, neurons and glial cells have successfully been created from stem cells such as embryonic stem cells (ESCs), mesenchymal stem cells (MSCs), and neural stem/progenitor cells (NPCs) with successful functional outcomes (Bareyre 2008, Coutts and Keirstead 2008). The board goals of cell replacement strategies are (1) transplantation of embryonic or NPCs into the lesioned SC with/without *ex vivo* manipulation and (2) reactivation and mobilization of endogenous spinal cord NPCs. The functional recovery is mediated not only by secretion of trophic factors or by remyelination of spared axons through newly created oligodendrocytes (Keirstead et al. 1998), but also by creation of new neurons (Cummings et al. 2005). We review here few notable experimental studies involving stem cell–based therapies for SCI, TBI, and PNI. For more exhaustive reviews of the different cell types and sources used experimentally following TBI and SCI, readers are referred to Longhi et al. (2005) and Enzmann et al. (2006). However, there are still many obstacles to be overcome before cell therapy can be adopted in a clinical setting. The key challenges include risk of immune rejection, the need for external sources of cells, poor cell survivability, and need to optimize cell characteristics before grafting.

Stem cells have the inherent capacity for self-renewal and capability of differentiation into various cell lineages under appropriate conditions. Thus, they represent an important building block for regenerative medicine and tissue engineering (Lindvall et al. 2004). Mammalian pluripotent stem cells, ESCs derived from the inner cell mass of blastocysts, and embryonic germ cells (EGCs) can create various organs and tissues (Thompson et al. 1998, Donovan and Gearhart 2001). Furthermore, tissue-specific stem cells can be isolated from tissues such as hematopoietic stem cells, bone marrow MSCs, adipose tissue–derived stem cells, amniotic fluid stem cells, and neural stem cells (NSCs). In particular, NSCs with indefinite growth and multipotent potential have been shown to differentiate into all three major CNS cells—neurons, astrocytes, and oligodendrocytes (McKay 1997, Gottlieb 2002). It is hoped that these NSCs will provide an inexhaustible source of neurons and glia for therapies aimed at cell replacement and/or neuroprotection in case of neural disorders. Even though ESCs have greater plastic potential compared to adult NSCs, ethical issues and unwanted growth potential and tumor formation limit their usability. Currently, when no long-term effective treatment is available for neural disorder or injury, cell therapy seems to be the most promising strategy. However, the development of effective stem cell therapies will require (1) detailed knowledge of neuronal disease pathology, (2) how specific cell types in CNS are affected, (3) cell survival, control of cell fate, and (4) maintenance of a defined differentiated phenotype and proper cell engraftment after transplantation.

Currently, there is no single effective therapeutic option to improve functional outcome after traumatic SCI. Stem cells for SCI can be used to achieve three broad goals: (1) regeneration to replace lost or damaged neurons and to induce plasticity; (2) repair or replace supportive cells such as oligodendrocytes in order to induce remyelination (Totoiu and Keirstead 2005); and (3) promote neuroprotection of endogenous cells to limit secondary injury (Eftekharpour et al. 2008). Since the first study that showed that transplantation of ESCs induces functional recovery (McDonald et al. 1999), several studies have been reported in literature showing functional improvement after either stem cell or progenitor cell transplantation into the injured SC, including ESCs, bone marrow MSCs, NSCs, and glia-restricted precursor cells (Hofstetter et al. 2002, Ogawa 2002, Teng et al. 2002, Cummings et al. 2005, Iwanami et al. 2005, Karimi-Abdolrezaee et al. 2006). However, there are still many obstacles to be overcome before stem cell–based therapy can be adopted for clinical use. The biggest challenge is massive cell death after stem cell transplantation into the injured SC. NSCs are multipotent stem cells with the capacity to differentiate into the major cells of the CNS and have many potential applications in transplantation. NSCs transplanted after experimental TBI have been shown to promote motor and cognitive recovery (Philips et al. 2001, Schouten et al. 2004). NSCs have also demonstrated benefit when implanted after experimental SCI (Faulkner and Keirstead 2005, Karimi-Abdolrezaee et al. 2006). For SCI, transplantation of ESC-derived oligodendrocyte precursors is being pursued for clinical trials (Faulkner and Keirstead 2005), where the resulting oligodendrocytes are expected to myelinate degenerated fibers, thereby providing a neuroprotective effect against degeneration. Olfactory ensheathing glia (OEG) have also shown to guide axon regeneration and to myelinate axons (Ramon-Cueto et al. 1998). In other studies, enhanced donor cell survival was observed for transplantations of intact tissue due to the presence of three-dimensional architecture and a higher accessibility of extracellular adhesive proteins to which the donor cells can attach (Sinson et al. 1996). Thus, tissue-engineering approaches that emulate tissue transplants are currently being explored to enhance survival and integration of donor cells in host tissue to further advance cell transplantation therapy. Other hurdles associated with translating cell transplantation to the clinic include the host immune response to the cells or shed antigens (Jones et al. 2004). The choice of cell type and source is critical in addressing these issues. In addition to determining the optimal cell type and source, the delivery time, location, and method (cell number, delivery vehicle) are important considerations. All of these factors will affect the efficacy of the treatment, and it is likely that multiple combinations of these parameters will prove to be beneficial at promoting complete functional recovery.

In the case of PNI, studies have been carried out using stem cells and their inherent potential to differentiate into cells that exhibit the Schwann cell phenotype. Skin-derived stem cells have been employed in conduits to bridge 16 mm gaps (Marchesi et al. 2007). The conduits with ecto-MSCs (EMSCs) produced sciatic functional index values that were statistically comparable to autografts (Nie et al. 2007). In a comparison study, MSCs were able to mimic Schwann cells but were unable to match their myelination capabilities (Keilhoff et al. 2006, Li et al. 2006). In another study, using 14 mm nerve conduits with MSC encapsulation had significantly better fibrin matrix compared to empty tubes (Kalbermatten et al. 2008). Similarly, bone marrow stromal cells transplanted into the nerve injury site were observed to have differentiated into Schwann cells (Zhang et al. 2004). In a 12 mm rat sciatic nerve model, bone marrow stem cell–derived Schwann cells significantly increased the number of regenerated axons compared to controls (Mimura et al. 2004). Dimos et al. (2008) showed for the first time that induced pluripotent stem (iPS) cells isolated from ALS patients can be directed to differentiate into motor neurons. To boost cell viability, collagen-immobilized nanofibers have been studied cortical NSCs as peripheral nerve scaffolds (Li et al. 2008).

12.5.1.4 Tissue Engineering and Biomaterial Strategies

Tissue-engineering approaches include incorporation of natural/synthetic biomaterials as well as combinations of cells, drugs, and scaffolds. The biomaterial scaffold itself has some therapeutic advantage or serves as a delivery vehicle for growth factors and/or extracellular matrix proteins, with the goal of recruiting host cells or enhancing axonal growth. Strategies for the PNS have primarily focused on finding alternatives to the nerve autografts, whereas efforts in SCI/TBI have focused on creating a "permissive" regenerative environment (Schmidt and Leach 2003). Various tissue-engineering strategies have been used to influence different aspects of the PNS regenerative process with an ultimate goal of complete functional recovery (Schmidt and Leach 2003, Mukhatyar et al. 2009). In particular, the formation of the peripheral nerve cable is influenced by a variety of factors, such as physical structure, composition (Aebischer et al. 1988), dimensions (Williams and Varon 1985), exogenous factors (Williams et al. 1987), and scaffolding within the tube (Ngo et al. 2003) or incorporation of cells (Koshimune et al. 2003). The readers are referred to exhaustive reviews for PNI repair and regeneration (Schmidt and Leach 2003, Mukhatyar et al. 2009). Specifically, several strategies have been developed to stimulate Schwann cell migration and axonal growth. Fabrication techniques such as microlithography, microcontact printing, and electrospinning have been used to manipulate synthetic scaffolds at micro- and nanoscale to fabricate structural features similar to naturally occurring matrix with relative ease. Bellamkonda group has used electrospun fiber films loaded into a semipermeable scaffold to promote nerve regeneration. Poly(acrylonitrile methacrylate) (PAN-MA) electrospun-aligned fibers have been loaded into a polysulfone tube to stimulate endogenous Schwann cell migration in 17 mm nerve gaps in rats (Kim et al. 2008). Compared to empty tubes and randomly oriented fibers, aligned fiber-based conduits were able to elicit nerve growth and improved functional recovery. These scaffolds have been shown to align glial cells and encourage organized ECM formation (Figure 12.5). Even though the function and minimal number of aligned fibers has not been elucidated, it has been hypothesized that they stimulate endogenous repair by sustaining, augmenting, or replacing the fibrin cable. In addition, the Bellamkonda group proposed a regenerative electrode scaffold (RES) using layered nanofiber scaffolds and thin-film electrode arrays (Figure 12.6). The underlying design principle is that axons regenerating from a nerve stump are guided along each nanofiber layer and then across the plane of an embedded electrode array to support high-resolution, closed-loop prosthetic control (Clements et al. 2007).

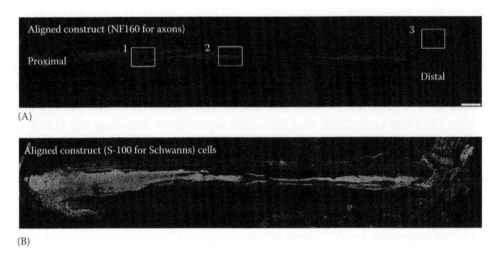

FIGURE 12.5 Immunohistochemical analysis of nerve regeneration through implants *in vivo* (longitudinal section, 17 mm nerve gap). (A) and (B) Representative nerve regeneration through aligned fiber-based polymeric construct. (A) and (B) Double immunostained nerve regeneration (A, NF160) and Schwann cell infiltration from both proximal and distal nerve stump (B, S-100). Scale bar = 1 mm. (Reproduced from *Biomaterials.* 29(21), Kim, Y.T., Haftel, V.K., Kumar, S., and Bellamkonda, R.V., The role of aligned polymer fiber-based constructs in the bridging of long peripheral nerve gaps, 3117–3127, Copyright 2008, with permission from Elsevier.)

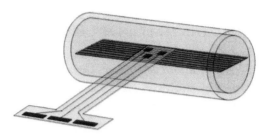

FIGURE 12.6 Illustration of the regenerative electrode scaffold (RES). A thin-film polyimide electrode array (32 channels) was integrated into a scaffold containing a single sheet of oriented nanofibers. The nanofiber layer directs regenerating axons through the tube and across the electrode surface. The electrode's connector end extends through the outside of the tube where it is enclosed in a silicone envelope and sutured beneath the skin. (Reproduced from Clements, I.P. et al., eds., *3rd International IEEE/EMBS Conference on Neural Engineering*, Kohala Coast, HI, 2007, with permission from IEEE.)

Next, when a biomaterial is used as a delivery vehicle for cells or drugs, the biomaterial must provide a suitable microenvironment for cell survival, regeneration, and host tissue integration. An approach in this regard is a hydrogel system injected in liquid form into the lesion cavity, which then forms a three-dimensional scaffold *in situ*, allowing for minimally invasive delivery into the lesion. The injectable hydrogel such as thermosensitive polymer systems can contain free or tethered drugs and/or suspended cells (Jeong et al. 2002, Yu and Bellamkonda 2003, Jain et al. 2006). Hollow fiber membranes filled with brain-derived neurotrophic factor have promoted axonal regeneration *in vivo* (Patist et al. 2004). In other approaches, scaffolds can be tailored to mimic the developing brain by promoting migration of endogenous stem cells, thereby enhancing plasticity and hence redevelopment following SCI/TBI. Cell-seeded polymer scaffolds have been shown to increase cell adhesion, survival, and host–implant integration in many physiological systems, including the CNS (Yu et al. 1999, Park et al. 2002, Silva et al. 2004). NSCs have also been used in combination with biomaterial scaffolds for enhanced delivery of cells following TBI (Tate et al. 2002) and enhanced regeneration following SCI (Lavik et al. 2002). To date, several efforts have been made to utilize tissue-engineering approaches in the CNS, ranging from implanting encapsulated nerve growth factor–secreting cells to treat Alzheimer's disease (Winn et al. 1996) to implanting NSCs within porous polyglycolic acid scaffolds to treat hypoxia–ischemia (Park et al. 2002). Furthermore, SCI regeneration using either peripheral nerve grafts or biomimetic nerve guidance channels have yielded interesting results, where Schwann cells likely contribute by cleaning up the degenerative debris that follows injury (Bunge 2002, Nomura et al. 2006). Nerve guidance channels, or nerve cuffs, are used clinically to repair PNIs, providing a permissive route through which severed axons can regrow. Connecting gray and white matter with a series of intercostal peripheral nerve grafts have also shown promising results (Cheng et al. 1996); however, these results have been difficult to replicate. The challenge with these biomimetic approaches is to stimulate a sufficient number of axons to regenerate within the defined environment. Another strategy is to combine the permissive channel environment with an enzyme, such as chondroitinase ABC (Rhodes and Fawcett 2004, Lee et al. 2010) or xylosyltransferase-1 (Grimpe and Silver 2004) or by targeting chondroitin-polymerizing factor (ChPF) (Laabs et al. 2007), which has been shown to degrade the glial scar, thereby improving the physical pathway for regeneration (Friedman et al. 2002).

However, in general approaches should not only guide axonal growth in CNS, but also improve survival and integration of cells implanted into the injured area. Cell survival limitations can be overcome by engineering a tissue-like construct based on core components of the developing brain tissue, such as by using NSCs, extracellular matrix proteins, and/or *in situ* forming three-dimensional structures. By attaching bioactive ligands, such as ECM motifs, to scaffold materials may positively influence cell behavior of transplanted cells. For example, NSCs transplanted in TBI animal models within a matrix-based scaffold showed improved cell survival and migration (Tate et al. 2002) in comparison to cells transplanted in the absence of the scaffold, because of the anti-apoptotic properties of ECM proteins (laminin and fibronectin) (Gu et al. 2005).

12.5.2 Neurorehabilitation

Despite substantial research, an effective long-term solution for SCI remains elusive. Locomotor rehabilitation training remains the only accepted and somewhat effective clinical treatment. The goal of locomotor training has been (1) to achieve activation of neurological levels located both above and below the injury site and (2) to promote inherent CNS plasticity, repair, and regeneration. It is hoped that by activating residual "uninjured" neural circuitry, the formation of functionally "meaningful" new connections can be enticed (Weidner et al. 2001). Particularly, rehabilitation training can reinforce efficacy of specific sensorimotor pathways, which could result in a more selective and stable neuronal network of neurons. However, because of the presence of endogenous inhibitors within the nervous system, the formation of such new connections is largely limited in an injured CNS (Fawcett 2006). In other approaches, spontaneous regeneration was observed by applying patterned sensory feedback to enhance neural activity. This was accomplished by use of partial weight–supported walking (PWSW), or passive limb movements, electrically stimulated stationary bicycling, and/or tendon transfers (Becker et al. 2003). The hand function loss, which is perceived by tetraplegic individuals as the biggest loss due to SCI, was partially regained by tendon transfer. In addition, tendon transfers are performed to improve grip strength, restore voluntary thumb pinch, active elbow, and wrist extension (Freehafer 1998). Similarly, PWSW improve gait in individuals with incomplete SCI (Protas et al. 2001).

In summary, the potential benefits of activity-dependent rehabilitation are (1) muscle mass increase which in turn reduces skin breakdown; (2) maintenance of bone density, thus preventing pathological bone fractures; (3) increase in blood flow, which reduces formation of blood clots; and (4) significant reduction in spasticity and potential enhancement of regeneration (Grill et al. 2001). However, by using rehabilitation training in conjunction with biological and/or electrical stimulation approaches (exogenous or endogenous), it is expected that the combinatorial intervention will be more effective for severe PNS or CNS injury (Garcia-Alias et al. 2009).

12.5.3 Neural Prostheses

The electrical activation of the nervous system is used to not only restore function, but also promote plasticity and learning while preventing secondary injury (Grill and Kirsch 2000). In spite of explosive success, the field of neuroprostheses is still far from being able to achieve full restoration of all able-bodied functions in the nervous system (Grill et al. 2001). Numerous reports indicate that applying DC electric fields can enhance axonal outgrowth, causing growth toward the cathode with alignment of axons along the electric field lines (Sisken et al. 1993, Borgens 1999). Electrical stimulation can also overcome the deficit produced by the lesion in the spinal cord and maintain the integrity of various bodily functions through direct neuromuscular stimulation. However, there are technical limitations to this approach; the use of chronic DC currents is known to damage potentially both the electrode and the underlying tissue (Agnew and McCreery 1990).

12.5.3.1 Functional Electrical Stimulation

Functional electrical stimulation (FES) is a technique of applying safe amounts of electric current to activate damaged or disabled neuromuscles in a coordinated manner in order to achieve lost function. The goal of FES devices is to provide greater mobility to SCI patients, assistance with respiration, bowel/bladder activity, or some return of upper or lower limb function (Hamid and Hayek 2008). External neuromuscular excitation has been attempted since the eighteenth century, when Luigi Galvani discovered that electric current can generate an action potential leading to muscular contractions. Both nerves and muscle fibers respond to electric currents. Recent experiments with an adult guinea pig model transected at mid-thoracic level and implanted with guidance channel containing electrodes indicate that DC fields can promote axonal regeneration following SCI (Mensinger et al. 2000). However, a better understanding of (1) the effects of electric fields on the growth cone machinery, (2) mechanism of regeneration, (3) electrode materials and electrochemistry at the electrode/tissue interface, and (4) effects of transient pulsing rather than DC currents is necessary to build an effective neuroprosthetic device (Grill et al. 2001). Clinically, there are two applications for FES devices in case of SCI—functional and therapeutic applications (Hamid and Hayek 2008). Functional applications aim to restore vital body functions lost due to SCI. For example, ambulation and locomotive support in cases of paraplegia, assistance with respiration or hand grasp in case of quadriplegia, in addition to electro-ejaculation, bowel, or bladder voiding. Of the several commercial and research FES devices, the only FDA-approved FES for short distance ambulation is the Parastep I (Graupe 2002). Presently for quadriplegia patients, two FDA-approved systems are available—Freehand System (Hobby et al. 2001, Taylor et al. 2001) and Handmaster (Snoek et al. 2000). The goal of these devices is to enable restoration of grasp for holding bigger/heavier objects and lateral grasp for smaller/thinner ones. The therapeutic applications for FES devices include cardiovascular conditioning and prevention of muscular atrophy. The most common FES system for lower extremity exercise is the bicycle ergometer. Gazula et al. (2004) demonstrated the significant effects of lower limb FES on spinal motor neurons. The different FES electrodes (both invasive and noninvasive) with their applications and limitations are discussed in detail elsewhere (Navarro et al. 2005, Giszter 2008).

Although the current development and advances in the design of FES system have made it possible to provide some mobility and function to the SCI patients, at present FES alone has multiple inherent limitations. To restore the lost function safely, completely, and efficaciously, further research or combinatorial strategies may be needed. There are multiple challenges that need to be met before FES can be utilized in a clinical setting (Hamid and Hayek 2008). An emerging line of research in the field of FES is intraspinal microstimulation (ISMS), where the SC locomotor circuits called Central Pattern Generators (CPG) are directly tapped for stimulation and restoration of limb movements (Sadowsky 2001). Future work on these neuroprosthetic devices is focusing on decoding the intended motion trajectories from the cerebral motor cortex and using this signal to control the FES devices. Hybrid neuroprosthetics is being investigated and may lead to the development of a cognitive link through cerebral motor cortex to these neural prosthetic devices (Musallam et al. 2004). Another recent effort is oscillating field stimulation (OFS), which potentially is safe and effective in enhancing functional outcomes after SCI. However, OFS is an invasive intervention with multiple associated risks such as surgical technique, immune reaction, infection, breakage of wires, battery life, etc. (Borgens et al. 2002).

12.6 FUTURE OUTLOOK: OPPORTUNITIES AND CHALLENGES

In the case of PNI, the opportunity is to develop a bioengineering or regenerative solution that is a clinically viable alternative to autografts. In the case of CNS, the long-standing belief that still lingers to some extent in the clinical setting is that CNS "once injured" could never be repaired. However, recent advances in experimental regenerative, electrical stimulation, and rehabilitative research have created optimism in the field that the spinal cord is not a rigid or unrepairable structure. Several studies have attempted to use combinatorial interventions, which can target multiple factors of repair and regeneration. For example, treatment with ChABC, which breaks down inhibitory molecules, promotes regeneration of injured axons in the CNS (Moon et al. 2001, Bradbury et al. 2002). This treatment has now been used to enhance axonal regrowth across the dorsal root in combination with (1) preconditioning methods (Steinmetz et al. 2005); (2) Schwann cell–seeded guidance channels (Chau et al. 2004); (3) transplanted NPCs (Ikegami et al. 2005); and (4) transplanted Schwann cells and OEG (Fouad et al. 2005). Similarly, other studies have combined treatments that induce regeneration (by elevating cyclic AMP levels) with treatments such as neurotrophic factors (Lu et al. 2004) and Schwann cell transplants (Pearse et al. 2004). Similarly, many other potential convergence strategies exist between electrical stimulation and regenerative medicine. For example, electrical stimulation has the potential to limit secondary injury and to regulate the efficacy of cell transplantation (Borgens 2003). Therefore, by using electrical activity axonal regeneration and guidance can be modulated along with spasticity (Grill et al. 2001). Cell therapy, with the possibility to repair the degenerated tissue, holds tremendous promise for the treatment of neurological disorders. However, the major challenges, which include cell survival, cell fate determination, and engraftment after transplantation, still remain. Tissue engineering may contribute to alleviate some or all of these issues and several proof-of-concept experiments have been reported with even some clinical trials. For example, advanced scaffold modifications, such as the biomimetic approaches, can allow for better control of cell survival, proliferation, migration, differentiation, and engraftment *in vivo*. An example of a combinatorial method is the transplantation of gel-based scaffolds with hMSCs (as delivery vehicle) for neuroprotection and repair of neural injury following TBI (Qu et al. 2009).

Neural regeneration following SCI is likely to become a clinical reality in the near future. However, the question still remains as to the level of functional recovery that can be attained within neural reconnectivity. Assistive neuroprosthetic devices, regenerative medicine, and rehabilitation will continue to play an important role in repair and regeneration. A combination of interventions would be significantly more effective than either alone, suggesting a synergistic action between biological, pharmacological, electrical stimulation, and rehabilitation communities. For example, locomotor rehabilitative training, in conjunction with pharmacological (Chau et al. 1998, Antri et al. 2003, Maier et al. 2009) and/or electrical stimulation (Edgerton et al. 2008, Ichiyama et al. 2008), promoted use-dependent plasticity in the sensorimotor circuits below the injury site (Cote and Gossard 2004, Petruska et al. 2007, Musienko et al. 2009) that lead to specific improvements of stepping patterns. These interventions, however, showed limited potential for promoting weight-bearing capacities. Recently, for the first time rats with chronic SCI showed the ability to generate full weight-bearing bipedal treadmill locomotion that was almost indistinguishable from voluntary stepping recorded in the same rats prior to injury. This was achieved by using combinations of specific pharmacological and electrical stimulation interventions, along with locomotor training (Courtine et al. 2009, Fong et al. 2009). Using kinematics, physiological, and anatomical analyses, the authors showed that combinatorial interventions recruit specific populations of spinal circuits, refine their control via sensory input, and functionally remodel the locomotor pathways. Further challenges with respect to neural interfacing include integration of electrodes and the brain, stability of such an interface, and the ability to bidirectionally communicate with the CNS or PNS. In addition, the understanding of the underlying "neural code" and how information may be "put in" to the nervous system is largely unknown. Furthermore, better understanding of how rehabilitation works in terms of the underlying molecular and systemic responses will be required in the future.

12.7 SUMMARY

In conclusion, the literature of neural injuries suggests that several therapeutic strategies are currently available to promote CNS and PNS repair and regeneration. However, the degree of regeneration and hence the functional recovery remains relatively modest. Neural deficit, in particular SCI being a multifaceted problem, will require a multifaceted or combinatorial intervention. The earlier discussion clearly shows that enhanced axonal regeneration can be achieved when two or more treatments are combined, in other words, an integrated, inter-disciplinary research that cuts across rehabilitation, regenerative medicine, and neuroprosthetics is required. If indeed combinatorial approaches are required, the question that arises is—what combination and on what spatial and temporal scales are they necessary? We postulate here that there exist convergent themes that form a common basis for a synergistic application of regenerative medicine, rehabilitation, and neuroprosthetics and future research: (1) modulating inflammation and secondary damage, (2) encouraging endogenous repair/regeneration (using scaffolds, cell transplantation, and drug delivery), (3) applying electrical fields to modulate healing and/or activity, and (4) modulating plasticity. The future of restoring function after neural injury may depend on our ability to target the earlier process in a combinatorial and yet simple approach that is safe, passes regulatory muster, and is efficacious.

ACKNOWLEDGMENT

Funding support from National Institutes of Health (R01 NS 044409 and R01 NS065109) and National Science Foundation (CBET 0651716) is gratefully acknowledged (RVB).

REFERENCES

Abbott A. (2006) Neuroprosthetics: In search of the sixth sense. *Nature.* 442(7099):125–127.

Ackery A, Tator C, Krassioukov A. (2004) A global perspective on spinal cord injury epidemiology. *J Neurotrauma.* 21(10):1355–1370.

Aebischer P, Winn SR, Galletti PM. (1988) Transplantation of neural tissue in polymer capsules. *Brain Res.* 448(2):364–368.

Agnew WF, McCreery DB. (1990) Considerations for safety with chronically implanted nerve electrodes. *Epilepsia.* 31(Suppl 2):S27–S32.

Ansselin AD, Davey DF. (1988) Axonal regeneration through peripheral nerve grafts: The effect of proximo-distal orientation. *Microsurgery.* 9(2):103–113.

Antri M, Mouffle C, Orsal D, Barthe JY. (2003) 5-HT1A receptors are involved in short- and long-term processes responsible for 5-HT-induced locomotor function recovery in chronic spinal rat. *Eur J Neurosci.* 18(7):1963–1972.

Bao F, Chen Y, Dekaban GA, Weaver LC. (2004) Early anti-inflammatory treatment reduces lipid peroxidation and protein nitration after spinal cord injury in rats. *J Neurochem.* 88(6):1335–1344.

Bareyre FM. (2008) Neuronal repair and replacement in spinal cord injury. *J Neurol Sci.* 265(1–2):63–72.

Bareyre FM, Kerschensteiner M, Raineteau O, Mettenleiter TC, Weinmann O, Schwab ME. (2004) The injured spinal cord spontaneously forms a new intraspinal circuit in adult rats. *Nat Neurosci.* 7(3):269–277.

Becker D, Sadowsky CL, McDonald JW. (2003) Restoring function after spinal cord injury. *Neurologist.* 9(1):1–15.

Bellamkonda RV. (2006) Peripheral nerve regeneration: An opinion on channels, scaffolds and anisotropy. *Biomaterials.* 27(19):3515–3518.

Borgens RB. (1999) Electrically mediated regeneration and guidance of adult mammalian spinal axons into polymeric channels. *Neuroscience.* 91(1):251–264.

Borgens RB. (2003) Restoring function to the injured human spinal cord. *Adv Anat Embryol Cell Biol.* 171:III–IV, 1–155.

Borgens RB, Shi R, Bohnert D. (2002) Behavioral recovery from spinal cord injury following delayed application of polyethylene glycol. *J Exp Biol.* 205(Pt 1):1–12.

Bracken MB. (1990) Methylprednisolone in the management of acute spinal cord injuries. *Med J Aust.* 153(6):368.

Bracken MB. (2001) Methylprednisolone and acute spinal cord injury: An update of the randomized evidence. *Spine (Phila Pa 1976).* 26(24 Suppl):S47–S54.

Bradbury EJ, Khemani S, Von R, King, Priestley JV, McMahon SB. (1999) NT-3 promotes growth of lesioned adult rat sensory axons ascending in the dorsal columns of the spinal cord. *Eur J Neurosci.* 11(11):3873–3883.

Bradbury EJ, McMahon SB. (2006) Spinal cord repair strategies: Why do they work? *Nat Rev Neurosci.* 7(8):644–653.

Bradbury EJ, Moon LD, Popat RJ, King VR, Bennett GS, Patel PN et al. (2002) Chondroitinase ABC promotes functional recovery after spinal cord injury. *Nature.* 416(6881):636–640.

Bregman BS, Kunkel-Bagden E, Schnell L, Dai HN, Gao D, Schwab ME. (1995) Recovery from spinal cord injury mediated by antibodies to neurite growth inhibitors. *Nature.* 378(6556):498–501.

Buchli AD, Schwab ME. (2005) Inhibition of Nogo: A key strategy to increase regeneration, plasticity and functional recovery of the lesioned central nervous system. *Ann Med.* 37(8):556–567.

Bunge MB. (1994) Transplantation of purified populations of Schwann cells into lesioned adult rat spinal cord. *J Neurol.* 242(1 Suppl 1):S36–S39.

Bunge MB. (2002) Bridging the transected or contused adult rat spinal cord with Schwann cell and olfactory ensheathing glia transplants. *Prog Brain Res.* 137:275–282.

Cajal SRy. (1928) *Degeneration and Regeneration of the Nervous System.* New York: Hafner.

Carlson GD, Gorden C. (2002) Current developments in spinal cord injury research. *Spine J.* 2(2):116–128.

Caroni P, Savio T, Schwab ME. (1988) Central nervous system regeneration: Oligodendrocytes and myelin as non-permissive substrates for neurite growth. *Prog Brain Res.* 78:363–370.

Chau C, Barbeau H, Rossignol S. (1998) Early locomotor training with clonidine in spinal cats. *J Neurophysiol.* 79(1):392–409.

Chau CH, Shum DK, Li H, Pei J, Lui YY, Wirthlin L et al. (2004) Chondroitinase ABC enhances axonal regrowth through Schwann cell-seeded guidance channels after spinal cord injury. *FASEB J.* 18(1):194–196.

Chaudhry V, Glass JD, Griffin JW. (1992) Wallerian degeneration in peripheral nerve disease. *Neurol Clin.* 10(3):613–627.

Chen MS, Huber AB, van der Haar ME, Frank M, Schnell L, Spillmann AA et al. (2000) Nogo-A is a myelin-associated neurite outgrowth inhibitor and an antigen for monoclonal antibody IN-1. *Nature.* 403(6768):434–439.

Cheng H, Cao Y, Olson L. (1996) Spinal cord repair in adult paraplegic rats: Partial restoration of hind limb function. *Science.* 273(5274):510–513.

Chuah MI, Choi-Lundberg D, Weston S, Vincent AJ, Chung RS, Vickers JC et al. (2004) Olfactory ensheathing cells promote collateral axonal branching in the injured adult rat spinal cord. *Exp Neurol.* 185(1):15–25.

Chvatal SA, Kim YT, Bratt-Leal AM, Lee H, Bellamkonda RV. (2008) Spatial distribution and acute anti-inflammatory effects of methylprednisolone after sustained local delivery to the contused spinal cord. *Biomaterials.* 29(12):1967–1975.

Clements IP, Kim YT, English AW, Lu X, Chung A, Bellamkonda RV. (2009) Thin-film enhanced nerve guidance channels for peripheral nerve repair. *Biomaterials.* 30(23–24):3834–3846.

Clements IP, Young-Tae K, Andreasen D, Bellamkonda RV, eds. (2007) A regenerative electrode scaffold for peripheral nerve interfacing. *3rd International IEEE/EMBS Conference on Neural Engineering,* Kohala Coast, HI, pp. 390–393.

Correale J, Villa A. (2004) The neuroprotective role of inflammation in nervous system injuries. *J Neurol.* 251(11):1304–1316.

Corso P, Finkelstein E, Miller T, Fiebelkorn I, Zaloshnja E. (2006) Incidence and lifetime costs of injuries in the United States. *Inj Prev.* 12(4):212–218.

Cote MP, Gossard JP. (2004) Step training-dependent plasticity in spinal cutaneous pathways. *J Neurosci.* 24(50):11317–11327.

Courtine G, Gerasimenko Y, van den Brand R, Yew A, Musienko P, Zhong H et al. (2009) Transformation of nonfunctional spinal circuits into functional states after the loss of brain input. *Nat Neurosci.* 12(10):1333–1342.

Courtine G, Song B, Roy RR, Zhong H, Herrmann JE, Ao Y et al. (2008) Recovery of supraspinal control of stepping via indirect propriospinal relay connections after spinal cord injury. *Nat Med.* 14(1):69–74.

Coutts M, Keirstead HS. (2008) Stem cells for the treatment of spinal cord injury. *Exp Neurol.* 209(2):368–377.

Cummings BJ, Uchida N, Tamaki SJ, Salazar DL, Hooshmand M, Summers R et al. (2005) Human neural stem cells differentiate and promote locomotor recovery in spinal cord-injured mice. *Proc Natl Acad Sci U S A.* 102(39):14069–14074.

Daar AS, Greenwood HL. (2007) A proposed definition of regenerative medicine. *J Tissue Eng Regen Med.* 1(3):179–184.

Dash PK, Mach SA, Moore AN. (2001) Enhanced neurogenesis in the rodent hippocampus following traumatic brain injury. *J Neurosci Res.* 63(4):313–319.

David S, Aguayo AJ. (1982) Axonal elongation into peripheral nervous system "bridges" after central nervous system injury in adult rats. *Science.* 214:931–933.

De Leon RD, Hodgson JA, Roy RR, Edgerton VR. (1999) Retention of hindlimb stepping ability in adult spinal cats after the cessation of step training. *J Neurophysiol.* 81(1):85–94.

Dimos JT, Rodolfa KT, Niakan KK, Weisenthal LM, Mitsumoto H, Chung W et al. (2008) Induced pluripotent stem cells generated from patients with ALS can be differentiated into motor neurons. *Science.* 321(5893):1218–1221.

Dodla MC, Bellamkonda RV. (2008) Differences between the effect of anisotropic and isotropic laminin and nerve growth factor presenting scaffolds on nerve regeneration across long peripheral nerve gaps. *Biomaterials.* 29(1):33–46.

Donovan PJ, Gearhart J. (2001) The end of the beginning for pluripotent stem cells. *Nature.* 414(6859):92–97.

Dunlop SA. (2008) Activity-dependent plasticity: Implications for recovery after spinal cord injury. *Trends Neurosci.* 31(8):410–418.

Eddleston M, Mucke L. (1993) Molecular profile of reactive astrocytes—Implications for their role in neurologic disease. *Neuroscience.* 54(1):15–36.

Edgerton VR, Courtine G, Gerasimenko YP, Lavrov I, Ichiyama RM, Fong AJ et al. (2008) Training locomotor networks. *Brain Res Rev.* 57(1):241–254.

Eftekharpour E, Karimi-Abdolrezaee S, Fehlings MG. (2008) Current status of experimental cell replacement approaches to spinal cord injury. *Neurosurg Focus.* 24(3–4):E19.

Enzmann GU, Benton RL, Talbott JF, Cao Q, Whittemore SR. (2006) Functional considerations of stem cell transplantation therapy for spinal cord repair. *J Neurotrauma.* 23(3–4):479–495.

Faulkner J, Keirstead HS. (2005) Human embryonic stem cell-derived oligodendrocyte progenitors for the treatment of spinal cord injury. *Transpl Immunol.* 15(2):131–142.

Fawcett JW. (2006) Overcoming inhibition in the damaged spinal cord. *J Neurotrauma.* 23(3–4):371–383.

Fawcett JW, Asher RA. (1999) The glial scar and central nervous system repair. *Brain Res Bull.* 49(6):377–391.

Fong AJ, Roy RR, Ichiyama RM, Lavrov I, Courtine G, Gerasimenko Y et al. (2009) Recovery of control of posture and locomotion after a spinal cord injury: Solutions staring us in the face. *Prog Brain Res.* 175:393–418.

Fouad K, Schnell L, Bunge MB, Schwab ME, Liebscher T, Pearse DD. (2005) Combining Schwann cell bridges and olfactory-ensheathing glia grafts with chondroitinase promotes locomotor recovery after complete transection of the spinal cord. *J Neurosci.* 25(5):1169–1178.

Fournier AE, Takizawa BT, Strittmatter SM. (2003) Rho kinase inhibition enhances axonal regeneration in the injured CNS. *J Neurosci.* 23(4):1416–1423.

Freehafer AA. (1998) Tendon transfers in tetraplegic patients: The Cleveland experience. *Spinal Cord.* 36(5):315–319.

Friedman JA, Windebank AJ, Moore MJ, Spinner RJ, Currier BL, Yaszemski MJ. (2002) Biodegradable polymer grafts for surgical repair of the injured spinal cord. *Neurosurgery.* 51(3):742–751; discussion 751–752.

Gaetz M. (2004) The neurophysiology of brain injury. *Clin Neurophysiol.* 115(1):4–18.

Galtrey CM, Fawcett JW. (2007) The role of chondroitin sulfate proteoglycans in regeneration and plasticity in the central nervous system. *Brain Res Rev.* 54(1):1–18.

Galvin J, Mandalis A. (2009) Executive skills and their functional implications: Approaches to rehabilitation after childhood TBI. *Dev Neurorehabil.* 12(5):352–360.

Garcia-Alias G, Barkhuysen S, Buckle M, Fawcett JW. (2009) Chondroitinase ABC treatment opens a window of opportunity for task-specific rehabilitation. *Nat Neurosci.* 12(9):1145–1151.

Garcia-Alias G, Lin R, Akrimi SF, Story D, Bradbury EJ, Fawcett JW. (2008) Therapeutic time window for the application of chondroitinase ABC after spinal cord injury. *Exp Neurol.* 210(2):331–338.

Gazula VR, Roberts M, Luzzio C, Jawad AF, Kalb RG. (2004) Effects of limb exercise after spinal cord injury on motor neuron dendrite structure. *J Comp Neurol.* 476(2):130–145.

Gerndt SJ, Rodriguez JL, Pawlik JW, Taheri PA, Wahl WL, Micheals AJ et al. (1997) Consequences of high-dose steroid therapy for acute spinal cord injury. *J Trauma.* 42(2):279–284.

Giles GM. (2009) Maximizing TBI rehabilitation outcomes with targeted interventions. *Arch Phys Med Rehabil.* 90(3):530.

Giszter SF. (2008) Spinal cord injury: Present and future therapeutic devices and prostheses. *Neurotherapeutics.* 5(1):147–162.

Gomes-Leal W, Corkill DJ, Freire MA, Picanco-Diniz CW, Perry VH. (2004) Astrocytosis, microglia activation, oligodendrocyte degeneration, and pyknosis following acute spinal cord injury. *Exp Neurol.* 190(2):456–467.

Gottlieb DI. (2002) Large-scale sources of neural stem cells. *Annu Rev Neurosci.* 25:381–407.

Graham DI, Maxwell WL, Adams JH, Jennett B. (2005) Novel aspects of the neuropathology of the vegetative state after blunt head injury. *Prog Brain Res.* 150:445–455.

GrandPre T, Li S, Strittmatter SM. (2002) Nogo-66 receptor antagonist peptide promotes axonal regeneration. *Nature.* 417(6888):547–551.

Graupe D. (2002) An overview of the state of the art of noninvasive FES for independent ambulation by thoracic level paraplegics. *Neurol Res.* 24(5):431–442.

Grill R, Murai K, Blesch A, Gage FH, Tuszynski MH. (1997) Cellular delivery of neurotrophin-3 promotes corticospinal axonal growth and partial functional recovery after spinal cord injury. *J Neurosci.* 17(14):5560–5572.

Grill WM, Kirsch RF. (2000) Neuroprosthetic applications of electrical stimulation. *Assist Technol.* 12(1):6–20.

Grill WM, McDonald JW, Peckham PH, Heetderks W, Kocsis J, Weinrich M. (2001) At the interface: Convergence of neural regeneration and neural prostheses for restoration of function. *J Rehabil Res Dev.* 38(6):633–639.

Grimpe B, Silver J. (2004) A novel DNA enzyme reduces glycosaminoglycan chains in the glial scar and allows microtransplanted dorsal root ganglia axons to regenerate beyond lesions in the spinal cord. *J Neurosci.* 24(6):1393–1397.

Groves ML, McKeon R, Werner E, Nagarsheth M, Meador W, English AW. (2005) Axon regeneration in peripheral nerves is enhanced by proteoglycan degradation. *Exp Neurol.* 195(2):278–292.

Gu Z, Cui J, Brown S, Fridman R, Mobashery S, Strongin AY et al. (2005) A highly specific inhibitor of matrix metalloproteinase-9 rescues laminin from proteolysis and neurons from apoptosis in transient focal cerebral ischemia. *J Neurosci.* 25(27):6401–6408.

Hagg T, Oudega M. (2006) Degenerative and spontaneous regenerative processes after spinal cord injury. *J Neurotrauma.* 23(3–4):264–280.

Hall ED. (1992) The neuroprotective pharmacology of methylprednisolone. *J Neurosurg.* 76(1):13–22.

Hall ED. (1993) Neuroprotective actions of glucocorticoid and nonglucocorticoid steroids in acute neuronal injury. *Cell Mol Neurobiol.* 13(4):415–432.

Hall ED, Sullivan PG, Gibson TR, Pavel KM, Thompson BM, Scheff SW. (2005) Spatial and temporal characteristics of neurodegeneration after controlled cortical impact in mice: More than a focal brain injury. *J Neurotrauma.* 22(2):252–265.

Hamid S, Hayek R. (2008) Role of electrical stimulation for rehabilitation and regeneration after spinal cord injury: An overview. *Eur Spine J.* 17(9):1256–1269.

Harkey HL, 3rd, White EA, 4th, Tibbs RE, Jr., Haines DE. (2003) A clinician's view of spinal cord injury. *Anat Rec B New Anat.* 271(1):41–48.

Hobby J, Taylor PN, Esnouf J. (2001) Restoration of tetraplegic hand function by use of the neurocontrol freehand system. *J Hand Surg Br.* 26(5):459–464.

Hofstetter CP, Schwarz EJ, Hess D, Widenfalk J, El Manira A, Prockop DJ et al. (2002) Marrow stromal cells form guiding strands in the injured spinal cord and promote recovery. *Proc Natl Acad Sci U S A.* 99(4):2199–2204.

Ichiyama RM, Courtine G, Gerasimenko YP, Yang GJ, van den Brand R, Lavrov IA et al. (2008) Step training reinforces specific spinal locomotor circuitry in adult spinal rats. *J Neurosci.* 28(29):7370–7375.

Ikegami T, Nakamura M, Yamane J, Katoh H, Okada S, Iwanami A et al. (2005) Chondroitinase ABC combined with neural stem/progenitor cell transplantation enhances graft cell migration and outgrowth of growth-associated protein-43-positive fibers after rat spinal cord injury. *Eur J Neurosci.* 22(12):3036–3046.

Iwanami A, Kaneko S, Nakamura M, Kanemura Y, Mori H, Kobayashi S et al. (2005) Transplantation of human neural stem cells for spinal cord injury in primates. *J Neurosci Res.* 80(2):182–190.

Jacobson S, Guth L. (1965) An electrophysiological study of the early stages of peripheral nerve regeneration. *Exp Neurol.* 11:48–60.

Jain A, Kim YT, McKeon RJ, Bellamkonda RV. (2006) *In situ* gelling hydrogels for conformal repair of spinal cord defects, and local delivery of BDNF after spinal cord injury. *Biomaterials.* 27(3):497–504.

Jennett B, Adams JH, Murray LS, Graham DI. (2001) Neuropathology in vegetative and severely disabled patients after head injury. *Neurology.* 56(4):486–490.

Jeong B, Kim SW, Bae YH. (2002) Thermosensitive sol–gel reversible hydrogels. *Adv Drug Deliv Rev.* 54(1):37–51.

Jones KS, Sefton MV, Gorczynski RM. (2004) *In vivo* recognition by the host adaptive immune system of microencapsulated xenogeneic cells. *Transplantation.* 78(10):1454–1462.

Kalbermatten DF, Kingham PJ, Mahay D, Mantovani C, Pettersson J, Raffoul W et al. (2008) Fibrin matrix for suspension of regenerative cells in an artificial nerve conduit. *J Plast Reconstr Aesthet Surg.* 61(6):669–675.

Karimi-Abdolrezaee S, Eftekharpour E, Wang J, Morshead CM, Fehlings MG. (2006) Delayed transplantation of adult neural precursor cells promotes remyelination and functional neurological recovery after spinal cord injury. *J Neurosci.* 26(13):3377–3389.

Keilhoff G, Goihl A, Langnase K, Fansa H, Wolf G. (2006) Transdifferentiation of mesenchymal stem cells into Schwann cell-like myelinating cells. *Eur J Cell Biol.* 85(1):11–24.

Keirstead HS, Levine JM, Blakemore WF. (1998) Response of the oligodendrocyte progenitor cell population (defined by NG2 labelling) to demyelination of the adult spinal cord. *Glia.* 22(2):161–170.

Kerns J. (2008) The microstructure of peripheral nerves. *Tech Reg Anesth Pain Manag.* 12(3):127–133.

Kim YT, Caldwell JM, Bellamkonda RV. (2009) Nanoparticle-mediated local delivery of methylprednisolone after spinal cord injury. *Biomaterials.* 30(13):2582–2590.

Kim YT, Haftel VK, Kumar S, Bellamkonda RV. (2008) The role of aligned polymer fiber-based constructs in the bridging of long peripheral nerve gaps. *Biomaterials.* 29(21):3117–3127.

Kim SU, de Vellis J. (2009) Stem cell-based cell therapy in neurological diseases: A review. *J Neurosci Res.* 87(10):2183–2200.

Koshimune M, Takamatsu K, Nakatsuka H, Inui K, Yamano Y, Ikada Y. (2003) Creating bioabsorbable Schwann cell coated conduits through tissue engineering. *Biomed Mater Eng.* 13(3):223–229.

Kubasak MD, Jindrich DL, Zhong H, Takeoka A, McFarland KC, Munoz-Quiles C et al. (2008) OEG implantation and step training enhance hindlimb-stepping ability in adult spinal transected rats. *Brain.* 131(Pt 1):264–276.

Laabs TL, Wang H, Katagiri Y, McCann T, Fawcett JW, Geller HM. (2007) Inhibiting glycosaminoglycan chain polymerization decreases the inhibitory activity of astrocyte-derived chondroitin sulfate proteoglycans. *J Neurosci.* 27(52):14494–14501.

Landon DN. (1975) *The Peripheral Nerve.* New York: Wiley.

Landry ES, Lapointe NP, Rouillard C, Levesque D, Hedlund PB, Guertin PA. (2006) Contribution of spinal 5-HT1A and 5-HT7 receptors to locomotor-like movement induced by 8-OH-DPAT in spinal cord-transected mice. *Eur J Neurosci.* 24(2):535–546.

Langer R, Vacanti JP. (1993) Tissue engineering. *Science.* 260(5110):920–926.

Lavik E, Teng YD, Snyder E, Langer R. (2002) Seeding neural stem cells on scaffolds of PGA, PLA, and their copolymers. *Methods Mol Biol.* 198:89–97.

Lee H, McKeon RJ, Bellamkonda RV. (2010) Sustained delivery of thermostabilized chABC enhances axonal sprouting and functional recovery after spinal cord injury. *Proc Natl Acad Sci U S A.* 107(8):3340–3345.

Lee SK, Wolfe SW. (2000) Peripheral nerve injury and repair. *J Am Acad Orthop Surg.* 8(4):243–252.

Lenzlinger PM, Morganti-Kossmann MC, Laurer HL, McIntosh TK. (2001) The duality of the inflammatory response to traumatic brain injury. *Mol Neurobiol.* 24(1–3):169–181.

Levin HS, Gary HE, Jr., Eisenberg HM, Ruff RM, Barth JT, Kreutzer J et al. (1990) Neurobehavioral outcome 1 year after severe head injury. Experience of the Traumatic Coma Data Bank. *J Neurosurg.* 73(5):699–709.

Li W, Guo Y, Wang H, Shi D, Liang C, Ye Z et al. (2008) Electrospun nanofibers immobilized with collagen for neural stem cells culture. *J Mater Sci Mater Med.* 19(2):847–854.

Li Y, Field PM, Raisman G. (1997) Repair of adult rat corticospinal tract by transplants of olfactory ensheathing cells. *Science.* 277(5334):2000–2002.

Li Q, Ping P, Jiang H, Liu K. (2006) Nerve conduit filled with *GDNF* gene-modified Schwann cells enhances regeneration of the peripheral nerve. *Microsurgery.* 26(2):116–121.

Lindvall O, Kokaia Z. (2006) Stem cells for the treatment of neurological disorders. *Nature.* 441(7097):1094–1096.

Lindvall O, Kokaia Z, Martinez-Serrano A. (2004) Stem cell therapy for human neurodegenerative disorders—How to make it work. *Nat Med.* 10(Suppl):S42–S50.

Lisak RP, editor. (2009) *International Neurology: A Clinical Approach.* Oxford, U.K.: Blackwell Publishing Ltd.

Liu Y, Kim D, Himes BT, Chow SY, Schallert T, Murray M et al. (1999) Transplants of fibroblasts genetically modified to express BDNF promote regeneration of adult rat rubrospinal axons and recovery of forelimb function. *J Neurosci.* 19(11):4370–4387.

Longhi L, Zanier ER, Royo N, Stocchetti N, McIntosh TK. (2005) Stem cell transplantation as a therapeutic strategy for traumatic brain injury. *Transpl Immunol.* 15(2):143–148.

Lu P, Jones LL, Snyder EY, Tuszynski MH. (2003) Neural stem cells constitutively secrete neurotrophic factors and promote extensive host axonal growth after spinal cord injury. *Exp Neurol.* 181(2):115–129.

Lu P, Yang H, Jones LL, Filbin MT, Tuszynski MH. (2004) Combinatorial therapy with neurotrophins and cAMP promotes axonal regeneration beyond sites of spinal cord injury. *J Neurosci.* 24(28):6402–6409.

Maier IC, Ichiyama RM, Courtine G, Schnell L, Lavrov I, Edgerton VR et al. (2009) Differential effects of anti-Nogo-A antibody treatment and treadmill training in rats with incomplete spinal cord injury. *Brain*. 132(Pt 6):1426–1440.

Mammis A, McIntosh TK, Maniker AH. (2009) Erythropoietin as a neuroprotective agent in traumatic brain injury Review. *Surg Neurol*. 71(5):527–531; discussion 531.

Marchesi C, Pluderi M, Colleoni F, Belicchi M, Meregalli M, Farini A et al. (2007) Skin-derived stem cells transplanted into resorbable guides provide functional nerve regeneration after sciatic nerve resection. *Glia*. 55(4):425–438.

McAllister TW. (2009) Psychopharmacological issues in the treatment of TBI and PTSD. *Clin Neuropsychol*. 23(8):1338–1367.

McDonald JW, Liu XZ, Qu Y, Liu S, Mickey SK, Turetsky D et al. (1999) Transplanted embryonic stem cells survive, differentiate and promote recovery in injured rat spinal cord. *Nat Med*. 5(12):1410–1412.

McIntosh TK, Juhler M, Wieloch T. (1998a) Novel pharmacologic strategies in the treatment of experimental traumatic brain injury. *J Neurotrauma*. 15(10):731–769.

McIntosh TK, Saatman KE, Raghupathi R, Graham DI, Smith DH, Lee VM et al. (1998b) The Dorothy Russell Memorial Lecture. The molecular and cellular sequelae of experimental traumatic brain injury: Pathogenetic mechanisms. *Neuropathol Appl Neurobiol*. 24(4):251–267.

McKay R. (1997) Stem cells in the central nervous system. *Science*. 276(5309):66–71.

Mensinger AF, Anderson DJ, Buchko CJ, Johnson MA, Martin DC, Tresco PA et al. (2000) Chronic recording of regenerating VIIIth nerve axons with a sieve electrode. *J Neurophysiol*. 83(1):611–615.

Mimura T, Dezawa M, Kanno H, Sawada H, Yamamoto I. (2004) Peripheral nerve regeneration by transplantation of bone marrow stromal cell-derived Schwann cells in adult rats. *J Neurosurg*. 101(5):806–812.

Moon LD, Asher RA, Rhodes KE, Fawcett JW. (2001) Regeneration of CNS axons back to their target following treatment of adult rat brain with chondroitinase ABC. *Nat Neurosci*. 4(5):465–466.

Morganti-Kossmann MC, Rancan M, Stahel PF, Kossmann T. (2002) Inflammatory response in acute traumatic brain injury: A double-edged sword. *Curr Opin Crit Care*. 8(2):101–105.

Mukhatyar V, Karumbaiah L, Yeh J, Bellamkonda RV. (2009) Tissue engineering strategies designed to facilitate the endogenous regenerative potential of peripheral nerves. *Adv Mater*. 21:4670–4679.

Mukhopadhyay G, Doherty P, Walsh FS, Crocker PR, Filbin MT. (1994) A novel role for myelin-associated glycoprotein as an inhibitor of axonal regeneration. *Neuron*. 13(3):757–767.

Musallam S, Corneil BD, Greger B, Scherberger H, Andersen RA. (2004) Cognitive control signals for neural prosthetics. *Science*. 305(5681):258–262.

Musienko P, van den Brand R, Maerzendorfer O, Larmagnac A, Courtine G. (2009) Combinatory electrical and pharmacological neuroprosthetic interfaces to regain motor function after spinal cord injury. *IEEE Trans Biomed Eng*. 56(11 Pt 2):2707–2711.

Narayan RK, Michel ME, Ansell B, Baethmann A, Biegon A, Bracken MB et al. (2002) Clinical trials in head injury. *J Neurotrauma*. 19(5):503–557.

Navarro X, Krueger TB, Lago N, Micera S, Stieglitz T, Dario P. (2005) A critical review of interfaces with the peripheral nervous system for the control of neuroprostheses and hybrid bionic systems. *J Peripher Nerv Syst*. 10(3):229–258.

Neumann S, Woolf CJ. (1999) Regeneration of dorsal column fibers into and beyond the lesion site following adult spinal cord injury. *Neuron*. 23(1):83–91.

Ngo TT, Waggoner PJ, Romero AA, Nelson KD, Eberhart RC, Smith GM. (2003) Poly(L-lactide) microfilaments enhance peripheral nerve regeneration across extended nerve lesions. *J Neurosci Res*. 72(2):227–238.

Nichols CM, Brenner MJ, Fox IK, Tung TH, Hunter DA, Rickman SR et al. (2004) Effects of motor versus sensory nerve grafts on peripheral nerve regeneration. *Exp Neurol*. 190(2):347–355.

Nie X, Zhang YJ, Tian WD, Jiang M, Dong R, Chen JW et al. (2007) Improvement of peripheral nerve regeneration by a tissue-engineered nerve filled with ectomesenchymal stem cells. *Int J Oral Maxillofac Surg.* 36(1):32–38.

Noble J, Munro CA, Prasad VS, Midha R. (1998) Analysis of upper and lower extremity peripheral nerve injuries in a population of patients with multiple injuries. *J Trauma.* 45(1):116–122.

Nomura H, Tator CH, Shoichet MS. (2006) Bioengineered strategies for spinal cord repair. *J Neurotrauma.* 23(3–4):496–507.

Ogawa M. (2002) Changing phenotypes of hematopoietic stem cells. *Exp Hematol.* 30(1):3–6.

Orive G, Anitua E, Pedraz JL, Emerich DF. (2009) Biomaterials for promoting brain protection, repair and regeneration. *Nat Rev Neurosci.* 10(10):682–692.

Oudega M, Hagg T. (1996) Nerve growth factor promotes regeneration of sensory axons into adult rat spinal cord. *Exp Neurol.* 140(2):218–229.

Park KI, Teng YD, Snyder EY. (2002) The injured brain interacts reciprocally with neural stem cells supported by scaffolds to reconstitute lost tissue. *Nat Biotechnol.* 20(11):1111–1117.

Patist CM, Mulder MB, Gautier SE, Maquet V, Jerome R, Oudega M. (2004) Freeze-dried poly(D,L-lactic acid) macroporous guidance scaffolds impregnated with brain-derived neurotrophic factor in the transected adult rat thoracic spinal cord. *Biomaterials.* 25(9):1569–1582.

Pearse DD, Pereira FC, Marcillo AE, Bates ML, Berrocal YA, Filbin MT et al. (2004) cAMP and Schwann cells promote axonal growth and functional recovery after spinal cord injury. *Nat Med.* 10(6):610–616.

Petruska JC, Ichiyama RM, Jindrich DL, Crown ED, Tansey KE, Roy RR et al. (2007) Changes in motoneuron properties and synaptic inputs related to step training after spinal cord transection in rats. *J Neurosci.* 27(16):4460–4471.

Philips MF, Mattiasson G, Wieloch T, Bjorklund A, Johansson BB, Tomasevic G et al. (2001) Neuroprotective and behavioral efficacy of nerve growth factor-transfected hippocampal progenitor cell transplants after experimental traumatic brain injury. *J Neurosurg.* 94(5):765–774.

Povlishock JT, Katz DI. (2005) Update of neuropathology and neurological recovery after traumatic brain injury. *J Head Trauma Rehabil.* 20(1):76–94.

Properzi F, Asher RA, Fawcett JW. (2003) Chondroitin sulphate proteoglycans in the central nervous system: Changes and synthesis after injury. *Biochem Soc Trans.* 31(2):335–336.

Protas EJ, Holmes SA, Qureshy H, Johnson A, Lee D, Sherwood AM. (2001) Supported treadmill ambulation training after spinal cord injury: A pilot study. *Arch Phys Med Rehabil.* 82(6):825–831.

Qian T, Guo X, Levi AD, Vanni S, Shebert RT, Sipski ML. (2005) High-dose methylprednisolone may cause myopathy in acute spinal cord injury patients. *Spinal Cord.* 43(4):199–203.

Qiu J, Cai D, Dai H, McAtee M, Hoffman PN, Bregman BS et al. (2002) Spinal axon regeneration induced by elevation of cyclic AMP. *Neuron.* 34(6):895–903.

Qu C, Xiong Y, Mahmood A, Kaplan DL, Goussev A, Ning R et al. (2009) Treatment of traumatic brain injury in mice with bone marrow stromal cell-impregnated collagen scaffolds. *J Neurosurg.* 111(4):658–665.

Raghupathi R. (2004) Cell death mechanisms following traumatic brain injury. *Brain Pathol.* 14(2):215–222.

Raineteau O, Fouad K, Bareyre FM, Schwab ME. (2002) Reorganization of descending motor tracts in the rat spinal cord. *Eur J Neurosci.* 16(9):1761–1771.

Raineteau O, Fouad K, Noth P, Thallmair M, Schwab ME. (2001) Functional switch between motor tracts in the presence of the mAb IN-1 in the adult rat. *Proc Natl Acad Sci U S A.* 98(12):6929–6934.

Ramon-Cueto A, Plant GW, Avila J, Bunge MB. (1998) Long-distance axonal regeneration in the transected adult rat spinal cord is promoted by olfactory ensheathing glia transplants. *J Neurosci.* 18(10):3803–3815.

Rhodes KE, Fawcett JW. (2004). Chondroitin sulphate proteoglycans: Preventing plasticity or protecting the CNS? *J Anat.* 204(1):33–48.

Richardson PM, Issa VM, Aguayo AJ. (1984) Regeneration of long spinal axons in the rat. *J Neurocytol.* 13(1):165–182.

Roberts I, Schierhout G, Alderson P. (1998) Absence of evidence for the effectiveness of five interventions routinely used in the intensive care management of severe head injury: A systematic review. *J Neurol Neurosurg Psychiatry.* 65(5):729–733.

Sadowsky CL. (2001) Electrical stimulation in spinal cord injury. *NeuroRehabilitation.* 16(3):165–169.

Schmidt CE, Leach JB. (2003) Neural tissue engineering: Strategies for repair and regeneration. *Annu Rev Biomed Eng.* 5:293–347.

Schouten JW, Fulp CT, Royo NC, Saatman KE, Watson DJ, Snyder EY et al. (2004) A review and rationale for the use of cellular transplantation as a therapeutic strategy for traumatic brain injury. *J Neurotrauma.* 21(11):1501–1538.

Schwab ME. (2004) Nogo and axon regeneration. *Curr Opin Neurobiol.* 14(1):118–124.

Schwab ME, Bartholdi D. (1996) Degeneration and regeneration of axons in the lesioned spinal cord. *Physiol Rev.* 76(2):319–370.

Schwab ME, Caroni P. (1988) Oligodendrocytes and CNS myelin are nonpermissive substrates for neurite growth and fibroblast spreading *in vitro. J Neurosci.* 8(7):2381–2393.

Schwab ME, Kapfhammer JP, Bandtlow CE. (1993) Inhibitors of neurite growth. *Annu Rev Neurosci.* 16:565–595.

Schwartz M, Yoles E. (2005) Macrophages and dendritic cells treatment of spinal cord injury: From the bench to the clinic. *Acta Neurochir Suppl.* 93:147–150.

Scott SH. (2008) Cortical-based neuroprosthetics: When less may be more. *Nat Neurosci.* 11(11):1245–1246.

Shoichet MS, Tate CC, Baumann MD, LaPlaca MC, eds. (2008) *Strategies for Regeneration and Repair in the Injured Central Nervous System.* Boca Raton, FL: CRC Press.

Silva GA, Czeisler C, Niece KL, Beniash E, Harrington DA, Kessler JA et al. (2004) Selective differentiation of neural progenitor cells by high-epitope density nanofibers. *Science.* 303(5662):1352–1355.

Silver J, Miller JH. (2004) Regeneration beyond the glial scar. *Nat Rev Neurosci.* 5(2):146–156.

Sinson G, Voddi M, McIntosh TK. (1996) Combined fetal neural transplantation and nerve growth factor infusion: Effects on neurological outcome following fluid-percussion brain injury in the rat. *J Neurosurg.* 84(4):655–662.

Sisken BF, Walker J, Orgel M. (1993) Prospects on clinical applications of electrical stimulation for nerve regeneration. *J Cell Biochem.* 51(4):404–409.

Snoek GJ, IJzerman MJ, in't Groen FA, Stoffers TS, Zilvold G. (2000) Use of the NESS Handmaster to restore handfunction in tetraplegia: Clinical experiences in ten patients. *Spinal Cord.* 38(4):244–249.

Stalhammar D, Starmark JE. (1986) Assessment of responsiveness in head injury patients. The Glasgow Coma Scale and some comments on alternative methods. *Acta Neurochir Suppl (Wien).* 36:91–94.

Steinmetz MP, Horn KP, Tom VJ, Miller JH, Busch SA, Nair D et al. (2005) Chronic enhancement of the intrinsic growth capacity of sensory neurons combined with the degradation of inhibitory proteoglycans allows functional regeneration of sensory axons through the dorsal root entry zone in the mammalian spinal cord. *J Neurosci.* 25(35):8066–8076.

Stoll G, Griffin JW, Li CY, Trapp BD. (1989) Wallerian degeneration in the peripheral nervous system: Participation of both Schwann cells and macrophages in myelin degradation. *J Neurocytol.* 18(5):671–683.

Tatagiba M, Brosamle C, Schwab ME. (1997) Regeneration of injured axons in the adult mammalian central nervous system. *Neurosurgery.* 40(3):541–546; discussion 546–547.

Tate MC, Shear DA, Hoffman SW, Stein DG, Archer DR, LaPlaca MC. (2002) Fibronectin promotes survival and migration of primary neural stem cells transplanted into the traumatically injured mouse brain. *Cell Transplant.* 11(3):283–295.

Tate CC, Tate MC, LaPlaca MC. (2007) Fibronectin and laminin increase in the mouse brain after controlled cortical impact injury. *J Neurotrauma.* 24(1):226–230.

Taylor P, Esnouf J, Hobby J. (2001) Pattern of use and user satisfaction of Neuro Control Freehand System. *Spinal Cord.* 39(3):156–160.

Tello F. (1911) La influencia del neurotropismo en la regeneracion de los centros nerviosos. *Trab Lab Invest Biol.* 9:123–159.

Teng YD, Lavik EB, Qu X, Park KI, Ourednik J, Zurakowski D et al. (2002) Functional recovery following traumatic spinal cord injury mediated by a unique polymer scaffold seeded with neural stem cells. *Proc Natl Acad Sci U S A.* 99(5):3024–3029.

Thallmair M, Metz GA, Z'Graggen WJ, Raineteau O, Kartje GL, Schwab ME. (1998) Neurite growth inhibitors restrict plasticity and functional recovery following corticospinal tract lesions. *Nat Neurosci.* 1(2):124–131.

Thompson JR, Register E, Curotto J, Kurtz M, Kelly R. (1998) An improved protocol for the preparation of yeast cells for transformation by electroporation. *Yeast.* 14(6):565–571.

Tillakaratne NJ, de Leon RD, Hoang TX, Roy RR, Edgerton VR, Tobin AJ. (2002) Use-dependent modulation of inhibitory capacity in the feline lumbar spinal cord. *J Neurosci.* 22(8):3130–3143.

Totoiu MO, Keirstead HS. (2005) Spinal cord injury is accompanied by chronic progressive demyelination. *J Comp Neurol.* 486(4):373–383.

Valentini RF, ed. (2000) *Nerve Guidance Channels.* Boca Raton, FL: CRC Press LLC.

Vavrek R, Girgis J, Tetzlaff W, Hiebert GW, Fouad K. (2006) BDNF promotes connections of corticospinal neurons onto spared descending interneurons in spinal cord injured rats. *Brain.* 129(Pt 6):1534–1545.

Velardo MJ, Burger C, Williams PR, Baker HV, Lopez MC, Mareci TH et al. (2004) Patterns of gene expression reveal a temporally orchestrated wound healing response in the injured spinal cord. *J Neurosci.* 24(39):8562–8576.

Wang KC, Koprivica V, Kim JA, Sivasankaran R, Guo Y, Neve RL et al. (2002) Oligodendrocyte-myelin glycoprotein is a Nogo receptor ligand that inhibits neurite outgrowth. *Nature.* 417(6892):941–944.

Weidner N, Ner A, Salimi N, Tuszynski MH. (2001) Spontaneous corticospinal axonal plasticity and functional recovery after adult central nervous system injury. *Proc Natl Acad Sci U S A.* 98(6):3513–3518.

Wells JE, Hurlbert RJ, Fehlings MG, Yong VW. (2003) Neuroprotection by minocycline facilitates significant recovery from spinal cord injury in mice. *Brain.* 126(Pt 7):1628–1637.

Wickelgren I. (2004) Neuroprosthetics. Brain–computer interface adds a new dimension. *Science.* 306(5703):1878–1879.

Williams LR, Danielsen N, Muller H, Varon S. (1987) Exogenous matrix precursors promote functional nerve regeneration across a 15-mm gap within a silicone chamber in the rat. *J Comp Neurol.* 264(2):284–290.

Williams LR, Varon S. (1985) Modification of fibrin matrix formation *in situ* enhances nerve regeneration in silicone chambers. *J Comp Neurol.* 231(2):209–220.

Winn SR, Lindner MD, Lee A, Haggett G, Francis JM, Emerich DF. (1996) Polymer-encapsulated genetically modified cells continue to secrete human nerve growth factor for over one year in rat ventricles: Behavioral and anatomical consequences. *Exp Neurol.* 140(2):126–138.

Yatsiv I, Grigoriadis N, Simeonidou C, Stahel PF, Schmidt OI, Alexandrovitch AG et al. (2005) Erythropoietin is neuroprotective, improves functional recovery, and reduces neuronal apoptosis and inflammation in a rodent model of experimental closed head injury. *FASEB J.* 19(12):1701–1703.

Yick LW, Cheung PT, So KF, Wu W. (2003) Axonal regeneration of Clarke's neurons beyond the spinal cord injury scar after treatment with chondroitinase ABC. *Exp Neurol.* 182(1):160–168.

Yu X, Bellamkonda RV. (2003) Tissue-engineered scaffolds are effective alternatives to autografts for bridging peripheral nerve gaps. *Tissue Eng.* 9(3):421–430.

Yu X, Dillon GP, Bellamkonda RB. (1999) A laminin and nerve growth factor-laden three-dimensional scaffold for enhanced neurite extension. *Tissue Eng.* 5(4):291–304.

Zasler ND. (2009) Long-term survival after severe TBI: Clinical and forensic aspects. *Prog Brain Res.* 177:111–124.

Zhang P, He X, Liu K, Zhao F, Fu Z, Zhang D et al. (2004) Bone marrow stromal cells differentiated into functional Schwann cells in injured rats sciatic nerve. *Artif Cells Blood Substit Immobil Biotechnol.* 32(4):509–518.

Ligament Regenerative Engineering*

Parimala S. Samuel, MS; Benjamin R. Mintz, BS;
Kristen L. Lee, BS; and James A. Cooper, Jr., PhD

CONTENTS

13.1 INTRODUCTION

As the elderly population continues to increase, the elderly will demand high quality-of-life standards and expect medical research to discover, develop, and implement strategies that address the challenges of disabling diseases and disorders. Therefore, therapeutic approaches are needed that are financially efficient, predictable, and have measurable clinical outcomes. New approaches to solve some of these problems include tissue

---

* Please note that James A. Cooper Jr., PhD, an author of Chapter 13, is retaining copyright of this chapter.

engineering and regenerative medicine. Tissue engineering uses three approaches for the development of new tissues (Bell, 1995; Deuel and Lanza, 1997; Langer and Vacanti, 1993; Morgan and Yarmush, 1999). These approaches include the use of isolated cells, the addition of biological tissue–inducing molecules such as growth factors, and biocompatible matrices, each used separately or as a combination of all three approaches. Regenerative medicine can be defined as medical therapies that will enable the body to repair, replace, restore, and regenerate damaged or diseased cells, tissues, and organs. It encompasses a variety of research and targeted therapies including cells, gene therapy, tissue engineering, biomaterials, growth factors, and transplantation. Regenerative medicine provides the promise of improved quality of life by supporting and activating the body's natural healing of previously untreatable injuries and diseases.

The need for surgical reconstruction or replacement of a damaged ligament is most often the result of trauma, pathological degeneration, or congenital deformity of the tissue (Jackson, 1995; Jackson and Arnoczky, 1993; Jackson et al., 1994; Johnson et al., 1992; Langer and Vacanti, 1993; Snook, 1983). Reconstructive surgery is based upon the principle of replacing defective tissues with viable alternatives. Tissue-engineered scaffolds have the potential to circumvent the problems shown with metals and nondegradable polymers by reducing the foreign body response and eliminating the need for implant retrieval (Bell, 1995; Deuel and Lanza, 1997; Langer and Vacanti, 1993; Morgan and Yarmush, 1999). These scaffolds can be made from bioceramics, collagen, and synthetic degradable materials that aim to reduce the immune response in both magnitude and duration (Bell, 1995; Deuel and Lanza, 1997; Langer and Vacanti, 1993; Morgan and Yarmush, 1999).

The most common health concern for athletes is musculoskeletal injury (Bernstein, 2003). The knee is one of the most frequently injured joints in sports; the anterior cruciate ligament (ACL), in particular, is at risk. The ACL is the most commonly injured ligament in the knee, with greater than 200,000 ACL ruptures documented each year in the United States (Iobst and Stanitski, 2000). Although many sports injuries result from contact with other players, ACL tears are usually noncontact injuries (Gwinn, 2000; Woo et al., 2000b, 2006). For example, while playing soccer, the athlete is required to constantly change directions with twisting and cutting movements. When these movements occur at high speeds, forces that are normally resisted by the ACL tend to partially dislocate the tibia on the femur. If the forces exceed the tensile strength of the ACL, the ligament ruptures (Bach and Boonos, 2001). In cutting sports, these high forces are exerted on the knee during hyperextension, when the knee is straightened more than 10° beyond its fully straightened position, or during pivoting of the knee, with excessive inward turning of the lower leg. Approximately 40% of individuals hear a "popping" sound or feel a tearing sensation at the time of the ACL rupture. Additionally, at least half of all ACL tears also cause injury to one of the menisci of the knee joint (Jackson and Arnoczky, 1993). The pivoting activities, especially with the knee hyperflexed, place sheer forces across the posterior horn of the meniscus contributing to meniscal tears. ACL injuries can cause persistent symptomatic instability, which becomes particularly problematic with continued high-speed athletic activities (Bernstein, 2003). With the continued use of an ACL-deficient knee, the risk of osteoarthritis also significantly increases (Noyes et al., 1983; Roos et al., 1995; Sherman et al., 1988). Therefore, strategies for ligament repair, functional replacement, and regeneration have included autograft and allograft implants along with augmentation devices, pharmacological treatments, stem cell–based therapies, tissue-engineering approaches, and advanced rehabilitation (Corsetti and Jackson, 1996; Petrigliano et al., 2006; Seedhom, 1992; Shelton et al., 1998a; Silver et al., 1991; Zavras et al., 1995; Zimmerman et al., 1994).

However, in spite of profound advances in bioengineering strategies and understanding ligament pathologies at the molecular scale, there is currently no effective long-term treatment available to restore complete function of the ligament. In this chapter, we will highlight approaches currently being investigated to achieve the common goal of restoring function after ligament damage.

13.2 ANATOMY AND PHYSIOLOGY OF THE LIGAMENT

The ACL of the knee is the major intra-articular ligament of the knee and is critical to normal kinematics and stability (Arnoczky, 1983; Miller, 1996; Miller et al., 1995; Müller, 1983; Nigg and Herzog, 1994; Silver et al., 1991). The ACL connects the posterior-lateral portion of the femur to the anterior-medial part of the tibia and is completely enveloped by the synovium within the knee joint capsule (Arnoczky, 1983; Miller, 1996; Miller et al., 1995; Müller, 1983; Nigg and Herzog, 1994). The synovium is a membrane that contains fluid designed to lubricate the joint and prevent clots. This geometry imposes limitations in fluid flow and nutrient diffusion that results in an environment with a very low capacity for healing, leaving a torn ACL incapable of self-repair (Feagin and Applewhite, 1994). There is an envelope that surrounds the ligament called the epiligament that contains cells, nerves, and blood vessels that branch into the region known as the mid-substance, while the main blood supply to the cruciate ligaments comes from the middle geniculate artery and fat pad (Amiel et al., 1990; Arnoczky, 1983; Feagin and Applewhite, 1994).

The tibial insertion of the ACL is broad and irregular at the front of the intercondylar area, whereas the femoral attachment is semicircular at the posteromedial part of the lateral femoral condylar area (Arnoczky, 1983; Miller, 1996; Miller et al., 1995; Müller, 1983; Nigg and Herzog, 1994). Working in conjunction with the posterior cruciate ligament (PCL), the ACL provides primary stabilization of anterior displacement of the tibia as well as secondary stabilization of tibial adduction and internal rotation (Frank, 1996; Frank and Jackson, 1997).

The human ACL is approximately 30–38 mm in length and 10–13 mm wide (Fischer and Ferkel, 1988; Harner et al., 1995; Jackson and Arnoczky, 1993; Miller, 1996; Miller et al., 1995; Müller, 1983; Silver et al., 1991; Smith et al., 1993; Yahia, 1997). It is composed of a network of collagen, elastin, structural glycoproteins such as fibronectin and laminin, and glycosaminoglycans, with each component contributing to the structural properties of the ligament; however, it is the helical organization of the collagen type I fiber network which imparts the necessary high tensile strength to the ligament (Arnoczky, 1983; Fischer and Ferkel, 1988; Yahia, 1997). The ACL consists of a large number of collagen fibers arranged into anteromedial, posterolateral, and intermedial bundles (Arnoczky, 1983; Miller, 1996; Miller et al., 1995; Müller, 1983; Nigg and Herzog, 1994). The arrangement of these fibers results in low friction and low tension during normal range of motion (Arnoczky, 1983; Miller, 1996; Miller et al., 1995; Müller, 1983; Nigg and Herzog, 1994).

The anteromedial bundle tightens during flexion and the posterolateral tightens during extension (Arnoczky, 1983; Miller, 1996; Miller et al., 1995; Müller, 1983; Nigg and Herzog, 1994). During the rotation of the human knee, the mode of attachment results in a 90° twist of the ACL and the peripheral fiber bundles. During flexion, the ACL fibers remain isometric in length, allowing equal distribution in load to all the fiber bundles, and maximizing its strength (Vunjak-Novakovic et al., 2004).

The ACL has a complex hierarchical structure defined by fiber architecture, orientation, and interaction. The fiber architecture of the ligament consists of collagen fibrils (5–100 nm in diameter) that are grouped into collagen fiber bundles (1–20 μm in diameter) that are gathered into larger bundles called fascicles (100–400 μm in diameter) in various orientations (Amiel et al., 1984; Clark and Sidles, 1990; Silver et al., 1991; Woo and Buckwalter, 1988; Yahia, 1997). Near the bone junction some fascicles are arranged into helical patterns, whereas in the internal area of the ligament these fascicles are arranged in a parallel pattern. The orientations of nonparallel fibers of varying lengths allow different areas of the ligament to be loaded at different times and by varying degrees (Arnoczky, 1983; Jackson and Arnoczky, 1993; Yahia, 1997). This characteristic contributes to the uniqueness and complexity of the ACL.

Ligaments also provide important sensory information, especially for the purpose of proprioception (Madey et al.). This relates to the nerves within the ligaments that have an afferent function to convey signals to the brain with regard to position, motion, and acceleration of the joint (Adachi et al., 2002; Schutte et al., 1987; Zimny et al., 1986). Therefore, lack of proprioception can contribute to inferior function of the knee joint in individuals with degenerative diseases and poor outcomes for patients of ACL-deficient joints or reconstructions (Hogervorst and Brand, 1998; Shimizu et al., 1999; Zimny, 1988).

13.2.1 Ligament and Bone Interface

There are two different ways in which a ligament is attached to the bone in the human body. The first manner of attachment, or enthesis, is called a fibrous enthesis or "periosteal insertion," where the ligament attaches indirectly to the bone by first connecting to the periosteum (Benjamin and Ralphs, 1998; Burdick and Mauck, 2011; Yang and Temenoff, 2009). Fibroblasts and collagen fibers, also known as Sharpey's fibers, comprise this type of tissue. These fibers are named after their first observer and describer William Sharpey in 1856 (Sharpey and Ellis, 1856).

The second type is considered a direct attachment and is more gradual in transition from ligament to bone. This attachment is called a fibrocartilagenous enthesis and is divided into four distinct zones (Benjamin and Ralphs, 1998; Woo et al., 2006; Yang and Temenoff, 2009). In the middle of the ligament, fibers are aligned in the same direction resulting in very high tensile strength, parallel to the direction of loading (Benjamin and Ralphs, 1998). This marks the first zone and type of tissue in the fibrocartilagenous enthesis. This area is mainly dense fibrous connective tissue composed of collagen and fibroblasts.

As the ligament transitions to bone, the second zone has tissue that consists of fibrocartilage. This fibrocartilage has a decreased population of fibroblast cells and an increased population of chondrocytes as compared to the midsection of the ligament.

The cells in the second zone are not as well aligned as the midsection and not as spindle-like in shape. The third zone is the transition of cartilagenous tissue to calcified fibrocartilage, where the cells are mostly chondrocytes and not aligned in the direction of loading. The third zone is often referred to as the "tide mark," an easily distinguished zone in histological samples. The fourth and last zone is comprised of bone and osteocytes, which marks the end of the tissue transition from ligament to bone and is the site of ligament to bone attachment. Most grafts and replacements cannot mimic the natural insertion and transition from ligament to bone, which creates another obstacle to finding a suitable graft substitute to repair damaged ligaments.

13.2.2 Mechanical Properties of the Ligament

The mechanical behavior of the ACL is viscoelastic, which suggests that with increasing strain rate there is a subsequent increase in stress in the ligament (see Figure 13.1). The initial portion of the stress–strain curve, the nonlinear toe region, corresponds to the crimping microstructure of the ligament's fascicles. This crimping is generally considered to be responsible for the mechanical behavior observed in ligaments at low loads and extensions. The crimp allows the ligament to straighten out a small amount under low loading before it is subjected to substantial force. This theoretically allows the joint surfaces and ligaments to passively move during common activities and to markedly stiffen under extreme motion to protect the joint. When at rest, these fascicles have a slight folding pattern as shown in the histological cross section of ACL tissue (see Figure 13.2). When a tensile load is applied, the crimping is straightened prior to direct loading of the fibrils as they are recruited. When loading is removed and the ligament relaxes, the elastin fibers in the ligament work to restore the crimping pattern (Buckwalter et al., 1987). This property enables elastic deformation in tension at physiological levels. Because ligaments exhibit

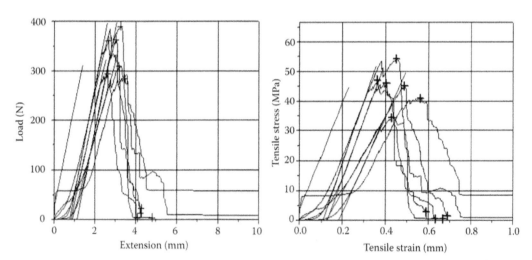

FIGURE 13.1 Examples of load–elongation and stress–strain curves of rabbit Femur-ACL-tibial complex demonstrating the toe region, the linear elastic region, yield point and failure region. (From Cooper, J.A. ed., Design, optimization and in vivo evaluation of a tissue-engineered anteriorcruciate ligament replacement, Dissertation, Drexel University, Philadelphia, PA, 2002.)

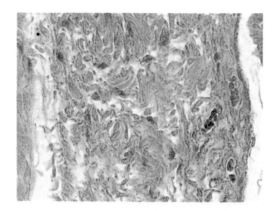

FIGURE 13.2 Histological cross-section of anterior cruciate ligament tissue (Masson's trichrome stain) which shows the fibrocytes (red) and crimped nature of the collagen tissue (blue–green).

viscoelastic properties, they behave in a time-dependent manner. The difference between a constant stress or deformation signal and deformation in the tissue over time is known as lag. If the ligament is loaded at a higher frequency than it can fully restore its initial conformation between cycles, its mechanical properties begin to change. This is called hysteresis. This important property of ligaments is especially difficult to reproduce with synthetic ligament reconstruction techniques but is critical to its physiological duties.

Table 13.1 lists the mechanical properties of human ligaments, human patellar tendons, and rabbit ligaments (Azangwe et al., 2001; Butler et al., 1978; Cabaud, 1983; Carlstedt and Nordin, 1989; Danto and Woo, 1993; Dunn et al., 1992; Feagin and Applewhite, 1994; Goulet et al., 1997; Hefti et al., 1991; Jones et al., 1995; Miller, 1996; Miller et al., 1995; Nigg and Herzog, 1994; Noyes and Grood, 1976; Noyes et al., 1983; Sekiguchi et al., 1998; Silver et al., 1991; Takai and Woo, 1993, 1984, 1990; Woo et al., 1991, 1999, 1992a–c). Loading magnitudes

TABLE 13.1　Mechanical Properties of ACL Relevant Connective Tissues

Connective Tissue	Human ACL	Human ACL	Human ACL	Human Patellar Tendon	Rabbit ACL	Rabbit ACL
Age (years)	Immature (22–35)	Mature (35–50)	Mature (60–97)	—	Immature (2.5)	Mature (4–5 kg)
Maximum tensile load (N)	1725–2200	1160–1503	495–734	2900 ± 260	218 ± 33	369 ± 53 (251 ± 47)
Ultimate tensile strength (MPa)	38 ± 4	13–46	13.3 ± 5	24–69	—	516 ± 69 (49 ± 20)
Maximum strain (%)	44.3 ± 9	9–44	30 ± 10	14–27	—	—
Stiffness (N/mm)	182–292	192–220	124–180	1154 ± 193	109 ± 10	130 ± 19
Activity loads (N)	—	67–700	—	—	—	—
Length (mm)	26.9 ± 1	33	27.5 ± 3	48.7 ± 4	8.2 ± 0.8	11.7 ± 1.0
Cross-sectional area (mm²)	44.4 ± 4	—	57.5 ± 16	50.5 ± 3	—	3.3–3.7 (5.3 ± 0.6)

Source: Cooper, J.A., ed., Design, optimization and in vivo evaluation of a tissue-engineered anterior cruciate ligament replacement, Dissertation, Drexel University, Philadelphia, PA, 2002.

and the rate of impact can affect the ultimate tensile strength that can lead to ligament injury. The ultimate tensile strength of the human ACL ranges between 1730 and 2200 N (Fischer and Ferkel, 1988; Jackson and Arnoczky, 1993; Yahia, 1997). Normal physiological loading of the human ACL as measured by Chen and Black is between 67 and 700 N (Black, 1992; Chen and Black, 1980), which corresponds to the stress on the human ACL when ascending and descending stairs, walking, and jumping. Additionally, the ACL is capable of withstanding cyclic loads of ~300 N 1–2 million times/year (Fischer and Ferkel, 1988). A replacement ligament would ideally mimic the natural ACL mechanical properties, creating another challenge for the field of tissue engineering and regenerative medicine.

13.3 LIGAMENT INJURIES

The cruciate ligaments control motion by connecting bones and bracing the joint against abnormal types of motion. Their main function is to support and strengthen joints in addition to preventing any excessive movements that would cause a dislocation and breakage of bones in the knee joint. A ligament can be injured when it is moved into a position for which it is not designed. The results of a tear or partial rupture in the ligament can be treated with cold compresses, immobilization, and elevation to allow fluid to drain from the joint. Surgery is required for a full rupture of the mid-substance of the ligament or if the ligament is severed from its point of insertion into the bone. If left untreated, some of the associated problems that can result include joint instability, meniscal tears, and degenerative joint disease. Additionally, the loading of the unstable joint produces abnormal stress on the articular cartilage, which can lead to early osteoarthritis (Ballock et al., 1989; Segawa et al., 2001).

Factors shown to correlate highly with ACL tears include genetic predisposition (Collins and Raleigh, 2009), specific ethnic groups, athletes (King et al., 2009), gender (women have demonstrated significantly higher injury rates than men in several studies) (Arendt and Dick, 1995; Arendt et al., 1999; Gwinn et al., 2000), and age with a bimodal distribution (peaks occur at 20 and 45 years old expectedly due to physical activity and degenerative musculoskeletal disorders, respectively) (Roos et al., 1995).

The number of surgical procedures for ligament repair has conservatively increased since 1995 to greater than 100,000 per year (Cameron et al., 2000).

Most ACL injuries occur during sporting activities such as skiing, basketball, soccer, and football. Athletes that wear cleated shoes are most susceptible to ACL and PCL injuries. Injuries and defects of the ACL and PCL frequently result in permanent disability (Miller, 1996; Miller et al., 1995; Ohno et al., 1995; Simon, 1994; Yahia, 1997).

13.4 LIGAMENT REPAIR: CLINICAL CHALLENGES AND OPPORTUNITIES

The ligament healing process is impacted by both aging and degree of mobilization following injury. Aging causes an alteration in collagen structure and decrease in cell metabolism that result in a decline in ligament mechanical properties. Mobilization allows the ligaments to remodel in response to mechanical stresses on the tissue via mechanotransduction. Ligaments in joints that are immobilized following injury do not receive these biomechanical stimuli and remodel in a less robust and weaker fashion. As mentioned earlier, both the

ACL and PCL have poor intrinsic healing capacities because they are enveloped by synovial fluid and lack vascularity (Lyon et al., 1991; Nickerson et al., 1992).

13.4.1 Ligament Healing

Ligament healing can be characterized by four distinct phases: inflammation, matrix, and cellular proliferation, remodeling, and maturation (Frank, 1996; Frank and Jackson, 1997; Miller, 1996; Miller et al., 1995; Page, 1959; Papageorgiou et al., 2001; Silver et al., 1991; Simon, 1994; Woo and Buckwalter, 1988; Woo et al., 1986, 2000a,b). The inflammation phase occurs during the first 3 days following injury with hypercellular activity and matrix synthesis. Within the first few hours, inflammatory cells and erythrocytes migrate to the injury site. Inflammatory cells such as polymorphonuclear leukocytes, lymphocytes, monocytes, and macrophages phagocytose necrotic tissue and cell debris. The shift in cell population from inflammatory cells to fibroblasts marks the transition from the inflammatory phase to the matrix and cellular proliferation stage. During this phase, there is an active proliferation of fibroblasts that become the predominant cell type actively synthesizing extracellular matrix. Other cell types present during this phase are macrophages and mast cells. In addition, over the ~6 week time period of the proliferation phase, a ligament scar tissue or fibrous capsule forms around the injured areas. This tissue aids in the development of vascularity in the wound. The ligament scar tissue is highly cellularized and comprises a much greater area than the normal ligament. Prior to remodeling, there is a high ratio of collagen type III to collagen type I. Collagen type III is associated with disorganized collagen fibrils, which are not as effective as collagen type I in resisting tensile loads along the length of the ligament. As the transition to the remodeling phase takes place over several months, there is a decrease in cellular density in the healing tissue. There is also a commensurate decrease in the fibrous capsule and vascularity of the tissue. As the proportion of collagen type I increases over collagen type III, the fibrils align along the primary axis of the ligament. The duration of the maturation phase of healing can vary from months to years. As the scar tissue slowly matures, slight disorganization and abnormalities in the tissue may remain due to environmental and mechanical factors.

13.4.2 Current Strategies for Repairing Ligaments

Robeson and Battle performed the first ACL repair in the late 1890s with silk and catgut sutures (Salamone, 1999; Snook, 1983). The first ligament reconstructions were performed between 1906 and 1966 using autogenous tissues such as fascia lata and tendon (Salamone, 1999; Snook, 1983). Post World War II, progression of the development of synthetic polymers led to the use of artificial materials in ACL replacement in the late 1950s and early 1960s. In the late 1950s, several researchers tested nylon ligament replacements (Johnson, 1960). These replacements were not well received due to their carcinogenic side effects and foreign body reactions (Jackson et al., 1990). During the 1970s, the FDA approved a polyethylene replacement called the POLYFLEX prosthesis but it was eventually retracted from the market in 1977 due to fatigue failure. Over the past 30 years, new procedures and devices have been developed to repair injured ligaments (Salamone, 1999; Snook, 1983).

TABLE 13.2 ACL Replacement Classifications

Biological Grafts		Non-Degradable Grafts			Biodegradable/ Tissue Engineered Grafts	
Autografts	Allografts	Permanent replacements	Augmentation devices	Scaffolds	Collagen/ protein based grafts	Biodegradable polymeric graftsL

Source: Cooper, J.A. ed., Design, optimization and in vivo evaluation of a tissue-engineered anterior cruciate ligament replacement, Dissertation, Drexel University, Philadelphia, PA, 2002.

Since the development of a guidance document for intra-articular prosthetic knee ligament devices by the FDA in 1987, the number of approved synthetic ligaments in the United States has been limited (Administration, 1993). The three approved ligaments are the Gore–Tex Cruciate Ligament Prosthesis by W.L. Gore and Associates, the Stryker Dacron Ligament Prosthesis by Meadox Medicals, Inc., and the 3M Kennedy Ligament Augmentation Device (LAD) by 3M for the Marshall–MacIntosh procedure (McPherson et al., 1985; Silver et al., 1991; Woods et al., 1991). This approval was expanded in 1992 to include the use of patellar tendon grafts of 10 mm or smaller in patients suffering more than 3 weeks after injury (Administration, 1993). Torn ligament is usually repaired by suture, whereas ruptured ligaments are reconstructed and replaced by biological grafts, biological grafts with augmentation, and nondegradable prostheses (Silver et al., 1991). Table 13.2 shows the various ACL replacement choices for ligament repair that are being used or under investigation.

The management of ACL injuries has advanced from nonoperative treatments to extracapsular augmentation and primary ligament repair to ACL reconstruction (Fu et al., 1999). Nonoperative treatments, in the form of coordinated rehabilitation and modification of activity, are recommended for individuals with ACL ruptures who have low athletic demand or sedentary occupations as well as for those who refuse ACL reconstruction (Casteleyn and Handelberg, 1996; Ciccotti et al., 1994; Segawa et al., 2001). However, due to the poor healing properties of the ACL, the injured ligament often requires reconstruction to restore stability to the knee. The standard clinical solution for ACL reconstruction utilizes tendon-based grafts. Today, these grafts represent the best clinical option with several advantages including biocompatibility, nontoxicity, and structural support to promote extracellular matrix (ECM) formation. There are many drawbacks including availability and donor site morbidity. Although grafts restore function, they have reduced performance when compared to healthy native ligament tissue.

The surgical technique for most graft replacement involves drilling bone tunnels into both the femur and the tibia, at the attachment sites of the original ACL, to serve as guides for the implantation and proper placement of the new graft (Fu et al., 2000). The graft is then pulled through the tunnels and anchored with metal or bioabsorbable screws. Postoperative care involves physical therapy to recover full range of motion and to strengthen the muscles around the reconstructed knee (Fu et al., 2000). The current reconstruction options include the use of biological, nondegradable, and bioabsorbable synthetic grafts.

13.4.2.1 Biological Grafts

Collagen is the major constituent of all autografts and allografts being used to reconstruct the ACL. Currently, autografts (tissue taken from the patient) of patellar tendon, hamstring tendon, and quadricep tendon are the most commonly used tissues for the repair of ruptured ACLs (Frank, 1996; Jackson et al., 1994; Johnson et al., 1992; Lane et al., 1993; Mendes et al., 1998; Schiavone Panni et al., 1993; Seedhom, 1992; Warren, 1983; Zavras et al., 1995). For example, a section of the patellar tendon has been frequently used to repair the ACL (Jackson et al., 1994). Success of these ligament grafts is largely dependent on the revascularization and remodeling of the transplanted tissue that is progressively surrounded by the synovial membrane. Most methods, regardless of graft choice, require drilling of bone tunnels in the femur and tibia for graft passage and fixation. First time ACL reconstructions are done with one of the three graft materials mentioned earlier.

Over the past 20 years, the central one-third or lateral one-third of the patellar tendon (8–11 mm wide) has been a gold standard choice for surgeons (Bell, 1995). This graft has been a popular ACL replacement graft primarily because of its high ultimate tensile load (~2300 N) and its stiffness (~620 N/mm) (Brody et al., 1988). It is usually harvested with a piece of bone from the patella along with the piece of bone from the patellar tendon insertion area of the tibia. This "bone-patellar tendon-bone" autograft is then channeled up through the tibia bone tunnel across the knee joint and into the femur tunnel where it is held in place. The advantage of this reconstruction is the strength of both the patellar tendon and bone–bone grafting interfaces that make this graft good at withstanding future stresses after proper rehabilitation. Usually, the bony attachment of the graft heals in approximately 6–8 weeks. For autografts, the key limitation is donor site morbidity where patients experience pain as tissue at the harvest site is damaged by harvesting of the graft. Other considerations include the limited amount of tendon available for harvesting, unpredictable resorption characteristics of the graft, increased recovery time, sensitivity to kneeling that can cause knee pain, and potential complication of subsequent patellar fracture.

Using hamstring grafts for ligament repair involves harvesting tendons from the posteromedial aspect of the thigh. This graft is also channeled through drill holes in the tibia, across the knee, and then fixed in the femur. Newer methods of implementing this graft involve folding the hamstring tendon over itself two to four times before securing it via buttons, staples, and screws that demonstrate suitable biomechanical strength of the graft. The tensile strength of this graft has been measured to failure at 4500 N (Hammer et al., 1999). This repair technique offers faster rehabilitation. Disadvantages associated with this graft include bone tunnel enlargement due to micromotion of graft ends and hamstring tendon loss from lack of regenerative capacity.

Quadricep tendon grafts consists of a bone block from the top surface of the patella that yields a graft with one bone end and one soft tissue end. The bone of the quadricep graft is fixed in the femur with an interference screw and the tibial end is fixed in accordance with soft tissue fixation. The tensile strength of this graft is 2376 N to failure (Staubli et al., 1996). The disadvantages of this graft are similar to those of the patellar tendon graft.

Allografts are tissues taken from another individual. In the case of ACL reconstruction, the patellar tendon, hamstring tendon, and Achilles tendon are taken from cadavers

(Arnoczky et al., 1986; Jackson et al., 1990, 1994; Johnson et al., 1992; Noyes et al., 1990; Shelton et al., 1998a,b; Shino et al., 1988; Vasseur et al., 1991; Zimmerman et al., 1994). The advantages of using cadaver tissue include the absence of donor site morbidity commonly associated with autograft procedures (Noyes et al., 1990; Shelton et al., 1998a,b; Zimmerman et al., 1994). Also, only performing one operative procedure equates to less time in surgery and less postoperative pain due to the lack of a donor site. Allografts are often the choice of replacement when there is a need for multiple grafts and revision surgeries where an autograft has previously been harvested and failed. The main limitation of allograft use is the risk of disease transmission with fatal outcomes (HIV, hepatitis, etc.), bacterial infection, and an immunogenic response to the foreign graft. Allografts cannot be sterilized without altering or degrading the tensile strength of the graft. Autoclaving the tissue, one potential sterilization technique, would be analogous to placing it in a pressure cooker. If the tissues are irradiated over 2.5 Mrads, another sterilization technique used with medical devices, the collagen tissue will be altered and reduce the graft's ultimate tensile strength (Shelton et al., 1998a; Yahia, 1997). In current practice tissue is harvested, cleaned, and frozen in liquid nitrogen after being screened for HIV and hepatitis. This gives the tissue a clearance of disease at approximately 1:1,000,000. Some grafts are additionally treated with lower doses of radiation in the 1–2 Mrad range to provide some degree of sterilization to the tissue without damaging the tissue properties (Fu et al., 1999, 2000). Freeze-drying procedures are typically used to preserve allografts, and have been shown to have no significant effect on the mechanical properties of the ligaments (Jackson et al., 1991; Woo et al., 1986). Conversely, the freeze–thaw process can alter or damage cells and matrices of the allograft resulting in decreased tensile properties, an increased risk of inflammatory reaction and bacterial infection, and overall immunological response (Fu et al., 1999; Woo et al., 1986). Other disadvantages include cost and availability due to high demand for low-risk grafts.

Both autografts and allografts are limited by certain uncontrollable factors. Revitalization and remodeling of ACL autografts occur by 8 weeks and are complete by 20 weeks postimplantation (Silver et al., 1991). The use of tendons as allografts has led to excellent clinical results. However, transplanted tendon does not remodel to become histologically identical to the native ACL and as a result does not completely recreate the ACL function (Fu et al., 1999; Shino et al., 1988; Silver et al., 1991). Disadvantages such as the limited supply of autogenous grafts and the potential of disease transfer of allografts have fueled the search for alternative repair options, including the use of synthetic materials in ligament reconstruction (Deuel and Lanza, 1997; Greco et al., 1994; Jackson and Arnoczky, 1993; Jackson et al., 1994; Yahia, 1997).

13.4.2.2 Nondegradable Grafts

Various methods have been employed to replace knee ligaments including autografts, allografts, and synthetic materials (Bolton and Bruchman, 1985; Deuel and Lanza, 1997; Friedman et al., 1985; Jackson and Arnoczky, 1993; Jackson et al., 1990, 1994; Johnson et al., 1992; McPherson et al., 1985; Shino et al., 1988; Thomas et al., 1987; Woo and Buckwalter, 1988; Yahia, 1997). Nondegradable synthetic prostheses evaluated for ACL repair include carbon fiber, Leeds–Keio ligament (polyethylene terephthalate), Gore–Tex (polytetrafluoroethylene [PTFE]), and the Kennedy LAD (polypropylene) (Bolton and Bruchman, 1985; Demmer et al., 1991; Fujikawa et al., 1989; Guidoin et al., 2000; Jackson and Arnoczky, 1993; McPherson et al., 1985; Neugebauer and Burri, 1985; Strover and Firer, 1985; Strum and Larson, 1985; Thomas et al., 1987). However, no synthetic ligaments have met the qualifications required for a long-term ACL substitute (Silver et al., 1991; Yahia, 1997). Although most synthetic grafts allow for return to physical activity, they gradually fragment due to repeated cycling and shedding at the edges of the bone tunnels to which they are anchored. Synthetic ligaments have been conditionally approved by the FDA for testing and augmentation but are not recommended for primary ACL repair (Guidoin et al., 2000; Silver et al., 1991).

Nondegradable grafts can be divided into three categories: permanent replacements, augmentation devices, and scaffolds (Yahia, 1997). Permanent synthetic ACL replacements must provide total function of the ligament they replace but are mostly not amenable to tissue ingrowth. As a result, they are prone to long-term mechanical failure due to creep and fatigue. Augmentation devices protect autografts and allografts from high loads during the early postoperative period of graft weakness. An area of concern with these grafts is stress shielding, so it is preferable to use devices with the approximate stiffness of the biological graft. When shielding occurs, insufficient mechanical signals are sent to the remodeling tissue resulting in poor long-term neoligament formation. Some nondegradable replacements are designed to protect the knee during early-stage remodeling and promote tissue ingrowth via porous structures. But like augmentation devices, replacements are sensitive to the effects of stress shielding. Additionally, these replacements inadequately transfer mechanical loads to the neoligament.

Nondegradable prostheses have mechanical properties that can be manipulated to match or exceed those of the normal ACL. Initially, these grafts provide sufficient strength and excellent short-term results; however, long-term results showed that many patients encountered fatigue failures and poor integration of the graft with the host tissue (Bartlett et al., 2001; Corsetti and Jackson, 1996; Thomas et al., 1987). One of the first FDA-approved synthetic grafts was the Gore–Tex ligament. The graft was made of braided PTFE consisting of a sheathed multifilament structure, which provided increased tensile strength (Dahlstedt et al., 1990). The device was used clinically for ~10 years after its introduction in 1982 (Roolker et al., 2000). However, due to poor performance, high rupture rates, painful side effects, and cost, the prosthesis was discontinued (Wilson et al., 1998). Other synthetic grafts and prostheses include carbon-based prostheses, the Leeds–Keio (polyethylene terephthalate) device, and the Stryker–Dacron ligament (Olson et al., 1988; Wredmark and Engstrom, 1993). The Stryker–Dacron ligament never received FDA approval due to its poor clinical trial results. In a 4 year follow-up study, it was determined that 28% of the Dacron prostheses ruptured (Barrett et al., 1993; Demmer et al., 1991). Additionally, degenerative arthritis was found in all the patients who had the ruptured replacement.

A more advanced synthetic prosthesis, the 3M Kennedy LAD, is an assist device designed to promote tissue growth within the graft (Dunn et al., 1993). The material was a hybrid of an intra-articular autograft and a piece of diamond-braided polypropylene

(Dunn, 1996; Dunn et al., 1993, 1994a). The purpose of the LAD was to provide internal protection for an autograft during its initial phase of weakness. However, due to the nondegradable nature of the scaffold and its relatively high rupture rates, the tissue developed an inflammatory response and painful side effects, similar to those of the previous synthetic grafts (Dunn, 1996; Dunn et al., 1993, 1994a). An additional mode of failure in this design was the disorganized tissue growth into the scaffold that resembled scar rather than native tissue. As the stiffness in the polymer was much higher than that in the growing tissue, stress-shielding effects were produced that prevented proper remodeling. In a 15 year study, 40%–78% of the 885 tested synthetic replacements failed due to one or more of the previously mentioned complications (Dunn et al., 1995).

The results of ACL reconstruction with nondegradable prostheses indicate many problems including long-term failure due to synovitis, arthritis, and mechanical deterioration (Jackson and Arnoczky, 1993; Yahia, 1997). This has led scientists to consider research in the development of tissue-engineered ligaments (Cooper et al., 2005, 2007; Koski et al., 2000; Laurencin et al., 1999b; Lu et al., 2005).

13.4.2.3 Biodegradable and Tissue-Engineered Grafts

Tissue-derived materials such as collagen and synthetic biodegradable materials show promise for the development of ACL replacements. Collagen type I is the major component of connective tissues and can be extracted from bovine and porcine sources (Goldstein et al., 1989; Jackson et al., 1996; McMaster, 1985, 1986; Lee et al., 2001; Liu et al., 1995; Van Steensel et al., 1987; Yahia, 1997). After extraction, these tissues can be processed into fibers to fabricate biodegradable scaffolds. Treatments include cross-linking to control collagen resorption rate, and additional processing such as lyophilization and decellularization to ensure that the collagen does not incite an immune response from cells involved in tissue repair. Collagen scaffolds experience an early loss in mechanical strength, followed by tissue remodeling between 10 and 20 weeks with a strength gain similar to autografts.

Dunn and associates present an example of a novel designed tissue-engineered approach using collagen (Dunn, 1996; Dunn et al., 1992, 1993, 1994a,b, 1995). They developed fibroblast-seeded collagen scaffolds for ACL reconstruction. These collagen scaffolds were seeded with rabbit fibroblasts of the ACL, synovium, patellar tendon, and skin. The fibroblasts' viability, adherence, spreading, proliferation, and deposition of collagen and protein were measured on the scaffolds. These scaffolds were made of collagen fibers (60 μm diameter), which have been made by an extrusion process rinsed and dried under tension. The collagen scaffolds were constructed from 225 aligned fibers treated with cyanamide vapor or glutaraldehyde vapor. They determined that collagen fibers used in the scaffold device for ACL reconstruction had to be thin, strong, and resorbable. By minimizing the diameter (<70 μm), they found that fiber strength increased without prolonging the fiber resorption rate. They also discovered that ACL fibroblasts adhered better than the other fibroblast types but proliferated at the slowest rate. In addition, patellar tendon fibroblasts proliferated at the fastest rate and all the fibroblast types secreted protein and collagen within the scaffolds. The *in vivo* studies suggested that fibroblast-seeded collagen scaffolds were viable after reimplantation into the donor rabbit. Therefore, future studies were needed to determine whether autogenous fibroblast-seeded scaffolds can be used in ligament formation/remodeling. These collagen scaffolds would be potentially useful in clinical ACL reconstruction in which fibroblasts would be obtained through a biopsy, cultured, seeded onto a collagen scaffold, and implanted as the ACL substitute in the same patient.

As mentioned previously, the development of tissue-engineered scaffolds incorporates *in vitro* seeding of scaffolds with cells or coating of scaffolds with tissue-regenerating factors before implantation. The goals of these manipulations are the promotion of early healing, and improved long-term remodeling and biomechanical function of the biodegradable grafts.

Brody and associates examined the effects of seeding canine fibroblast cells onto the surface of knitted Dacron ligament prostheses prior to implantation (Brody et al., 1988). Results showed that prostheses seeded with fibroblast cells demonstrated a more uniform and abundant encapsulation with connective tissue than did unseeded prostheses.

As an alternative to the currently used nondegradable polymers, investigators have begun to examine biodegradable materials that would provide immediate stabilization to the repaired ligament and also act as a scaffold for the ingrowth and/or replacement by host cells (Brighton et al., 1999; Cooper et al., 2005; Deuel and Lanza, 1997; Dunn, 1996; Dunn et al., 1995; Greco, 1994; Ito et al., 1992; Jackson and Simon, 1999; Koski et al., 2000; Laurencin et al., 1999a,b; Lin et al., 1999; McCarthy et al., 1993; Mooney et al., 1992; Naughton et al., 1995; Shieh et al., 1990; Weiler et al., 2000; Yahia, 1997). These polymers can be fabricated to have tensile strengths between 0.6 and 500 MPa and modulate between 10 and 6500 MPa (Jackson and Arnoczky, 1993; Silver et al., 1991; Yahia, 1997). In addition, the biodegradation times of the polymer can be controlled to last for days or months (Silver et al., 1991). Cabaud et al. (1982) characterized Dexon poly(glycolic) acid sutures no. 2.0 (PGA, Davis & Geck, River, NJ) as a Y-shaped reinforcement device for a transected dog ACL. The PGA reinforcement device provided excellent support to the healing ligament and had been completely resorbed at 5 week postimplantation. Rodkey and associates also investigated a woven ligament composite of Dacron and Dexon (Yahia, 1997).

Auger and associates have developed a bioengineered ligament (bACL) model. The significant differences between the bACL and other ligament models are the addition of ACL fibroblasts to the structure, the absence of cross-linking agents (previously used in Dunn's group work), and the use of bone to anchor the bioengineered tissue (Deuel and Lanza, 1997; Yahia, 1997). Bone is introduced in the beginning of the processing to facilitate transplantation *in vivo*. Briefly, fibroblasts were isolated from ACL biopsies of patients undergoing total knee arthroplasty (ages 60–67 years). bACLs were cultured vertically and horizontally; from their histological sections and immunofluorescence analysis they showed that under elongation, tension induced an alignment of collagen type I fibers parallel to the applied load. These studies demonstrate that the bACL has a histological organization that is progressively modulated by the fibroblasts seeded into its structure and the tension applied *in vitro* during its development.

An L-polylactic acid resorbable LAD (3M, MN) that consisted of parallel-oriented fiber cords covered with a braid of six yarns (two-dimensional [2D] architecture) has been investigated (Kobayashi et al., 1995; Salamone, 1999). Briefly, they studied this device for a 2 year follow-up, which is the time of resorption of L-PLA, and reported no major complications. They did observe seroma around the L-PLA osteosynthesis devices (pins and screws) that were used for fixation. This effect was attributed to a release of acidic products from the degradation. They also obtained mechanical data from a subcutaneous L-PLA implantation study in rabbits for 2.0 and 3.2 mm devices with maximum loads of 262 and 545 N, respectively, which was reduced by γ-irradiation to 223 and 375 N. After 16 weeks implantation, the 2.0 mm device had strength retention of 205 N.

Laitinen et al. (1992, 1993) investigated another experimental L-PLA LAD implanted in rabbits and sheep. In the rabbit model, the LAD devices were implanted in the subcutaneous tissue and after 48 weeks the implant lost 97% of its tensile load strength. In the sheep model, a fascia lata poly-L-lactide (PLLA) LAD (fascia lata wrapped around implant device) and primary suture LAD device were implanted in the intra-articular joint of the knee. After 6 weeks, the maximum load observed for the reconstructed ACL using the fascia lata PLLA group and primary suture PLLA group was 9% and 6% of the contralateral control, respectively. At 12 weeks, the fascia lata became stronger and reached 13% of the maximum load of the control. In addition at 48 weeks, the maximum load was 21% and 12% for the fascia lata and primary suture group, respectively. These results were shown to be comparable to fascia lata grafts used alone in ACL repair where the maximum load is 9%–15% of the contralateral control at 8 weeks postoperatively. These investigators suggested that weakest remodeling of the graft occurred at 12 weeks with increased mechanical properties beyond that time point due to increased fibrous tissue maturation. Also, they had acceptable mechanical properties at the end of a 1 year follow-up period (Laitinen et al., 1993).

Another biodegradable, polymeric LAD was investigated by ETHICON (Puddu et al., 1993; Salamone, 1999). Briefly, cords and flat braids were fabricated from Vicryl (Polyglactin 910, ETHICON, NJ) with PDS (Polyparadioxanone, ETHICON, NJ) used as a resorbable suture material. During clinical application of PDS, seroma and local infections were observed and the material was not fully covered with a deep layer of soft tissue. Much like the L-PLA resorbable ligament, it was surmised that some of the nonbacterial inflammation was due to degradation products that caused a change in the pH. In addition, they observed a total loss in mechanical strength in the augmentation devices at the weakest tendon graft mechanical strength remodeling (<8 weeks), which does not fully remodel until after 8 weeks postoperation.

Biodegradable polymeric and collagen scaffolds have recently been developed for ligament tissue regeneration. There are few investigations of in vivo applications performed that show controlled and genuine ligament regeneration in the knee joint (Fan et al., 2009; Vunjak-Novakovic et al., 2004).

13.5 FUTURE OF LIGAMENT REPAIR AND REGENERATION

Tissue engineering is a multidisciplinary field that incorporates the principles of biochemistry, engineering, and materials science to develop substitutes that replace injured or diseased tissues (Cooper et al., 2005; Petrigliano et al., 2006; Vunjak-Novakovic et al., 2004; Weitzel et al., 2002). The development of a functional tissue-engineered ligament is based on a system that uses (1) reparative cells with the capacity for proliferation and matrix synthesis, (2) a structural scaffold that facilitates cell adaptation, and (3) an environment that provides sufficient nutrient transport and appropriate regulatory stimuli (Petrigliano et al., 2006).

13.5.1 Tissue-Engineering and Biomaterial Strategies

Typically, *in vivo* ligament tissue engineering uses a scaffold that is designed to be implanted into the host tissue and promotes both tissue ingrowth and neoligament formation (Cooper et al., 2005, 2007; Lu et al., 2005; Petrigliano et al., 2006). The scaffolds are seeded with either autogenic or allogenic cells and are modified to enhance biocompatibility and host cellular response with the incorporation of adhesion molecules and growth factors. *Ex vivo* systems use a bioreactor, in which the ligament is developed on a structural scaffold for subsequent host implantation by replicating the physiological conditions presented during normal ligament development and repair (Vunjak-Novakovic et al., 2004). The potential tissue replacement would allow for immediate implantation of a functional ligament that would undergo physiological remodeling within the host knee. *In vivo* and *ex vivo* ligament tissue engineering require cells seeded onto the scaffold to synthesize collagen and other ECM proteins in an organized fashion, thus mimicking the native ligament structure, both mechanically and biochemically, for proper functioning during physiological loading after implantation (Cooper et al., 2007; Petrigliano et al., 2006; Vunjak-Novakovic et al., 2004; Weitzel et al., 2002).

As an alternative to biological tissues and nondegradable materials, investigators have begun to examine biodegradable materials that would provide immediate stabilization to the repaired ligament, but would also act as a scaffold for the ingrowth and/or replacement by host cells (Rodkey, 1994). Although the only completely degradable material currently reported to be under investigation for ACL repair is poly(glycolic acid) (PGA) (Cabaud et al., 1982), researchers have begun to examine other polymers in conjunction with ligament cells (fibroblasts) (Cooper, 2006). Cooper and associates used fibers from the polyester family of PLLA, PGA, and poly(lactide-*co*-glycolide) to develop tissue-engineered ligament scaffolds (Laurencin–Cooper Ligament [L-C Ligament™]) (Cooper, 2002; Cooper et al., 2005, 2007; Lu et al., 2005). Multifilament yarns of these biodegradable polymers were utilized in the range of 60–70 denier size, which corresponds to a filament size between 15 and 25 μm. This fiber size is close to that of natural collagen fibers, which allows the cells to readily adjust to the hierarchical fiber architecture of the synthetic ligament, as shown in Figure 13.3. The L-C Ligament model differs from other ligament models by (1) the use of >50% porous scaffold, (2) the use of a three-dimensional (3D)-braided structure, and (3) the use of a two braiding angle designs to form the tissue-engineered ligament. Previously, it has been reported on the use of cells seeded and cultured onto 3D-braided scaffolds (Cooper, 2002; Cooper et al., 2005, 2007; Laurencin et al., 1999b; Lu et al., 2005). A 3D braid differs from the other textile structures in that there are more than three braiding yarn systems in the through-thickness direction of the braid (Ko, 1987, 1989; Ko and Pastore, 1985; Ko et al., 1988, 1989). This braid is considered 3D because of its appearance at the macroscopic level, as compared to many 2D, or flat-braided, ligament replacements that are considered 3D because they have a measurable length in the third dimension, regardless of how small that measured length may be as Figure 13.4 shows examples of a 5×5 PLLA 3D square

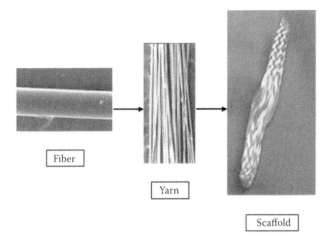

FIGURE 13.3 Scaffold designed to biomimic the hierarchical structure of anterior cruciate ligament starting from single fiber to mimic the collagen fibril, the yarn to mimic the fascicles and scaffold 3-D braid (L-C ligament) to mimic the ligament structure with sections for ligament bone integration in the bone tunnels. (From Cooper, J.A. ed., Design, optimization and in vivo evaluation of a tissue-engineered anterior cruciate ligament replacement, Dissertation, Drexel University, Philadelphia, PA, 2002.)

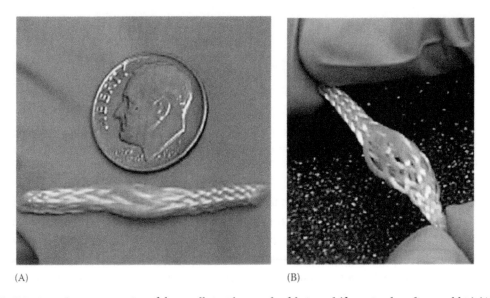

(A)   (B)

FIGURE 13.4 Is representative of the small size that can be fabricated (for animal studies—rabbit) (A); shows the crimped nature of the middle intra-articular region of the tissue-engineered ligament (L-C Ligament) and the tightly braided ends for insertion within the bone tunnels (B).

braid (L-C Ligament prototype) designed for implantation into a rabbit model. The tissue-engineered ligament is a continuous 3D-braided structure that creates three-dimensionality and is not layered or stitched together as is commonly used to create a 2D braid and woven structure. The ends of the three dimensional (3-D) structure have high braiding angles for resistance to bone tunnel wear while the central region has a low braiding angle that

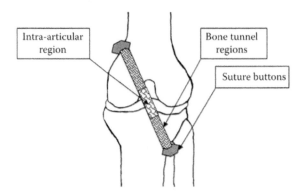

FIGURE 13.5 Schematic diagram of L-C tissue-engineered ligament replacement (L-C Ligament) after ACL reconstruction.

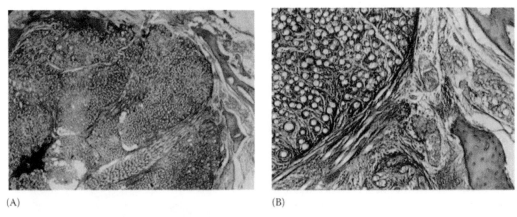

(A)　　　　　　　　　　　　　　　　　　　(B)

FIGURE 13.6 Histological cross-section shows integration of the tissue engineered ligament (L-C ligament) within intra-articular zone after 12 weeks implantation. (Masson's trichrome stain, A—1×, B—4×.)

produces an open crimp-like structure to allow for tissue ingrowth and remodeling within the intra-articular zone of the knee. An example of the placement of the tissue-engineered ligament within the knee joint is represented by the schematic in Figure 13.5. Cooper and associates developed this biomimetic ligament replacement by using 3D braiding technology. *In vivo* studies have been conducted in which ACL cell-seeded or -unseeded tissue engineered Ligament prototypes were implanted into New Zealand white rabbits (Cooper et al., 2007). Histological sections of the intra-articular zone showed excellent tissue infiltration throughout the implants at the end of the implantation period of 12 weeks as shown in Figure 13.6. In addition, 6 months after implantation the histological cross section in the femur bone tunnel showed the integration of the tissue-engineered ligament scaffold (L-C Ligament) with the bone (Figure 13.7). The 3D-braided tissue-engineered ligament was designed to gradually transfer the load of the intra-articular joint to the cells and to allow for collagen infiltration into the tissue-engineered ligament to eliminate stress shielding (Cooper et al., 2007). As healing occurred, the braided structure became weaker,

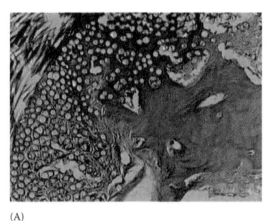 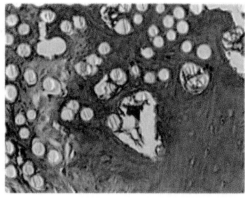

(A)   (B)

FIGURE 13.7   Histological cross-section shows integration of the tissue engineered ligament (L-C ligament) in the bone tunnel of the rabbit Femur after 6 months. (hematoxylin and eosin stain, A—4×, B—10×)

and tensile loads were gradually supported by both the braid and the neoligament tissue. During this study, the seeded tissue-engineered ligament ruptured in the intra-articular zone in three out of six replacements, which was better than the results of the unseeded scaffolds (Cooper et al., 2007). Despite the failures of the grafts at 12 weeks, other studies have shown that the strength retention of the maximum tensile loads of the 12 week seeded ligament scaffolds was much greater when compared with the "gold standard replacement" of autografts in previous animal model studies for the same time period (Ballock et al., 1989). As further studies are performed, the success of this particular tissue-engineered ligament study will be realized and may provide orthopedic surgeons with another option in ACL repair without the risk of donor site morbidity or disease transmission.

Recently, silk has become an increasingly studied scaffold material for ligament tissue engineering due to its good biocompatibility, slow degradability, and remarkable mechanical capability (Altman et al., 2002, 2003; Fan et al., 2008). Silk fibers have been woven into a "wire–rope" scaffold that has been shown to possess similar mechanical properties to that of the native ACL (Altman et al., 2002). Fan and associates fabricated a silk scaffold in which a knitted silk mesh was rolled up around a braided silk cord and seeded with mesenchymal stem cells (MSCs) (Fan et al., 2008; Liu et al., 2008). The tissue-engineered scaffold has already been implanted into a rabbit model to reconstruct the ACL. The regenerated ligament exhibited abundant ECM production and direct ligament–bone insertion. Additionally, its tensile strength could meet the mechanical requirements for daily activities (Fan et al., 2008; Liu et al., 2008). Larger animal models are now being used to evaluate the efficacy of the ACL replacement scaffold before starting clinical trials. Fan and associates conducted an *in vivo* study to regenerate the ACL in a pig model using the silk scaffold seeded with porcine MSCs (Fan et al., 2009). The MSC-seeded scaffold was implanted in a pig model where the host knee joint served as a functional bioreactor providing various cytokines and physiological cyclic loading on implants to induce the differentiation of the MSCs (Fan et al., 2009). The regenerated ligament, at 24 weeks postoperatively, showed histological, mechanical, and physical similarities to the native pig ACL. The microporous silk mesh had sufficient pore size (20–100 μm) and a large surface area that facilitated cell adhesion, proliferation, and ECM production, resulting in excellent tissue infiltration. There were a few limitations of this study, such as not tracking the MSCs on the scaffold after implantation; however, this preliminary study shows the potential possibilities of this silk scaffold for ACL regeneration (Fan et al., 2009).

13.5.2 Cell-Based Gene Therapy Applied to Ligament Healing

Current research trends aim at using both physical and chemical means of cell signaling to promote phenotypes of cells. Changes to physical properties of the extracellular environment such as scaffold stiffness, loading, and topography can control the way cells interact and grow. Chemical signaling can include growth factors and cytokines, which also effect the growth and phenotype of cells in the environment. Scientists have started to use these signaling methods to promote different cell lines, such as MSCs, to differentiate and synthesize matrix to mimic native tissue. These methods are considered to be cell-based therapy techniques.

In the case of ligament tissue engineering, natural or synthetic biomaterial scaffolds can be seeded with cells and then cultured in a specific environment with added signaling molecules to promote a phenotype comparable to those of native tissue. Taking this one step further, cell-based gene therapy is a technique that utilizes the alteration of genes within the cells to direct their growth. *In vitro* and *in situ* experiments have shown that inserting cDNA-encoding growth factors controls cell division and matrix synthesis (Evans et al., 2007, 2008). The cDNA can encode for different growth factors such as transforming growth factor β1 (TGF-β1), insulin-like growth factor (IGF), platelet-derived growth factor (PDGF), and vasculoendothelial growth factor (VEGF) (Evans et al., 2007, 2008; Hilderbrand et al., 2004; Hoffmann and Gross, 2007; Pascher et al., 2004; Scherping et al., 1997). Although these growth factors promote the phenotype of ligament tissue, it has yet to be reproduced *in vivo* with confidence (Menetrey et al., 1999; Nakamura et al., 2000). Many studies now focus on determining what growth factors are up-regulated naturally in wound repair and then focus on applying that knowledge to culturing replacement tissues. These factors would serve to mimic the same factors that would potentially accelerate healing and matrix production (Hilderbrand et al., 2004; Pascher et al., 2004). By inserting these genes into the cells themselves, the seeded scaffolds would self-regulate what is needed for optimal generation of replacement tissue (Noth et al., 2010). The future of gene-based therapy is growing and interest in utilizing this technique in combination with environmental culture conditions may hold the answer to creating a substitute ligament tissue suitable for replacing injured tissue.

13.6 SUMMARY

In summary, the literature discussing ligament injuries suggests that several therapeutic strategies are currently available to promote repair and regeneration. However, the degree of regeneration, and hence the functional recovery, remains relatively modest. To date, the clinical repair of ACL ruptures is still routinely accomplished using autografts and allografts.

These grafts can be considered biodegradable scaffolds of collagen that stimulate wound healing from chemotactic properties derived from peptides released during degradation and remodeling. Nondegradable synthetic grafts have high mechanical strength to withstand the loads seen in the intra-articular joint but cause stress-shielding scar tissue and granulomatous tissue rather than organized collagen fibers typical of a normal ligament (Guidoin et al., 2000; Koski et al., 2000). As a result, combining the advantages of biological and synthetic grafts has led to the development of biodegradable tissue-engineered ligaments such as the L-C Ligament. ACL injury is a multifaceted problem that requires a multifaceted approach. Enhanced regeneration can be achieved when two or more treatments are combined, in other words, using an integrated, interdisciplinary regenerative medicine–based approach is required. As progress is being made in biotechnology and biomaterials, tissue engineering is becoming the chosen strategy to solve the musculoskeletal problems in orthopedic surgery. 3D scaffolds for ACL reconstruction surgery have been developed and are now undergoing *in vitro* and *in vivo* studies. However, to fabricate optimal ACL replacements, a thorough understanding of the interaction between specific cell types and their tissue-engineered matrices is needed. Growth factors, such as basic fibroblast growth factor, transforming growth factor β, and PDGF, have been shown both *in vitro* and *in vivo* to influence the maturation and homeostasis of the healing response of ligament tissue (Laurencin et al., 1999b; Scherping et al., 1997); thus, their use in ligament regeneration is being considered. Other future works include studying the role of gene therapy and its use in the delivery of genetic information coding for stimulatory agents for ligament regeneration (Evans and Robbins, 1995). We postulate that a synergistic application of regenerative medicine will include the modulation of inflammation and encouragement of endogenous regeneration (using scaffolds, cell transplantation, and drug delivery) to modulate healing and regeneration. The future of restoring function after ligament injury may depend on our ability to target the earlier process with an interdisciplinary approach.

ACKNOWLEDGMENTS

The authors would like to thank Dr. Cato Laurencin, Dr. Yusuf Khan, and Dr. Stephen S. Doty for their advice and support in addition to the members of Musculoskeletal & Translational Tissue Engineering Research (MATTER) Lab. Dr. Cooper would like to particularly recognize his mentors and advisors over the years, which include Dr. Cato Laurencin, Dr. Frank Ko, Dr. Christopher S. Chen, Dr. Rustum Roy, Dr. Walter Yarbrough, Dr. Saligrama SubbaRao, and Dr. Robert Langley.

REFERENCES

Adachi, N., Ochi, M., Uchio, Y. et al. 2002. Mechanoreceptors in the anterior cruciate ligament contribute to the joint position sense. *Acta Orthopaed*, 73: 330–334.

Administration, United States Food and Drug. 1993. *Guidance Document for the Preparation of Investigational Device Exemptions and Premarket Approval Applications for Intra-Articular Prosthetic Knee Ligament Devices.* U.S. Department of Health and Human Services.

Altman, G. H., Diaz, F., Jakuba, C. et al. 2003. Silk-based biomaterials. *Biomaterials*, 24: 401–416.

Altman, G. H., Horan, R. L., Lu, H. H. et al. 2002. Silk matrix for tissue engineered anterior cruciate ligaments. *Biomaterials*, 23: 4131–4141.

Amiel, D., Billings, E., and Akeson, W. H. 1990. Ligament structure, chemistry, and physiology. In: Daniel, D. M., Akeson, W. H., and O'Connor, J. J. (eds.), *Knee Ligaments: Structure, Function, Injury and Repair*. Raven Press, New York.

Amiel, D., Frank, C., and Harwood, F. 1984. Tendons and ligaments. A morphological and biochemical comparison. *J Orthop Res*, 1: 257–265.

Arendt, E., Agel, J., and Dick, R. 1999. Anterior cruciate ligament injury patterns among collegiate men and women. *J Athl Train*, 34: 86–92.

Arendt, E. and Dick, R. 1995. Knee injury patterns among men and women in collegiate basketball and soccer. *Am J Sports Med*, 23: 694–701.

Arnoczky, S. P. 1983. Anatomy of the anterior cruciate ligament. *Clin Orthop Relat Res*, 172: 19–25.

Arnoczky, S., Warren, R., and Ashlock, M. 1986. Replacement of the anterior cruciate ligament using a patellar tendon allograft. An experimental study. *J Bone Joint Surg Am*, 68: 376–385.

Azangwe, G., Mathias, K., and Marshall, D. 2001. Preliminary comparison of the rupture of human and rabbit anterior cruciate ligaments. *Clin Biomech*, 16: 913–917.

Bach, B. R., Jr. and Boonos, C. L. 2001. Anterior cruciate ligament reconstruction. *AORN J*, 74: 152–164; quiz 166–171, 173–174.

Ballock, R. T., Woo, S. L., Lyon, R. M., Hollis, J. M., and Akeson, W. H. 1989. Use of patellar tendon autograft for anterior cruciate ligament reconstruction in the rabbit: A long-term histologic and biomechanical study. *J Orthop Res*, 7: 474–485.

Barrett, G. R., Line, L. L., Jr., Shelton, W. R., Manning, J. O., and Phelps, R. 1993. The Dacron ligament prosthesis in anterior cruciate ligament reconstruction. A four-year review. *Am J Sports Med*, 21: 367–373.

Bartlett, R. J., Clatworthy, M. G., and Nguyen, T. N. 2001. Graft selection in reconstruction of the anterior cruciate ligament. *J Bone Joint Surg Br*, 83: 625–634.

Bell, E. 1995. Strategy for the selection of scaffolds for tissue engineering. *Tissue Eng*, 1: 163–179.

Benjamin, M. and Ralphs, J. 1998. Fibrocartilage in tendons and ligaments—An adaptation to compressive load. *J Anat*, 193: 487–494.

Bernstein, J. 2003. Special concerns of the athlete. In: *Musculoskeletal Medicine*, 1st ed. American Academy of Orthopaedic Surgeons, Rosemont, IL.

Black, J. 1992. *Biological Performance of Materials*. Marcel Dekker, New York.

Bolton, C. W. and Bruchman, W. C. 1985. The GORE-TEX expanded polytetrafluoroethylene prosthetic ligament. An *in vitro* and *in vivo* evaluation. *Clin Orthop Relat Res*, 202–213.

Brody, G. A., Eisinger, M., Arnoczky, S. P., and Warren, R. F. 1988. *In vitro* fibroblast seeding of prosthetic anterior cruciate ligaments. *Am J Sports Med*, 16: 203.

Buckwalter, J. A., Einhorn, T. A., and Simon, S. R. 2000. *Orthopaedic Basic Science: Biology and Biomechanics of the Musculoskeletal System*. American Academy of Orthopaedic Surgeons, Rosemont, IL.

Buckwalter, J., Maynard, J., and Vailas, A. 1987. Skeletal fibrous tissue: Tendon, joint capsule, and ligament. In: Albright, J. A. and Brand, R. A. (eds.), The Scientific Basis of Orthopedics. Appleton & Lange, Norwalk, CT, pp. 387–405.

Burdick, J. A. and Mauck, R. L. (eds.) 2011. *Biomaterials for Tissue Engineering Applications—A Review of the Past and Future Trends*. Springer Wien, New York.

Butler, D., Grood, E., Noyes, F., and Zernicke, R. 1978. Biomechanics of ligaments and tendons. *Exerc Sport Sci Rev*, 6: 125.

Cabaud, H. E. 1983. Biomechanics of the anterior cruciate ligament. *Clin Orthop Relat Res*, 172: 26.

Cabaud, H. E., Feagin, J. A., and Rodkey, W. G. 1982. Acute anterior cruciate ligament injury and repair reinforced with a biodegradable intraarticular ligament. Experimental studies. *Am J Sports Med*, 10: 259–265.

Cameron, M., Mizuno, Y., and Cosgarea, A. 2000. Diagnosing and managing anterior cruciate ligament injuries. *J Musculoskeletal Med*, 17: 47–53.

Caplan, A. I. and Goldberg, V. M. (eds.). 1999. *Association of Bone and Joint Surgeons Workshop Supplement: Orthopaedic Tissue Engineering: Clinical Orthopaedics and Related Research*, Vol. 367. Lippincott Williams & Wilkins, Philadelphia, PA, pp. S2–S423.

Carlstedt, C. A. and Nordin, M. 1989. Biomechanics of tendons and ligaments. In: M. Nordin and V. H. Frankel (eds.), *Basic Biomechanics of the Musculoskeletal System*, 2nd edn. Lea & Febiger, Philadelphia, PA, pp. 59–74.

Casteleyn, P. P. and Handelberg, F. 1996. Non-operative management of anterior cruciate ligament injuries in the general population. *J Bone Joint Surg Br*, 78: 446–451.

Chen, E. H. and Black, J. 1980. Materials design analysis of the prosthetic anterior cruciate ligament. *J Biomed Mater Res*, 14: 567–586.

Ciccotti, M. G., Lombardo, S. J., Nonweiler, B., and Pink, M. 1994. Non-operative treatment of ruptures of the anterior cruciate ligament in middle-aged patients. Results after long-term follow-up. *J Bone Joint Surg Am*, 76: 1315–1321.

Clark, J. M. and Sidles, J. A. 1990. The interrelation of fiber bundles in the anterior cruciate ligament. *J Orthop Res*, 8: 180–188.

Collins, M. and Raleigh, S. 2009. Genetic risk factors for musculoskeletal soft tissue injuries. *Med Sport Sci*, 54: 136–149.

Cooper, J. A. (ed.) 2002. Design, optimization and *in vivo* evaluation of a tissue-engineered anterior cruciate ligament replacement, Dissertation. Drexel University, Philadelphia, PA.

Cooper, J. A. 2006. Evaluation of the anterior cruciate ligament, medial collateral ligament, Achilles tendon and patellar tendon as cell sources for tissue-engineered ligament. *Biomaterials*, 27: 2747–2754.

Cooper, J. A., Lu, H. H., Ko, F. K., Freeman, J. W., and Laurencin, C. T. 2005. Fiber-based tissue-engineered scaffold for ligament replacement: Design considerations and *in vitro* evaluation. *Biomaterials*, 26: 1523–1532.

Cooper, J. A., Sahota, J. S., Gorum, W. J. et al. 2007. Biomimetic tissue-engineered anterior cruciate ligament replacement. *Proc Natl Acad Sci*, 104: 3049–3054.

Corsetti, J. R. and Jackson, D. W. 1996. Failure of anterior cruciate ligament reconstruction: The biologic basis. *Clin Orthop Relat Res*, 325: 42–49.

Dahlstedt, L., Dalen, N., and Jonsson, U. 1990. Goretex prosthetic ligament vs. Kennedy ligament augmentation device in anterior cruciate ligament reconstruction. A prospective randomized 3-year follow-up of 41 cases. *Acta Orthop Scand*, 61: 217–224.

Danto, M. I. and Woo, S. L. 1993. The mechanical properties of skeletally mature rabbit anterior cruciate ligament and patellar tendon over a range of strain rates. *J Orthop Res*, 11: 58–67.

Demmer, P., Fowler, M., and Marino, A. A. 1991. Use of carbon fibers in the reconstruction of knee ligaments. *Clin Orthop Relat Res*, 271: 225–232.

Deuel, T. and Lanza, R. 1997. *Principles of Tissue Engineering*. Academic Press, Austin RG Landes, San Diego, CA, pp. 133–134.

Dunn, M. G. 1996. Tissue-engineering strategies for ligament reconstruction. *MRS Bull*, 21: 43–46.

Dunn, M. G., Avasarala, P. N., and Zawadsky, J. P. 1993. Optimization of extruded collagen fibers for ACL reconstruction. *J Biomed Mater Res*, 27: 1545–1552.

Dunn, M. G., Leish, J. B., Tiku, M. L., Maxian, S. H., and Zawadsky, J. P. 1994a. The tissue engineering approach to ligament reconstruction. In: *Proceedings of the Materials Research Society Symposium*, Boston, MA, pp. 13–18.

Dunn, M. G., Liesch, J. B., Tiku, M. L., and Zawadsky, J. P. 1995. Development of fibroblast-seeded ligament analogs for ACL reconstruction. *J Biomed Mater Res*, 29: 1363–1371.

Dunn, M. G., Maxian, S. H., and Zawadsky, J. P. 1994b. Intraosseous incorporation of composite collagen prostheses designed for ligament reconstruction. *J Orthop Res*, 12: 128–137.

Dunn, M. G., Tria, A. J., Kato, Y. P. et al. 1992. Anterior cruciate ligament reconstruction using a composite collagenous prosthesis. A biomechanical and histologic study in rabbits. *Am J Sports Med*, 20: 507–515.

Evans, C. H., Ghivizzani, S. C., and Robbins, P. D. 2008. Orthopedic gene therapy in 2008. *Mol Ther*, 17: 231–244.

Evans, C. H., Palmer, G. D., Pascher, A. et al. 2007. Facilitated endogenous repair: Making tissue engineering simple, practical, and economical. *Tissue Eng*, 13: 1987–1993.

Evans, C. H. and Robbins, P. D. 1995. Possible orthopaedic application of gene therapy. *J Bone Joint Surg*, 77A: 1103–1114.

Fan, H., Liu, H., Toh, S. L., and Goh, J. C. 2009. Anterior cruciate ligament regeneration using mesenchymal stem cells and silk scaffold in large animal model. *Biomaterials*, 30: 4967–4977.

Fan, H., Liu, H., Wong, E. J., Toh, S. L., and Goh, J. C. 2008. *In vivo* study of anterior cruciate ligament regeneration using mesenchymal stem cells and silk scaffold. *Biomaterials*, 29: 3324–3337.

Feagin, J. A. and Applewhite, L. B. 1994. *The Crucial Ligaments: Diagnosis and Treatment of Ligamentous Injuries about the Knee.* Churchill Livingstone, New York.

Fischer, S. and Ferkel, R. 1988. *Prosthetic Ligament Reconstruction of the Knee.* W.B. Saunders Company, Philadelphia, PA, pp. 3–10.

Frank, C. B. 1996. Ligament healing: Current knowledge and clinical applications. *J Am Acad Orthop Surg*, 4: 74–83.

Frank, C. B. and Jackson, D. W. 1997. The science of reconstruction of the anterior cruciate ligament. *J Bone Joint Surg Am*, 79: 1556–1576.

Friedman, M. J., Sherman, O. H., Fox, J. M. et al. 1985. Autogeneic anterior cruciate ligament (ACL) anterior reconstruction of the knee. A review. *Clin Orthop Relat Res*, 9–14.

Fu, F. H., Bennett, C. H., Lattermann, C., and Ma, C. B. 1999. Current trends in anterior cruciate ligament reconstruction. Part 1: Biology and biomechanics of reconstruction. *Am J Sports Med*, 27: 821–830.

Fu, F. H., Bennett, C. H., Ma, C. B., Menetrey, J., and Lattermann, C. 2000. Current trends in anterior cruciate ligament reconstruction. Part II. Operative procedures and clinical correlations. *Am J Sports Med*, 28: 124–130.

Fujikawa, K., Iseki, F., and Seedhom, B. B. 1989. Arthroscopy after anterior cruciate reconstruction with the Leeds–Keio ligament. *J Bone Joint Surg Br*, 71: 566–570.

Goldstein, J., Tria, A., Zawadsky, J. et al. 1989. Development of a reconstituted collagen tendon prosthesis. A preliminary implantation study. *J Bone Joint Surg Am*, 71: 1183–1191.

Goulet, F., Germain, L., Rancourt, D., Caron, C., Normand, A., and Auger, Fa. 1997. Tendons and ligaments. In: Lanza, R. P. and L. R., and Chick, W. L. (eds.), *Principles of Tissue Engineering*. RG Landes Company, Austin, TX, pp. 909–918.

Greco, R. S. 1994. *Implantation Biology: The Host Response and Biomedical Devices.* CRC Press, Boca Raton, FL.

Guidoin, M. F., Marois, Y., Bejui, J. et al. 2000. Analysis of retrieved polymer fiber based replacements for the ACL. *Biomaterials*, 21: 2461–2474.

Gwinn, D., Wilckens, J., McDevitt, E., Ross, G., and Kao, T. 2000. The relative incidence of anterior cruciate ligament injury in men and women at the United States Naval Academy. *Am J Sports Med*, 28: 98.

Hammer, D., Brown, C., Jr., Steiner, M., Hecker, A., and Hayes, W. 1999. Hamstring tendon grafts for reconstruction of the anterior cruciate ligament: Biomechanical evaluation of the use of multiple strands and tensioning techniques. *J Bone Joint Surg Am*, 81: 549–557.

Harner, C., Livesay, G., Kashiwaguchi, S. et al. 1995. Comparative study of the size and shape of human anterior and posterior cruciate ligaments. *J Orthop Res*, 13: 429–434.

Hefti, F., Kress, A., Fasel, J., and Mprscher, E. 1991. Healing of the transected anterior cruciate ligament in the rabbit. *J Bone Joint Surg Am*, 73: 373–383.

Hilderbrand, K. A., Frank, C. B., and Hard, D. A. 2004. Gene intervention in ligament and tendon: Current status, challenges, future directions. *Gene Ther*, 11: 368–387.

Hoffmann, A. and Gross, G. 2007. Tendon and ligament engineering in the adult organism: Mesenchymal stem cells and gene-therapeutic approaches. *Int Orthop*, 31: 791–797.

Hogervorst, T. and Brand, R. A. 1998. Mechanoreceptors in joint function. *J Bone Joint Surg Am*, 80: 1365–1378.

Iobst, C. A. and Stanitski, C. L. 2000. Acute knee injuries. *Clin Sports Med*, 19: 621–635.

Ito, K., Fujisato, T., and Ikada, Y. 1992. Implantation of cell-seeded biodegradable polymers for tissue reconstruction. In: *Materials Research Society Symposium Proceedings*. Materials Research Society, San Francisco, CA, pp. 359–364.

Jackson, D. W. 1995. Reconstructive knee surgery. *J Orthop Trauma*, 9: 277.

Jackson, D. W. and Arnoczky, S. P. 1993. *The Anterior Cruciate Ligament: Current and Future Concepts*. Lippincott Williams & Wilkins, Philadelphia, PA.

Jackson, D. W., Grood, E. S., Cohn, B. T. et al. 1991. The effects of *in situ* freezing on the anterior cruciate ligament. An experimental study in goats. *J Bone Joint Surg Am*, 73: 201–213.

Jackson, D. W., Heinrich, J. T., and Simon, T. M. 1994. Biologic and synthetic implants to replace the anterior cruciate ligament. *Arthroscopy*, 10: 442–452.

Jackson, D. W. and Simon, T. M. 1999. Tissue engineering principles in orthopaedic surgery. *Clin Orthop Relat Res*, (367 Suppl): S31–S45.

Jackson, D. W., Simon, T. M., Lowery, W., and Gendler, E. 1996. Biologic remodeling after anterior cruciate ligament reconstruction using a collagen matrix derived from demineralized bone. An experimental study in the goat model. *Am J Sports Med*, 24: 405–414.

Jackson, D. W., Windler, G. E., and Simon, T. M. 1990. Intraarticular reaction associated with the use of freeze-dried, ethylene oxide-sterilized bone-patella tendon-bone allografts in the reconstruction of the anterior cruciate ligament. *Am J Sports Med*, 18: 1–10; discussion 10–11.

Johnson, F. 1960. Use of braided nylon as a prosthetic anterior cruciate ligament of the dog. *J Am Veterinary Med Assoc*, 137: 646–647.

Johnson, R. J., Beynnon, B. D., Nichols, C. E., and Renstrom, P. A. 1992. The treatment of injuries of the anterior cruciate ligament. *J Bone Joint Surg Am*, 74: 140–151.

Jones, R., Nawana, N., Pearcy, M. et al. 1995. Mechanical properties of the human anterior cruciate ligament. *Clin Biomech*, 10: 339–344.

King, D., Hume, P., Milburn, P., and Gianotti, S. 2009. Rugby league injuries in New Zealand: Variations in injury claims and costs by ethnicity, gender, age, district, body site, injury type and occupation. *NZ J Sports Med*, 36: 48–55.

Ko, F. 1987. *Braiding Engineering Materials Handbook*. ASM International, Metals Park, OH.

Ko, F. K. 1989. Three-dimensional fabrics for composites. In: *Textile Structural Composites*. Elsevier Science Publishers, New York, pp. 129–171.

Ko, F. K. and Pastore, C. M. 1985. Structure and properties of an integrated 3-D fabric for structural composites. In: *ASTM STP 864*. ASTM International, Philadelphia, PA, p. 428.

Ko, F. K., Pastore, C. M., and Head, A. A. 1989. Tsu Wei Chou and Frank K. Ko (eds.), *Atkins & Pearce Handbook of Industrial Braiding*. Atkins & Pearce, Covington, KY.

Ko, F. K., Soebroto, H. B., and Lei, C. 1988. 3-D net shaped composites by the two-step braiding process. In: *Proceedings of 33rd International SAMPE Symposium*. Society for the Advancement of Material and Process Engineering, Covina, CA, pp. 912–921.

Kobayashi, H., Kawamoto, Y., Hara, S. et al. 1995. Study on bioresorbable poly-L-lactide (PLLA) ligament augmentation device (LAD). In: *Japan Chapter of SAMPE*, pp. 583–588.

Koski, J. A., Ibarra, C., and Rodeo, S. A. 2000. Tissue-engineered ligament: Cells, matrix, and growth factors. *Orthop Clin North Am*, 31: 437–452.

Laitinen, O., Pohjonen, T., Tormala, P. et al. 1993. Mechanical properties of biodegradable poly-L-lactide ligament augmentation device in experimental anterior cruciate ligament reconstruction. *Arch Orthop Trauma Surg*, 112: 270–274.

Laitinen, O., Tormala, P., Taurio, R. et al. 1992. Mechanical properties of biodegradable ligament augmentation device of poly(L-lactide) *in vitro* and *in vivo*. *Biomaterials*, 13: 1012–1016.

Lane, J., McFadden, P., Bowden, K., and Amiel, D. 1993. The ligamentization process: A 4 year case study following ACL reconstruction with a semitendinosis graft. *Arthroscopy: J Arthros Relat Surg*, 9: 149–153.

Langer, R. and Vacanti, J. P. 1993. Tissue engineering. *Science*, 260: 920–926.

Laurencin, C., Ko, P., Borden, M. et al. 1999a. Fiber based tissue engineered scaffolds for musculoskeletal applications: *In vitro* cellular response. In *MRS Proceedings*. Materials Research Society, Boston, MA, pp. 127–136.

Laurencin, C. T., Ambrosio, A. M., Borden, M. D., and Cooper, J. A., Jr. 1999b. Tissue engineering: Orthopedic applications. *Annu Rev Biomed Eng*, 1: 19–46.

Lee, C. H., Singla, A., and Lee, Y. 2001. Biomedical applications of collagen. *Int J Pharm*, 221: 1–22.

Lin, V. S., Lee, M. C., O'neal, S., McKean, J., and Sung, K. L. 1999. Ligament tissue engineering using synthetic biodegradable fiber scaffolds. *Tissue Eng*, 5: 443–452.

Liu, H., Fan, H., Toh, S. L., and Goh, J. C. 2008. A comparison of rabbit mesenchymal stem cells and anterior cruciate ligament fibroblasts responses on combined silk scaffolds. *Biomaterials*, 29: 1443–1453.

Liu, S. H., Yang, R. S., Al-Shaikh, R., and Lane, J. M. 1995. Collagen in tendon, ligament, and bone healing. A current review. *Clin Orthop Relat Res*, 318: 265–278.

Lu, H. H., Cooper, J. A., Jr., Manuel, S. et al. 2005. Anterior cruciate ligament regeneration using braided biodegradable scaffolds: *In vitro* optimization studies. *Biomaterials*, 26: 4805–4816.

Lyon, R. M., Akeson, W. H., Amiel, D., Kitabayashi, L. R., and Woo, S. L. 1991. Ultrastructural differences between the cells of the medical collateral and the anterior cruciate ligaments. *Clin Orthop Relat Res*, 279–286.

Madey, S. M., Cole, K. J., and Brand, R. A. 1993. The sensory role of the anterior cruciate ligament. In: *The Anterior Cruciate Ligament. Current and Future Concepts*. Raven Press Ltd., New York, pp. 23–33.

McCarthy, D. M., Tolin, B. S., Schwendeman, L., Friedman, M., and Woo, S. 1993. Prosthetic replacement for the anterior cruciate ligament. In: DW Jackson and SP Amocsky (eds.), *The Anterior Cruciate Ligament: Current and Future Concepts*. Raven Press Ltd., New York, pp. 343–356.

McMaster, W. C. 1985. A histologic assessment of canine anterior cruciate substitution with bovine xenograft. *Clin Orthop Relat Res*, 196–201.

McMaster, W. 1986. Mechanical properties and early clinical experience with xenograft biomaterials. *Bull Hosp Joint Dis Orthop Inst*, 46: 174–184.

McPherson, G. K., Mendenhall, H. V., Gibbons, D. F. et al. 1985. Experimental mechanical and histologic evaluation of the Kennedy ligament augmentation device. *Clin Orthop Relat Res*, 186–195.

Mendes, E., Lopes, J. M., Castro, C., and Oliveira, J. 1998. Time of remodeling of the patellar tendon graft in anterior cruciate ligament surgery: An histological and immunohistochemical study in a rabbit model. *Knee*, 5: 9–19.

Menetrey, J., Kasemkijwattana, C., Day, C. S., Bosch, P., Fu, F. H., Moreland, M. S., and Huard, J. 1999. Direct-, fibroblast- and myoblast-mediated gene transfer to the anterior cruciate ligament. *Tissue Eng*, 5: 435–442.

Miller, M. D. 1996. *Review of Orthopaedics*. W.B. Saunders Company, Philadelphia, PA.

Miller, M. D., Cooper, D. E., and Warner, J. J. P. 1995. *Review of Sports Medicine and Arthroscopy*. W.B. Saunders Company, Philadelphia, PA.

Mooney, D. J., Cima, L., Langer, R., Johnson, L., Hansen, L. K., Ingber, D. E., and Vacanti, J. P. 1992. Principles of tissue engineering and reconstruction using polymer–cell constructs. In: *Materials Research Society Symposium Proceedings*, Materials Research Society, San Francisco, CA, pp. 345–352.

Morgan, J. R. and Yarmush, M. L. 1999. *Tissue Engineering Methods and Protocols*. Humana Press Inc., Totowa, NJ.

Müller, W. 1983. *The Knee: Form, Function, and Ligament Reconstruction.* Springer-Verlag, Berlin, Germany.

Nakamura, N., Hart, D. A., Boorman, R. S., Kaneda, Y., Shrive, N. G., Marchuk, L. L., Shino, K., Ochi, T., and Frank, C. B. 2000. Decorin antisense gene therapy improves functional healing of early rabbit ligament scar with enhanced collagen fibrillogenesis *in vivo. J Orthopaed Res,* 18: 517–523.

Naughton, G. K., Tolbert, W. R., and Grillot, T. M. 1995. Emerging developments in tissue engineering and cell technology. *Tissue Eng,* 1: 211–219.

Neugebauer, R. and Burri, C. 1985. Carbon fiber ligament replacement in chronic knee instability. *Clin Orthop Relat Res,* 118–123.

Nickerson, D. A., Joshi, R., Williams, S., Ross, S. M., and Frank, C. 1992. Synovial fluid stimulates the proliferation of rabbit ligament. Fibroblasts *in vitro. Clin Orthop Relat Res,* 294–299.

Nigg, B. M. and Herzog, W. 1994. *Biomechanics of the Musculo-Skeletal System.* John Wiley & Sons, New York.

Noth, U., Rackwitz, L., Steinert, A. F., and Tuan, R. S. 2010. Cell delivery therapeutics for musculoskeletal regeneration. *Adv Drug Deliv Rev,* 62: 765–793.

Noyes, F., Butler, D., Grood, E., Zernicke, R., and Hefzy, M. 1984. Biomechanical analysis of human ligament grafts used in knee–ligament repairs and reconstructions. *J Bone Joint Surg Am,* 66: 344–352.

Noyes, F. R., Barber, S. D., and Mangine, R. E. 1990. Bone-patellar ligament–bone and fascia lata allografts for reconstruction of the anterior cruciate ligament. *J Bone Joint Surg Am,* 72: 1125–1136.

Noyes, F. R. and Grood, E. S. 1976. The strength of the anterior cruciate ligament in humans and rhesus monkeys. *J Bone Joint Surg Am,* 58: 1074–1082.

Noyes, F. R., Matthews, D. S., Mooar, P. A., and Grood, E. S. 1983. The symptomatic anterior cruciate-deficient knee. Part II: The results of rehabilitation, activity modification, and counseling on functional disability. *J Bone Joint Surg Am,* 65: 163–174.

Ohno, K., Pomaybo, A. S., Schmidt, C. C. et al. 1995. Healing of the medial collateral ligament after a combined medial collateral and anterior cruciate ligament injury and reconstruction of the anterior cruciate ligament: Comparison of repair and nonrepair of medial collateral ligament tears in rabbits. *J Orthop Res,* 13: 442–449.

Olson, E. J., Kang, J. D., Fu, F. H. et al. 1988. The biochemical and histological effects of artificial ligament wear particles: *In vitro* and *in vivo* studies. *Am J Sports Med,* 16: 558–570.

Page, I. 1959. *Connective Tissue Thrombosis and Atherosclerosis.* Academic Press, New York.

Papageorgiou, C. D., Ma, C. B., Abramowitch, S. D., Clineff, T. D., and Woo, S. L. 2001. A multidisciplinary study of the healing of an intraarticular anterior cruciate ligament graft in a goat model. *Am J Sports Med,* 29: 620–626.

Pascher, A., Steinert, A. F., Palmer, G. D., Betz, O., Gouze, J. N., Gouze, E., Pilapil, C., and Ghivizzani, S. C., Evans, C. H., and Murray, M. M. 2004. Enhanced repair of the anterior cruciate ligament by *in situ* gene transfer: Evaluation in an *in vitro* model. *Mol Ther,* 10: 327–336.

Petrigliano, F. A., McAllister, D. R., and Wu, B. M. 2006. Tissue engineering for anterior cruciate ligament reconstruction: A review of current strategies. *Arthroscopy,* 22: 441–451.

Puddu, G., Cipolla, M., Cerullo, G., Franco, V., and Gianni, E. 1993. Anterior cruciate ligament reconstruction and augmentation with PDS graft. *Clin Sports Med,* 12: 13–24.

Rodkey, W. 1994. *The Cruciate Ligaments: Diagnosis and Treatment of Ligamentous Injuries about the Knee.* Churchill Livingstone, New York.

Roolker, W., Patt, T. W., Van Dijk, C. N., Vegter, M., and Marti, R. K. 2000. The Gore-Tex prosthetic ligament as a salvage procedure in deficient knees. *Knee Surg Sports Traumatol Arthrosc,* 8: 20–25.

Roos, H., Adalberth, T., Dahlberg, L., and Lohmander, L. S. 1995. Osteoarthritis of the knee after injury to the anterior cruciate ligament or meniscus: The influence of time and age. *Osteoarthritis Cartilage,* 3: 261–267.

Salamone, J. C. 1999. *Concise Polymeric Materials Encyclopedia*. CRC Press, Boca Raton, FL.

Scherping, S. C., Jr., Schmidt, C. C., Georgescu, H. I. et al. 1997. Effect of growth factors on the proliferation of ligament fibroblasts from skeletally mature rabbits. *Connect Tissue Res*, 36: 1–8.

Schiavone Panni, A., Fabbriciani, C., Delcogliano, A., and Franzese, S. 1993. Bone–ligament interaction in patellar tendon reconstruction of the ACL. *Knee Surg Sports Traumatol Arthrosc*, 1: 4–8.

Schutte, M. J., Dabezies, E., Zimny, M., and Happel, L. 1987. Neural anatomy of the human anterior cruciate ligament. *J Bone Joint Surg Am*, 69: 243.

Seedhom, B. B. 1992. Reconstruction of the anterior cruciate ligament. *Proc Inst Mech Eng H*, 206: 15–27.

Segawa, H., Omori, G., and Koga, Y. 2001. Long-term results of non-operative treatment of anterior cruciate ligament injury. *Knee*, 8: 5–11.

Sekiguchi, H., Post, W., Han, J., Ryu, J., and Kish, V. 1998. The effects of cyclic loading on tensile properties of a rabbit femur–anterior cruciate ligament–tibia complex (FATC). *Knee*, 5: 215–220.

Sharpey, W. and Ellis, G. 1856. *Elements of Anatomy*. Walton and Moberly, London, U.K.

Shelton, W. R., Treacy, S. H., Dukes, A. D., and Bomboy, A. L. 1998a. Use of allografts in knee reconstruction: I. Basic science aspects and current status. *J Am Acad Orthopaed Surg*, 6: 165–168.

Shelton, W. R., Treacy, S. H., Dukes, A. D., and Bomboy, A. L. 1998b. Use of allografts in knee reconstruction: II. Surgical considerations. *J Am Acad Orthopaed Surg*, 6: 169–175.

Sherman, M. F., Warren, R. F., Marshall, J. L., and Savatsky, G. J. 1988. A clinical and radiographical analysis of 127 anterior cruciate insufficient knees. *Clin Orthop Relat Res*, 227: 229–237.

Shieh, S. J., Zimmerman, M. C., and Parsons, J. R. 1990. Preliminary characterization of bioresorbable and nonresorbable synthetic fibers for the repair of soft tissue injuries. *J Biomed Mater Res*, 24: 789–808.

Shimizu, T., Takahashi, T., Wada, Y. et al. 1999. Regeneration process of mechanoreceptors in the reconstructed anterior cruciate ligament. *Arch Orthopaed Trauma Surg*, 119: 405–409.

Shino, K., Inoue, M., Horibe, S., Nagano, J., and Ono, K. 1988. Maturation of allograft tendons transplanted into the knee. An arthroscopic and histological study. *J Bone Joint Surg Br*, 70: 556–560.

Silver, F. H., Tria, A. J., Zawadsky, J. P., and Dunn, M. G. 1991. Anterior cruciate ligament replacement: A review. *J Long Term Eff Med Implants*, 1: 135–154.

Simon, S. R. 1994. *Orthopaedic Basic Science*. American Academy of Orthopaedic.

Smith, B. A., Livesay, G. A., and Woo, S. L. 1993. Biology and biomechanics of the anterior cruciate ligament. *Clin Sports Med*, 12: 637–670.

Snook, G. A. 1983. A short history of the anterior cruciate ligament and the treatment of tears. *Clin Orthop Relat Res*, 11–13.

Staubli, H. U., Schatzmann, L., Brunner, P., Rincon, L., and Nolte, L. P. 1996. Quadriceps tendon and patellar ligament: Cryosectional anatomy and structural properties in young adults. *Knee Surg Sports Traumatol Arthrosc*, 4: 100–110.

Strover, A. E. and Firer, P. 1985. The use of carbon fiber implants in anterior cruciate ligament surgery. *Clin Orthop Relat Res*, 196: 88–98.

Strum, G. M. and Larson, R. L. 1985. Clinical experience and early results of carbon fiber augmentation of anterior cruciate reconstruction of the knee. *Clin Orthop Relat Res*, 124–138.

Takai, S. and Woo, S. L. 1993. Determination of the *in situ* loads on the human anterior cruciate ligament. *J Orthopaed Res*, 11: 686–695.

Thomas, N. P., Turner, I. G., and Jones, C. B. 1987. Prosthetic anterior cruciate ligaments in the rabbit. A comparison of four types of replacement. *J Bone Joint Surg Br*, 69: 312–316.

Van Steensel, C. J., Schreuder, O., Van Den Bosch, B. F. et al. 1987. Failure of anterior cruciate-ligament reconstruction using tendon xenograft. *J Bone Joint Surg Am*, 69: 860–864.

Vasseur, P. B., Stevenson, S., Gregory, C. R. et al. 1991. Anterior cruciate ligament allograft transplantation in dogs. *Clin Orthop Relat Res*, 295–304.

Vunjak-Novakovic, G., Altman, G., Horan, R., and Kaplan, D. L. 2004. Tissue engineering of ligaments. *Annu Rev Biomed Eng*, 6: 131–156.

Warren, R. F. 1983. Primary repair of the anterior cruciate ligament. *Clin Orthop Relat Res*, 65–70.

Weiler, A., Hoffmann, R. F. G., Stähelin, A. C., Helling, H. J., and Südkamp, N. P. 2000. Biodegradable implants in sports medicine: The biological base. *Arthroscopy J Arthros Relat Surg*, 16: 305–321.

Weitzel, P. P., Richmond, J. C., Altman, G. H., Calabro, T., and Kaplan, D. L. 2002. Future direction of the treatment of ACL ruptures. *Orthoped Clin North Am*, 33: 653–661.

Wilson, A. G., Plessas, S. J., Gray, T., and Forster, I. W. 1998. Lymphadenopathy after GORE-TEX anterior cruciate ligament reconstruction. *Am J Sports Med*, 26: 133–135.

Woo, S. L., Abramowitch, S. D., Kilger, R., and Liang, R. 2006. Biomechanics of knee ligaments: Injury, healing and repair. *J Biomech*, 39: 1–20.

Woo, S. L. Y. and Buckwalter, J. A. 1988. Injury and repair of the musculoskeletal soft tissues. Savannah, Georgia, June 18–20, 1987. *J Orthopaed Res*, 6: 907–931.

Woo, S. L. Y., Debski, R. E., Withrow, J. D., and Janaushek, M. A. 1999. Biomechanics of knee ligaments. *Am J Sports Med*, 27: 533–543.

Woo, S. L. Y., Debski, R. E., Zeminski, J. et al. 2000b. Injury and repair of ligaments and tendons. *Annu Rev Biomed Eng*, 2: 83–118.

Woo, S. L. Y., Hollis, J. M., Adams, D. J., Lyon, R. M., and Takai, S. 1991. Tensile properties of the human femur–anterior cruciate ligament–tibia complex. *Am J Sports Med*, 19: 217.

Woo, S., Livesay, G., and Engle, C. 1992a. Biomechanics of the human anterior cruciate ligament. ACL structure and role in knee motion. *Orthopaed Rev*, 21: 835–842.

Woo, S., Livesay, G., and Engle, C. 1992b. Biomechanics of the human anterior cruciate ligament. Muscle stabilization and ACL reconstruction. *Orthopaed Rev*, 21: 935–941.

Woo, S. L. Y., Newton, P. O., Mackenna, D. A., and Lyon, R. M. 1992c. A comparative evaluation of the mechanical properties of the rabbit medial collateral and anterior cruciate ligaments. *J Biomech*, 25: 377–386.

Woo, S. L., Orlando, C. A., Camp, J. F., and Akeson, W. H. 1986. Effects of postmortem storage by freezing on ligament tensile behavior. *J Biomech*, 19: 399–404.

Woo, S. L., Vogrin, T. M., and Abramowitch, S. D. 2000a. Healing and repair of ligament injuries in the knee. *J Am Acad Orthop Surg*, 8: 364–372.

Woods, G. A., Indelicato, P. A., and Prevot, T. J. 1991. The Gore-Tex anterior cruciate ligament prosthesis. Two versus three year results. *Am J Sports Med*, 19: 48–55.

Wredmark, T. and Engstrom, B. 1993. Five-year results of anterior cruciate ligament reconstruction with the Stryker Dacron high-strength ligament. *Knee Surg Sports Traumatol Arthrosc*, 1: 71–75.

Yahia, H. 1997. *Ligaments and Ligamentoplasties*. Springer, Berlin, Heidelberg.

Yang, P. J. and Temenoff, J. S. 2009. Engineering orthopedic tissue interfaces. *Tissue Eng Pt B Rev*, 15: 127–141

Zavras, T., Mackenney, R., and Amis, A. 1995. The natural history of anterior cruciate ligament reconstruction using patellar tendon autograft. *Knee*, 2: 211–217.

Zimmerman, M. C., Contiliano, J. H., Parsons, J. R., Prewett, A., and Billotti, J. 1994. The biomechanics and histopathology of chemically processed patellar tendon allografts for anterior cruciate ligament replacement. *Am J Sports Med*, 22: 378–386.

Zimny, M. L. 1988. Mechanoreceptors in articular tissues. *Am J Anat*, 182: 16–32.

Zimny, M. L., Schutte, M., and Dabezies, E. 1986. Mechanoreceptors in the human anterior cruciate ligament. *Anatom Record*, 214: 204–209.

CHAPTER 14

Skeletal Muscle Regenerative Engineering

Shaun W. McLaughlin, BS;* Michael N. Wosczyna, PhD;*
Cato T. Laurencin, MD, PhD; and David J. Goldhamer, PhD

CONTENTS

---

* Shared first authorship.

14.1 INTRODUCTION

Skeletal muscle has a robust regenerative capacity, and minor injuries are effectively repaired by the action of resident muscle stem cells. However, the loss of muscle from trauma, surgery, or disease, in the amount of ~20% or more, interrupts the natural repair mechanisms of the body, induces excessive scar tissue formation, and severely hinders muscle function (Turner and Badylak, 2012). At present, there are limited interventional options to improve clinical outcomes, necessitating the development of innovative regenerative engineering strategies that consider both cell-based and cell/material-based approaches. After introducing the basic biology of skeletal muscle and normal regenerative processes, this chapter will focus on current concepts in skeletal muscle engineering with a focus on interdisciplinary approaches that bridge cell biology and biomedical engineering. Specific attention will be given to existing technologies with the potential to treat localized injuries, since such treatments are probably on the horizon. Unrealized challenges of treating pathologies that broadly affect the entire skeletal muscle system, such as certain muscular dystrophies, will also be discussed.

14.2 BASIC ANATOMY AND PHYSIOLOGY OF SKELETAL MUSCLE

The fundamental cellular unit of skeletal muscle is the muscle fiber, a multinucleated syncytium that results from fusion of myogenic precursor cells (myoblasts). Depending on the muscle type, muscle fibers can contain hundreds to thousands of myoblast-derived nuclei, which are aligned along the periphery of the fiber in undamaged muscle (Ross and Pawlina, 2006). The canonical muscle stem cell, the satellite cell (SC), lies just outside the fiber plasma membrane (sarcolemma), and it is this population of cells that is responsible for the inherent regenerative capacity of skeletal muscle. Although the basic organization of skeletal muscle is similar in most anatomical locations, muscles vary dramatically in size, reflecting variability in the length, diameter, and number of constituent muscle fibers. For example, in the sartorius muscle of the leg, muscle fibers can reach lengths of up to nearly 600 mm, whereas in the stapedius muscle of the middle ear, individual fibers are no more than a few millimeters in length (Harris et al., 2005; Aristeguieta et al., 2010). Muscle fiber diameter can range from 5 to 100 μm in width depending on the muscle, and alterations in fiber diameter are associated with aging, exercise, and myopathic conditions. Each muscle fiber is surrounded by a sarcolemma, which is attached to a thin layer of connective tissue known as the endomysium (Mauro and Adams, 1961; Borg and Caulfield, 1980; Taylor and Koohmaraie, 1998). It is within the endomysium where small-diameter blood vessels and neurons run parallel to the muscle fiber, providing nutrients and innervation to the adjacent structure (Figure 14.1).

These neuronal branches infiltrate the transverse tubular system, or T system. Each T tubule surrounds individual muscle fibers and is responsible for directing the activity of the functional contractile unit of the muscle fiber, the sarcomere (Ezerman and Ishikawa, 1967). These functional units are made up of myofilaments, or individual polymers of myosin II (thick filaments) and actin (thin filaments) (Keynes et al., 2011). It is the specific arrangement and appearance of these proteins under light microscopy that gives

Gross organization of skeletal muscle

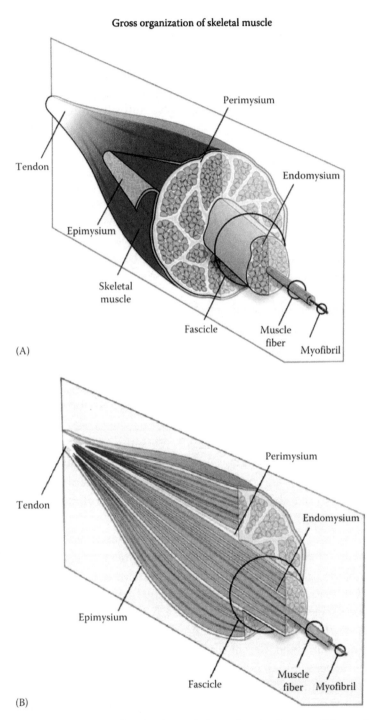

(A)

(B)

FIGURE 14.1   Gross organization of skeletal muscle from the attachment of the tendon down to the single myofibril. Skeletal muscle in cross section shows the organization of the muscle fascicle with individual myofibers (A). Skeletal muscle in longitudinal section shows the length of the muscle fibers, which can vary greatly between muscles from its origin at the tendon (B). (Reprinted from Gillies, A.R., *Muscle Nerve*, 44, 3, 2011. With permission.)

skeletal muscle its more colloquial name, *striated* skeletal muscle (Huxley, 1953). Driven by the motor domain of myosin, actin and myosin filaments slide relative to each other, contracting the muscle and generating force. Muscle fiber sarcomeres are all arranged in a parallel fashion with no syncytial bridges between cells (Barrett et al., 2010). If a force is produced in the x–y plane and some of the muscle fibers are oriented in the x–y plane but others are oriented in the y–z plane, the force and direction of contraction will be significantly altered.

14.3 SKELETAL MUSCLE REGENERATION

Skeletal muscle has a remarkable inherent ability to regenerate following injury, a process that is driven by muscle stem cells resident in muscle tissue. However, the nature and severity of muscle injury can greatly impact the regenerative process, resulting in a broad spectrum of outcomes. In order to effectively treat disorders in which regeneration has failed, the normal injury and repair process must be understood. The typical stages following injury are discussed below.

14.3.1 Degeneration and Inflammation

During muscle injury, the integrity of the sarcolemma as well as the basal lamina can become compromised (Armstrong et al., 1991). A cascade of events, which include the disruption of calcium homeostasis and the activation of the immune system, follow this initial insult. Muscle tissue integrity is highly dependent on a tightly regulated balance of intracellular and extracellular calcium levels (Delbono, 2002). Increased cytosolic calcium leads to decreased mitochondrial function, reduced ATP production, and dysregulated and impaired muscle contraction (Orrenius et al., 2003). Further, calcium is a key activator of many intracellular enzymes including endonucleases (digests DNA), proteases (digests proteins), and phospholipases (digests membrane phospholipids), and elevated calcium levels thereby contribute to the destruction of muscle cells from within (Kristian and Siesjo, 1998).

Immediately following muscle damage, leukocyte extravasation from the vasculature and free radical generation occurs (Tidball, 2005). Neutrophils and macrophages are some of the first inflammatory cells on the scene of injured muscle tissue. These cells utilize reactive oxygen species (ROS) to cause necrotic cells to release their contents extracellularly and be eliminated. Macrophages are also involved in clearing necrotic debris and release a variety of cytokines such as IL-1 and IL-12, which can lead to pathological inflammation (Jovanovic et al., 1998; Zhang et al., 2009). Recent studies indicate that macrophage-activating signals may dictate the generation of fibrosis (excessive accumulation of connective tissues) versus regeneration (Villalta et al., 2009); macrophages produce significant amounts of the cytokine, transforming growth factor β (TGF-β), which can lead to excessive fibrosis within the regenerating muscle if not appropriately controlled (Shen et al., 2008).

14.3.2 Regeneration

The process of muscle regeneration begins in the first week of muscle injury. Phagocytic cells clear the necrotic debris from the initial injury and area of inflammation, while SCs become

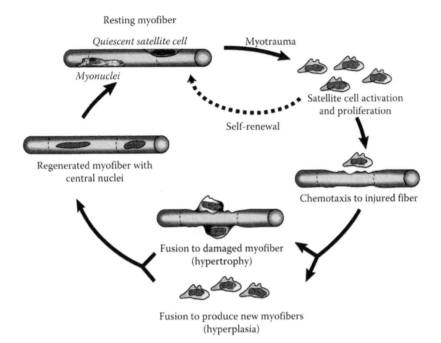

Resting myofiber

Quiescent satellite cell

Myotrauma

Myonuclei

Satellite cell activation
and proliferation

Self-renewal

Regenerated myofiber with
central nuclei

Chemotaxis to injured fiber

Fusion to damaged myofiber
(hypertrophy)

Fusion to produce new myofibers
(hyperplasia)

FIGURE 14.2   Satellite cell-mediated fiber regeneration following injury. (Reprinted with minor modifications from Hawke, T.J. and Garry, D.J., *J. Appl. Physiol.*, 91(2), 534, 2001. With permission.)

activated and proliferate to generate a population of daughter cells (Figure 14.2). These descendants contribute to nascent myotube formation through cell fusion, recapitulating many aspects of embryonic myogenesis, while self-renewal ensures maintenance of the SC niche for subsequent rounds of muscle repair (Collins et al., 2005). Various growth factors are thought to be involved at this stage, many of which belong to the fibroblast growth factor (FGF) family, hepatocyte growth factor (HGF) family, and TGF-β superfamily (Charge and Rudnicki, 2004). It is commonly accepted that both FGF and HGF promote SC proliferation and which delays their differentiation, acting as a positive regulator of regeneration. TGF-β and myostatin (a member of the TGF-β superfamily) may act as negative regulators of regeneration by inhibiting the proliferation of SCs (Allen and Rankin, 1990).

Insulin-like growth factors (IGFs), particularly IGF-1, are known to have both proliferative and pro-differentiative effects on SCs (Chakravarthy et al., 2000). During regeneration, IGF-1 can also promote cell fusion, an important step in muscle regeneration (Engert et al., 1996). As such, IGF-1 may be a key player when designing regenerative engineering systems for skeletal muscle. It is interesting to note that increased muscle loading increases IGF-1 secretion (Bamman et al., 2001), a result that merits further investigation into the use of physical tension to initiate regenerative effects. On the other hand, myostatin, a negative regulator of quiescent stem cell activation, has been found at elevated levels when a muscle is unloaded (Carlson et al., 1999) and may play a vital role in the intricate design of the complex muscle–tendon junction (MTJ). For example, in an engineered system, the incorporation of myostatin into a continuous junction may allow for the healing of this tissue in a fashion that mimics native tissue.

14.3.3 Fibrosis

When severe or chronic muscle injury occurs, the regenerative process can become perturbed, resulting in the deposition of dense connective tissue between regenerating and damaged muscle fibers—a pathological process known as fibrosis (Sato et al., 2003). As mentioned earlier, the macrophages that migrate out of the vasculature into the damaged muscle tissue release growth factors and cytokines and can cause a decrease in metalloproteinase activity. FGF and TGF-β cause the proliferation of fibroblast and endothelial cells, which in combination with specific cytokines causes an increase in collagen synthesis within the muscle (Mourkioti and Rosenthal, 2005). Increased TGF-β levels have also been noted in Duchenne muscular dystrophy (DMD) and dermatomyositis, two pathologies affecting skeletal muscle (Ishitobi et al., 2000; Funauchi et al., 2006). When metalloproteinase activity is inhibited, excess collagen accumulates, as the balance between synthesis and degradation is perturbed. Ruptured blood vessels in the injured muscle can be replaced initially by type III collagen and then type I collagen, as early as 3 days after injury. Fibrosis not only causes a decreased functionality of muscle from a structural standpoint but can also prevent the muscle from accessing vital nutrients and cells. Further, dense fibrotic tissue can inhibit reinnervation of damaged muscle resulting in the loss of contractile activity and ultimately muscle atrophy (Kaariainen et al., 2000).

14.4 DEFECTS IN SKELETAL MUSCLE

The complexity of skeletal muscle—from the neurons that innervate muscle to the vasculature that provides blood supply—makes effective repair strategies challenging, as a complex tissue organization must be rebuilt. In fact, certain injuries or physiological disorders exhaust the intrinsic regenerative capacity of skeletal muscle and thus require intervention to return to normal function. An area that can feasibly benefit in the near future from skeletal muscle engineering is likely to be in the treatment of localized injuries—for example, in the amelioration of the fatty degeneration associated with rotator cuff tendon tears or in the reconstruction of the tissue mass absent in large skeletal muscle defects. While these types of wounds present clinically challenging scenarios, as both cellular and structural support is needed to effectively regenerate tissue and alleviate secondary degenerative effects, they impact discrete areas of the body and thus are ideal candidates for regenerative engineering-based therapeutics. Conversely, diseases, such as the muscular dystrophies, which broadly affect skeletal muscle throughout the body, still present an ever-challenging situation, as successful therapies will require the targeting of numerous and anatomically distant tissues. A brief description of examples of these pathologies and defects follows.

14.4.1 Systemic Skeletal Muscle Defects

The muscular dystrophies are an example of genetic disorders that can have severe consequences on muscle structure, often beginning in early childhood. The most common and severe form, DMD, is an X-linked recessive disease that results in progressive muscle weakness and wasting (Koenig et al., 1989). The incidence of DMD is ~1 in 3500 live births, and patients are normally confined to a wheelchair by the age of 10 (Kumar et al., 2010). The gene that is mutated in this pathology normally encodes a 427 kDa protein known as dystrophin, a rod-shaped cytoplasmic protein (Fabbrizio et al., 1995) that provides a structural link between the muscle cytoskeleton and the extracellular matrix (ECM). Mutations in dystrophin can cause loss of muscle integrity, which ultimately results in muscle degeneration. Histology of muscle biopsies shows progressive deterioration of muscle architecture. Early in disease progression, muscle is characterized by foci of necrotic fibers, regenerating fibers arising from the activity of SC, and areas of fibrosis. During the final stages of the disease, muscle tissue becomes completely replaced by adipose and connective tissue leading to the total loss of normal muscle function (Haslett et al., 2002). The origin of infiltrating fat and fibrotic tissue within skeletal muscle, which affects muscle architecture and function and is associated with a poor prognosis, is a topic of significant debate. As indicated earlier, pathologies like DMD that affect muscle groups throughout the body cannot be cured by localized tissue regeneration strategies, and systemic delivery of stem cells to treat the muscular dystrophies is currently being tested in animal models (see later).

14.4.2 Localized Skeletal Muscle Defects

Large skeletal muscle defects or volumetric muscle loss (VML) can result from traumatic injuries or surgical interventions (e.g., tumor resection). Extremity wounds that result in VML and significant damage to bone are prevalent among combat personnel and are extremely difficult to treat effectively. Such severe injuries often result in permanent functional and anatomical deficits (Grogan and Hsu, 2011). Secondary to the initial injury, functional impairment of the muscle unit results in further tissue degeneration and scar tissue formation, which complicates treatment. Currently, the most prescribed treatment is the transplantation of skeletal muscle from other areas of the body, which can provide limited functional improvement (DiEdwardo et al., 1999). When VML occurs and permanent functional impairment results, many patients elect to have the injured limb amputated to avoid various complications that can occur with a functionless limb (Huh et al., 2011).

Another pathological abnormality with significant clinical implications is known as fatty degeneration of the rotator cuff muscles. Fatty degeneration is a common problem that orthopedic surgeons have been trying to understand and prevent since it was first reported (Goutallier et al., 1994; Fuchs et al., 1999). When a tendon is damaged or detached from its bony insertion, as in rotator cuff injuries, there is a subsequent increase in the presence of fat and atrophy of the corresponding muscle (Rowshan et al., 2010). Data suggest that up to 50% of asymptomatic individuals over the age of 50 have a rotator cuff tear (Tempelhof et al., 1999); infiltration of adipose tissue and atrophy also occurs in these asymptomatic individuals. When patients present clinically and the tendon is repaired, the infiltration of fat stops but is not reversed. This infiltration of fat is eventually accompanied by fibrosis, restricting movement of the shoulder joint and leading to re-tears, which are estimated to occur in as many as 70% of patients (Galatz et al., 2004).

14.5 CELL-BASED THERAPIES FOR SKELETAL MUSCLE REGENERATION

The syncytial nature of skeletal muscle—formed by myoblast fusion—lends itself to cell-based therapeutic interventions. Thus, transplanted stem cells can participate in muscle repair by fusing with host muscle cells, potentially supplying missing gene products to diseased muscle. Proof-of-principle studies in mouse models of DMD have documented the production of dystrophin-positive fibers comprised of both donor and host nuclei (Partridge et al., 1989). Many subsequent studies have demonstrated the efficacy of cell transplantation for repair of diseased and injured muscle, and the remaining sections of this chapter will highlight some of the successes, challenges, and critical parameters in skeletal muscle regenerative engineering.

When discussing possible cellular sources for skeletal muscle regenerative engineering, by far the most investigated and understood myogenic precursor is the SC—the canonical myogenic stem cell. Thus, the majority of this section will discuss the SC in the context of anatomical, molecular, and functional characteristics, all with the overarching goal of addressing its current potential in cellular therapeutics. However, in regard to practical clinical applications, direct SC therapies, as currently applied, have significant limitations. As such, the characteristics and potential therapeutic feasibility of other myogenic precursors resident in skeletal muscle tissue will also be addressed. Finally, this section will close with a discussion of prospective combined therapies, exploiting myogenic precursors with engineered materials to achieve the full potential of cell-based regenerative remedies.

14.5.1 Characteristics of Skeletal Muscle Satellite Cells

SC are derived from an embryonic pool of progenitors that express the paired box transcription factors, Pax3 and Pax7, and originate in an early dorsal structure of the somite, the dermomyotome. In the early muscle fields of the limb, these initial progenitors eventually downregulate Pax3 expression but remain Pax7+, as they inhabit their characteristic sublaminar anatomical location on nascent muscle fibers (Buckingham and Relaix, 2007). This intimate association with the muscle fiber, sharing the fiber's basal lamina but separated from the fibers, cytoplasm by its own cell membrane, is a defining feature of the SC niche and allows for unequivocal anatomical identification (Figure 14.3; Mauro, 1961). SCs remain mitotically quiescent until an activating stimulus, such as exercise or injury, disrupts the myofiber sarcolemma. Following this provocation, SCs proliferate and contribute myogenic cells to repair existing fibers and build new ones. Importantly, SCs can divide asymmetrically, contributing cells for myogenic differentiation and self-renewal, thereby replenishing the niche, a hallmark of a therapeutically effective stem cell (Charge and Rudnicki, 2004). The robust proliferative potential of SCs renders them capable of contributing enough cells to regenerate multiple fibers. An elegant study by Collins et al. (2005) showed that when single fibers with intact SCs (~7 SCs per extensor digitorum longus (EDL) muscle fiber) were transplanted into damaged muscle, the donor SCs could regenerate greater than 100 myofibers ($\geq 2.5 \times 10^4$ donor-derived nuclei) (Collins et al., 2005). Due to this pronounced proliferative and myogenic potential, SCs considered the preeminent myogenic precursors. In fact, recent studies in which SCs were selectively

Fiber associated Pax7 + satellite cell

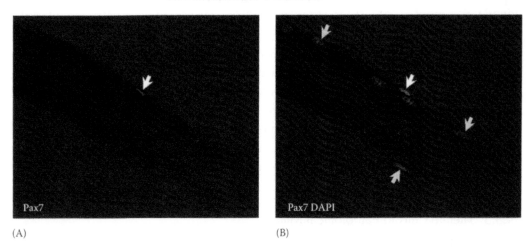

(A)   (B)

FIGURE 14.3   A single muscle fiber from the EDL muscle of the mouse hindlimb was immunostained for the satellite cell marker Pax7 (red; white arrows), and counterstained with DAPI to reveal the nuclei (blue; three shown with yellow arrows.) (Courtesy of M. D. Wienhold.)

ablated confirmed their essential role for effective muscle regeneration (Lepper et al., 2011; Murphy et al., 2011; Sambasivan et al., 2011). However, until recently, SCs were difficult to characterize or functionally test due to the inability to isolate these cells or target them with *in vivo* labeling techniques, as exclusive and specific markers were lacking.

SCs in their sublaminar niche express cell surface antigens CD34, Syndecan 3/4, and CD29, antigens often associated with stemness, as well as M-cadherin and CD56, bona fide markers of the myogenic program (Tedesco et al., 2010). While these markers label the majority of cells in the sublaminar niche, none are exclusive to SCs. Complicating SC identification and purification is the noted molecular and functional heterogeneity of cells residing in the sublaminar niche and the fluctuation in antigen expression upon removal from this location (Beauchamp et al., 2000). Typically, SCs are isolated by cell-sorting techniques using multiple cell surface markers (e.g., CD34 and α7 integrin) for positive identification, while simultaneously removing contaminating cell types such as endothelium (CD31+) and hematopoietic (CD45+) cells (Blanco-Bose et al., 2001; Sacco et al., 2008). As the ability to mark and isolate SCs becomes more effective, the opportunity to better understand their role in development, skeletal muscle–associated pathologies, and regeneration will be forthcoming.

14.5.2 Satellite Cell Self-Renewal

As mentioned earlier, a cell needs to meet two criteria to be considered a stem cell: the cell must be able to produce daughter cells capable of tissue-specific differentiation, and the cell must be able to self-renew, thereby sustaining its niche. While numerous studies over several decades have documented the robust proliferative and differentiative capacity of SCs (see earlier), the ability of SCs to self-renew has been a matter of considerable debate. Research over the past several years, however, has now clearly established the capacity of SCs to self-renew following transplantation (Collins et al., 2005; Sacco et al., 2008). Interestingly, molecular and functional heterogeneity among cells occupying the SC compartment suggests that only a fraction of these cells are true stem cells capable of self-renewal (Kuang et al., 2007), underscoring the importance of additional studies to molecularly define and purify the self-renewing subfraction for regenerative engineering applications. While the specific mechanisms underlying SC asymmetric self-renewal remain unknown, convincing evidence for the essential role of Notch signaling, a pathway commonly associated with asymmetrical stem cell division, has been reported (Conboy et al., 2002; Shinin et al., 2006; Kuang et al., 2007). Manipulation of Notch signaling and associated pathways may provide a means of producing "better" stem cells for regenerative engineering.

14.5.3 Satellite Cells in Pathological Milieus

SCs have typically been considered committed myogenic precursors due to their robust myogenic potential (Figure 14.4) and their presumed derivation from embryonic myoblasts (Armand et al., 1983; Bischoff, 1994; Kanisicak et al., 2009). In fact, over the past decade results from intensive investigations into SC potential have been consistent with its commitment to the myogenic program (Joe et al., 2010; Starkey et al., 2011). Recent evidence strongly suggests that the cellular origins of non-myogenic tissue in skeletal muscle–associated pathologies, such as that of muscular dystrophy and heterotopic ossification, are not from SCs, but instead from non-myogenic multipotent progenitor cells located in the interstitial space of muscle (Joe et al., 2010; Uezumi et al., 2010, 2011; Wosczyna et al., 2012).

Transplanted GFP + satellite cells contribute to nascent fibers
of regenerating muscle

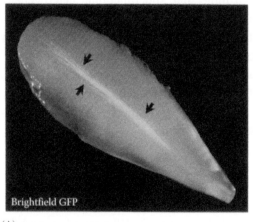 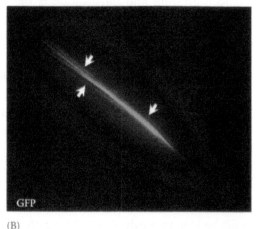

(A)   (B)

FIGURE 14.4   GFP+ murine satellite cells were isolated by fluorescence-activated cell sorting (FACS) and transplanted into an injured tibialis anterior (TA) muscle of the mouse hind leg. (A and B) Fourteen days following injury and 12 days after cell transplantation, GFP+ fibers (arrows) are observed in whole mount images of the TA.

However, SCs continue to receive attention as possible contributors to the fibrotic response associated with aging. In fact, SCs from older mice are more likely to become fibrogenic when compared to their younger counterparts (Conboy et al., 2005; Brack et al., 2007). Additionally, as the SC compartment ages with normal development, notable changes intrinsic to the muscle stem cell influence the cell's capacity to self-renew and contribute differentiated cells for maintenance and repair (Shay and Wright, 2005; Partridge, 2009). Therefore, it is reasonable to assume that SCs derived from younger donors are most desirable as a cell source for engineered skeletal muscle, as they would be better at sustaining tissue over time and less likely to stray from the myogenic program. However, the greater fibrogenic tendency of older regenerating muscle has also been attributed to an aged environment—specifically an increase in TGF-β serum levels and an increase in the activation of the Wnt signaling pathway (Brack et al., 2007; Carlson et al., 2008). Thus, using SCs from young donors may be ideal but not sufficient for effective regenerative therapies in older patients, as the recipient's systemic environment may dominate the inherent cues of a transplanted cell. In light of these cell autonomous and nonautonomous effects on the myogenic capacity and commitment of SCs future regenerative therapies must strive to mitigate donor and recipient influences on transplanted cells, thereby providing effective and lasting treatments.

14.5.4 Potential of Satellite Cell Therapies

As noted earlier, SCs have several important properties for regenerative engineering, including potent myogenic capacity (Figure 14.4), the ability to self-renew, robust proliferative capacity in culture and *in vivo*, and the availability of sufficient marker profiling data for purification by cell-sorting methodologies. Nevertheless, initial clinical trials showed minimal success (Law et al., 1990; Gussoni et al., 1992; Huard et al., 1992; Karpati et al., 1993), probably for multifactorial reasons that include the following. First, survival of transplanted SCs into diseased or injured tissue is usually very low. Immunological differences between donor and host contribute to poor survival; however, the recent development of induced pluripotent stem cell technologies (iPSC) (Takahashi and Yamanaka, 2006), in which immunologically identical, patient-derived stem cells can be produced, should eliminate this complicating factor and spare patients from lifelong immunosuppression therapy. Interestingly, in mouse models, cultured SCs show poor survival and engraftment following transplantation (Montarras et al., 2005) even when donor and host cells are genetically identical. This is due, in part, to the loss of "stemness" during SC expansion in culture, although the reasons for phenotypic changes of cultured SCs are not clear. Second, SC migration is limited, and engraftment is typically restricted to areas close to the transplantation site. Thus, poor survival and migratory properties would necessitate numerous injections of a single muscle to achieve therapeutic benefit (Peault et al., 2007; Price et al., 2007), although even multiple injections may be insufficient for effective engraftment for muscle masses encountered in clinical settings. As such, an essential goal will be the design of engineered scaffolds that provide an optimized environment for progenitor cell survival, migration, and functional integration. Interestingly, recent reports of *in vitro* culture systems that apparently help counteract the loss of stemness (Page et al., 2011; Gilbert et al., 2012) may provide an important compliment to advances in delivery methodologies. Additionally, noncanonical myogenic precursors (see below), which survive better when transplanted and can travel throughout the tissue or even hone to sites of injury when delivered systemically, may provide a viable alternative to SC therapeutics.

14.5.5 Noncanonical Myogenic Progenitors

The current limitations of SC therapeutics have fostered the search for noncanonical myogenic progenitors. We will discuss the most notable noncanonical myogenic progenitors as follows.

14.5.5.1 Mesoangioblasts and Pericytes

De Angelis et al. identified progenitors in the embryonic dorsal aorta, which upon transplantation exhibit multilineage mesodermal differentiation, including skeletal muscle differentiation (De Angelis et al., 1999; Minasi et al., 2002). These vascular-associated progenitors, termed mesoangioblasts (De Angelis et al., 1999), may have access to the circulatory system, suggesting the intriguing possibility that this progenitor population could be used for systemic delivery. In fact, transplantation of the mesoangioblast revealed the ability of these cells to travel through the circulation and engraft in skeletal muscle, distant from the site of injection—a characteristic not observed with skeletal muscle SCs (Minasi et al., 2002; Sampaolesi et al., 2003). Interestingly, cells with a similar functional capacity were identified in a perivascular location in adult skeletal muscle and express markers consistent with a pericyte phenotype. These cells, when delivered systemically, also can hone to damaged tissue and regenerate damaged muscle (Dellavalle et al., 2007). Recent large animal studies, in which mesoangioblasts/pericytes were delivered intravenously to dystrophic recipients, revealed the potential of these cells to mitigate skeletal muscle degeneration and improve overall mobility (Sampaolesi et al., 2006). Thus, the pericytes may have advantages over SCs for conditions where systemic delivery is likely to be advantageous, such as for muscular dystrophy and other diseases affecting muscles in many anatomical locations.

14.5.5.2 Additional Noncanonical Myogenic Precursors

In addition to mesoangioblasts and pericytes, there are other notable noncanonical progenitors, which warrant mentioning, namely, myoendothelial cells (Zheng et al., 2007), the muscle side population (mSP) (Jackson et al., 1999), and muscle-derived stem cells (MDSCs) (Lee et al., 2000; Qu-Petersen et al., 2002). All harbor great myogenic capacity *in vitro* and *in vivo*, although the ability to migrate through the circulatory system is unknown at this time. Like SCs, mSPs, and MDSCs are known to be heterogeneous in regard to marker profiles and functional capacity (Peng and Huard, 2004; Motohashi et al., 2008; Uezumi et al., 2011), and further investigation is needed to fully address the molecular and functional characteristics of these cells and their possible use in clinical applications.

As advances are made in cell-based therapies for skeletal regeneration, parallel advances are being made in materials science and scaffold-based tissue repair. As new viable cell populations for muscle regeneration are identified and their function better understood, new strategies for harboring, supporting, and guiding these cells both before and after implantation continue to emerge in the biomaterials realm. Muscle regenerative engineering will rely on the advances that can be made by artfully combining these two strategies. Following is a summary of some recent advances in biomaterial-based approaches to skeletal muscle regeneration.

14.6 MATERIALS-BASED THERAPIES FOR SKELETAL MUSCLE REGENERATIVE ENGINEERING

The paradigm of direct injection of cells into mouse models of muscle disease has been instrumental in identifying and validating sources of cells for possible clinical application. These studies, however, have highlighted the challenges and limitations of direct cellular injection, as noted in the earlier sections. The challenge of engineering more effective delivery systems has been undertaken by tissue engineers, who have made considerable progress in the design of artificial structures that may prove effective in facilitating muscle growth and regeneration. This section will highlight recent advances in skeletal muscle regenerative engineering.

In any complex biological system, scaffolds must mimic the native environment into which they will be implanted. Several parameters have been identified as important for tissue-engineered constructs, such as biodegradability, biocompatibility, and ability to facilitate cellular ingrowth. Scaffolds can act as delivery vehicles for implanting cells, providing a template for cell adhesion, that allows for controlled delivery to specific areas. Their surface can be modified with various cell-specific functional groups, such as integrins (Yu and Shoichet, 2005). Biodegradable scaffolds that the body eventually metabolizes have shown the most promise for regenerative engineering thus far. Once these scaffolds have been removed from the body, natural processes and host cells must create their own endogenous ECM for the strategy to be successful. Material composition can be varied so that when scaffolds degrade, little to no immune response is elicited from the body. For skeletal muscle there are additional parameters that need to be considered when designing scaffolds, including their ability to facilitate flexion and stretch, the two fundamental functions of skeletal muscle (Hidalgo-Bastida et al., 2007). Another parameter to consider with skeletal muscle tissue engineering is the highly organized structure within each muscle fiber. From myoblast fusion to the orientation of the sarcomere, directionality in skeletal muscle is highly conserved. One way to design skeletal muscle tissue-engineered scaffolds that confer directionality is through modified electrospinning techniques. Early work in this area demonstrated that aligned nanofibers can facilitate cellular adhesion and cytoskeletal protein spreading in an oriented fashion (Huang et al., 2006). Conductivity of the material is also a parameter that should be considered when designing a skeletal muscle scaffold (McKeon-Fischer and Freeman, 2011). When scaffolds containing engineered skeletal muscle become innervated, a material that conducts and propagates charge down its length could potentially synchronize skeletal muscle contractions at an early time point.

One of the seminal publications in this area demonstrated that myoblasts derived from neonatal rats could be seeded on polyglycolic acid (PGA) meshes, implanted in tissue within the abdomen wall, and cultured. The biodegradability of PGA allowed the scaffold to be hydrolyzed by the body while the myoblasts fused to form more mature myotubes. These results were confirmed by positive staining of their recovered cell–polymer scaffolds for α-sarcomeric actin and desmin at days 30 and 45 post-implantation (Saxena et al., 1999). There are many limitations to this approach, but the novelty of this research at the time led to the emergence of novel engineering approaches to design artificial skeletal muscle. Since these early studies, a wide variety of materials have been used in engineering skeletal muscle, with collagen and fibrin being two of the most common (Koning et al., 2009). These materials and some of the most promising scaffold synthesis methods are described next.

14.6.1 Electrospun Scaffolds

The technique of electrospinning utilizes a high voltage electrofield to create a scaffold with fibers ranging from 500 to 800 nm in diameter. Li et al. (2002) conducted pioneering work in electrospinning scaffolds for tissue engineering. It was demonstrated that the electrospinning technique yields scaffolds capable of supporting cellular proliferation, attachment, and growth, which was directly dependent on nanofiber orientation (Li et al., 2002). Since this initial publication, electrospun scaffolds for tissue-engineering purposes have been well studied (Pham et al., 2006). A major breakthrough was the realization that fiber orientation can be controlled by mechanically manipulating the electrospinning system. As mentioned earlier, one of the criteria for a suitable scaffold for skeletal muscle tissue engineering is its ability to facilitate cellular orientation. Using different approaches, researchers have developed methods to create oriented nanofibers that mimic skeletal muscle orientation (Wang et al., 2009). Parallel oriented electrospun scaffolds can provide the necessary ECM cues to guide cell growth and behavior (Figure 14.5).

Generated fibers are collected on a grounded plate. If the grounding plate is placed on a rotating mandrel, the collected fibers spanning the cylinder will be aligned in a parallel fashion. This technique has been utilized by Aviss et al. (2010) to spin highly oriented poly(lactic-*co*-glycolic acid) (PLGA) nanofibers. The choice of this polymer is ideal for application in skeletal muscle engineering because of its elastic nature. When using stiff polymers, myoblasts tend to spontaneously contract and detach from the fiber as they differentiate (Engler et al., 2004). PLGA at a ratio of 75:25 has been shown to enable myotube formation since its Young's modulus is great enough to support myotube forces (Levy-Mishali et al., 2009). The aligned fibers that Aviss and colleagues generated induced a phenomenon known as contact guidance, which can act as a template for alignment of myoblasts (Figure 14.6). Although these scaffolds are two-dimensional, further research has shown that cells on aligned scaffolds can be transferred into a 3D hydrogel and still maintain alignment (Lam et al., 2009).

The PLGA-aligned fibers also significantly increased mature skeletal muscle tissue differentiation markers, providing evidence that contact guidance is essential for proper myogenic differentiation. Another advantage of electrospinning is the ability to spin blended structures. Choi et al. (2008) showed that aligned electrospun poly(ε-caprolactone) (PCL) blended with type I collagen enhances biocompatibility of the scaffold and cellular adhesion

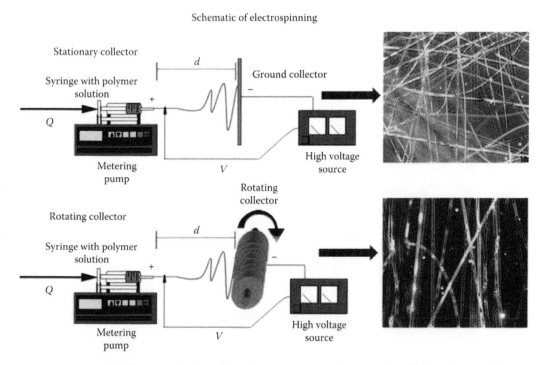

Schematic of electrospinning

FIGURE 14.5 Nanofiber morphology depends on the type of grounded collector used. A stationary collector (top) results in nanofibers that are randomly oriented. A rotating collector (bottom) results in nanofibers that are aligned with the direction of rotation. Nanofiber morphology depends also on the flow rate (Q) of the polymer from the syringe, the voltage (V) applied to the tip of the needle, and the distance (d) between the needle and the grounded collector.

of human skeletal muscle cells. In this study, it was demonstrated that oriented, nanofiber-blended meshes can facilitate growth and fusion of myotubes along their longitudinal axis (Choi et al., 2008). Other composite electrospun scaffolds have been created that incorporate metal nanoparticles, such as gold, into their structure. These scaffolds have unique conductive and electrical properties that may prove useful in regenerative engineering of skeletal muscle (McKeon-Fisher and Freeman, 2011).

14.6.2 Hydrogels

Approaches have been designed to incorporate growth factors such as FGF-2 into engineered scaffolds for muscle regeneration. One of these includes encapsulating myoblasts that overexpress FGF-2 into alginate microsphere hydrogels, a system that is useful for studying the effects of FGF-2 signaling *in vivo*. Using the alginate microspheres, one can direct the delivery of the encapsulated content to specific area. FGF-2-encapsulated microspheres were shown to increase the proliferation and decrease the rate of apoptosis in muscle cells (Stratos et al., 2011). As such, functionalizing scaffolds with FGF-2 and other growth factors may prove particularly important for effective treatment of VML and significant muscle loss associated with other conditions, where maximizing efficiency of engraftment will be critical.

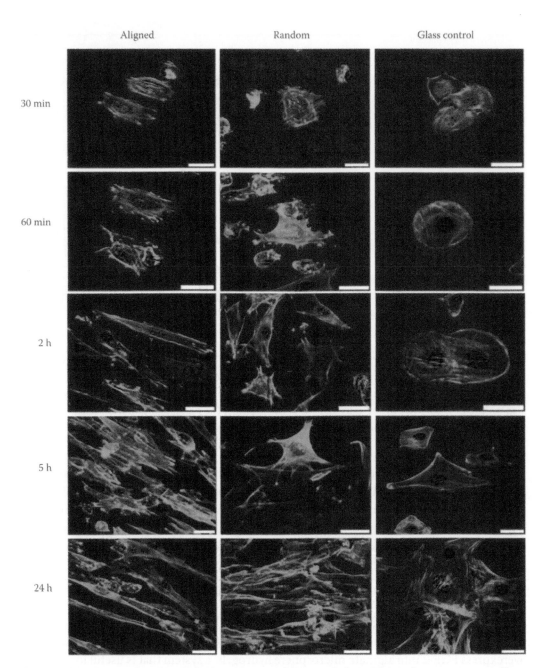

FIGURE 14.6 Image showing C2C12 murine myoblast seeded on PLGA electrospun nanofibers that were either mandrel aligned or randomly oriented. For comparison, the myoblasts are also shown growing on a glass control. At different time points, the degree of elongation of the myoblasts can be quantified, and after 24 h, there is a significant increase in elongation of the myoblasts on the aligned fibers versus the random and glass control. The actin cytoskeleton was revealed by immunofluorescence. (Reprinted from Aviss, K.J., *Eur. Cells Mater.*, 19, 2010. With permission.)

Hydrogels have several advantages for regenerative engineering applications. Depending on the material composition of the gel, its modulus can be modified to match that of the native tissue it is replacing. These gels are hydrophilic networks that absorb water throughout their structure allowing for the delivery of nutrients throughout the scaffold. Rossi et al. (2011) demonstrated functional and histological reconstruction of ablated skeletal muscle when SCs were embedded within photopolymerizable hydrogels. Over the initial 8 days of implantation *in vivo*, the hydrogels were confined to the implantation site and degraded completely. For this study, hyaluronic acid (HA) was used as the major component of the hydrogel. HA is known for its role in cell growth and differentiation and also influences many aspects of wound healing and inflammation (Leach et al., 2004). Of note, decreased fibrosis was observed, which likely facilitated revascularization and growth of nerve fibers into the regenerated area (Rossi et al., 2011). Although potentially useful for regenerative engineering, hydrogel cross-linking was accomplished using a photoinitiator compound that may have cytotoxic effects.

14.6.3 Decellularized Scaffolds

Decellularized scaffolds have been demonstrated to promote tissue formation in organs such as heart, skeletal muscle, urinary bladder, and small intestinal submucosa (Yoo and Meng, 1998; Conconi et al., 2005; De Coppi et al., 2006; Ott et al., 2008). These decellularized scaffolds provide several advantages for regenerative purposes. For example, they are often nonimmunogenic since the host cells have been removed. Further, these scaffolds may retain mechanical and chemical properties that closely resemble their tissue of origin. Gillies et al. (2011) recently published a novel method of decellularizing skeletal muscle without the use of detergents or proteolytic enzymes. Prior to this report, decellularizing skeletal muscle required harsh conditions that resulted in ECM degradation and compromised the mechanical and structural support that native ECM normally provides. The novel protocol utilized osmotic shock and actin and myosin depolymerization to decellularize skeletal muscle while preserving the mechanical integrity of the scaffold. Earlier work by Borschel et al. (2004) demonstrated that myoblasts reseeded on decellularized skeletal muscle undergo fusion, and resulting myofibers can assemble a force-generating contractile apparatus. Merritt et al. (2010) tested the ability of a decellularized muscle-derived ECM seeded with bone-marrow-derived mesenchymal stem cells (MSCs) to facilitate repair of traumatic skeletal muscle injury. They reported near-normal functional recovery of injuries that would not otherwise heal on their own. After 42 days, there were signs of blood vessel and myofiber regeneration within the structure. The MSCs may have directly contributed to regeneration or served as a suitable environment to facilitate the endogenous reparative response (Merritt et al., 2010). In a related approach, Machingal et al. (2011) used myoblasts seeded on an acellular porcine bladder matrix to functionally restore skeletal muscle after injury. Two months after these scaffolds were implanted, 72% of maximal tetanic force generation was observed as compared to 50% if the defect was left unrepaired or repaired with scaffold alone (Machingal et al., 2011).

14.6.4 Collagen-Based Scaffolds

Collagen is an ideal material for regenerative engineering because it forms a highly porous, spongelike lattice structure capable of supporting the growth and functionalization of many cell types, including myoblasts (Glowacki and Mizuno, 2008). The porosity of collagen sponges can be controlled and allows for ideal delivery of nutrients and growth factors through the entirety of the structure. It has also been demonstrated that the orientation of the pores can be controlled using a technique known as "unidirectional freezing" (Kroehne et al., 2008). This process resulted in a parallel arrangement of myotubes within the collagen sponge when implanted into recipient mice that were engineered to express GFP. When analyzed after surgery, the host muscle cells had incorporated into the implanted sponge structure and were capable of producing contractile forces. This technique holds significant promise for clinical situations where host myoblasts are genetically normal, such as tumor excision or trauma. However, the use in hereditary diseases such as DMD would be limited, as effective cell-based treatment will likely require that the regenerative response is dominated by wild-type, transplanted cells.

Another technique utilizing collagen's unique properties as a scaffold is collagen fiber painting. In this technique, type I collagen fibers are allowed to polymerize on culture dishes after a collagen-containing substrate is painted across the surface in an oriented fashion. Yan et al. (2007) seeded SCs on a thin layer of parallel-aligned fibers and allowed the cells to adhere for a week. In order to recreate the 3D architecture of muscle, the researchers increased the thickness of their construct by applying a thin layer of collagen to the top of their painted fibers. This resulted in a construct with many layers of skeletal myocytes, which display physiological force length behavior similar to native tissue (Yan et al., 2007). Collagen also has the ability to be functionalized with different substituents, such as FGF-2. Yun et al. (2012) found that FGF-2 stimulates C2C12 adhesion, enhances myoblast migratory ability, and enhances wound healing activity after injury. This functionalization may prove to be critical in regulating the initial phases of muscle injury and regeneration.

14.6.5 Fibrin-Based Scaffolds

Fibrin-based systems, including fibrin hydrogels, arrays, and microthreads, have also been used in skeletal muscle engineering applications. Fibrin gels have several advantages when used for muscle tissue engineering. Within 3–4 weeks of implantation, muscle progenitor cells produce their own ECM, replacing the fibrin gel scaffold (Ross and Tranquillo, 2003). This native ECM allows the myoblasts to freely migrate and proliferate within the gel, which aids in cell survival and regeneration. Fibrin also has the ability to bind to the growth factors mentioned earlier in this chapter, which can aid in the regenerative process. Huang et al. (2005) used a fibrin gel system to produce 3D skeletal muscle constructs that produced measurable forces up to 805 μN. This system also allows for the delivery of the growth factor IGF-1, which increased the force generated in their fibrin gel construct by nearly 50% (Huang et al., 2005).

In order to facilitate alignment of a fibrin scaffold, *in vitro* manipulation can be performed to form a microthreaded structure. This technique generates fibrin threads averaging 100 μm in diameter that have been shown to facilitate directional growth down the length of the threads (Proulx et al., 2011). Page et al. (2011) showed that fibrin threads can be altered chemically to provide enough stability to be anchored into a muscle defect site with fibrin glue. Host cell ingrowth and biocompatibility were found at the wound margin, where the scaffold interfaced with native tissue. Fibrin microthreads decreased the amount of collagen deposition at this margin and facilitated endogenous muscle cell ingrowth. Moreover, the cell-loaded fibrin microthread scaffolds appeared to restore 100% of muscle function compared to 50% with the non-implanted controls at 90 days, as demonstrated by maximum tetanic force measurements (Page et al., 2011). Significant potential exists for clinical translation with these scaffolds although rapid *in vivo* degradation may limit their application.

14.7 FUTURE OF SKELETAL MUSCLE REGENERATIVE ENGINEERING

Given recent progress in stem cell and biomaterials research, successful treatment of localized muscle injuries such as VML and fatty degeneration of the shoulder using a combination of progenitor cells and functionalized biomaterials can now be envisioned. Treatment of pathologies that affect larger muscle areas, such as the muscular dystrophies, will require development of new regenerative engineering approaches that may include systemic delivery of progenitor cells and the use of functionalized biomaterials that optimize cell survival and honing to peripheral muscle targets. Biomaterial-mediated delivery of noncellular, genetic reagents (such as inhibitory RNAs to modify the cellular splicing machinery and remove the mutant portion of dystrophin, creating a functional protein) may also be feasible in the future. Still further in the future is the ultimate goal of regenerating complex biological structures, such as the limb. While salamanders exhibit a remarkable capacity to regenerate limbs and other complex structures, this capacity has been lost or rendered dormant in humans. Better understanding of natural regenerative processes in lower vertebrates, together with development of engineered materials that provide precise spatiotemporal control of cellular interactions and cell differentiation, is the first step toward this ambitious goal.

REFERENCES

Allen, R. E. and L. L. Rankin. Regulation of satellite cells during skeletal muscle growth and development. *Proc Soc Exp Biol Med* 194(2) (1990): 81–86.

Aristeguieta, L. M. R. Tensor veli palatine and tensor tympani muscles: Anatomical, functional and symptomatic links. *Acta Otorrinolaringol Esp* (61) (2010): 26–33.

Armand, O., A. M. Boutineau, A. Mauger, M. P. Pautou, and M. Kieny. Origin of satellite cells in avian skeletal muscles. *Arch Anat Microsc Morphol Exp* 72(2) (1983): 163–181.

Armstrong, R. B., G. L. Warren, and J. A. Warren. Mechanisms of exercise-induced muscle fibre injury. *Sports Med* 12(3) (1991): 184–207.

Aviss, K. J., J. E. Gough, and S. Downes. Aligned electrospun polymer fibres for skeletal muscle regeneration. *Eur Cell Mater* 19 (2010): 193–204.

Bamman, M. M., J. R. Shipp, J. Jiang, B. A. Gower, G. R. Hunter, A. Goodman, C. L. McLafferty, Jr., and R. J. Urban. Mechanical load increases muscle Igf-I and androgen receptor mRNA concentrations in humans. *Am J Physiol Endocrinol Metab* 280(3) (2001): E383–E390.

Barrett, K. E., S. Boitano, S. M. Barman, and H. L. Brooks. *Ganong's Review of Medical Physiology*, 23rd edn. McGraw Hill Medical, New York, 2010, pp. 93–94.

Beauchamp, J. R., L. Heslop, D. S. Yu, S. Tajbakhsh, R. G. Kelly, A. Wernig, M. E. Buckingham, T. A. Partridge, and P. S. Zammit. Expression of Cd34 and Myf5 defines the majority of quiescent adult skeletal muscle satellite cells. *J Cell Biol* 151(6) (2000): 1221–1234.

Bischoff, R. The satellite cell and muscle regeneration. *Myology*, 1st edn. (1994): 97–118.

Blanco-Bose, W. E., C. C. Yao, R. H. Kramer, and H. M. Blau. Purification of mouse primary myoblasts based on alpha 7 integrin expression. *Exp Cell Res* 265(2) (2001): 212–220.

Borg, T. K. and J. B. Caulfield. Morphology of connective tissue in skeletal muscle. *Tissue Cell* 12(1) (1980): 197–207.

Borschel, G. H., R. G. Dennis, and W. M. Kuzon, Jr. Contractile skeletal muscle tissue-engineered on an acellular scaffold. *Plast Reconstr Surg* 113(2) (2004): 595–602; discussion 603–604.

Brack, A. S., M. J. Conboy, S. Roy, M. Lee, C. J. Kuo, C. Keller, and T. A. Rando. Increased Wnt signaling during aging alters muscle stem cell fate and increases fibrosis. *Science* 317(5839) (2007): 807–810.

Buckingham, M. and F. Relaix. The role of *Pax* genes in the development of tissues and organs: Pax3 and Pax7 regulate muscle progenitor cell functions. *Annu Rev Cell Dev Biol* 23(2007): 645–673.

Carlson, C. J., F. W. Booth, and S. E. Gordon. Skeletal muscle myostatin mRNA expression is fiber-type specific and increases during hindlimb unloading. *Am J Physiol* 277(2 Pt 2) (1999): R601–R606.

Carlson, M. E., M. Hsu, and I. M. Conboy. Imbalance between Psmad3 and Notch induces Cdk inhibitors in old muscle stem cells. *Nature* 454(7203) (2008): 528–532.

Chakravarthy, M. V., T. W. Abraha, R. J. Schwartz, M. L. Fiorotto, and F. W. Booth. Insulin-like growth factor-I extends *in vitro* replicative life span of skeletal muscle satellite cells by enhancing G1/S cell cycle progression via the activation of phosphatidylinositol 3′-kinase/Akt signaling pathway. *J Biol Chem* 275(46) (2000): 35942–35952.

Charge, S. B. and M. A. Rudnicki. Cellular and molecular regulation of muscle regeneration. *Physiol Rev* 84(1) (2004): 209–238.

Choi, J. S., S. J. Lee, G. J. Christ, A. Atala, and J. J. Yoo. The influence of electrospun aligned poly(epsilon-caprolactone)/collagen nanofiber meshes on the formation of self-aligned skeletal muscle myotubes. *Biomaterials* 29(19) (2008): 2899–2906.

Collins, C. A., I. Olsen, P. S. Zammit, L. Heslop, A. Petrie, T. A. Partridge, and J. E. Morgan. Stem cell function, self-renewal, and behavioral heterogeneity of cells from the adult muscle satellite cell niche. *Cell* 122(2) (2005): 289–301.

Conboy, I. M. and T. A. Rando. The regulation of notch signaling controls satellite cell activation and cell fate determination in postnatal myogenesis. *Dev Cell* 3(3) (2002): 397–409.

Conboy, I. M., M. J. Conboy, A. J. Wagers, E. R. Girma, I. L. Weissman, and T. A. Rando. Rejuvenation of aged progenitor cells by exposure to a young systemic environment. *Nature* 433(7027) (2005): 760–764.

Conconi, M. T., P. De Coppi, S. Bellini, G. Zara, M. Sabatti, M. Marzaro, G. F. Zanon, P. G. Gamba, P. P. Parnigotto, and G. G. Nussdorfer. Homologous muscle acellular matrix seeded with autologous myoblasts as a tissue-engineering approach to abdominal wall-defect repair. *Biomaterials* 26(15) (2005): 2567–2574.

De Angelis, L., L. Berghella, M. Coletta, L. Lattanzi, M. Zanchi, M. G. Cusella-De Angelis, C. Ponzetto, and G. Cossu. Skeletal myogenic progenitors originating from embryonic dorsal aorta coexpress endothelial and myogenic markers and contribute to postnatal muscle growth and regeneration. *J Cell Biol* 147(4) (1999): 869–878.

De Coppi, P., S. Bellini, M. T. Conconi, M. Sabatti, E. Simonato, P. G. Gamba, G. G. Nussdorfer, and P. P. Parnigotto. Myoblast–acellular skeletal muscle matrix constructs guarantee a long-term repair of experimental full-thickness abdominal wall defects. *Tissue Eng* 12(7) (2006): 1929–1936.

Delbono, O. Calcium homeostasis and skeletal muscle alterations in aging. *Adv Cell Aging Gerontol* (10) (2002): 167–173.

Dellavalle, A., M. Sampaolesi, R. Tonlorenzi, E. Tagliafico, B. Sacchetti, L. Perani, A. Innocenzi et al. Pericytes of human skeletal muscle are myogenic precursors distinct from satellite cells. *Nat Cell Biol* 9(3) (2007): 255–267.

DiEdwardo, C. A., P. Petrosko, T. O. Acarturk, P. A. DiMilla, W. A. LaFramboise, and P. C. Johnson. Muscle tissue engineering. *Clin Plast Surg* 26(4) (1999): 647–656, ix–x.

Engert, J. C., E. B. Berglund, and N. Rosenthal. Proliferation precedes differentiation in Igf-I-stimulated myogenesis. *J Cell Biol* 135(2) (1996): 431–440.

Engler, A. J., M. A. Griffin, S. Sen, C. G. Bonnemann, H. L. Sweeney, and D. E. Discher. Myotubes differentiate optimally on substrates with tissue-like stiffness: Pathological implications for soft or stiff microenvironments. *J Cell Biol* 166(6) (2004): 877–887.

Ezerman, E. B. and H. Ishikawa. Differentiation of the sarcoplasmic reticulum and T system in developing chick skeletal muscle *in vitro*. *J Cell Biol* 35(2) (1967): 405–420.

Fabbrizio, E., A. Bonet-Kerrache, F. Limas, G. Hugon, and D. Mornet. Dystrophin, the protein that promotes membrane resistance. *Biochem Biophys Res Commun* 213(1) (1995): 295–301.

Fuchs, B., D. Weishaupt, M. Zanetti, J. Hodler, and C. Gerber. Fatty degeneration of the muscles of the rotator cuff: Assessment by computed tomography versus magnetic resonance imaging. *J Shoulder Elbow Surg* 8(6) (1999): 599–605.

Funauchi, M., H. Shimadsu, C. Tamaki, T. Yamagata, Y. Nozaki, M. Sugiyama, S. Ikoma, and K. Kinoshita. Role of endothelial damage in the pathogenesis of interstitial pneumonitis in patients with polymyositis and dermatomyositis. *J Rheumatol* 33(5) (2006): 903–906.

Galatz, L. M., C. M. Ball, S. A. Teefey, W. D. Middleton, and K. Yamaguchi. The outcome and repair integrity of completely arthroscopically repaired large and massive rotator cuff tears. *J Bone Joint Surg Am* 86-A(2) (2004): 219–224.

Gilbert, P. M., S. Corbel, R. Doyonnas, K. Havenstrite, K. E. Magnusson, and H. M. Blau. A single cell bioengineering approach to elucidate mechanisms of adult stem cell self-renewal. *Integr Biol (Camb)* 4(4) (2012): 360–367.

Gillies, A. R., L. R. Smith, R. L. Lieber, and S. Varghese. Method for decellularizing skeletal muscle without detergents or proteolytic enzymes. *Tissue Eng Part C Methods* 17(4) (2011): 383–389.

Glowacki, J. and S. Mizuno. Collagen scaffolds for tissue engineering. *Biopolymers* 89(5) (2008): 338–344.

Goutallier, D., J. M. Postel, J. Bernageau, L. Lavau, and M. C. Voisin. Fatty muscle degeneration in cuff ruptures. Pre- and postoperative evaluation by CT scan. *Clin Orthop Relat Res* (304) (1994): 78–83.

Grogan, B. F. and J. R. Hsu. Volumetric muscle loss. *J Am Acad Orthop Surg* 19(Suppl 1) (2011): S35–S37.

Gussoni, E., G. K. Pavlath, A. M. Lanctot, K. R. Sharma, R. G. Miller, L. Steinman, and H. M. Blau. Normal dystrophin transcripts detected in Duchenne muscular dystrophy patients after myoblast transplantation. *Nature* 356(6368) (1992): 435–438.

Harris, A. J., M. J. Duxson, J. E. Butler, P. W. Hodges, J. L. Taylor, and S. C. Gandevia. Muscle fiber and motor unit behavior in the longest human skeletal muscle. *J Neurosci* 25(37) (2005): 8528–8533.

Haslett, J. N., D. Sanoudou, A. T. Kho, R. R. Bennett, S. A. Greenberg, I. S. Kohane, A. H. Beggs, and L. M. Kunkel. Gene expression comparison of biopsies from Duchenne muscular dystrophy (Dmd) and normal skeletal muscle. *Proc Natl Acad Sci U S A* 99(23) (2002): 15000–15005.

Hawke, T. J. and D. J. Garry. Myogenic satellite cells: Physiology to molecular biology. *J Appl Physiol* 91(2) (2001): 534–551.

Hidalgo-Bastida, L. A., J. J. Barry, N. M. Everitt, F. R. Rose, L. D. Buttery, I. P. Hall, W. C. Claycomb, and K. M. Shakesheff. Cell adhesion and mechanical properties of a flexible scaffold for cardiac tissue engineering. *Acta Biomater* 3(4) (2007): 457–462.

Huang, Y. C., R. G. Dennis, L. Larkin, and K. Baar. Rapid formation of functional muscle *in vitro* using fibrin gels. *J Appl Physiol* 98(2) (2005): 706–713.

Huang, N. F., S. Patel, R. G. Thakar, J. Wu, B. S. Hsiao, B. Chu, R. J. Lee, and S. Li. Myotube assembly on nanofibrous and micropatterned polymers. *Nano Lett* 6(3) (2006): 537–542.

Huard, J., R. Roy, J. P. Bouchard, F. Malouin, C. L. Richards, and J. P. Tremblay. Human myoblast transplantation between immunohistocompatible donors and recipients produces immune reactions. *Transplant Proc* 24(6) (1992): 3049–3051.

Huh, J., D. J. Stinner, T. C. Burns, and J. R. Hsu. Infectious complications and soft tissue injury contribute to late amputation after severe lower extremity trauma. *J Trauma* 71(1 Suppl) (2011): S47–S51.

Huxley, H. E. Electron microscope studies of the organization of the filaments in striated muscle. *Biochim Biophys Acta* (12) (1953): 357.

Ishitobi, M., K. Haginoya, Y. Zhao, A. Ohnuma, J. Minato, T. Yanagisawa, M. Tanabu, M. Kikuchi, and K. Iinuma. Elevated plasma levels of transforming growth factor beta1 in patients with muscular dystrophy. *Neuroreport* 11(18) (2000): 4033–4035.

Jackson, K. A., T. Mi, and M. A. Goodell. Hematopoietic potential of stem cells isolated from murine skeletal muscle. *Proc Natl Acad Sci U S A* 96(25) (1999): 14482–14486.

Joe, A. W., L. Yi, A. Natarajan, F. Le Grand, L. So, J. Wang, M. A. Rudnicki, and F. M. Rossi. Muscle injury activates resident fibro/adipogenic progenitors that facilitate myogenesis. *Nat Cell Biol* 12(2) (2010): 153–163.

Jovanovic, D. V., J. A. Di Battista, J. Martel-Pelletier, F. C. Jolicoeur, Y. He, M. Zhang, F. Mineau, and J. P. Pelletier. IL-17 stimulates the production and expression of proinflammatory cytokines, IL-beta and TNF-alpha, by human macrophages. *J Immunol* 160(7) (1998): 3513–3521.

Kaariainen, M., T. Jarvinen, M. Jarvinen, J. Rantanen, and H. Kalimo. Relation between myofibers and connective tissue during muscle injury repair. *Scand J Med Sci Sports* 10(6) (2000): 332–337.

Kanisicak, O., J. J. Mendez, S. Yamamoto, M. Yamamoto, and D. J. Goldhamer. Progenitors of skeletal muscle satellite cells express the muscle determination gene, Myod. *Dev Biol* 332(1) (2009): 131–141.

Karpati, G., S. Carpenter, G. E. Morris, K. E. Davies, C. Guerin, and P. Holland. Localization and quantitation of the chromosome 6-encoded dystrophin-related protein in normal and pathological human muscle. *J Neuropathol Exp Neurol* 52(2) (1993): 119–128.

Keynes, R. D., D. J. Aidley, C. L. Huang. *Nerve and Muscle*, 4th edn. Cambridge University Press, New York, 2011, pp. 101–102.

Koenig, M., A. H. Beggs, M. Moyer, S. Scherpf, K. Heindrich, T. Bettecken, G. Meng et al. The molecular basis for Duchenne versus Becker muscular dystrophy: Correlation of severity with type of deletion. *Am J Hum Genet* 45(4) (1989): 498–506.

Koning, M., M. C. Harmsen, M. J. van Luyn, and P. M. Werker. Current opportunities and challenges in skeletal muscle tissue engineering. *J Tissue Eng Regen Med* 3(6) (2009): 407–415.

Kristian, T. and B. K. Siesjo. Calcium in ischemic cell death. *Stroke* 29(3) (1998): 705–718.

Kroehne, V., I. Heschel, F. Schugner, D. Lasrich, J. W. Bartsch, and H. Jockusch. Use of a Novel collagen matrix with oriented pore structure for muscle cell differentiation in cell culture and in grafts. *J Cell Mol Med* 12(5A) (2008): 1640–1648.

Kuang, S., K. Kuroda, F. Le Grand, and M. A. Rudnicki. Asymmetric self-renewal and commitment of satellite stem cells in muscle. *Cell* 129(5) (2007): 999–1010.

Kumar V., K. Abbas, D. Fausto, and J. C. Aster. *Robbins and Cotran: Pathological Basis of Disease*, 8th edn., Saunders Elsevier, Philadelphia, PA, 2010, pp. 2079–2080.

Lam, M. T., Y. C. Huang, R. K. Birla, and S. Takayama. Microfeature guided skeletal muscle tissue engineering for highly organized 3-dimensional free-standing constructs. *Biomaterials* 30(6) (2009): 1150–1155.

Law, P. K., T. E. Bertorini, T. G. Goodwin, M. Chen, Q. W. Fang, H. J. Li, D. S. Kirby, J. A. Florendo, H. G. Herrod, and G. S. Golden. Dystrophin production induced by myoblast transfer therapy in Duchenne muscular dystrophy. *Lancet* 336(8707) (1990): 114–115.

Leach, J. B., K. A. Bivens, C. N. Collins, and C. E. Schmidt. Development of photocrosslinkable hyaluronic acid–polyethylene glycol–peptide composite hydrogels for soft tissue engineering. *J Biomed Mater Res A* 70(1) (2004): 74–82.

Lee, J. Y., Z. Qu-Petersen, B. Cao, S. Kimura, R. Jankowski, J. Cummins, A. Usas et al. Clonal isolation of muscle-derived cells capable of enhancing muscle regeneration and bone healing. *J Cell Biol* 150(5) (2000): 1085–1100.

Lepper, C., T. A. Partridge, and C. M. Fan. An absolute requirement for Pax7-positive satellite cells in acute injury-induced skeletal muscle regeneration. *Development* 138(17) (2011): 3639–3646.

Levy-Mishali, M., J. Zoldan, and S. Levenberg. Effect of scaffold stiffness on myoblast differentiation. *Tissue Eng Part A* 15(4) (2009): 935–944.

Li, W. J., C. T. Laurencin, E. J. Caterson, R. S. Tuan, and F. K. Ko. Electrospun nanofibrous structure: A novel scaffold for tissue engineering. *J Biomed Mater Res* 60(4) (2002): 613–621.

Machingal, M. A., B. T. Corona, T. J. Walters, V. Kesireddy, C. N. Koval, A. Dannahower, W. Zhao, J. J. Yoo, and G. J. Christ. A tissue-engineered muscle repair construct for functional restoration of an irrecoverable muscle injury in a murine model. *Tissue Eng Part A* 17(17–18) (2011): 2291–2303.

Mauro, A. Satellite cell of skeletal muscle fibers. *J Biophys Biochem Cytol* 9 (1961): 493–495.

Mauro, A. and W. R. Adams. The structure of the sarcolemma of the frog skeletal muscle fiber. *J Biophys Biochem Cytol* 10(4 Suppl) (1961): 177–185.

McKeon-Fischer, K. D. and J. W. Freeman. Characterization of electrospun poly(L-lactide) and gold nanoparticle composite scaffolds for skeletal muscle tissue engineering. *J Tissue Eng Regen Med* 5(7) (2011): 560–568.

Merritt, E. K., M. V. Cannon, D. W. Hammers, L. N. Le, R. Gokhale, A. Sarathy, T. J. Song et al. Repair of traumatic skeletal muscle injury with bone-marrow-derived mesenchymal stem cells seeded on extracellular matrix. *Tissue Eng Part A* 16(9) (2010): 2871–2881.

Minasi, M. G., M. Riminucci, L. De Angelis, U. Borello, B. Berarducci, A. Innocenzi, A. Caprioli et al. The meso-angioblast: A multipotent, self-renewing cell that originates from the dorsal aorta and differentiates into most mesodermal tissues. *Development* 129(11) (2002): 2773–2783.

Montarras, D., J. Morgan, C. Collins, F. Relaix, S. Zaffran, A. Cumano, T. Partridge, and M. Buckingham. Direct isolation of satellite cells for skeletal muscle regeneration. *Science* 309(5743) (2005): 2064–2067.

Motohashi, N., A. Uezumi, E. Yada, S. Fukada, K. Fukushima, K. Imaizumi, Y. Miyagoe-Suzuki, and S. Takeda. Muscle Cd31(−) Cd45(−) side population cells promote muscle regeneration by stimulating proliferation and migration of myoblasts. *Am J Pathol* 173(3) (2008): 781–791.

Mourkioti, F. and N. Rosenthal. Igf-1, inflammation and stem cells: Interactions during muscle regeneration. *Trends Immunol* 26(10) (2005): 535–542.

Murphy, M. M., J. A. Lawson, S. J. Mathew, D. A. Hutcheson, and G. Kardon. Satellite cells, connective tissue fibroblasts and their interactions are crucial for muscle regeneration. *Development* 138(17) (2011): 3625–3637.

Orrenius, S., B. Zhivotovsky, and P. Nicotera. Regulation of cell death: The calcium-apoptosis link. *Nat Rev Mol Cell Biol* 4(7) (2003): 552–565.

Ott, H. C., T. S. Matthiesen, S. K. Goh, L. D. Black, S. M. Kren, T. I. Netoff, and D. A. Taylor. Perfusion-decellularized matrix: Using nature's platform to engineer a bioartificial heart. *Nat Med* 14(2) (2008): 213–221.

Page, R. L., C. Malcuit, L. Vilner, I. Vojtic, S. Shaw, E. Hedblom, J. Hu, G. D. Pins, M. W. Rolle, and T. Dominko. Restoration of skeletal muscle defects with adult human cells delivered on fibrin microthreads. *Tissue Eng Part A* 17(21–22) (2011): 2629–2640.

Partridge, T. Developmental biology: Skeletal muscle comes of age. *Nature* 460(7255) (2009): 584–585.

Partridge, T. A., J. E. Morgan, G. R. Coulton, E. P. Hoffman, and L. M. Kunkel. Conversion of Mdx myofibres from dystrophin-negative to -positive by injection of normal myoblasts. *Nature* 337(6203) (1989): 176–179.

Peault, B., M. Rudnicki, Y. Torrente, G. Cossu, J. P. Tremblay, T. Partridge, E. Gussoni, L. M. Kunkel, and J. Huard. Stem and progenitor cells in skeletal muscle development, maintenance, and therapy. *Mol Ther* 15(5) (2007): 867–877.

Peng, H. and J. Huard. Muscle-derived stem cells for musculoskeletal tissue regeneration and repair. *Transpl Immunol* 12(3–4) (2004): 311–319.

Pham, Q. P., U. Sharma, and A. G. Mikos. Electrospinning of polymeric nanofibers for tissue engineering applications: A review. *Tissue Eng* 12(5) (2006): 1197–1211.

Price, F. D., K. Kuroda, and M. A. Rudnicki. Stem cell based therapies to treat muscular dystrophy. *Biochim Biophys Acta* 1772(2) (2007): 272–283.

Proulx, M. K., S. P. Carey, L. M. Ditroia, C. M. Jones, M. Fakharzadeh, J. P. Guyette, A. L. Clement et al. Fibrin microthreads support mesenchymal stem cell growth while maintaining differentiation potential. *J Biomed Mater Res A* 96(2) (2011): 301–312.

Qu-Petersen, Z., B. Deasy, R. Jankowski, M. Ikezawa, J. Cummins, R. Pruchnic, J. Mytinger et al. Identification of a novel population of muscle stem cells in mice: Potential for muscle regeneration. *J Cell Biol* 157(5) (2002): 851–864.

Ross, M. H. and W. Pawlina. *Histology a Text and Atlas*, 5th edn.. Lippincott Williams & Wilkins, Baltimore, MD, 2006, pp. 281–282.

Ross, J. J. and R. T. Tranquillo. *Ecm* gene expression correlates with *in vitro* tissue growth and development in fibrin gel remodeled by neonatal smooth muscle cells. *Matrix Biol* 22(6) (2003): 477–490.

Rossi, C. A., M. Flaibani, B. Blaauw, M. Pozzobon, E. Figallo, C. Reggiani, L. Vitiello, N. Elvassore, and P. De Coppi. *In vivo* tissue engineering of functional skeletal muscle by freshly isolated satellite cells embedded in a photopolymerizable hydrogel. *FASEB J* 25(7) (2011): 2296–2304.

Rowshan, K., S. Hadley, K. Pham, V. Caiozzo, T. Q. Lee, and R. Gupta. Development of fatty atrophy after neurologic and rotator cuff injuries in an animal model of rotator cuff pathology. *J Bone Joint Surg Am* 92(13) (2010): 2270–2278.

Sacco, A., R. Doyonnas, P. Kraft, S. Vitorovic, and H. M. Blau. Self-renewal and expansion of single transplanted muscle stem cells. *Nature* 456(7221) (2008): 502–506.

Sambasivan, R., R. Yao, A. Kissenpfennig, L. Van Wittenberghe, A. Paldi, B. Gayraud-Morel, H. Guenou, B. Malissen, S. Tajbakhsh, and A. Galy. Pax7-expressing satellite cells are indispensable for adult skeletal muscle regeneration. *Development* 138(17) (2011): 3647–3656.

Sampaolesi, M., S. Blot, G. D'Antona, N. Granger, R. Tonlorenzi, A. Innocenzi, P. Mognol et al. Mesoangioblast stem cells ameliorate muscle function in dystrophic dogs. *Nature* 444(7119) (2006): 574–579.

Sampaolesi, M., Y. Torrente, A. Innocenzi, R. Tonlorenzi, G. D'Antona, M. A. Pellegrino, R. Barresi et al. Cell therapy of alpha-sarcoglycan null dystrophic mice through intra-arterial delivery of mesoangioblasts. *Science* 301(5632) (2003): 487–492.

Sato, K., Y. Li, W. Foster, K. Fukushima, N. Badlani, N. Adachi, A. Usas, F. H. Fu, and J. Huard. Improvement of muscle healing through enhancement of muscle regeneration and prevention of fibrosis. *Muscle Nerve* 28(3) (2003): 365–372.

Saxena, A. K., J. Marler, M. Benvenuto, G. H. Willital, and J. P. Vacanti. Skeletal muscle tissue engineering using isolated myoblasts on synthetic biodegradable polymers: Preliminary studies. *Tissue Eng* 5(6) (1999): 525–532.

Shay, J. W. and W. E. Wright. Use of telomerase to create bioengineered tissues. *Ann N Y Acad Sci* 1057 (2005): 479–491.

Shen, W., Y. Li, J. Zhu, R. Schwendener, and J. Huard. Interaction between macrophages, Tgf-beta1, and the Cox-2 pathway during the inflammatory phase of skeletal muscle healing after injury. *J Cell Physiol* 214(2) (2008): 405–412.

Shinin, V., B. Gayraud-Morel, D. Gomes, and S. Tajbakhsh. Asymmetric division and cosegregation of template DNA strands in adult muscle satellite cells. *Nat Cell Biol* 8(7) (2006): 677–687.

Starkey, J. D., M. Yamamoto, S. Yamamoto, and D. J. Goldhamer. Skeletal muscle satellite cells are committed to myogenesis and do not spontaneously adopt nonmyogenic fates. *J Histochem Cytochem* 59(1) (2011): 33–46.

Stratos, I., H. Madry, R. Rotter, A. Weimer, J. Graff, M. Cucchiarini, T. Mittlmeier, and B. Vollmar. Fibroblast growth factor-2-overexpressing myoblasts encapsulated in alginate spheres increase proliferation, reduce apoptosis, induce adipogenesis, and enhance regeneration following skeletal muscle injury in rats. *Tissue Eng Part A* 17(21–22) (2011): 2867–2877.

Takahashi, K. and S. Yamanaka. Induction of pluripotent stem cells from mouse embryonic and adult fibroblast cultures by defined factors. *Cell* 126(4) (2006): 663–676.

Taylor, R. G. and M. Koohmaraie. Effects of postmortem storage on the ultrastructure of the endomysium and myofibrils in normal and callipyge longissimus. *J Anim Sci* 76(11) (1998): 2811–2817.

Tedesco, F. S., A. Dellavalle, J. Diaz-Manera, G. Messina, and G. Cossu. Repairing skeletal muscle: Regenerative potential of skeletal muscle stem cells. *J Clin Invest* 120(1) (2010): 11–19.

Tempelhof, S., S. Rupp, and R. Seil. Age-related prevalence of rotator cuff tears in asymptomatic shoulders. *J Shoulder Elbow Surg* (84) (1999): 296–299.

Tidball, J. G. Inflammatory processes in muscle injury and repair. *Am J Physiol Regul Integr Comp Physiol* 288(2) (2005): R345–R353.

Turner, N. J. and S. F. Badylak. Regeneration of skeletal muscle. *Cell Tissue Res* 347(3) (2012): 759–774.

Uezumi, A., S. Fukada, N. Yamamoto, S. Takeda, and K. Tsuchida. Mesenchymal progenitors distinct from satellite cells contribute to ectopic fat cell formation in skeletal muscle. *Nat Cell Biol* 12(2) (2010): 143–152.

Uezumi, A., T. Ito, D. Morikawa, N. Shimizu, T. Yoneda, M. Segawa, M. Yamaguchi et al. Fibrosis and adipogenesis originate from a common mesenchymal progenitor in skeletal muscle. *J Cell Sci* 124(Pt 21) (2011): 3654–3664.

Villalta, S. A., H. X. Nguyen, B. Deng, T. Gotoh, and J. G. Tidball. Shifts in macrophage phenotypes and macrophage competition for arginine metabolism affect the severity of muscle pathology in muscular dystrophy. *Hum Mol Genet* 18(3) (2009): 482–496.

Wang, H. B., M. E. Mullins, J. M. Cregg, A. Hurtado, M. Oudega, M. T. Trombley, and R. J. Gilbert. Creation of highly aligned electrospun poly-L-lactic acid fibers for nerve regeneration applications. *J Neural Eng* 6(1) (2009): 016001.

Wosczyna, M. N., A. A. Biswas, C. A. Cogswell, and D. J. Goldhamer. Multipotent progenitors resident in the skeletal muscle interstitium exhibit robust Bmp-dependent osteogenic activity and mediate heterotopic ossification. *J Bone Miner Res* 27(5) (2012): 1004–1017.

Yan, W., S. George, U. Fotadar, N. Tyhovych, A. Kamer, M. J. Yost, R. L. Price, C. R. Haggart, J. W. Holmes, and L. Terracio. Tissue engineering of skeletal muscle. *Tissue Eng* 13(11) (2007): 2781–2790.

Yoo, J. J., J. Meng, F. Oberpenning, and A. Atala. Bladder augmentation using allogenic bladder submucosa seeded with cells. *Urology* 51(2) (1998): 221–225.

Yu, T. T. and M. S. Shoichet. Guided cell adhesion and outgrowth in peptide-modified channels for neural tissue engineering. *Biomaterials* 26(13) (2005): 1507–1514.

Yun, Y. R., S. Lee, E. Jeon, W. Kang, K. H. Kim, H. W. Kim, and J. H. Jang. Fibroblast growth factor 2-functionalized collagen matrices for skeletal muscle tissue engineering. *Biotechnol Lett* 34(4) (2012): 771–778.

Zhang, L., L. Ran, G. E. Garcia, X. H. Wang, S. Han, J. Du, and W. E. Mitch. Chemokine Cxcl16 regulates neutrophil and macrophage infiltration into injured muscle, promoting muscle regeneration. *Am J Pathol* 175(6) (2009): 2518–2527.

Zheng, B., B. Cao, M. Crisan, B. Sun, G. Li, A. Logar, S. Yap et al. Prospective identification of myogenic endothelial cells in human skeletal muscle. *Nat Biotechnol* 25(9) (2007): 1025–1034.

CHAPTER 15

Engineering Limb Regeneration

Lessons from Animals That Can Regenerate

David M. Gardiner, PhD; Susan V. Bryant, PhD;
and Ken Muneoka, PhD

CONTENTS

15.1 INTRODUCTION

The goal of regenerative engineering is to restore the structure and function of a complex organ. To this end, a focus on the translation of discoveries from the lab into the clinic has led to considerable progress in the areas of biomaterials, tissue engineering, and stem cell biology. Ultimately, the goal is to induce an endogenous regenerative response to replace damaged tissues with regenerated tissues that become functionally integrated into the host tissues. This vision of activating an endogenous regenerative potential is based on the realization that many animals exhibit this remarkable ability. These animals provide evidence that endogenous regeneration is a basic biological property that we as humans can learn to activate therapeutically. Although this has been little more than a dream up to this point, the remarkable progress in our ability to discover and manipulate biological processes has provided the tools and resources needed to make human regeneration a reality. In this chapter, we argue that all that is now standing in the way of successful regeneration is the lack of a feasible strategy to achieve that outcome. In theory, there may be many ways to develop such a strategy; however, we already know of one way that works extraordinarily well, which is the way that highly regenerative animals such as the salamander do it. Therefore, we argue that the strategy that is most likely to achieve success is to understand how salamanders are able to regenerate so well.

15.2 STRATEGY

In spite of efforts over many decades to induce regeneration in mammals, little progress has been realized in terms of devising regeneration therapies for humans. The underlying experimental strategy of most investigations has been to attempt to induce regeneration in animals that have limited regenerative abilities (e.g., mammals). Since there is no regenerative response to study, it is not possible to identify any key steps to target in order to enhance the nonresponse. This strategy thus requires the investigator to make a reasonable guess as to what might stimulate a regenerative response and then test whether or not it works. In the early days, such approaches focused on manipulation of the physiology of the cells within the wound, for example, manipulation of electrical currents that arise at the site of wounds (e.g., Becker and Selden, 1985; Rose, 1970). As would be expected, the response of the cells to injury is altered, including regeneration-associated behaviors such as proliferation; however, none have led to success in inducing regeneration. In recent years, this same approach has been adapted so as to manipulate specific molecular signaling pathways that respond to injury and thus might be involved in regeneration. Identification of complex injury-associated gene regulatory networks has led to an abundance of candidate pathways to target; however, to date the "reasonable candidate" approach to manipulating signaling pathways has not led to the discovery of how to divert the injury response toward an enhanced regenerative response. The "reasonable candidate" strategy can only be successful if the problem is simple, which it is not. A fundamental lesson that we have learned from studies of salamanders is that regeneration progresses through a sequence of multiple, interdependent steps and thus the failure to progress beyond any one step results in regenerative failure of all subsequent steps (Figures 15.1 and 15.2; Bryant et al., 2002; Endo et al., 2004; Muller et al., 1999).

An alternative approach to focusing on wound-healing genes has been to focus on the relationship between regeneration and embryonic development. It seems reasonable to consider that since developmental mechanisms lead to the formation of complex organs in the embryo, these same mechanisms could be used in the adult to regenerate (i.e., redevelopment) these same organs. The abundance of data-identifying gene regulatory networks that regulate embryonic development provides a very long list of "reasonable candidate" pathways to target in order to induce regeneration. One approach to the "developmental candidate" strategy would be to generate a population of undifferentiated cells that could be directed to redevelop (regenerate) the various tissues. This could be done by inducing resident cells at the site of injury to become pluripotent by using reprogramming

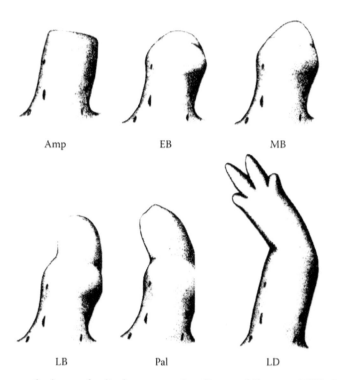

FIGURE 15.1 Stages of salamander limb regeneration (Iten and Bryant, 1973). Over the course of about a month, an amputated limb (Amp) regenerates to reform the missing limb structures (LD, late digit stage of regeneration). This process occurs by the formation of a blastema at the amputation plane. The blastema is equivalent to a developing limb bud and grows from an early stage (EB, early bud), elongates (MB, medium bud; LB, late bud), flattens along the dorsal–ventral axis, and begins to form digit condensations distally (Pal, palette).

strategies similar to those used to generate iPS (induced pluripotent stem) cells *in vitro* (e.g., Takahashi and Yamanaka, 2006). Alternatively, pluripotent or multipotent stem cells (e.g., ES [embryonic stem] cells or adult stem cells) could be directed along developmental pathways *in vitro* in order to create a population of appropriately differentiated cells to be used in cell-based therapies for the repair/replacement of the damaged tissue. These approaches are promising but challenging in terms of directing highly multipotent/pluripotent cells through many developmental steps in order to recapitulate the desired developmental outcome.

An alternative to starting with undifferentiated stem cells would be to start with differentiated cells and direct them backward step by step to an earlier developmental state. Presumably, it would only be necessary to go back a few steps to generate the population of regeneration-competent cells required to replace the specific tissues they were derived from. Starting with the adult tissues and reverting them back to a more embryonic state in order to then redevelop the missing structure(s) would restrict the cells to the lineage of the original progenitor cells, which is what is observed during regeneration of both salamander limbs and mouse digit tips (Fernando et al., 2011; Kragl et al., 2009; Lehoczky et al., 2011; Muneoka et al., 1986; Rinkevich et al., 2011).

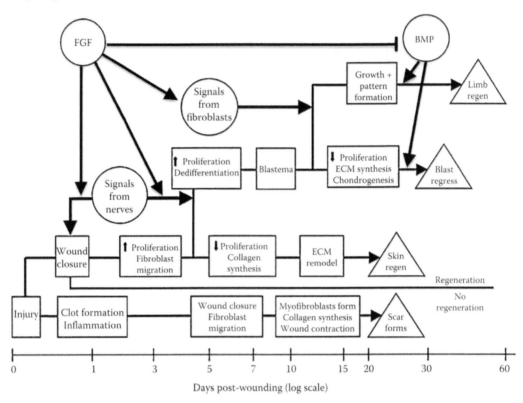

FIGURE 15.2 Stepwise model for limb regeneration. This model is based largely on the accessory limb model (Figure 15.3) that demonstrated that an ectopic limb can be induced to form at the site of a full-thickness skin wound on the side of the arm of an axolotl. If additional signals are not provided, the wound heals and regenerates the skin, in contrast to the wound-healing response in mammals which leads to scar formation and no regeneration. In response to signals from a surgically deviated nerve, the wound is induced to form an ectopic blastema. Additional signals from fibroblasts derived from a graft of dermal tissue from the side of the arm that is opposite to the wound site induce the ectopic blastema to form an ectopic limb. The early steps of this cascade of signaling events are mediated in part by FGF signaling (Mullen et al., 1996; Satoh et al., 2008a,b, 2010b) and repress the later events associated with differentiation that are mediated by BMP signaling (Satoh et al., 2008a).

The second alternative strategy to engineering regeneration is to utilize experimental models based on successful regeneration. One success to date in terms of inducing regeneration in a mammal has come from studies of the regenerative response of amputated digit tips (Fernando et al., 2011; Yu et al., 2010). In mammals, including humans, amputated digit tips regenerate, whereas amputations at more proximal levels fail to regenerate. The identification of BMP signaling as a critical pathway in the regenerative response guided subsequent investigations leading to the recent success in inducing regeneration from a normally non-regenerating, proximal amputation site via enhancing BMP signaling (Fernando et al., 2011; Yu et al., 2010). This result argues for a strategy that involves studying wounds that regenerate in order to gain mechanistic insights in order to induce regeneration of wounds that do not regenerate.

The strategy of studying regenerating wounds is based on the recognition that regeneration is a basic biological property that has evolved and been selected for over the course of evolution. Thus the nature-driven experiments to select for regenerative ability have been done for us already, they have been successful, and the next step is to use the results to guide our efforts in the field of regenerative engineering. Although it might be possible to discover alternative and novel ways to manipulate physiological and/or developmental pathways to stimulate regeneration, there is the reality that it might not be possible. For example, although the later stages of salamander limb regeneration recapitulate limb development, the early stages of regeneration are unique and different from development (Bryant et al., 2002), and thus the redevelopment approach would not be successful for inducing these early events. Therefore, it is appropriate and pragmatic to recognize that we already know of one way that regeneration works well, which is the way that salamanders (as well as other animals) do it.

If we approach the challenge of regenerative engineering based on the principle of starting with what works, then there are two ways to proceed. Both strategies are likely to be successful, and therefore we would argue that efforts be put into both. The first is most directly amenable to an engineering approach, which is to reverse engineer a regeneration blastema (Figure 15.1). The blastema is structurally and functionally equivalent to the limb bud of the embryo in that it grows and eventually reforms the missing limb structures. It is generated by migration of cells from the amputated stump that become covered by a specialized epithelium (apical epithelial cap) that functions to maintain the mesenchymal cells in an undifferentiated, proliferative state. As the blastema grows, it reaches a developmental stage (Figure 15.1; late bud) at which it can autonomously give rise to a regenerated limb when grafted to an ectopic host site. This would presumably be the stage to reverse engineer in order to reduce this system to its component parts and then reassemble it in order to create a regenerated limb. Having accomplished this initial goal, it would then be possible to create each of the component parts and test their ability to function as part of the reengineered whole. Although this is a promising approach, and likely to provide mechanistic insights over a relatively short period of time, to our knowledge it has not been systematically attempted with salamander limb regeneration.

The alternative approach is to start at the beginning of regeneration, and work forward step by step. As discussed later, this requires gain-of-function assays in order to test the ability of candidate signaling molecules to induce the appropriate regenerative responses. Although an incremental forward approach has been attempted repeatedly throughout the history of regeneration research, almost all studies have been limited to descriptions of the anatomy and patterns of gene expression associated with the regeneration process. Attempts to understand the function of candidate genes have been limited by the lack of gain-of-function models for regeneration. It is paradoxical that you cannot directly test the function of a candidate regeneration-inducing factor in an animal that can already regenerate perfectly. It is possible to test for inhibition of regeneration (loss of function), but how can you induce regeneration when it is the default response? As discussed in detail later, it is possible to design gain-of-function experiments in the axolotl by creating wounds that do not regenerate until additional signals are provided.

When comparing the two basic strategies of starting with either non-regenerating or regenerating experimental models, it is clear that the "reasonable candidate" approach has a very low probability of success given the large number of possible guesses; however, success would happen instantly if the correct factor was tested. A quick, instant success would also require a good guess as to the functional concentration of the factor(s), as well as the appropriate time(s) of delivery to the wound, which further decreases the probability of success. If regeneration involves more than one signaling event (which is a reasonable expectation), then the probability of success approaches zero as the number of required factors increases. Although the "reasonable candidate" approach is logical, it makes the assumption that the regeneration problem is simple, when we know that it is complex. In contrast, the stepwise forward approach (Figure 15.2) based on gain-of-function assays could take a long time but has a high probability of success.

15.3 CHALLENGES OF REGENERATION

There are a number of technical challenges to regenerative engineering, but it is important to first recognize that there is a fundamental conceptual challenge to be addressed. Although everyone agrees that successful regeneration is a desired goal, we do not share a unified view of what "regeneration" is.

15.3.1 Regeneration Is a Process and Not a Trait

The word "regeneration" is used to refer to very different processes, many of which are clearly unrelated, yet we talk about them as if they were all the same. For example, regeneration of the tail of a salamander and a lizard appear the same in that the lost tail is replaced. However, the two regenerated tails differ significantly from each other in structure. In the salamander, a perfect replacement tail is regrown, whereas in the lizard, a "good enough" tail is regenerated, which differs from the original in numerous ways, but nevertheless serves as a replacement tail (Alibardi, 2010; Bellairs and Bryant, 1985).

This is the issue of semantics famously raised in Lewis Carroll's *Through the Looking-Glass* (1872); "'When I use a word', Humpty Dumpty said, in rather a scornful tone, 'it means just what I choose it to mean—neither more nor less.'" There are at least two important consequences of our failure to agree upon the definition of "regeneration." The first is that it is difficult to have scientifically critical discussions about the principles and mechanisms of regeneration. For example, since we do not yet understand regenerative mechanisms, it is difficult to make comparisons between regenerative abilities in different organisms, and thus conclusions about how such mechanisms arose and diverged or converged over time are at best tentative (see Bely, 2010; Bely and Nyberg, 2010; Garza-Garcia et al., 2010). Regenerative abilities vary between species, and thus, presumably the underlying mechanisms and genes also exhibit variability associated with how they have evolved. However, regeneration is not itself a trait with genetic variation, but rather it is a complex and diverse process. The lack of a mechanistic definition of "regeneration" opens the door for speculation about what might or might not be conserved between species. Simply put, what is referred to as "regeneration" in one organism may or may not be related mechanistically to "regeneration" in another organism.

An appreciation of the diversity of regenerative responses leads to the recognition that "regeneration" is not something special that only special animals can do. Rather it is a process that works better, and differently, in some animals rather than in others. Lack of such an appreciation leads to the naive conclusion that since humans do not have exactly the same genes as a salamander, we will never be able to regenerate an amputated limb. The wide distribution and variability of regenerative responses imply that regeneration is an emergent property of the conserved mechanisms regulating the behavior of cells in response to injury, comparable to the conserved mechanisms regulating the behavior of cells during embryonic development (see Gilbert, 2010). Thus, we can utilize these mechanisms in the same way that they work to regenerate a salamander limb in order to achieve the same outcome in a human.

The second negative consequence of talking about regeneration as a trait rather than a process is that we fail to appreciate that there are many different ways to go about regenerating tissues and organs. Thus, there are multiple possible outcomes, and we need to consider what the desired outcome is. It is likely and reasonable that regenerative engineering should lead to multiple desirable and thus successful outcomes. For example, it would be a desirable outcome to regenerate articular cartilage without having to amputate the limb and in the process of regeneration grow an entire new joint. Achieving the desired outcome is dependent on first recognizing that there are multiple possible outcomes and then designing appropriate experiments and assays that target that specific outcome.

By recognizing that "regeneration" is complex, variable, and diverse, we have cause to be encouraged that engineering regenerative therapies will be successful. Given how widespread regenerative abilities are among plants and animals, it is as if regeneration in one form or another is a common biological response to injury. Although there may never be a "Eureka!" moment breakthrough, the diversity of regenerative responses encourages us to believe that we can achieve incremental advances that will bring positive therapeutic benefits over time. Nevertheless, we envision that in the end, we will be able to activate and regulate our intrinsic regenerative abilities in order to regenerate organs like a salamander can.

Aside from the conceptual challenge of defining what we mean when referring to "regeneration" and "regenerative mechanisms," we consider there to be three immediate scientific and technical challenges. Admittedly there likely will be further problems to solve as we progress toward the goal of perfect endogenous regeneration. However, until we can address and surmount these immediate challenges, we cannot move forward to discover what lies beyond. For the sake of clarity, we focus on regeneration of the salamander (axolotl) limb, and thus we consider the behavior of cells present in a typical tetrapod vertebrate limb and their role in regeneration via the formation of a blastema.

15.3.2 Origin of the Regeneration-Competent Cells

Regeneration is by definition the replacement of lost structure, and the new structure is built by cells. Thus, it is essential to understand where the cells involved in regeneration come from and how their behavior is regulated. For some cells, it is evident that they are derived from adult stem cells, and their biology is well understood, for example, satellite cells of the muscle (see Chapter XX). In other cases, very little is known. This question of the origin of regeneration-competent cells has been asked repeatedly since the earliest day of regeneration research, and in spite of suggestions to the contrary, it is far from resolved (Kragl et al., 2009; Lehoczky et al., 2011; Muneoka et al., 1986; Rinkevich et al., 2011). Early studies based on detailed histological analyses established the view that there is a one-to-one relationship between the number of cells of a particular tissue type in the stump and their contribution to the blastema as it forms and grows. By this view, the regenerated limb forms as a distal extension of a template of the stump tissues (Chalkley, 1954; Hay and Fischman, 1961). With the subsequent development of techniques for the quantitative analysis of cell contribution, it was discovered that this is not the case (Muneoka et al., 1986). Although all the tissues of the stump eventually contribute cells to the regenerated structure, some progenitor tissues over-contribute cells to the blastema relative to their availability in the stump, whereas other tissues under-contribute. For example, the cells of the dermis contributed on average half of all the cells of the early blastema, but account for less than 20% of the cells in the stump (Muneoka et al., 1986; Tank and Holder, 1979). In contrast, muscle that accounts for more than 50% of the stump contributes less than 20% of the cells of the early blastema (Echeverri et al., 2001; Tank and Holder, 1979). There is also considerable spatial mixing of cells as the blastema grows such that on average 25% of the cells on one side of the blastema originated from progenitors that resided on the opposite side of the limb at the time of amputation (Tank et al., 1985). Eventually, the relative abundance and patterns of the various tissues are reestablished such that again the muscle accounts for more than 50% and connective tissue less than 20% of the stump.

Since regeneration is a dynamic process whereby the early blastema creates the microenvironment necessary to allow the transition to the later stages of blastema development, the ability to engineer regeneration will require creating the appropriate early conditions that will allow for progression to progressively later stages. These changes over time will involve dynamic changes in the contribution and participation of cells derived from different tissues. Recent, nonquantitative contribution studies are consistent with the view that cell contribution to the blastema is largely, or entirely lineage-restricted (Kragl et al., 2009; Lehoczky et al., 2011; Muneoka et al., 1986; Rinkevich et al., 2011), and there is little or no transdifferentiation. However, these results should not lead us to come full circle in thinking that cells of the stump contribute to the regenerate in a mosaic fashion such that the identity and fate of cells are fixed from their origin in the stump, through their residence in the blastema, and differentiation into the regenerated structures. This is particularly important when considering the contribution and function of dermal fibroblasts, which can give rise to multiple tissue types as discussed later. We stress the necessity of conducting contribution studies that are quantitative rather than qualitative, and temporal as well as spatial if the results are to be insightful for efforts in regenerative engineering.

Much is known about the regenerative response of several cell types in the limb, and most of them actually regenerate well under permissive conditions. For example, nerves cannot regenerate axons across gaps, but do regenerate axons well when provided appropriate guidance cues from the nerve sheath (see Bryant et al., 2002). Similarly, satellite cells can regenerate muscle, but do not in response to injuries that result in scarring (see Bryant et al., 2002). Angiogenesis is regulated dynamically, and epithelia, blood cells, and skeletal tissues are continuously renewed throughout life. For these tissues, the question is not whether or not they can regenerate, but what happens such that they do not. Presumably they fail to regenerate because the environment is not permissive for a regenerative response. For example, wounds that result in a muscle tissue defect likely fail to regenerate new muscle because of the formation of scar tissue. The tissue that consistently fails to regenerate in mammals is the loose connective tissue that forms scar tissue when injured. In contrast, the connective tissue is regenerated in salamanders, and scars are not formed (Bryant et al., 2002; Endo et al., 2004). We consider this difference in the regenerative response of the connective tissue cells (generally referred to as fibroblasts) to be important, and we discuss this issue later in the context of designing assays for functional studies.

Although some tissues regenerate by the mechanism of adult stem cells, for other tissues it is unclear how regeneration-competent cells are generated. Historically, the term "dedifferentiation" has been used to refer to a mechanism for generating blastema cells. There is no mechanistic definition of "dedifferentiation" and it thus is defined operationally as the process whereby cells in adult tissues revert to an early developmental state as evidenced by the reexpression of embryonic genes and the acquisition of enhanced developmental potential (Han et al., 2005; Satoh et al., 2008b). By this definition, dedifferentiation appears to occur during salamander limb regeneration, as well as during mouse digit tip regeneration. It is important to note that dedifferentiation does not necessarily involve lineage switching, also referred to as transdifferentiation. These are related but distinctly different processes, and the absence of transdifferentiation is not evidence against the presence of dedifferentiation. Whether or not cells switch lineages, it is clear that progenitor cells in the dermis of salamanders can differentiate into multiple cell types within the connective tissue lineage, including cartilage, ligaments, tendons, and muscle fascia (Dunis and Namenwirth, 1977; Holder, 1989; Lheureux, 1983).

An additional source of confusion when considering the origin of regeneration-competent cells is the use of the term "blastema cell" as if this is a specific cell type, which it is not. The blastema is an assemblage of cells of different tissue origins and developmental histories that are colocalized in the structure that is called the "blastema" that is changing from one moment to the next. Therefore, declarative statements and definitive conclusions about "blastema cells" are misleading at best.

From the perspective of engineering regeneration of a complex structure, it is essential to face the reality that although cell contribution is complex, we still need to understand it. The engineering approach is built on the principle of cell theory that cells are specialized for specific functions, and therefore we need to regenerate the specialized cells required for restoration of function. It is relatively simple to recognize most of the specialized cells and their corresponding functions in a limb, skin, muscle, bone, connective tissues, nerves, and blood vessels. However, we do not know how to regulate the function of regeneration of the limb, and therefore we must not know about the cells that function to control regeneration.

Studies of regenerating salamander limbs have demonstrated that there are specialized cells that function to control the growth and pattern of all the other cell types (see Bryant et al., 2002). Successful regeneration requires that the replaced structural components be arranged in such a way as to be functional. For example, muscles have to have spatially appropriate origins and insertions that span the elbow joint in order to flex and extent the lower arm. In the salamander, the cells that function to arrange the pattern and location of the other tissues are derived from connective tissue fibroblasts (see Bryant et al., 2002). The origin, behavior, and contribution of fibroblasts to regeneration have been understudied in recent years, mainly because we do not have the markers and reagents to identify and study the behavior of those cells.

15.3.3 Tools to Identify Subpopulations of Regeneration Progenitor Cells

The essential function of connective tissue fibroblasts in controlling pattern formation during salamander limb regeneration has been recognized for decades. These cells are the progenitors of the early blastema cell population (Kragl et al., 2009; Muneoka et al., 1986), and are the cells that induce formation of supernumerary limb structures when grafted to the opposite side of the limb (Bryant et al., 1981; Endo et al., 2004; French et al., 1976). Nevertheless, we understand less about the biology of these cells than most other cell types in our bodies. This lack of understanding is due largely to the lack of markers for these cells. These blastema progenitor cells in the dermis have information about spatial position along the limb axes (positional information), and use this information to interact with each other to stimulate growth and to reestablish the new limb pattern during regeneration (see Bryant et al., 2002). This positional information is fine-grained and continuous along the limb axes such that if a limb is amputated at any level along the proximal–distal axis, only the pattern that was lost is replaced. When these cells are surgically relocated so as to establish novel interactions between cells from the opposite side of the limb, entire supernumerary limbs with normal pattern are induced (Bryant et al., 1981; Endo et al., 2004; French et al., 1976). These cells establish a grid-like network of information that is distributed as two-dimensional sheets that wrap around all of the tissues within the limb, and thus we refer to them as the "grid" cells.

The ability of the connective tissue grid cells to control limb regeneration has been most directly demonstrated in experiments in which skin from an unirradiated limb is grafted to replace the skin on an x-irradiated limb (Dunis and Namenwirth, 1977; Holder, 1989; Lheureux, 1983). X-irradiation blocks regeneration, which is then rescued by cells from the grafted skin. During regeneration, the epidermis is lineage-restricted and only gives rise to new epidermis (Kragl et al., 2009; Lehoczky et al., 2011; Rinkevich et al., 2011), whereas blastema formation is rescued by cells from the grafted dermis. Regenerating muscle also is lineage-restricted (Cameron et al., 1986; Kragl et al., 2009; Morrison et al., 2006), and migration of myoprogenitor cells from the stump is not rescued by the skin graft, resulting in limbs that lack muscle. However, all other tissues are formed whether by migration from the stump (nerves and blood vessels) or from progenitor cells within the grafted dermis that give rise to a normally patterned limb with a skeleton, ligaments, tendons, muscle fascia, and dermis (Dunis and Namenwirth, 1977; Holder, 1989; Lheureux, 1983).

It is remarkable that we know so little about the grid cells. This presumably is due to the fact that the functional importance of grid cells has only been appreciated in the context of salamander limb regeneration. Nevertheless, they provide the information that is required to regulate and integrate the growth and pattern of the regenerated structures. From the regeneration perspective, fibroblasts are not relatively undifferentiated spindle-shaped cells as they have been characterized historically; rather they encode complex positional information, and their function is required for regeneration. The challenge is to develop the reagents necessary to isolate these cells and identify the subpopulation(s) of dermal dells that have this function. Discovering how to regulate the behavior of these cells will be critical to success in regenerative engineering whether the goal is to induce an endogenous regenerative response or to integrate engineered constructs into the host tissues.

Having markers to identify, isolate, and describe cells is not enough. Without functional assays, we cannot understand and regulate the activities of those cells. Since the challenge is to induce regeneration, we need assays for the cells that function to regulate regeneration. As discussed earlier, it is essential that these assays be gain of function, which is obviously the situation when trying to induce regeneration in an animal that does not regenerate. However, in these non-regenerating models, taking a "reasonable guess" approach has a very low probability of success that approaches zero as the complexity of the cellular response increases. We therefore have argued for the need to design gain-of-function assays for model systems that can regenerate, such as the salamander.

15.3.4 Models of Limb Regeneration

Most studies of salamander limb regeneration have been limited to descriptions of the anatomy and patterns of gene expression associated with the regeneration process. Although it is possible to test for ways to inhibit regeneration (loss of function), it is hard to think of ways to induce a regenerative response in an animal that already regenerates. Since the control limb always regenerates, it is not possible to test whether a candidate factor can induce a regenerative response. The traditional gain-of-function approach in regeneration research has been to couple it with loss of function to get rescue. Most often this has involved severing the nerves to the limb in order to inhibit regeneration and then adding back a factor to try to rescue regeneration. For example, denervation of a late stage regenerating limb blastema results in a loss of Dlx-3 expression and regenerative failure, both of which are rescued by the delivery of exogenous FGF2 (Mullen et al., 1996). This approach requires that we would need to understand how we rescued a process we did not understand in the first place, after having inhibited it by some unknown mechanism. It is not surprising that this strategy has yielded limited success today. For example, newt anterior gradient protein (nAG) rescues regeneration of limbs that are in transition to the point of becoming reinnervated enough to regenerate endogenously without the delivery of nAG (Kumar et al., 2007; Salley and Tassava, 1981; Salley-Guydon and Tassava, 2006). Overall, this gain-of-function strategy has not led to insights into how to initiate formation and sustain development of a blastema that is capable of progressing to regenerate a limb.

We have approached this challenge by designing and validating two gain-of-function models, the ALM (accessory limb model) and the ERM (excisional regeneration model), for axolotl regeneration. In both models, a regenerative response can be induced by signaling from a nerve and a specialized wound epithelium that forms in response to signaling from the nerve. This signaling cascade recruits cells from the surrounding tissues to form a blastema and regenerate the limb/defect. In both models, there is minimal damage (in contrast to an amputation), and thus only those cells required for regeneration are recruited to participate, and events that are extraneous to regeneration *per se* are eliminated. The important point is that the axolotl is an animal that we know is able to regenerate perfectly when the appropriate signals are provided, and thus we can assay for those signals. This is not the same as the "reasonable guess" approach in a non-regenerating animal in which there might be multiple steps that cause regenerative failure, and thus regeneration will not occur even if an important signal is provided early in the cascade.

In the case of the ALM, a full-thickness skin wound on the arm of an axolotl regenerates the skin but does not form a blastema (Figure 15.3). In response to signals from a surgically deviated nerve, cells at the wound site are recruited to form an ectopic blastema that is equivalent to an amputation-induced blastema (Endo et al., 2004; Satoh et al., 2007). If additional signals are provided by grafting dermal cells (fibroblasts with the appropriate

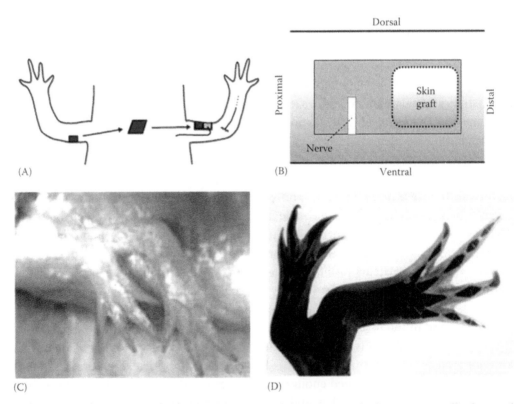

FIGURE 15.3 The accessory limb model (Endo et al., 2004). Signals from a surgically deviated nerve and a skin graft from the opposite side of the limb (A and B) induce a wound on the side of the arm of an axolotl to form a limb *de novo* (C and D). Contralateral skin graft is colored red in (A). The skeletal patterns of the host (right) and ectopic (left) limbs in (D) are visualized by staining with Victoria Blue.

positional information as discussed earlier) from the opposite side of the arm to the wound site, the ectopic blastema forms an ectopic arm (Figure 15.3C and D). This induced arm has all of the limb tissues and they are organized in a normal limb pattern. By identifying the signals that regulate each of these steps involved in making an ectopic arm, we have learned about how nerve signaling regulates dedifferentiation of the blastema apical epithelium that is required for blastema formation and growth (Satoh et al., 2008b). We also have discovered that nerve signaling negatively regulates redifferentiation of the dermis and thus appears to maintain blastema cells in an undifferentiated state (Satoh et al., 2008a).

The ERM is based on the observation that although an axolotl can regenerate an amputated arm, a critical size defect (CSD) in the radius does not regenerate, as is the case in humans (Figure 15.4). However, if signals from a wound epithelium and surgically deviated nerve are provided, like in the ALM, the defect is regenerated *in situ* (Figure 15.4F). This regenerative response is due at least in part by signaling that induces connective tissue fibroblasts to dedifferentiate and participate in regeneration of the skeletal defect (Satoh et al., 2010a). Since regeneration also can be induced by grafting undifferentiated cells from a blastema (Figure 15.4C) or treating the wound to enhance BMP signaling (Figure 15.4E), it is possible to use the ERM as an assay for the induction of both fibroblast dedifferentiation and the acquisition of regeneration competency.

Finally, we note that not all functional assays will provide the same information about how cells can participate in regeneration. Different assays will provide insights into different aspects of regeneration (e.g., the regulation of migration, proliferation, or differentiation/dedifferentiation), all of which are important regeneration mechanisms. However, it may or may not be appropriate to extrapolate the results from one assay or experimental model to another, particularly if the assays involve different animal species. As discussed at length earlier, regenerative mechanisms are diverse and not all regenerative responses are the same.

15.4 WAY FORWARD

If we assume that the field will eventually be successful in overcoming the challenges we have presented, we consider the following to be the immediate goals of regenerative engineering.

15.4.1 We Need Regeneration-Competent Cells

By definition, regeneration is the replacement of lost structure, and the structure is made by cells. Therefore, we need appropriate sources of progenitor cells suitable for the regeneration of the various components of the limb. There are two approaches: the first being to generate these cells exogenously (e.g., ES cells, adult stem cells, or iPS cells). The second approach is to recruit cells endogenously, which is what occurs in an animal that can regenerate (e.g., a salamander). Producing cells exogenously may be more successful over the shorter terms given the ability to grow these cells *in vitro*. Regeneration therapies are likely to require large numbers of cells, and the ability to expand cultures of regeneration-competent cells will be essential. The challenge for stem cell/iPS therapies lies in being able to control their differentiation into the appropriate tissue types. Though likely to be

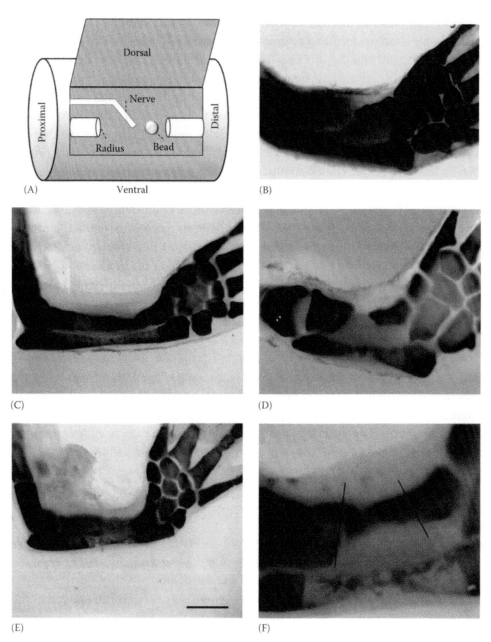

FIGURE 15.4   The excisional regeneration model (Satoh et al., 2010a). When a critical size defect is created surgically so as to remove the middle third of the radius of an axolotl arm (A), the defect is not regenerated (B) even though the entire limb will regenerate if it is amputated. This non-regenerating wound can be induced to regenerate by grafting regeneration-competent blastema cells (C), but is not regenerated if the blastema progenitor cells (differentiated dermal fibroblasts) are engrafted (D). The ERM also can be used to assay for signaling molecules that induce a regenerative response by implantation of microcarrier beads (A) soaked in a candidate factor, for example, BMP2 as illustrated in (E). The defect also is regenerated when dedifferentiation of cells at the wound site are induced to dedifferentiate *in situ* in response to signals from a surgically deviated nerve (A and F). Scale bar is 2 mm in (B–E) and 0.5 mm in (F).

a longer-term achievement, being able to recruit cells from the patient directly to the site of injury and induce them to expand and replace the lost tissues directly would be the ultimate goal.

15.4.2 We Need to Control Differentiation

Given that it will be possible to acquire regeneration-competent cells, we are then faced with the goal of how to get these cells to do what we want them to do, and equally important, where we want them to do it. In part, this raises questions about how to regulate the differentiation of regeneration-competent cells, which are going to be relatively undifferentiated. Although ES and iPS cells can differentiate into various lineages in response to specific stimuli, we have very limited experience with these cells and thus do not presently have experience with regards to the best paths along which to direct pluripotent cells into multipotent progenitors that can give rise to specific tissues. One reasonable approach is to direct these cells from an embryonic state to the differentiated state along the same pathways that are used in the embryo.

From a regeneration perspective, there is a second and equally or more reasonable approach, which is to use the pathways that already work for regeneration in animals that can actually regenerate. In this case, you start from the adult tissues and generate a population of regeneration-competent cells and then use them to remake the missing structures. There are at least two possible advantages for this approach over the developmental recapitulation approach. First, we know that these regeneration pathways already work (i.e., there is a proof of principle), whereas the developmental pathway approach may not work for rebuilding complex tissues and organs. Second, if you start back with embryonic stage cells (highly multipotent), you have to lead them along many steps to recapitulate the desired developmental outcome. Thus, there are multiple steps where the process could fail, particularly with regard to retaining pluripotent cells with the potential to generate tumors when grafted into the host. In contrast, by stating at the end and taking the regeneration approach of generating cells by dedifferentiation, one would only need to take these cells back a couple of steps in development to a state that is not far away from the desired differentiated cell type. This latter approach is dependent on understanding the details of the source and lineage of the cells in the adult limb/digit that participate in making the regenerate, and how they respond to endogenous signaling to become recruited and subsequently differentiate into the appropriate cell type(s).

15.4.3 We Need to Control the Information That Leads to the Right Tissues Being in the Right Place

Two things are essential for regeneration: the cells and the information to direct the cells about where to go and what to become relative to each other. The consequence of having only regeneration-competent cells without information is most dramatically observable in teratomas, which are tumors composed of disorganized, multiple differentiated cell types that are lacking the overall organization required for function. For the time being, the information to coordinate and integrate the multiple structural components of an engineered regenerate will be provided by the people who are doing the engineering.

Therein lies the promise of regenerative engineering. Given our appreciation of the role of the extracellular environment in regulating the behavior of cells in general and regeneration-competent cells in particular, the goal of regenerative engineering is to provide the matrix with the appropriately patterned cues for the cells, be they pluripotent stem cells or lineage-restricted cells. This hybrid approach is dependent on our understanding of these cues based on studies of animals such as the salamander. Ultimately, the goal is to figure out how to induce this information to regenerate itself, which would be equivalent to making an endogenous scaffold. Accomplishing this goal will require an understanding of the grid cells and how the information grid is established, maintained, and repaired.

In conclusion, we need to remember that although regeneration is a diverse and complex process, we do not need to know all of the facts and details from all of the regeneration models in order to achieve the goal of human regeneration. This is the most important lesson that biologists can learn from engineers, which is that you only need to know enough to build it and to make it work. If it does not work, then there must be something that we did not know was missing, and we can go back and search for the missing piece. Once we get it to work, it will be possible to focus future research efforts to optimize each of the steps in order to increase the quality of the regenerative outcome. On the other side, in spite of all the skill and elegance of engineering, it is informed by the biology. We can realize the potential of this "beautiful friendship" by building on the lessons to be learned from regenerating animals to inform the engineering and achieve the ultimate goal of regenerative engineering.

REFERENCES

Alibardi, L., 2010. *Morphological and Cellular Aspects of Tail and Limb Regeneration in Lizards.* Springer, New York.

Becker, R.O. and Selden, G., 1985. *The Body Electric: Electromagnetism and the Foundation of Life.* William Morrow, New York.

Bellairs, A.d'A. and Bryant, S.V., 1985. Autotomy and regeneration in reptiles. In: Gans, C. and Billett, F., Eds., *Biology of the Reptilia,* Vol. 15B. John Wiley & Sons, New York, pp. 301–410.

Bely, A.E., 2010. Evolutionary loss of animal regeneration: Pattern and process. *Integr Comp Biol* 50, 515–527.

Bely, A.E. and Nyberg, K.G., 2010. Evolution of animal regeneration: Re-emergence of a field. *Trends Ecol Evol* 25, 161–170.

Bryant, S.V., Endo, T., and Gardiner, D.M., 2002. Vertebrate limb regeneration and the origin of limb stem cells. *Int J Dev Biol* 46, 887–896.

Bryant, S.V., French, V., and Bryant, P.J., 1981. Distal regeneration and symmetry. *Science* 212, 993–1002.

Cameron, J.A., Hilgers, A.R., and Hinterberger, T.J., 1986. Evidence that reserve cells are a source of regenerated adult newt muscle *in-vitro. Nature* 321, 607–610.

Chalkley, D.T., 1954. A quantitative histological analysis of forelimb regeneration in *Triturus viridescens. J Morphol* 94, 21–70.

Dunis, D.A. and Namenwirth, M., 1977. The role of grafted skin in the regeneration of X-irradiated axolotl limbs. *Dev Biol* 56, 97–109.

Echeverri, K., Clarke, J.D., and Tanaka, E.M., 2001. *In vivo* imaging indicates muscle fiber dedifferentiation is a major contributor to the regenerating tail blastema. *Dev Biol* 236, 151–164.

Endo, T., Bryant, S.V., and Gardiner, D.M., 2004. A stepwise model system for limb regeneration. *Dev Biol* 270, 135–145.

Fernando, W.A., Leininger, E., Simkin, J., Li, N., Malcom, C.A., Sathyamoorthi, S., Han, M., and Muneoka, K., 2011. Wound healing and blastema formation in regenerating digit tips of adult mice. *Dev Biol* 350, 301–310.

French, V., Bryant, P.J., and Bryant, S.V., 1976. Pattern regulation in epimorphic fields. *Science* 193, 969–981.

Garza-Garcia, A.A., Driscoll, P.C., and Brockes, J.P., 2010. Evidence for the local evolution of mechanisms underlying limb regeneration in salamanders. *Integr Comp Biol* 50, 528–535.

Gilbert, S.F., 2010. *Developmental Biology*. Sinauer Associates, Inc., Sunderland, MA.

Han, M., Yang, X., Taylor, G., Burdsal, C.A., Anderson, R.A., and Muneoka, K., 2005. Limb regeneration in higher vertebrates: Developing a roadmap. *Anat Rec B New Anat* 287, 14–24.

Hay, E.D. and Fischman, D.A., 1961. Origin of the blastema in regenerating limbs of the newt *Triturus viridescens*. An autoradiographic study using tritiated thymidine to follow cell proliferation and migration. *Dev Biol* 3, 26–59.

Holder, N., 1989. Organization of connective tissue patterns by dermal fibroblasts in the regenerating axolotl limb. *Development* 105, 585–594.

Iten, L. and Bryant, S.V., 1973. Forelimb regeneration from different levels of amputation in the newt, *Notophthalmus viridescens*. *Wilhelm Roux Archiv* 173, 263–282.

Kragl, M., Knapp, D., Nacu, E., Khattak, S., Maden, M., Epperlein, H.H., and Tanaka, E.M., 2009. Cells keep a memory of their tissue origin during axolotl limb regeneration. *Nature* 460, 60–65.

Kumar, A., Godwin, J.W., Gates, P.B., Garza-Garcia, A.A., and Brockes, J.P., 2007. Molecular basis for the nerve dependence of limb regeneration in an adult vertebrate. *Science* 318, 772–777.

Lehoczky, J.A., Robert, B., and Tabin, C.J., 2011. Mouse digit tip regeneration is mediated by fate-restricted progenitor cells. *Proc Natl Acad Sci U S A* 108, 20609–20614.

Lheureux, E., 1983. The origin of tissues in the x-irradiated regenerating limb of the newt *Pleurodeles waltilii*. In: Fallon, J.F. and Caplan, A.I., Eds., *Limb Development and Regeneration*, Part A. Alan R. Liss, Inc., New York, pp. 455–465.

Morrison, J.I., Loof, S., He, P., and Simon, A., 2006. Salamander limb regeneration involves the activation of a multipotent skeletal muscle satellite cell population. *J Cell Biol* 172, 433–440.

Mullen, L., Bryant, S.V., Torok, M.A., Blumberg, B., and Gardiner, D.M., 1996. Nerve dependency of regeneration: The role of *Distal-less* and FGF signaling in amphibian limb regeneration. *Development* 122, 3487–3497.

Muller, T.L., Ngo-Muller, V., Reginelli, A., Taylor, G., Anderson, R., and Muneoka, K., 1999. Regeneration in higher vertebrates: Limb buds and digit tips. *Semin Cell Dev Biol* 10, 405–413.

Muneoka, K., Fox, W., and Bryant, S.V., 1986. Cellular contribution from dermis and cartilage to the regenerating limb blastema in axolotls. *Dev Biol* 116, 256–260.

Rinkevich, Y., Lindau, P., Ueno, H., Longaker, M.T., and Weissman, I.L., 2011. Germ-layer and lineage-restricted stem/progenitors regenerate the mouse digit tip. *Nature* 476, 409–413.

Rose, S. M., 1970. *Regeneration*. Appleton-Century-Crofts, New York.

Salley, J.D. and Tassava, R.A., 1981. Responses of denervated adult newt limb stumps to reinnervation and reinjury. *J Exp Zool* 215, 183–189.

Salley-Guydon, J.D. and Tassava, R.A., 2006. Timing the commitment to a wound-healing response of denervated limb stumps in the adult newt, *Notophthalmus viridescens*. *Wound Repair Regen* 14, 479–483.

Satoh, A., Bryant, S.V., and Gardiner, D.M., 2008a. Regulation of dermal fibroblast dedifferentiation and redifferentiation during wound healing and limb regeneration in the axolotl. *Dev Growth Differ* 50, 743–754.

Satoh, A., Cummings, G.M., Bryant, S.V., and Gardiner, D.M., 2010a. Neurotrophic regulation of fibroblast dedifferentiation during limb skeletal regeneration in the axolotl (*Ambystoma mexicanum*). *Dev Biol* 337, 444–457.

Satoh, A., Cummings, G.M., Bryant, S.V., and Gardiner, D.M., 2010b. Regulation of proximal–distal intercalation during limb regeneration in the axolotl (*Ambystoma mexicanum*). *Dev Growth Differ* 52, 785–798.

Satoh, A., Gardiner, D.M., Bryant, S.V., and Endo, T., 2007. Nerve-induced ectopic limb blastemas in the axolotl are equivalent to amputation-induced blastemas. *Dev Biol* 312, 231–244.

Satoh, A., Graham, G.M., Bryant, S.V., and Gardiner, D.M., 2008b. Neurotrophic regulation of epidermal dedifferentiation during wound healing and limb regeneration in the axolotl (*Ambystoma mexicanum*). *Dev Biol* 319, 321–335.

Takahashi, K. and Yamanaka, S., 2006. Induction of pluripotent stem cells from mouse embryonic and adult fibroblast cultures by defined factors. *Cell* 126, 663–676.

Tank, P.W., Connelly, T.G., and Bookstein, F.L., 1985. Cellular behavior in the anteroposterior axis of the regenerating forelimb of the axolotl, *Ambystoma mexicanum*. *Dev Biol* 109, 215–223.

Tank, P.W. and Holder, N., 1979. The distribution of cells in the upper forelimbs of the axolotl. *J Exp Zool* 209, 435–442.

Yu, L., Han, M., Yan, M., Lee, E.C., Lee, J., and Muneoka, K., 2010. BMP signaling induces digit regeneration in neonatal mice. *Development* 137, 551–559.

Index